Principles and Practice of Research
Strategies for Surgical Investigators

Second Edition

AF897645

Principles and Practice of Research

Strategies for Surgical Investigators

Second Edition

Edited by

H. Troidl W.O. Spitzer B. McPeek D.S. Mulder
M.F. McKneally A.S. Wechsler C.M. Balch

With Forewords by R.L. Cruess and J.C. Goligher

With 98 Illustrations

Springer-Verlag
New York Berlin Heidelberg London
Paris Tokyo Hong Kong Barcelona

Hans Troidl, Department of Surgery, University of Cologne, Surgical Clinic Merheim, D-5000 Cologne 91, Federal Republic of Germany

Walter O. Spitzer, Department of Epidemiology and Biostatistics, McGill University, Montreal, Quebec, Canada H3A 1A2

Bucknam McPeek, Department of Anaesthesia, Harvard University, Massachusetts General Hospital, Boston, Massachusetts 02114-2696, U.S.A.

David S. Mulder, Department of Surgery, McGill University, Montreal General Hospital, Montreal, Quebec, Canada H3G 1A4

Martin F. McKneally, Division of Thoracic Surgery, Eaton North 10-226, Toronto General Hospital, Toronto, Ontario, Canada M5G2C4

Andrew S. Wechsler, Department of Surgery, Medical College of Virginia, Virginia Commonwealth University, Richmond, Virginia 23298-0645, U.S.A.

Charles M. Balch, Department of General Surgery, MD Anderson Cancer Center, Houston, Texas 77030, U.S.A.

Library of Congress Cataloging-in-Publication Data
Principles and practice of research : strategies for surgical
investigators. – 2nd ed. / edited by Hans Troidl . . . [et al.]
p. cm.
Includes bibliographical references.
Includes index.
ISBN-13: 978-1-4684-0373-2
paper)
1. Surgery—Research— Methodology. I. Hans Troidl
[DNLM: 1. Research. 2. Surgery. WO 20 P957]
RD29.P75 1991
617'.0072—dc20
DNLM/DLC
for Library of Congress 90-9945

© 1991 Springer-Verlag New York Inc.
Softcover reprint of the hardcover 2nd edition 1991

Copyright is not claimed for works by U.S. Government employees.
All rights reserved. This work may not be translated or copied in whole or in part without the written permission of the publisher (Springer-Verlag New York, Inc., 175 Fifth Avenue, New York, NY 10010, USA), except for brief excerpts in connection with reviews or scholarly analysis. Use in connection with any form of information storage and retrieval, electronic adaptation, computer software, or by similar or dissimilar methodology now known or hereafter developed is forbidden.
The use of general descriptive names, trade names, trademarks, etc., in this publication, even if the former are not especially identified, is not to be taken as a sign that such names, as understood by the Trade Marks and Merchandise Marks Act, may accordingly be used freely by anyone.
While the advice and information in this book are believed to be true and accurate at the date of going to press, neither the authors nor the editors nor the publisher can accept any legal responsibility for any errors or omissions that may be made. The publisher makes no warranty, express or implied, with respect to the material contained herein.

Typeset by Publishers Service of Montana, Bozeman, Montana.

9 8 7 6 5 4 3 2 1

ISBN-13: 978-1-4684-0373-2 e-ISBN-13: 978-1-4684-0371-8
DOI: 10.1007/978-1-4684-0371-8

This book is dedicated to our students, who have added enormously to our lives. By their questions they have encouraged us to ask *why* rather than only *what*. They have not been satisfied with simplistic answers, but have forced us to examine what we know and how well we know it. Their inquiring minds have encouraged us to improve our own knowledge that we might better meet their hunger for honest, forthright help as they build their lives and careers.

Foreword to Second Edition

R.L. Cruess

This book addresses problems that are fundamental to the future of surgical practice. Although the enormous impact of technology on the practice of medicine has broadened the types of therapy that are possible, it has tended to re-emphasize the age-old pressures to make surgeons into technicians rather than compassionate physicians or scientists. Nevertheless, without an ongoing and regularly updated scientific basis for surgical practice, surgeons do indeed become mere technicians.

John Hunter became a surgeon in the late 18th century when surgery was a craft rather than a science. By the time he died, he had incorporated science as an essential part of surgery and had founded a tradition of investigation that has remained unbroken ever since. The pride of surgeons in their skills and knowledge and the intellectual satisfaction they gain from the surgical act are derived from this tradition.

It is surgeons who must pose the questions about the surgical aspects of the diseases they treat. The nutritional problems and requirements of surgical patients were not defined until they were investigated by surgeons and the therapeutic intravenous solutions we now use were developed in surgical research laboratories.

Modern joint replacements are the result of surgeons' investigations of the problems posed by arthritic patients and surgeons have participated actively in identifying the causes of arthritis. Much of our present understanding of epilepsy developed in response to questions posed by neurosurgeons and a host of other examples demonstrate how patients have benefitted from the questions surgeons ask.

Shifts in the academic centers of surgery during the last 150 years have been uniformly based on surgeons' perceptions of the state of the surgical sciences throughout the world. Surgeons have travelled for their training and intellectual enrichment to the centers at the forefront at any given time. The European centers that had such great influence in the late 19th and early 20th centuries, the renowned teaching hospitals in the United Kingdom, and the great academic centers in North America have all been built around research laboratories and inquiring surgical minds.

No operating surgeon or anaesthetist is satisfied with all aspects of contemporary surgical and clinical management. Accordingly, research is not just desirable, it is a necessity imposed upon us. The authors of this book are attempting to lay down a proper framework for the organization of surgical research. The benefits will not be for surgeons but for mankind.

McGill University
Montreal, Canada

Foreword to First Edition

J.C. Goligher

For some readers, the title of this book will immediately raise the question, what exactly is meant by surgical research? In the very broadest sense the term can be taken to include all endeavors, however elementary or limited in scope, to advance surgical knowledge. Ideally, it refers to well-organized attempts to establish on a proper scientific basis (i.e., to place beyond reasonable doubt) the truth or otherwise of any concepts, old or new, within the ambit of surgery, and, of course, anaesthesia.

The methods used to achieve that end vary enormously, depending on the issue being investigated. They comprise a wide range of activities in the wards, outpatient clinics, operating rooms, or laboratories, such as simple clinical or operative observations and clinical or laboratory investigations involving biophysics, biochemistry, pathology, bacteriology, and other disciplines. Well-planned animal experimentation is exceedingly important, and it is well to remember the old truism that every surgical operation is a biological experiment whose results, unfortunately, are not always as carefully documented and analyzed as they should be. When the findings of any clinical, operative, or laboratory study are being considered, stringent statistical methods must be applied to ensure that any conclusions rest on a statistically sound basis.

Surgery provides an almost unlimited range of topics for research. Much of what is practiced and taught in surgery consists of traditional concepts passed from surgical teacher to surgical trainee by example, by word of mouth, or by standard texts, without ever having been submitted to really objective assessment. Every year we see scores of promising new ideas emerging on the surgical scene to challenge orthodoxy. Although these innovations are often greeted with great optimism, a factual basis for that enthusiasm is sometimes far from secure and much further work is frequently required to discover whether we are dealing with genuine advances.

The most exciting and attractive scenario for surgical research is unquestionably one that depicts a successful attempt by a researcher to establish the accuracy of some bold innovation for which he himself is responsible. Joseph Lister, demonstrating by clinical trial that wound suppuration could be combated by antiseptic measures, comes to mind, along with Lester Dragstedt showing by experimental and clinical studies that vagotomy could play a valuable role in the treatment of peptic ulcer disease.

In all well-developed countries, and most notably in the United States, there is now strong pressure on surgeons in training to engage in a period of research in order to foster a critical attitude towards the appraisal of the results of surgical treatment, and to stimulate a continuing interest in combining investigative work with clinical practice.

Hitherto, acquainting the tyro researcher with the methods appropriate to his or her particular project has usually depended on the guidance of more experienced colleagues working in the same field, and on the acquisition of a gradually increasing understanding of how to conduct research as the result of being in a research environment. It is very surprising that there has been no textbook to which the young researcher could turn to secure a more systematic presentation of the various matters of importance in undertaking surgical research. Hans Troidl, David Mulder, Martin McKneally, Walter Spitzer, and Bucknam McPeek are to be congratulated most warmly on their great perspicacity in recognizing the claimant need for a work providing this sort of information and, even more, on the supremely effective way in which they have met that need by the production of their new book.

Principles and Practice of Research covers its subject in an unusually comprehensive way that includes not only the conduct of research in general, but also the special facilities and problems encountered in several personal attributes that are conducive to success in research, such as a certain amount of open-mindedness combined with the enthusiasm and determination needed to carry a project through to its ultimate conclusion despite the various obstacles that may be encountered en route. Not to be forgotten in this connection is the decisive role played by sheer good luck in achieving a successful outcome in research—as is true of many other activities in life. An important subsidiary matter in the prosecution of investigative work is how to present an account of that work and its results, most effectively, at subsequent meetings or discussion groups and in publications; this book offers very helpful advice on all these points. Very appropriately, a concluding section affords an inspiring appraisal of future prospects in surgical research by that great surgeon-researcher, Francis Moore of Boston, whose contributions to surgical knowledge are legion.

I have no doubts that *Principles and Practice of Research* will be very widely read and greatly appreciated, not only by surgical trainees starting on research work, but also by experienced researchers and established surgeons who will welcome the wealth of information it provides on every facet of surgical research. Since research follows essentially the same principles in anaesthesia, medicine, obstetrics, gynecology, and other fields of clinical activity, this book should prove equally helpful to beginning or established investigators in other branches of health care. It cannot, in my judgment, fail to secure an assured place in the libraries of all medical schools, departments of surgery, and clinical departments the world over, as well as in the studies of many individual purchasers.

University of Leeds
Leeds, England

Acknowledgments

Our families have supported us in so many ways.

As editors, we owe a special debt to the authors of this textbook. They have cheerfully given us their time to share their experience in diverse fields with us and with you, the reader. Like almost all truly able people, they are busy; most are overcommitted with active lives of scientific inquiry.

Our special thanks and deepest gratitude must go to our dear colleague the distinguished Canadian scientist and editor, Dr. N.J.B. Wiggin. Each part of this book from the initial planning to the writing and editing to the preparation of the final manuscript bears his stamp. We cannot adequately express how much we have enjoyed his wit, wisdom, and good fellowship. Most of the uniformity and clarity of expression are due to his artistic sense of the English language and his insightful clarity of thought.

We are especially grateful for the foresight and generosity of Wolfgang Schmidt von Roshide, who has worked so hard to support the science of surgery.

We are particularly grateful to our colleagues at the University of Cologne, Harvard University, Albany Medical College, McGill University, Virginia Commonwealth University, and the University of Texas who have generously assumed some of our duties and thus have made it possible for us to work on this project during the last 18 months.

We have benefited from thoughtful discussions and the sound advice of many of our many of colleagues: in particular, Dr. Edmund Neugebauer, Professor Frederick Mosteller, Dr. Sharon Wood-Dauphinée, Mr. Alan V. Pollock, Miss Mary Evans, and Professor Sir Karl Popper.

We want to especially acknowledge the grace and skill of Elna Stacey. In addition to managing the preparation of the manuscript and dealing with so many authors and editors from across the globe, Mrs. Stacey has taught us each more than we can imagine about organizational skills, the differential importance of tasks, and how to maintain a completely even keel in the presence of computer failures, scholars who do not return phone calls, authors who are late with promised manuscripts, and editors who want to redo work long since completed.

The final organization and checking of the manuscript were performed in Boston by Jeanette Cohan. Ever the perfectionist, unfailingly cheerful, Mrs. Cohan coped with three different computer programs and innumerable final changes as authors and editors descended on her with last minute improvements.

Mesdames Karen Naskau, Barbara Becker, Rosemary Lombardo, Therese Papineau, Emma Lisi, Gwen Peard, and Randa Srouji worked tirelessly to prepare the manuscript.

Acknowledgments

Contents

Contributors

Jean-Henri Alexandre
Professor of Surgery, University of Paris, Clinique de l'Hopital Broussais, Paris 75014, France

Teruaki Aoki
Professor and Chairman, Department of Surgery II, Jikei University School of Medicine, Minato-ku, Tokyo 105, Japan

John Christian Bailar III
Professor of Epidemiology and Biostatistics, McGill University, Montreal, Quebec H3A 1A2, Canada

Charles M. Balch
Professor of Surgery, University of Texas, Chairman, Department of General Surgery, M.D. Anderson Cancer Center, Houston, Texas 77030 U.S.A.

Alan N. Barkun
Assistant Professor of Medicine, McGill University, Montreal General Hospital, Montreal, Quebec H3G 1A4, Canada

Jeffery S. Barkun
Clinical Associate, Department of Surgery, Toronto General Hospital, Instructor, University of Toronto, Toronto, Ontario M5G 2C4 Canada

Renaldo N. Battista
Associate Professor of Epidemiology, Biostatistics, and Medicine, McGill University, and Director, Division of Clinical Epidemiology, Montreal General Hospital, Montreal, Quebec H3G 1A4, Canada

James A. Bennett
Associate Professor of Pharmacology, Division of Cardiothoracic Surgery, and Department of Pharmacology, Albany Medical College of Union University, ME 702, A-61, Albany, New York 12208, U.S.A.

Gary G. Bernstein
Telecommunications Manager, McGill University, Montreal, Quebec H3A 1A4, Canada

Peter McL. Black
Professor of Surgery, Harvard Medical School, and Chief of Neurosurgery, Brigham and Women's Hospital, Boston, Massachusetts 02115, U.S.A.

Bertil Bouillon
II. Department of Surgery, University of Cologne, Surgical Clinic Merheim, D-5000 Cologne 91, Federal Republic of Germany

Murray F. Brennan
Professor of Surgery, Cornell University Medical College, and Chairman, Department of Surgery, Memorial Sloan Kettering Cancer Center, New York, New York, 10021, U.S.A.

Gert H. Brieger
William H. Welch Professor and Director, Institute of the History of Medicine, The Johns Hopkins University School of Medicine, Baltimore, Maryland 21205, U.S.A.

Emery N. Brown
Department of Anesthesia, Harvard University, and Massachusetts General Hospital, Boston, Massachusetts 02114, U.S.A.

Natale Cascinelli
Director, Division of Surgical Oncology B, Istituto Nazionale Tumori, 20133 Milano, Italy

Mary E. Charlson
Associate Professor of Medicine, Cornell University Medical Center, and Attending Physician and Director, The Clinical Epidemiology Unit, New York Hospital, New York, New York 10021, U.S.A.

Ray Chu-Jeng Chiu
Professor of Surgery, McGill University, Montreal General Hospital, Montreal, Quebec H3G 1A4, Canada

George T. Christakis
Division of Cardiovascular Surgery, Sunnybrook Health Science Centre, North York, Toronto, Ontario M4N 3M5, Canada

James Coleman
Professorial Unit, Department of Surgery, Royal College of Surgeons in Ireland, Beaumont Hospital, Dublin 9, Ireland

Richard L. Cruess
Dean, Faculty of Medicine, Professor of Surgery, McGill University, McIntyre Medical Sciences Building, Montreal, Quebec H3A 1Y6, Canada

H. Brendan Devlin
Consultant Surgeon, North Tees General Hospital, Hardwick Stockton-on-Tees, Cleveland TS19 8PE, United Kingdom

Jeffrey A. Drebin
Department of Surgical Oncology, The Johns Hopkins University School of Medicine, Baltimore, Maryland 21205, U.S.A.

Stanley W. Dziuban, Jr.
Associate Professor of Cardiothoracic Surgery and Physiology, and Director of Medical Informatics, Department of Surgery, Albany Medical College of Union University, Albany, New York 12203, U.S.A.

Mary E. Evans
Research Coordinator and Freelance Technical Editor, Scarborough Hospital, Scarborough, North Yorkshire Y012 6QL, United Kingdom

Ernst Eypasch
II. Department of Surgery, University of Cologne Surgical Clinic Merheim, D-5000 Cologne 91, Federal Republic of Germany

Stig Fasth
Associate Professor, Department of Surgery II, University of Goeteborg, Sahlgrenska Sjukhuset, Goeteborg S/413 45, Sweden

David M. Fleiszer
Associate Professor of Surgery, Division of General Surgery, Montreal General Hospital, Montreal, Quebec H3G 1A4, Canada

Henrietta L. Galiana
Associate Professor of Biomedical Engineering, Faculty of Engineering, McGill University, Lymann Duff Medical Building, Montreal, Quebec H3A 2B4, Canada

John C. Goligher
Emeritus Professor of Surgery, University of Leeds, Leeds, United Kingdom

Dietrich Götze
Professor, Springer-Verlag, D-6900 Heidelberg, Federal Republic of Germany

Stephen W. Hartzell
Department of Oncology, The Johns Hopkins University School of Medicine, Baltimore, Maryland 21205, U.S.A.

Christian Herfarth
Dean of the Faculty of Medicine, Professor, and Head of the Department of Surgery, University of Heidelberg, D-6900 Heidelberg, Federal Republic of Germany

Peg Hewitt
Director, Peg Hewitt Information Services, 27 Stanton Road, Brookline, Massachusetts 02146, U.S.A.

Koshiro Hioki
Associate Professor of Surgery, Kansai Medical University, Fumizonocho Moriguchi, Osaka 570 Japan

Sarah McCue Horwitz
Assistant Professor of Public Health, Department of Epidemiology and Public Health, Yale University School of Medicine, New Haven, Connecticut 06510, U.S.A.

Leif Hultén
Professor of Surgery, Department of Surgery II, University of Goeteborg, Sahlgrenska Sjukhuset, Goeteborg S-41345, Sweden

Wolf H. Isselhard
Dean of the Faculty of Medicine, Professor of Experimental Surgery, and Director, Institute of Experimental Medicine, University of Cologne, D-5000 Cologne 41, Federal Republic of Germany

Norman A. Johanson
Professor of Orthopaedic Surgery, Cornell University Medical College, and Chief of Orthopaedics, Bronx Veterans Administration Medical Center, New York, New York 10021, U.S.A.

Michael S. Kramer
Professor of Pediatrics and of Epidemiology and Biostatistics, McGill University, Montreal, Quebec H3A 1A3, Canada

Jürgen Kusche
Professor, Madaus GmbH, D-5000 Cologne-Merheim, Federal Republic of Germany

Felix Largiadèr
Professor of Surgery, University of Zürich, Director of Visceral Surgery, University Hospital, Ch-8091 Zürich, Switzerland

Valerie A. Lawrence
Assistant Professor, Department of Medicine, The University of Texas, Health Science Center at San Antonio, San Antonio, Texas 78284-7879, U.S.A.

Francis E. LeBlanc
Professor and Chairman, Division of Neurosurgery, Foothills Hospital, Calgary, Alberta T2N 2T9, Canada

Rolf Lefering
Biochemical and Experimental Division, II. Department of Surgery University of Cologne, D-5000 Cologne 91, Federal Republic of Germany

Bernhard Lewerich
Springer-Verlag, D-6900 Heidelberg, Federal Republic of Germany

Wilfried Lorenz
Professor of Theoretical Surgery, and Head, Institute of Theoretical Surgery, Philipps-University of Marburg, Centre of Operative Medicine, Klinikum Lahnberge, D-3550 Marburg, Federal Republic of Germany

Daniel Marelli
Department of Surgery, McGill University Montreal, Quebec H3A 1Y6, Canada

Richard G. Margolese
Herbert Black Professor of Surgical Oncology, McGill University, and Director, Division of Oncology, Department of Surgery, Sir Mortimer B. Davis–Jewish General Hospital, Montreal, Quebec H3T 1E2, Canada

Stephen A. Marion
Assistant Professor, Department of Health Care and Epidemiology, University of British Columbia, Vancouver, British Columbia V6T 1W5, Canada

Arthur D. Mason, Jr.
Chief of Laboratory Division, U.S. Army Institute of Surgical Research, Fort Sam Houston, San Antonio, Texas 78234-6200, U.S.A.

Martin F. McKneally
Professor of Surgery, University of Toronto, Chief and Head, Division of Thoracic Surgery, Toronto General Hospital, Toronto, Ontario M5G 2C4, Canada

Bucknam McPeek
Associate Professor of Anaesthesia, Harvard University, and Anesthetist to the Massachusetts General Hospital, Boston, Massachusetts 02114, U.S.A.

Francis D. Moore
Moseley Professor of Surgery, Emeritus, Harvard Medical School, Countway Library of Medicine, Harvard Medical School, and Surgeon-in-Chief, Emeritus, Peter Bent Brigham Hospital, Boston, Massachusetts 02115, U.S.A.

Frederick Mosteller
Roger I. Lee Professor of Mathematical Statistics, Emeritus, Harvard School of Public Health, Boston, Massachusetts 02115, U.S.A.

C. Barber Mueller
Professor of Surgery, Emeritus, McMaster University, Hamilton, Ontario L8N 3Z5, Canada

David S. Mulder
H. Rocke Robertson Professor of Surgery, McGill University, Surgeon-in-Chief, Department of Surgery, Montreal General Hospital, Montreal, Quebec H3G 1A4, Canada

Terukakazu Muto
Professor and Chairman, First Department of Surgery, Niigata University School of Medicine, Niigata 951, Japan

Edmund A. M. Neugebauer
Assistant Professor of Theoretical Surgery, and Head, Biochemical and Experimental Division, II. Department of Surgery, University of Cologne, D-5000 Cologne 91, Federal Republic of Germany

John E. Niederhuber
Professor of Surgery, Johns Hopkins University School of Medicine, Baltimore, Maryland 21205, U.S.A.

Lisa Oxley-Droter
Department of Surgery, Medical College of Virginia, Richmond, Virginia 23298, U.S.A.

Andreas Paul
II. Department of Surgery, Surgical Clinic Merheim, University of Cologne, D-5000 Cologne 91, Federal Republic of Germany

Alan V. Pollock
Honorary Consultant Surgeon, Scarborough Hospital, Scarborough, North Yorkshire Y012 6QL, United Kingdom

Raphael E. Pollock
Associate Professor of Surgery, Department of General Surgery, M. D. Anderson Cancer Center, Houston, Texas 77030, U.S.A.

Basil A. Pruitt, Jr.
Commander and Director, U. S. Army Institute of Surgical Research, Fort Sam Houston, Texas, San Antonio, Texas 78234-6200, U.S.A.

H. David Reines
Associate Professor of Surgery, and Director of Critical Care/Trauma, Medical College of Virginia, Richmond, Virginia 23298, U.S.A.

Jack Roth
Professor and Chairman, Department of Thoracic Surgery, M. D. Anderson Cancer Center, Houston, Texas 77030, U.S.A.

Mathias Rothmund
Professor of Surgery and Chairman of the Department of Surgery, Philipps-University of Marburg, Centre of Operative Medicine, D-3550 Marburg, Federal Republic of Germany

David J. Roy
Director, Center for Bioethics, Clinical Research Institute of Montreal, Montreal, Quebec H2W 1R7, Canada

David C. Sabiston, Jr.
James B. Duke Professor of Surgery and Chairman, Department of Surgery, Duke University Medical Center, Durham, North Carolina 27710, U.S.A.

David L. Sackett
Professor of Medicine and of Clinical Epidemiology and Biostatistics, McMaster University, Hamilton, Ontario L8N 3Z5, Canada

Pedro A. Sanchez
Clinical Chief of Pediatric Cardiac Surgery, Centro Especial Ramon y Cajal, Madrid 28034, Spain

Martin T. Schechter
Associate Professor, Chairman of the Division of Epidemiology and Biostatistics, Department of Health Care and Epidemiology, University of British Columbia, Vancouver, British Columbia V6T 1W5, Canada

Sir Robert Shields
Professor and Head, Department of Surgery, University of Liverpool, and Consultant Surgeon, Royal Liverpool Hospital and Broadgreen Hospital, Liverpool L69 3BX, United Kingdom

Margot Siminovitch
Department of Audio-Visuals, Montreal General Hospital, Montreal, Quebec H3G 1A4, Canada

Walter O. Spitzer
Strathcona Professor of Epidemiology and Biostatistics, Professor of Medicine, and Chairman, Department of Epidemiology and Biostatistics, McGill University, Montreal, Quebec H3A 1A2, Canada

Patricia Steele
Director, Department of Audio-Visuals, Montreal General Hospital, Montreal, Quebec H3G 1A4, Canada

Christian Troidl
Unterlehmbach 22, Rösrath, D-5064 Hoffnungsthal, Federal Republic of Germany

Hans Troidl
Professor of Surgery and Chairman, II. Department of Surgery, Director, Surgical Clinic Merheim, University of Cologne, D-5000 Cologne 91, Federal Republic of Germany

Beverly C. Walters
Assistant Professor of Surgery, Division of Neurosurgery and Department of Preventive Medicine and Biostatistics, University of Toronto, Sunnybrook Health Science Centre, North York, Ontario M4N 3M5, Canada

Andrew S. Wechsler
Stuart McGuire Professor of Surgery and Chairman, Department of Surgery, Professor of Physiology, Medical College of Virginia, Richmond, Virginia, 23298-0645, U.S.A.

Richard D. Weisel
Professor and Director of Surgical Research and Centre for Cardiovascular Research, Toronto General Hospital, Toronto, Ontario M5G 2C4, Canada

Norman J.B. Wiggin
Biomedical Science Editor, 82 Rothwell Dr, Ottawa, Ontario K1J 7G6, Canada

J. Ivan Williams
Professor, Department of Family and Community Medicine, and Department of Preventive Medicine and Biostatistics, University of Toronto, and Deputy Director, Clinical Epidemiology Unit, Sunnybrook Health Science Centre, North York, Ontario M4N 3M5, Canada

Pamela G. Williams
The Clinical Epidemiology Unit, Cornell University Medical Center—New York Hospital, and Assistant Attending Physician, New York Hospital and the Hospital for Special Surgery, New York, New York 10021, U.S.A.

Sharon Wood-Dauphinée
Associate Professor of Physical and Occupational Therapy, and of Medicine, and Epidemiology and Biostatistics, and Associate Director, School of Physical and Occupational Therapy, McGill University, and Medical Scientist, Royal Victoria Hospital, Montreal, Quebec H3G 1Y5, Canada

Thomas Yeh, Jr.
Division of Cardiac and Thoracic Surgery, Department of Surgery, Medical College of Virginia, Richmond, Virginia 23298, U.S.A.

Introduction to Second Edition

H. Troidl

My colleagues and I have been most pleased at the reception given to the first edition of this book. We conceived the idea for *Principles and Practice of Research* because we could not find in one volume a clear exposition of research methods for clinical disciplines. We saw a need to cover the principles of experimental design, biostatistics, epidemiology, strategies for beginning and finishing research, and finally the diffusion of results. We sought a book in which a clinician–scholar could find an introduction to specific research methods, an introduction that would start at square one and give a complete overview of each issue, ending with suggestions for further readings on special topics. We deliberately tried to keep our chapters rather brief, to permit them to be comfortably read by a tired clinician between dinner and bedtime. We carefully sought authors who were good at exposition, who shared with us a special concern for helping others develop careers in clinical science.

The first edition was favorably reviewed in journals across the world, and their reviewers made many helpful suggestions. In the preparation of this second edition, we have tried to respond to them.

We have been particularly pleased by the letters received from readers in many countries, some from old friends, many from well-known clinical scholars and teachers. Perhaps the most heartening have been letters from young men and women just starting to build careers of practice and research. Most of our correspondents offered helpful suggestions for future revisions. They kindly pointed out important topics we failed to cover, issues we touched on too briefly, or explanations that seemed unclear. Their comments have been of prime importance in planning, writing, and editing this present edition.

When our publisher, Springer-Verlag, first approached us about preparing a second edition we were eager to do so. After all, we read the book too, and while we were proud of what had been done and pleased that both reviewers and individual readers liked it and found it met their needs, we could see ways to improve it even before our friends helped us by pointing out some of the warts and blemishes.

After a series of planning meetings, Professor David Mulder from Montreal, Professor Martin McKneally from Albany, Professor Jack McPeek from Boston, and I sat down together in Chicago during a meeting of the American College of Surgeons to discuss the best way of approaching a second edition. All of us were busy, none more so than Professor Walter Spitzer, who had just committed himself to a year's sabbatical in the United Kingdom coordinating a major research project in epidemiology. The temptation to do only a quick revision, a cosmetic job, was strong, but our hearts were not in that. We and Springer knew that our readers deserved something more. More meant a larger, more complete volume. To do this, we needed help and turned to two of the most respected and innovative clinical scholars in North America: Professor Andrew Wechsler, chairman of the Department of Surgery at Virginia Commonwealth University in Richmond, and Professor Charles Balch, chairman of the Division of General Surgery at the University of Texas–M.D. Anderson Cancer Institute in Houston. Andy and

Charles agreed without hesitation. This edition shows the effect of their outstanding teaching and editorial skills.

Thus began a busy 2-year process, at planning meetings in the United States, Canada, and Europe, research seminars in Boston, Montreal, and Cologne, and correspondence with methodologists and clinical scholars across the world to decide on a choice of emphasis, topics, and authors. We were indeed fortunate in again enlisting the collaboration of the distinguished Canadian editor, clinician, and research administrator, Dr. N.B.J. Wiggin. Authors and editors circulated drafts and redrafts of chapters by telefax, courier, and occasionally, by mail. Gradually a new book took shape.

Over the last 6 months, as we had been putting the final touches on this second edition, I reread each of the letters sent in by readers. I wanted to make sure that we have responded seriously to readers' suggestions. We have retained the format you liked, revised chapters that needed to be strengthened, and completely rewritten others that required more help. We have added new chapters to cover areas you felt got short shrift before. Especially helpful have been a series of research seminars held for budding academicians at Harvard University, McGill University, and the University of Cologne. These young academicians and their teachers offered many practical suggestions.

We hope that this second edition meets your needs and expectations. I am truly grateful to my friends, both old and new, who have helped in its preparation as critics and reviewers, authors, editors, and now to you as readers.

Cologne, Germany
August 1990

Introduction to First Edition

H. Troidl

Early in my career as an academic surgeon, Professor H. Hamelmann encouraged me to venture from my home department at the University of Marburg to visit other academic surgical departments in Germany. I was immediately struck by the variety of approaches to similar clinical challenges and surgical research problems. When my good fortune took me to other university centers in Europe, I was particularly impressed by Professor John Goligher's philosophy and approach to surgical scholarship in Leeds. During the several months I subsequently spent working with him in 1973, I learned as much as I could about his way of doing clinical research and found his and other British perspectives especially valuable because my previous experience in Germany had been largely confined to basic laboratory research. The following year, Professor Wilfried Lorenz of Marburg accompanied me to North America to visit basic research laboratories, clinical departments of surgery and anesthesia, and clinical research centers. We consulted researchers at the National Institutes of Health, Cornell University, and the University of California at Los Angeles, and clinicians at Albany, Chicago, and the Mayo Clinic.

When I left Marburg to become first assistant to Professor Hamelmann in the Department of Surgery at Kiel, I continued my laboratory research activities while I acquired further experience as a clinical surgeon. During this period, the necessity for an academic surgeon to be an exemplary clinician, a skilled and uncompromising technician in the operating theater, an inspiring teacher, and a competent researcher, *simultaneously*, was brought home to me.

Once again, I was struck by the similarity of the unanswered questions in surgery and anesthesia, no matter where they arose in the world. The problems had common themes, but the solutions proposed were very different in different cities and countries, whether they were related to the organization of medical care, levels and sources of funding, or the design of research studies. Even the organization of research facilities varies not only between countries, but within countries; differences among the individual units of a single university or hospital are the rule, not the exception.

As I traveled and corresponded with friends in other centers, I realized that some of the ideas and solutions developed in Sweden had relevance to the problems we faced in Marburg and Kiel. Some of the ideas I discovered in North America, the United Kingdom, or Japan could be profitably brought home to Germany. My colleagues at home showed me that only a little modification was sometimes required to make them applicable and useful in Marburg. I was delighted to find that colleagues around the world were curious to know how we cope with problems in Germany, and that new friends in Boston and Montreal were not only open to sharing their problems but very receptive to ideas and potential solutions that my colleagues and I had worked out in Germany.

When I became Professor of Surgery at Cologne, I instituted an open-door policy. I invited senior scholars to visit us in Cologne and arranged for my younger colleagues to be exposed to leaders and new ideas elsewhere. A number were able to present the results of their own work and to learn, firsthand, the techniques that I had discovered for myself, earlier.

My most trusted colleagues and I gradually recognized that while research problems had much in common around the world and many scientists had developed fruitful strategies and tactics for dealing with the problems associated with surgical research, there was no readily accessible source of information about much of the methodology that was evolving so rapidly. The idea of a book on feasible technology for research in surgery and other clinical disciplines became compelling. It would cover the principles of experimental design, biostatistics, epidemiology, starting and finishing research, and the diffusion of results.

Many a scholarly undertaking, whether it is a book or a research project, starts with an idea. Taking the idea from conception to fruition is often aided by interactions with friends—with whom I am still blessed!

The first step toward converting my idea of a book into a reality took place on October 14, 1984, in a chalet nestled in the hills near St. Adolphe, north of Montreal. My friend and host, Professor Walter Spitzer, spent half the night arguing with me about a possible table of contents. Early in the morning, we reached a consensus and quickly wrote down the headings and subheadings. When we called our mutual friend, Professor Jack McPeek in Boston, he immediately pronounced a benediction on our plan and agreed to work on it with us without hesitation. Professor Martin McKneally was the next to hear from us at four in the morning—it's hard to contact busy surgeons at any other time of the day. He was already up preparing slides for a paper and enthusiastically joined our growing team as soon as he had heard the details. Within a few hours, Walter and I succeeded in reaching Professor David Mulder in Montreal to find that he needed no persuasion before volunteering to contribute his considerable effort and resources.

Over a period of years, most clinical scholars develop an appreciation of the elements of experimental design and the recruitment and management of research resources. The acquisition of this knowledge is unpredictable in different academic settings and all too often is a matter of trial and error learning under the supervision of senior colleagues who have also learned by the trial and error method. It need not be so, because a much better understanding and consensus about scientifically acceptable methodology has been developing around the world.

The editors of this book share my concern about this state of affairs and my commitment to doing something about it. Each is a scholar with a special responsibility for advancing research. Three of us are clinical surgeons charged with the care of patients, the supervision of research laboratories, and the development of younger surgical research colleagues in Albany, Cologne, and Montreal. One is a professor with a long track record of clinical epidemiologic research and teaching who now directs the affairs of the major Department of Epidemiology and Biostatistics at McGill University. One is an anesthetist, clinician–teacher, and research administrator at the Massachusetts General Hospital and Harvard University. Each is single-minded about helping colleagues with research problems and establishing an atmosphere and facilities to advance applied science. The underlying motive of all is to improve the care of patients through better understanding of relevant biological phenomena. We all give priority to the task of nurturing the academic growth of younger associates. A significant number of individuals who are world experts in their fields have joined our undertaking. Investigators in clinical disciplines, epidemiology, biostatistics, and the basic medical sciences have created a complementary ensemble of chapters giving advice on how to make research the creative, exciting, stimulating, intellectual endeavor it should be.

We offer practical suggestions and describe approaches and methods that have a proven record of success. The treatments prescribed for some of the most common ailments that afflict many well-intended clinical research endeavors are straightforward, but not simplistic or superficial. Most chapters are the product of collaborative efforts among clinicians and methodologists. Although the exposition of each topic is by no means exhaustive, sources of additional information are provided.

I sincerely hope that this book will help many of my colleagues, especially those who are newer in the field of clinical investigation, to avoid the errors and frustrations I have encountered in my search for a deeper understanding of clinical surgical research. The rewards and excitement of seeking and finding new knowledge can only be accelerated and enhanced by having a roadmap in hand when you start on your journey of discovery.

Cologne, Germany
August 1986

Section I

Investigators and Investigation

The daily array of unsolved clinical problems presented by our patients remains the major stimulus for all medical research. Societal expectation from physicians makes research a vital and increasing function for all clinical departments in our universities. The future health of our population depends upon the full spectrum of research methods in human biology, including basic laboratory studies, clinical trials, population based investigation and more recently health technology assessment.

This section correctly begins with the historical evolution of research in general and of surgical research in particular. Pollock describes the development and importance of clinical trials in any clinical discipline. Sabiston provides a succinct summary of important milestones in the development of surgery as a scientific discipline. He emphasizes the pivotal role of scholarly activity in the training and development of all surgeons. Chiu describes a spectrum of roles for the investigator in a department of surgery.

The editors re-define the clinical researcher of the 1990s using the pentathlete as an illustrative analogy. Emphasis is placed on changes necessary in training programs, both clinical and laboratory in order to achieve these new goals. Many suggestions are provided to strengthen the research environment.

The final chapter in this section will introduce North American readers to the new concept of theoretical surgery through the "Marburg Experiment." Lorenz describes the value of a collaborative relationship between an academic clinician and a basic scientist. Several examples of the beneficial effects of this integration in the solution of common clinical problems are most convincing.

This introductory section on the development of investigators and investigation will pave the way for reading of subsequent sections on commencing the research process, methodology and finally communicating the results of your work to the scientific community.

1

Historical Evolution: Methods, Attitudes, Goals

A.V. Pollock

Research! A mere excuse for idleness; it has never achieved and will never achieve any results of the slightest value.

Benjamin Jowett[1]

Surgical research, whether in the laboratory, the animal house, the wards, or the community, relies first and foremost on accurate and honest observation and description.

> . . . it is not easy to be accurate in an account of anything, however simple. Zoologists often disagree in their descriptions of the curve of a shell, or the plumage of a bird, though they may lay their specimen on the table and examine it at their leisure; how much greater becomes the likelihood of error in the description of things which must be in many parts observed from a distance, or under unfavorable circumstances . . . I believe few people have an idea of the cost of truth in these things; of the expenditure of time necessary to make sure of the simplest facts, and of the strange way in which separate observations will sometimes falsify each other, incapable of reconcilement, owing to some imperceptible inadvertency.[2]

Observation, alone, can lead to fallacies. We still say the sun rises in the east and sets in the west. What could be more natural to medieval observers than to suppose that the sun travels around a stationary earth? It took the genius of Nicolaus Copernicus to refute this theory. The observation was correct, but the ancient proposition ignored the movements of the planets – a new hypothesis was needed, and Copernicus supplied it.

The essence of a scientific statement is that it can be falsified by further observation and be replaced by a new statement. Newton gave the world several propositions that explained nearly all astronomical events. Einstein sought the exceptions and propounded the theory of relativity to explain more observations than those supported by Newton's hypotheses. In Einstein's words:

> . . . [T]he new theory of gravitation diverges widely from that of Newton with respect to its basic principle. But in practical application, the two agree so closely that it has been difficult to find cases in which the actual differences could be subjected to observation.[3]

The Philosophy of Research

Two living philosophers of science stand out – Karl Popper and Thomas Kuhn – and their views conflict to some extent.[4] Popper proposed that the distinction between science and nonscience is that it is possible to falsify a scientific proposition. "God created the universe" is a statement of faith – a proposition that cannot be refuted; but "The world was created 7000 years ago" is a falsifiable hypothesis and therefore a scientific statement.

Popper sees criticism as a chief function of a scientist and has traced logical argument back to the pre-Socratic philosophers of Greece – Thales, Anaximander, and Anaximenes – who initiated the tradition of subjecting speculation to critical discussion that is the basis of the scientific method. In Popper's view, the scientific method comprises the following steps:

1. Seek a problem.
2. Propose a solution.
3. Formulate a testable hypothesis from that proposal.
4. Attempt to refute the hypothesis by observations and experiments.
5. Establish preference between competing theories.

> All this means that a young scientist who hopes to make discoveries is badly advised if his teacher tells him: "Go round and observe" and that he is well advised if his

teacher tells him: "Try to learn what people are discussing nowadays in science. Find out where difficulties arise, and take an interest in disagreements. These are the questions which you should take up." In other words, you should study the problems of the day. This means that you pick up, and try to continue, a line of inquiry which has the whole background of the earlier development of science behind it.[5]

Kuhn, in contrast, wrote that scientific knowledge does not progress steadily by criticism of established hypotheses and claimed that *ordinary* research seeks only to solve puzzles within the framework ("paradigm") of the existing accumulation of scientific knowledge. This steady state of puzzle solving is interrupted from time to time by *revolutions* that arrive suddenly, irrationally, and intuitively to establish a new paradigm within which the new scientists do their ordinary research and attempt to solve new puzzles.

Neither Popper nor Kuhn took much interest in biological or medical research, but we can accept both their philosophies. We can try to solve puzzles, and we can also set up hypotheses and devise observations and experiments to refute them. McIntyre and Popper[6] suggested the following 10 rules for medical practice and research:

1. Our present conjectural knowledge far transcends what any person can know, even in his own specialty. It changes quickly and radically and, in the main, not by accumulation but by the correction of erroneous doctrines and ideas. There can be no authorities; there can be better and worse scientists. More often than not, the better the scientist, the more aware he or she will be of personal limitations.
2. We are all fallible; nobody can avoid even all avoidable mistakes. The old idea that we must avoid them has to be revised. It is mistaken and has led to hypocrisy.
3. Nevertheless, it remains our task to avoid errors. But to do so we must recognize the difficulty. It is a task in which nobody succeeds fully—not even the great creative scientist who is led, but quite often misled, by intuition.
4. Errors may lurk even in our best-tested theories and it is the responsibility of the professional to search for them. The proposal of new alternative theories can help us greatly; we should be tolerant of ideas that differ from the dominant theories of the day and not wait until those theories are in trouble. The discovery that a well-tested and corroborated theory, or a commonly used procedure, is erroneous may be a most important discovery.
5. Our attitude toward mistakes must change because it is here that ethical reform must begin. The old attitude leads us to hide our mistakes and to forget them as quickly as we can.
6. The principle that we must learn from our mistakes, so that we avoid them in future, must take precedence even over the acquisition of new information. Hiding mistakes must be regarded as a deadly sin. Such errors as operating on the wrong patient or removing a healthy limb are inevitably exposed. Although the injury may be irreversible, exposure of the error can lead to the adoption of practices designed to prevent its recurrence. Other errors may be equally regrettable, but not so easily exposed. Those who commit them may not wish to have them brought to light, but they should not be concealed because discussion and analysis may change practice and prevent their repetition.
7. We must search for our mistakes, investigate them fully, and train ourselves to be self-critical.
8. We must recognize that self-criticism is best, but criticism by others is necessary and especially valuable if they approach problems from a different background. We must learn to be graceful, and even grateful, in accepting criticism from those who draw our attention to our errors.
9. When we draw the attention of others to their mistakes, we should remind ourselves of the similar errors we have made; it is human to err and even the greatest scientists make mistakes.
10. Rational criticism should be directed to definite, clearly identified mistakes. It should contain reasons and should be expressed in a form that allows its refutation. It should make clear which assumptions are being challenged and why. It should never contain insinuations, mere assertions, or only negative evaluations. It should be inspired by the aim of getting nearer to the truth; and, for this reason, it should be impersonal.

The surgeon, whether solving puzzles or refuting hypotheses, can seek help from three interdependent disciplines: bench work, animal experiments, and clinical practice. Many problems in clinical practice can be solved only in the biochemical and microbiological laboratories. Some questions can be answered ethically only by animal experiments, but laboratory and animal research is sterile unless it has a potential for affecting clinical practice. The historical development of clinical research is outlined here, that of laboratory research in Section III, Chapter 33.

The Social Responsibility of Scientists

Prometheus was punished for bringing knowledge into the world, and Faust for wanting it too much. Scientists should be aware that they are held responsible for the outcome of the knowledge they generate and must face up to their special responsibilities.

The word "eugenics" was coined by Francis Galton in 1883, and it generated the idea of producing "a highly gifted race of men by judicious marriages during several consecutive generations."[7] In 1904 Charles Davenport persuaded the Carnegie Foundation to set up the Cold Spring Harbor Laboratories to study human evolution. All these activities were undertaken by worthy scientists, but Hitler took up the idea of eliminating undesirable genes from the human stock, only 30 years later.

We can now insert genes into human cells. Inserting them into somatic cells gives little cause for argument about the desirability of such research, but inserting new genes into germ cells raises issues of such importance that the public must participate in the debate on its acceptability.

Wolpert[8] advocated letting the community share the responsibility for developing scientific advances, and quoted Thomas Jefferson:

> I know no safe depository of the ultimate powers of the society but the people themselves, and if we think them not enlightened enough to exercise that control with a wholesome discretion, the remedy is not to take it from them, but to inform their discretion.

The History of Clinical Research

The following statement is unscientific because it cannot be refuted: our forefathers, at least as far back as the fifth century BC, were no less intelligent than we are. Why, then, is biological and medical research, with a few exceptions, a product of the last century?

Respect for the Doctor–Patient Relationship

There was a time when a doctor was almost universally regarded as being all-seeing and all-knowing, and this attitude persists in some parts of the world. As a consequence, a physician could never admit that his diagnosis was conjectural or his treatment ineffective. He could never confess ignorance; but the acknowledgment of ignorance is the first step toward research.

Inaccurate Diagnoses

You cannot do clinical research unless you can make precise diagnoses. Diagnostic accuracy improved following the discovery of the causative role of microorganisms in certain diseases, the introduction of diagnostic radiology, and the more recent advances in biochemistry, immunology, and diagnostic imaging techniques.

Ineffective Remedies

When physicians were powerless to influence the course of most diseases, they did not think of doing research. One placebo was as good as the next, and it was merely discourteous to question the practice of colleagues.

Reverence for Authority

Until the late nineteenth century, the task of scholars was to study and interpret the writings of others; reverence for authority was the outstanding virtue. The approach to learning was conceptual rather than empirical. Sir Dominic John Corritan,[9] writing in *The Lancet*, in 1829, said about Harvey's discovery of the circulation of the blood: "Such, however, is the power of prejudice that no physician past the age of forty believed in Harvey's doctrine, and that his practice declined from the moment he published this ever-memorable discovery."[9] Although a few original thinkers have challenged authority in every age, in spite of opposing social pressures, it is only recently that respect for logical thinking has generated skepticism and the pursuit of pragmatism.

Lack of Statistical Tests

In therapeutics, scientific testing of remedies is one of the strongest forces for change. The fundamental requirement of a proper clinical trial is the evaluation of the outcome of a treatment regimen by the application of methods based on the mathematics of probability.

Evolution of Population Statistics

During the eight centuries between the compilation of the *Doomsday Book*—an inventory of King William's newly conquered English kingdom—and the nineteenth century, vital statistics were not systematically collected anywhere in Europe. In 1776 the Société Royale de Médicine made one of the first attempts to record births and deaths throughout France, but a reliable system was not introduced until the early 1800s, and later still in other European countries. By 1880, individual cards had taken the place of highly fallible lists in the compiling of statistics, and the Hollerith punch card sorting machine was first used in a national census in the United States in 1890.

It soon became evident that epidemiological studies were stultified by the inaccuracy of death certificates. Even as late as the beginning of the twentieth century, Sir Josiah Stamp was able to write:

> The government are very keen on amassing statistics. They collect them, add them, raise them to the *n*th power, take the cube root, and prepare wonderful diagrams. But you must never forget that every one of these figures comes in the first instance from the village watchman, who puts down what he damn well pleases.[10]

In 1853 William Farr, who had been a student of Pierre Charles Alexandre Louis, inventor of the "numerical method," in Paris, cooperated with Marc d'Espine in developing the anatomically based system of classification of diseases that formed the foundation of today's *International Classification of Diseases*.

Louis's numerical method received no acclaim until relatively recently. In 1835 he published a paper translated as "Research on the effect of blood-letting in several inflammatory maladies"; his main conclusion was that blood letting had little therapeutic value.[11] The paper attracted adverse comment in the French Academy of Sciences, and François Double issued a report condemning the use of statistical methods in clinical method and extolling Morgagni's aphorism: *Non numerandae sed perpendendae*—facts must be weighed, not counted. Nevertheless, in 1837 Simon Denis Poisson wrote that if a medication had been successfully used in a large number of similar cases, and if the number of cases in which it had not succeeded was small compared with the total number of cases, it was probable that the medication would succeed in a new trial.

Mathematics of Probability

Games of chance were the original stimulus to sixteenth-century philosophers, including Galileo, to attempt to give mathematical expression to probabilities.[12,13] In the following century, Blaise Pascal corresponded regularly with a fellow mathematician, Pierre de Fermat, on probabilities in relation to card games. The first inkling of modern methods of statistical analysis appeared in 1713 when Jacob Bernoulli's *Ars conjectandi* was published. He proved that the more often a test is repeated, the greater is the probability that the result will be within certain limits.

In eighteenth-century France, Abraham de Moivre published *Doctrines of Chance*, and "The Petersburg Problem" was widely discussed (i.e., if a coin toss comes up tails several times, is it more likely to come up heads the next time?). In 1785 the Marquis de Condorcet declared, in his Essay on the Application of Mathematics to the Theory of Decision Making, that probability calculus "weighs the grounds for belief and calculates the probable truth of testimony or decisions."

The French mathematical philosopher Pierre Simon, Marquis de Laplace, published his *Analytical Theory of Probabilities* in 1812 and wrote: "The theory of probabilities is fundamentally only good sense reduced to calculation."

By 1870, statistical analysis of whole populations was well advanced, but the problems of sampling had not been tackled. Then, the new science of microbiology temporarily eclipsed interest in the application of statistics in medicine, and the development of statistical methods for analyzing samples shifted to brewing and agriculture. The term "random" was first applied in a statistical sense at the end of the nineteenth century.

The Development of Clinical Trials

Historical Controls

Most great advances in therapeutics have been made by contrasting the results of a new regimen with those of previously documented treatment. The enormous benefits of general anesthesia, the reduction of surgical infection rates by asepsis, the cure of many infections by penicillin, and numerous other advances, have needed only careful documentation and comparison with previous experience to become accepted.

If a new treatment is immeasurably better than the old, historical controls are not only sufficient, they are the only ones that are ethical. Once it had been shown that penicillin could cure bacterial endocarditis—previously uniformly lethal—not treating all cases with penicillin was unacceptable. Random control trials are justified only if there is a therapeutic dilemma. Ignorance is essential.

The inappropriate use of historical controls can, however, lead to false conclusions. This is particularly true if the results of surgical treatment are compared with previous experience with medical treatment of the same disease. There is a selection bias in such a study; the surgeon operates only on patients who are fit enough to have the operation. The results cannot be compared with those of *all* patients in a previous series treated medically.

An example of this bias was published in the *New England Journal of Medicine* in 1948.[14] Among patients with bleeding esophageal varices, caused by cirrhosis of the liver, Linton reported better survival figures for those who were treated by portacaval shunts than in a control group treated medically in previous years. The surgical patients were those who survived long enough to be operated on; those who never became fit for surgery or died before it could be performed were not reported. Linton's conclusions were subsequently repudiated by the Boston Liver Group,[15] who randomized patients fit enough for operation to standard medical treatment or to portacaval shunting. The results were not significantly different in the two groups, but vastly superior to those in a group of patients not fit enough to be recruited into the trial.

Contemporary Nonrandom Controls

Many questions about etiology and epidemiology can be answered only by comparing a group of people subject to certain risks with another group that is not. Sometimes, the evidence from such comparisons is sufficiently compelling to demand acceptance (e.g., the association between cigarette smoking and bronchial carcinoma, or of exposure to asbestos dust and mesothelioma). Epidemiological research using case controls can, however, produce more questions than answers; witness the confusion about the connection between diet and atherosclerosis, or between oral contraceptives and breast cancer.

A carefully conducted case-control study showed a significant influence of prolonged use of oral contraceptives on the development of breast cancer in women under the age of 35 years.[16] The authors were careful to minimize biases, but their conclusions are at odds with those of other epidemiological studies and with the absence of a rise in the overall incidence of breast cancer during the years of wide usage of oral contraceptives.

In therapeutics, all contemporary nonrandom comparative studies are suspect because outcomes depend on so many factors. The population sample in the study group may differ from that in the control group in the incidence of risk factors, in an uneven distribution of the variables associated with treatment, and in variations in the methods of assessment of events. Although the conclusions reached in such studies can be tentative only, they may form the basis for hypotheses to be tested in random control trials.

Normann et al.[17] published an example of such a study. The two surgical departments of Ulleval Hospital, in Oslo, followed different regimens for the treatment of perforated appendicitis. In one, appendicectomy was completed by inserting a drain into the appendix fossa; in the other, it was followed by two days of peritoneal dialysis. The drainage group recorded 1 death, 6 pelvic abscesses, 1 intraperitoneal abscess, 4 cases of paralytic ileus, 4 repeat laparotomies, and 1 fecal fistula, for a total complication rate of 17 in 77 patients. In the lavage group, the complications comprised 1 death, 3 pelvic abscesses, 1 paralytic ileus, and 1 repeat laparotomy: a total rate 6 in 78. Firm conclusions about the superiority of peritoneal dialysis are not justified, however, because of the strong likelihood of important undisclosed variables.

Random Control Clinical Trials

Ronald Aylmer Fisher was the first to recognize that many pitfalls in nonrandom trials can be avoided by allocating subjects to each arm of a trial strictly by chance and allowing the investigator no control over the randomization process.[18]

Fisher was a mathematician and biologist who studied physics under James Jeans at Cambridge, but he chose a career in biology. In 1919 he became statistician to Rothamsted Agricultural Experimental Station, where field trials had been carried out since 1843 without ever being subjected to statistical analyses. Fisher undertook the task of analyzing earlier trials and designing new trials free from bias. He wrote widely on the statistical analysis of trials and worked out the exact probability test that bears his name. In 1925 he published *Statistical Methods for Research Workers*,[19] which dealt with the design and analysis of controlled trials. His second book, *The Design of Experiments*,[20] appeared in 1935 when he was Galton Professor at University College, London.

In 1937 Austin Bradford Hill published in *The Lancet* a series of papers that were reprinted in a book entitled *Principles of Medical Statistics*. Its tenth edition is renamed *A Short Textbook of Medical Statistics*.[21] Hill's name has become synonymous with the proper ethical and statistical design of clinical trials. One of his greatest achievements was the organization in 1947 of the Medical Research Council cooperative trial on the treatment of pulmonary tuberculosis by streptomycin.[22] Because the short supply of streptomycin in Britain precluded its being offered to all patients with tuberculosis, a random control trial in which the control group was treated by the best current standard methods was ethically justifiable. Central randomization was used for the first time, and the trial was a brilliant success.

Ethical Standards

The ethical obligation always and entirely outweighs the experimental.[23]

The doctor's duty to each patient must always come first. It is only within the framework of this duty that controlled trials are proper, and numerous measures exist to safeguard the welfare of patients. National and international rules are laid down for the conduct of clinical trials; financial support will not be provided for unethical trials; and lastly, peer review bodies judge, and if necessary, amend protocols of clinical trials to ensure their ethical acceptability.

Ethical principles in surgical research, including the ethical requirements of informed consent for the various forms of clinical trials, are discussed in Chapter 12, Section II.

In any trial, patients must be retained in the arm to which they were randomized, even if they do not get the treatment prescribed for that arm. This may dilute the results, and the outcomes in these patients may have to be analyzed separately, but such analysis must treat them as part of their allocated group and not as part of the alternative group. Publishing the results of a biased trial is just as unethical as failing to obtain consent to a trial.

Random Control Trials Can Be Misleading

The future of the random control trial in surgery is threatened by the recent refinements of ethical principles and by practising surgeons' doubts about the relevance of trials in small self-selected groups of patients. The low proportion of women with breast cancer who enrolled in the trial of total versus segmental mastectomy illustrates this.

A similar problem of selective enrollment came to light when the Extracranial–Intracranial Bypass Study Group reported that such bypasses failed to reduce the risk, compared with medical treatment, of ischemic stroke in patients with otherwise inoperable extracranial vascular disease.[24] The trial recruited 1377 patients in 71 centers and cost $9 million. After the report was published, T. Sundt, a physician at the Mayo Clinic, made extensive enquiries of the contributors and estimated (a) that less than half of all eligible patients had been entered into the trial and (b) that the conclusion that surgical versus medical treatment conferred no benefit could not be applied to all patients with the disease.[25]

Two statisticians took issue with Sundt's strictures and wrote that failure to randomize eligible patients was "not really a defect at all . . . A randomized trial implies merely random division between the group allocated to treatment and that allocated to control, not random selection of those to be included in the study."[26] Dudley had the last word in this debate; he wrote: ". . . tosh. Much more open and less adversarial debate is needed about how we acquire new, and particularly treatment related, information."[27]

Where Do We Go from Here?

Ethical restraints and resistance by patients and surgeons to allowing chance to decide the choice of operation—or the choice of operative versus nonoperative treatment—mean that we will have to rely increasingly on complete, accurate, and honest audit of the outcome of diseases treated in different ways. There must be no exclusions, no excuses, and no concealments.

Selective publication is one reason why techniques may be adopted uncritically, or not at all, or why old techniques are abandoned. Surgeons are generally reluctant to publish poor results, and fear of litigation may inhibit honest reporting, particularly in the United States. This is illustrated by the doubts recently cast on neutron treatment of cancer.[28] Although initially hailed as an important advance in the treatment of certain patients, particularly those with head and neck cancers, it is now regarded with considerable skepticism following reports of severe damage to normal tissues. Eli Glatstein, head of the radiation oncology branch of the National Cancer Institute in the United States, concluded: "My reading of the results is that neutrons have a slightly better effect on some tumors than x-rays, but that this is offset by severe side effects on normal tissues."

Reports of trials of new techniques must always include comparisons with the results in a control group. The selection of the control group may be biased: by choosing the worst published results of an alternative technique, authors sometimes exaggerate the excellence of their own results. Surgeons have a lot to learn from epidemiologists who, denied the possibility of doing random control trials, have evolved other methods of minimizing bias.

References

1. Sutherland J, ed. The Oxford Book of Literary Anecdotes. Oxford: Clarendon Press, 1975:253.
2. Ruskin J. The Stones of Venice. Boston: Dana Estes, 1851.
3. Einstein A. Einstein on his theory. The Times, November 28, 1919; quoted in The Times, November 28, 1985.
4. Lakatos I. Falsification and the methodology of scientific research programmes. In: Criticism and the Growth of Knowledge, Lakatos I, Musgrave A, eds. Cambridge: Cambridge University Press, 1970.
5. Popper K. Conjectures and Refutations: The Growth of Scientific Knowledge, 4th ed. London: Routledge & Kegan Paul, 1972:129.
6. McIntyre N, Popper K. The critical attitude in medicine: the need for a new ethics. Br Med J 1983;287: 1919–23.
7. Pearson K, Quoted by Wolpert L.[8]
8. Wolpert L. The social responsibility of scientists: moonshine and morals. Br Med J 1989;289:941–43.
9. Corrigan DJ. Aneurysm of the aorta. Singular pulsation of the arteries—necessity of the employment of the stethoscope. Lancet 1829;i:586–90.
10. Stamp J. Quoted by: Dunea G. Swallowing the golden ball. Br Med J 1983;286:1962–63.
11. Gaines WJ, Langford HG. Research on the effect of blood-letting in several inflammatory maladies. Arch Intern Med 1960;106:571–79.
12. Murphy TD. Medical knowledge and statistical methods in early nineteenth century France. Med Hist 1981;25:301–9.
13. Westergaard H. Contributions to the History of Statistics. London: PS King & Son Ltd, 1932.
14. Linton RR. Porta-caval shunts in the treatment of portal hypertension, with special reference to patients previously operated upon. N Engl J Med 1948;238:723–27.
15. Garceau AJ, Donaldson RM, O'Hara ET, Callow AD,'Muench H, Chalmers TC, and the Boston Inter-Hospital Liver Group. A controlled trial of prophylactic portacaval shunt surgery. N Engl J Med 1964;270:496–500.
16. UK National Case-Control Study Group. Oral contraceptive use and breast cancer risk in young women. Lancet 1989;i:973–82.
17. Normann E, Korvald E, Lotveit T. Perforated appendicitis—lavage or drainage? Ann Chir Gynaecol Fenn 1975;64:195–97.
18. Yates F, Mather K. Ronald Aylmer Fisher 1890–1962. Biographical Memoirs of Fellows of the Royal Society 1963;9:91–129.
19. Fisher RA. Statistical Methods for Research Workers. Edinburgh: Oliver & Boyd, 1925.
20. Fisher RA. The Design of Experiments. Edinburgh: Oliver & Boyd, 1935.
21. Hill AB. A Short Textbook of Medical Statistics. London: Hodder & Stoughton, 1977.
22. Medical Research Council. Streptomycin treatment of pulmonary tuberculosis. Br Med J 1948;2: 769–82.
23. Zelen M. A new design for randomized clinical trials. N Engl J Med 1979;300:1242–45.
24. EC/IC Bypass Study Group. Failure of extracranial–intracranial bypass to reduce the risk of ischaemic stroke: result of an international randomized study. N Engl J Med 1985;313:1191–200.
25. Sundt T. Was the international randomized trial of extracranial–intracranial arterial bypass representative of the population at risk? N Engl J Med 1987;316:814–16.
26. Warlow C, Peto R. Extracranial–intracranial bypass, one; clinical trials, nil. Br Med J 1987;295:211.
27. Dudley HAF. Extracranial–intracranial bypass, one; clinical trials, nil. Br Med J 1987;295:389.
28. Smith R. Neutron treatment: the international perspective. Br Med J 1989;298:347.

2

Roles for the Surgical Investigator

R.C.-J. Chiu and D.S. Mulder

A surgical investigator is a bridge tender, channelling knowledge from biological science to the patient's bedside and back again. He traces his origin from both ends of the bridge. He is thus a bastard and is called this by everybody. Those at one end of the bridge say he is not a very good scientist, and those at the other say that he does not spend enough time in the operating room. If only he is willing to live with this abuse, he can continue to do his job effectively.[1]

The observation above, attributed to Francis D. Moore, captures the essence of both the role and the dilemma of the surgical investigator. The increasing difficulty experienced by the surgical investigator in fulfilling this role well is partially responsible for what C. Rollins Hanlon, past director of the American College of Surgeons, has called a "deteriorating situation in surgical research that has been troublesome for some years and is now verging on crisis."[2]

The Dilemma of the Surgical Investigator

A surgeon who wishes to pursue active research faces many difficult questions, the foremost being how to maintain excellence both in the practice of surgery and in investigation. It is now generally accepted that to maintain operative competence, especially in performing such complex procedures as open heart surgery, a surgeon has to have a certain minimal case load. This requirement, combined with the increasing sophistication of technology and of competition for research funding, makes it difficult for the surgeon-investigator to dedicate enough time and effort to research to remain competitive. These conflicting time demands are aggravated by changing patterns of medical financing that may pressure investigators to generate funds by expanding their clinical practice. The administrative chores associated with government intervention in the practice of medicine compound the problem. Resolving this chronic and deepening time dilemma requires joint efforts by surgical investigators, themselves, and by the institutions that nurture surgical research.

Another common question surgical investigators face is: How "basic" should their research orientation be? A researcher studying transplantation immunology—a surgically relevant problem—may quickly find it necessary to study the function of suppressor T-lymphocytes; to understand that, he must appreciate the nature of cell surface receptors; to grasp the function of the receptors fully, and to convince the grant review committee that he possesses the necessary scientific depth, he finds himself learning to analyze the molecular structure of the protein components of receptors. At this point, he may wonder whether he is stretching the limits of his competence too far. At what point will whatever results he obtains become decreasingly cost-effective in relation to his investment of time and effort? No one denies the importance of basic and fundamental research to advances in surgery, but how basic should the research of an individual surgical investigator be?

Walter F. Ballinger denies the existence of "basic" research in surgery. He defines surgical research as a type of applied physiology. A surgical investigator uses biochemistry, biophysics, mathematics, or electronics and "may flirt with problems of radiation physics, but he will not become an expert radiologist or physicist because of his flirtation, and for this he may be criticized."[3] Moore has also cautioned against allowing surgical research to become too basic and has written about "the very urgent and elegant work of applied science." These outstanding leaders in surgical research have emphasized the role of surgical investigators as "bridge tenders" and have warned them not to go so far from the bridge that they lose sight of it.

The adoption of much more liberal definitions of surgical research by many institutions in recent years, despite the admonitions just cited, has given rise to some perplexing questions about what "surgical research" really is. The term surgical investigation may now be used to describe:

1. Research done by anyone on any subject, provided it is done within the jurisdiction of a department of surgery. The rationale is that virtually everything can be ultimately shown to have some relation to surgery. Accordingly, surgical research could include a study of the molecular structure of a cortisol-binding protein by someone with a Ph.D. in molecular biology, who has an appointment as an assistant professor in surgery and publishes the research results in journals of biochemistry. Is this really "surgical" research?
2. Research on any subject provided it is done by a surgeon. Would a surgeon's work on improving the safety of sailboats qualify as surgical research?
3. Research done by anyone, provided the subject is relevant to surgical problems. An individual with a Ph.D. in nutrition and an appointment in the Department of Medicine might make an important contribution by studying the nutritional support of patients with major burns. Does the work qualify as "surgical research"?
4. Research done by surgeons on such surgical problems as the devising of new instruments for operative procedures. Is this not excessively narrow to be called surgical research?

Any discussion of the role of the surgical investigator must reflect this wide range of current views about the meaning of "surgical research."

The Spectrum of Surgical Investigators

Several categories of surgical investigator play specialized roles in large departments of surgery:

1. *Tightrope walkers* are the real bridge tenders, trying to balance a commitment to clinical surgery with a research effort. They miss the operating theater if they are in the research laboratory every day, but if they operate all the time they feel guilty about ignoring the laboratory. Administrators or colleagues may feel that these people do not generate sufficient income for the department or institution, while grant review committees wonder whether these "part-time" investigators should be supported, as opposed to those who spend all their time in research. This dual pressure makes "tightrope walkers" the most endangered species among scholars, although they best fit the classical description of academic surgeons and play the most important and indispensable role of bridging the gap between patient care and basic science.
2. *Benchmen* are basic scientists or clinicians who devote their time exclusively to investigation. They have established, or are able to develop, the requisite expertise to pursue an in-depth program that may lead to important advances in surgery. They are indispensable in major projects, where a team approach is necessary. They function best in an environment offering good interaction between clinicians and scientists, and they may be more competitive in obtaining research grants; but they are more dependent on the institutions for personal support. Lack of clinical input and isolation from their colleagues, however, may make benchmen nominal "surgical" investigators, even if they work within a department of surgery.
3. *Occasional surgeon-investigators* are found among the many busy "cutting" surgeons who try to find the time and money to do some research. They have no difficulty in maintaining clinical competence, and their research efforts, although limited, bring mental stimulation to and promote interaction among other scientists, to their mutual benefit. Their research efforts enhance their ability to follow advances in surgical science and to be more critical and effective teachers. They, too, must constantly struggle to find time for research. The few hours they reserve each week for the lab will be constantly interrupted by emergency calls, unscheduled meetings, and similar demands. They have difficulty in winning peer-reviewed grants and may find that they can do meaningful research only by proxy, through research assistants, residents, and fellows. An extraordinary effort must be made by very busy, often exhausted, clinical surgeons even to provide adequate supervision for their trainees. It might be more practical for them to devote themselves to clinical research that can be coordinated or integrated with clinical practice. Alternatively, they could join forces with benchmen.

4. *The organizer and the team leader.* Some investigators are best suited to the role of organizer, either in a department or in a laboratory. Wise organizers follow the dictum of Detley Bronk, former president of Rockefeller University, to "find the right man, back him up, and stay out of the way."[4] In contrast, team leaders must be able to commit enough time to supervise their research teams properly and also be able to contribute actively to the formulation of research ideas. Lack of adequate time for supervision, especially of trainees who are too anxious to get ahead in a "publish or perish" milieu, produces a fertile environment for scientific fraud and scandal.[5,6] Team leaders who wish to receive credit for the achievements of team members must also be prepared to share the blame for their misconduct. The time demands on team leaders and senior investigators are heavy, since they usually carry a multitude of responsibilities and administrative duties, within and outside their institutions, in addition to their clinical work. They are also frequently in demand as visiting professors, lecturers, or consultants, and the number of scientific meetings they have to attend multiplies every year. Nevertheless, the team leader who provides strong leadership galvanizes his research team and provides a role model for his associates and trainees.

Some academic surgeons go through many metamorphoses as their careers move from one to another of the categories listed above. They may devote much of their time to research as benchmen after their training but, as their clinical practices grow, they move to being tightrope walkers, then to occasional surgeon–investigators, eventually becoming organizers or team leaders. This procession of roles has both positive and negative consequences, but it illustrates the dynamic changes a surgical investigator can undergo.

The Scope of Research by a Surgical Investigator

The research orientation of surgeons who are not basic scientists is likely to be determined by a number of influences. Scientific curiosity, of itself, may lead an investigator toward increasingly basic issues. The truism that "the results raise more questions than answers" holds for surgical research, and the desire to have answers to an accumulation of result-prompted questions tends to lead the investigator further away from clinical surgery. This urge should not be categorically discouraged, because doing so may not only risk dampening healthy scientific curiosity but may also forestall the discovery of a fundamental phenomenon of nature that could become the basis for a major breakthrough in surgery. The lure of probing ever deeper, however, should be tempered by an awareness of the danger of reaching beyond the limits of one's own expertise into an area best left to scientists trained specifically for that field.

Recognition by one's peers is desirable. If a surgeon–investigator's work is published mostly in basic science journals, it may not receive peer recognition from surgical colleagues who do not read such journals. Lack of surgical peer recognition may fix the investigator's research orientation and alter the path of his or her career. Consequently, surgical investigators must consider their own expertise and career objectives to determine how "basic" they wish to go in carrying out their own research.

The Role of Surgical Investigators in Research Grant and Journal Reviews

The quality of reviews for surgical grant applications and journal manuscripts is closely related to some of the problems discussed above. For a number of reasons, applications and manuscripts by surgeons are described as "often of low scientific merit" by our detractors. In some instances, "peer review" of the grant application is not carried out by a real "peer." A surgical investigator who wishes to study post-trauma sepsis may find that his application for grant support was sent to a "Committee on Infectious Disease and Immunology" and subsequently reviewed by a bacteriologist whose area of expertise is the bacterial cell wall.

It is recognized that, although the peer review process cannot be perfect, it is the best method available for assuring the quality of scientific research. Nevertheless, it should, at the very least, be performed by real "peers" who have experience with and understanding of surgical problems.

Surgeons are often underrepresented on review committees, partly because they are too busy. The devotion of time and effort to reviewing grant applications requires a very strong commitment by overburdened senior surgical investigators, but the surgical point of view must be presented to ensure the support of good surgical investigations.

It must be conceded that many surgical grant applications are prepared in haste and do not embody the principles of good experimental design and analysis outlined in this book. The experienced surgical investigator can play an important role in ensuring adequate funding for young researchers by providing advisors, by arranging prior internal reviews of applications, and by personally asking whether the proposal is a well-focused project with a clear hypothesis or merely a diffuse "fishing expedition" using a "shotgun approach" in its search for results.

Does the applicant document his or her capability to carry out the proposed work by citing previous training or a track record of publications? If not, does the application provide evidence of collaboration with appropriate experts? The reviewers want to be assured that the project is feasible in the applicant's hands. Is the experimental protocol appropriate and, most important, will it produce an answer to the question posed in the hypothesis? Does the applicant clearly describe how the sample size was calculated and how the data will be analyzed? Are the possible difficulties and pitfalls recognized? Does the application provide sufficient detail to justify the budgetary requests and include all required documents from appropriate ethics committees? And finally, has the applicant properly emphasized the originality, clinical relevance, and scientific significance of the proposed project?

Some of the negative scientific criticism of certain surgical journal articles may arise from the excessive proliferation of journals, but it may also reflect the difficulty in obtaining appropriately qualified reviewers for manuscripts, given the many demands on the time of senior surgical investigators. Lack of careful attention to the elements of rigorous scientific methodology is undoubtedly a factor. For many investigators, a thoughtful and detailed comment by grant and manuscript reviewers is a very useful and educational experience. Constructive criticisms and suggestions by recognized experts can clarify a hypothesis, improve an experimental design, sharpen the accuracy of data analysis, and contribute to an investigator's continuing research training and maturation.

Surgeons or surgical investigators who are so pressed for time that they reject an application or manuscript with a cursory paragraph, or an abusive note, deeply discourage and embitter rejected authors. It is the responsibility of granting agencies and journal editors to evaluate their reviewers and drop those with inadequate commitment or competence.

Peer review duties are generally undertaken by senior scientists on a voluntary basis. Although such devotion is desirable and praiseworthy, remuneration of reviewers may have to be considered in the future if it will lead to better reviews and enlarge this important channel of continuing education for investigators. This issue is receiving increasing attention from scientists in all disciplines,[7] but the problem may be more acute for many surgical clinical scientists, given the especially heavy and urgent demands on their time.

The Role of the Surgical Investigator in Surgical Education

Surgical investigators play a vital role in the education and training of students, surgical residents, and surgeons. They are uniquely qualified and situated to instill the critical scientific attitude that trainees will need to analyze, select, and absorb the expanding quantities of new information they will encounter during their careers. Surgical investigators serve not only as bridge tenders bringing surgical and scientific training together, but also as mentors, discovering and guiding their protégés—the future surgical investigators.

George T. Moore once commented on the lack of creativity among surgeons.[8] He felt that the surgical training environment is unfavorable for creative endeavor because it pressures residents to develop clinical skills and to become master technicians. John Gibbon advocated having surgical trainees spend at least a year working in a laboratory, under supervision, to give them the opportunity to discover whether research holds any particular appeal. Supervisors quickly learn whether such beginners are self-starters.

> The man with potentialities as an investigator will see problems that need solution and will outline methods of approaching them. The methods he proposes may be inadequate because of his experience, but the fact [that] he recognizes the incompleteness of his knowledge in a certain area, and that he formulates an attack upon the problems indicates that he is a potential investigator. On the other hand, the individual who spends the year intelligently and faithfully carrying out the suggestions of his supervisor, adding little or nothing of his own to the solution of the problem under consideration is not the man to continue to do research . . . both he and his mentor will have a good idea at the end of the period as to whether he has the capacity for research. If he has not, the time will not have been misspent, because the year's experience will enable him to be a more critical reader of surgical literature during the rest of his professional life.[9]

These insights are as valid today as they were when uttered more than two decades ago.

Few surgical investigators have been such successful mentors as Owen Wangensteen. One of his students, Clarence Dennis, became a pioneer in cardiac surgery and described the role of his mentor most succinctly:

> Early in Wangensteen's career as Chairman of Surgery, it became clear that, although he was desperately proud of his contributions to the science of surgery, he was even more devoted to the thesis that he could do more for mankind by training men in the cradle of free inspiration, with courage to express new and sometimes revolutionary ideas, with the greater courage to expose them to the tests of experimental verification and clinical application, and finally by becoming themselves leaders in teaching and developing other generations of imaginative investigators in their turn.[10]

The Role of the Surgical Investigator in a Department of Surgery

The primary role of surgical investigators is to improve the surgical care of patients by advancing the frontier of knowledge; their three functions of giving care, teaching, and leading research in an academic surgical department are the expression of this fact. To make such important contributions, they require support from their departmental chairmen and colleagues.

The research productivity of a surgical department is largely determined by how committed its chairman is to research. A young surgical department attempting to establish excellence in research will quickly discover what an expensive undertaking it is. The clinical service and staff generate funds as a by-product of their activities, but research and research investigators are a financial burden and will likely be the first to suffer when the monetary resources of a department are acutely strained. A mutually supportive, collaborative rapport between the clinical staff and investigators prevents jealousy, competition, and isolation. The department can nurture the productivity and excellence of surgical investigators by recognizing the dilemma they face in apportioning adequate time to both surgery and research. Surgical investigators must avoid arrogance and recognize that their best results will be achieved by working in partnership with their clinical colleagues. If they do not, they may be investigators, but not "surgical investigators."

The Ideals of a Complete Surgical Investigator

The ideal of surgical investigators is to be superb tenders of the bridge joining the science and the art of surgery. To be investigators, they must be good scientists who recognize that research starts with an idea—a working hypothesis. Claude Bernard pointed out many years ago, that an idea comes as a particular feeling, a quid proprium that constitutes the originality, the inventiveness, or the genius of each individual. A new idea appears as a new or unexpected relation that the mind perceives among different things. Surgeons with such gifts should be encouraged, and they do lean toward research. Research ideas, however, are not innate; they do not arise spontaneously. They arise only, a priori, from an event or problem observed by chance in the course of caring for patients, or following some experimental venture, or as corollaries of an accepted theory.

To be able to develop and pursue ideas that will bring benefit to patients, the investigator must be exposed to problems and be able to discover them. Once an idea or hypothesis has crystallized, a background of proper scientific training will enable the investigator to reason logically, develop appropriate experimental designs, carry out an investigation, and analyze and interpret the results. These matters are covered in other chapters of this book, but it is important to bear in mind that

> an experimenter puts questions to Nature, but as soon as she speaks, he must hold his peace; he must note her answer, hear her out and in every case accept her decision . . . he must never answer for her nor listen partially to her answers by taking, from the results of an experiment, only those which support or confirm his hypothesis . . . this is one of the great stumbling blocks . . . .[11]

The results obtained by research are brought back to the operating room or the patient's bedside, or they become the basis for further research.

In summary, the life of a surgical investigator is demanding and beset by competing priorities and dilemmas. And yet, the consummate surgical investigator is blessed with a career that encompasses the humanity associated with care of the sick, the artistic satisfaction of delicate surgical operations, and the joy of creation and discovery.

References

1. Moore FD. The university in American surgery. Surgery 1958;44:1–10.
2. Hanlon CR. Decline of surgical research. Bull Am Coll Surg 1985;70:1–2.
3. Ballinger WF, II. Surgical research as a discipline. In: Research Methods in Surgery, Ballinger WF II, editor, Boston: Little, Brown, 1964:3.
4. Bronk D (quoted from Genest J). Ann R Coll Physicians Surg Canada 1985;18:323–28.
5. Culliton BJ. Emery reports on Darsee's fraud. Science 1983;220:936.

6. Genest J. Clouds threatening medical research. Ann R Coll Physicians Surg Canada 1985;18: 323–28.
7. Bailar JC, III, Patterson K. Journal peer review: the need for a research agenda. N Engl J Med 1985;312: 654.
8. Moore GE. Surgeons: age, training and creativity. Surg Gynecol Obstet 1960;110:105–7.
9. Gibbon JH, Jr. The road ahead for thoracic surgery. J Thorac Cardiovasc Surg 1961;42:141–49.
10. Dennis C. A heart–lung machine for open-heart operations. How it came about. Trans Am Soc Artif Intern Organs 1989;35:767–77.
11. Bernard C. An Introduction to the Study of Experimental Medicine, Green HC, transl. New York: Dover, 1957:33.

3

The Development of Surgical Investigation

D.C. Sabiston, Jr.

The discipline of surgery has been fortunate in having had a number of investigators who have made significant basic scientific contributions with practical clinical application. The great medical historian, Garrison, considered Ambroise Paré, John Hunter, and Joseph Lister, to be the three greatest surgeons of all time (Fig. 3.1). Paré reintroduced and popularized the ancient use of the ligature to control hemorrhage and placed it on a firm basis. He also introduced the concept of the controlled experiment, when treating two soldiers with similar wounds lying side by side in a tent near the battlefield. The first soldier's wound was managed by the standard method of cauterization with boiling oil. The second was managed by debridement, cleansing, and the application of a clean dressing. Paré wrote that he spent a restless night, worrying that the second patient would do very poorly since his treatment defied the standard therapy of that time. The following morning, however, he found the second patient to be essentially without systemic symptoms, whereas the other had high fever, tachycardia, and disorientation. When he was congratulated on the outcome of this new approach, Paré very humbly replied: "Je le pansay, Dieu le guarit" (I treated him, God cured him"), a quotation subsequently inscribed on his statue.

To John Hunter is due the primary credit for introducing the *experimental method* by using animals to develop surgical techniques prior to their application to humans. His philosophy and practice are appropriately summarized in his often-quoted response to a question from Edward Jenner, the developer of smallpox vaccination. When Jenner was speculating about hibernation in the hedgehog, Hunter responded tersely, "I think your solution is just; but why *think*? Why not *try* the experiment?"[1]

Joseph Lister will be forever remembered for his great concern with wound infections and their hazard to the expansion of surgery. He was confident that wound infections could be prevented and was the first to apply the bacteriological studies of Louis Pasteur by initiating aseptic surgery in clinical practice.

The Development of Formal Training Programs

The original patterns of surgical training were established in Europe during the latter half of the nineteenth century, particularly in the university clinics of Germany, Austria, and Switzerland. The surgical masters, who were all-powerful in their respective hospitals, established the principle of stepwise assumption of responsibility in residency training programs, culminating in the concept of fully completing the training during the chief residency. Bernhard von Langenbeck, professor of surgery at the University of Berlin, is regarded as the father of modern training programs (Fig. 3.2). An extraordinary teacher, clinical investigator, and master surgeon, he is credited with devising 33 original operative procedures.[2] At the famed Charité Hospital in Berlin, he attracted a remarkable group of trainees, including Billroth, Kocher, Trendelenburg, and many others (Fig. 3.3). Each became a leader of his own school and a great contributor in his own right. Langenbeck was also the first to initiate a journal devoted solely to surgery, *Archiv für klinische Chirurgie*, also known as "*Langenbeck's Archiv*" (Fig. 3.4). After completing Langenbeck's program, Billroth became professor of surgery at Zurich and later at the University of Vienna, where he was chief

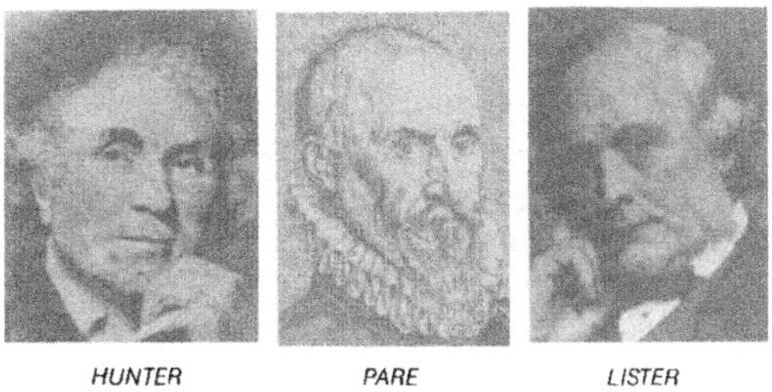

FIGURE 3.1. John Hunter, Ambroise Paré and Joseph Lister.

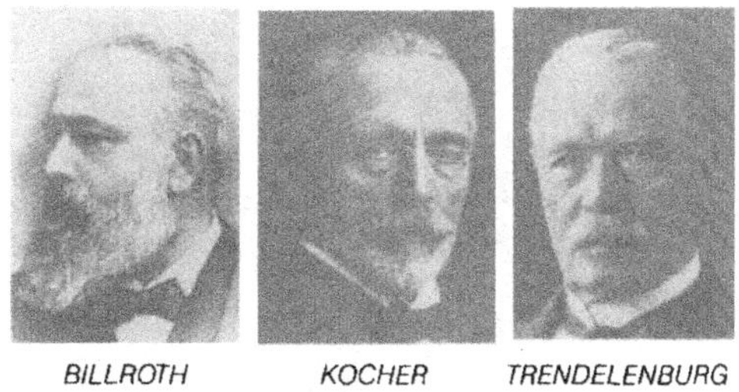

FIGURE 3.3. Students of Professor Bernhard von Langenbeck.

surgeon to Allegemeines Krankenhaus. Theodor Kocher was appointed professor at the University of Berne at the amazing age of 31; Trendelenburg was appointed to the chair in Leipzig.

In the United States, the development of surgical residency training programs followed the Langenbeck–Billroth schools, as introduced by William Stewart Halsted (Fig. 3.5). Generally regarded as the most outstanding surgeon in North America, Halsted regularly visited the major surgical clinics in Europe from 1878 until the end of his life. He was impressed by the progressive system of surgical training and completely devoted to the concept that highly selected, bright young trainees should begin as interns and gradually progress through the residency with increasing responsibility. He believed that, upon completion of the chief residency, the trainee should have essentially the same abilities as the teachers in the university clinic. Consequently, many trainees were appointed to

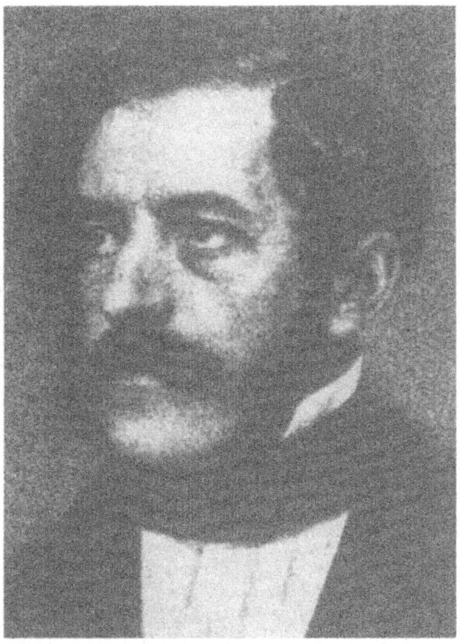

FIGURE 3.2. Bernhard von Langenbeck, professor of surgery at the University of Berlin.

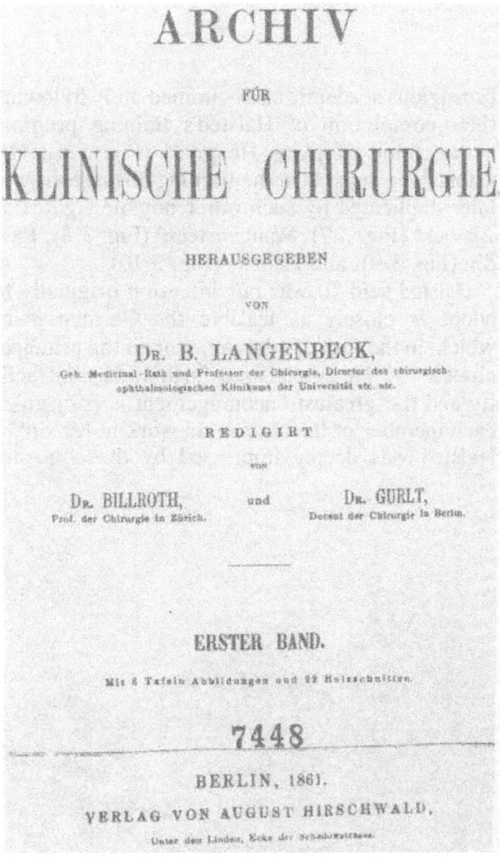

ARCHIV

FÜR

KLINISCHE CHIRURGIE

HERAUSGEGEBEN

VON

DR. B. LANGENBECK,

Geh. Medicinal-Rath und Professor der Chirurgie, Director des chirurgisch-ophthalmologischen Klinikums der Universität etc. etc.

REDIGIRT

VON

DR. BILLROTH, Prof. der Chirurgie in Zürich. und DR. GURLT, Docent der Chirurgie in Berlin.

ERSTER BAND.

Mit 6 Tafeln Abbildungen und 22 Holzschnitten.

7448

BERLIN, 1861.

VERLAG VON AUGUST HIRSCHWALD,

Unter den Linden, Ecke der Schadowstrasse.

FIGURE 3.4. Title page of first issue of Langenbeck's *Archiv für klinische Chirurgie*.

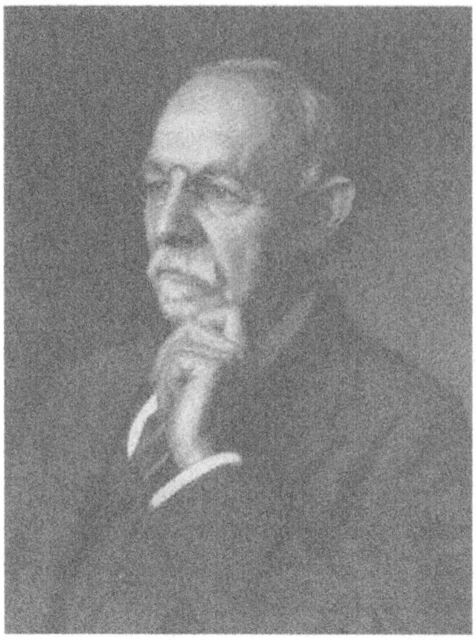

FIGURE 3.5. William Stewart Halsted.

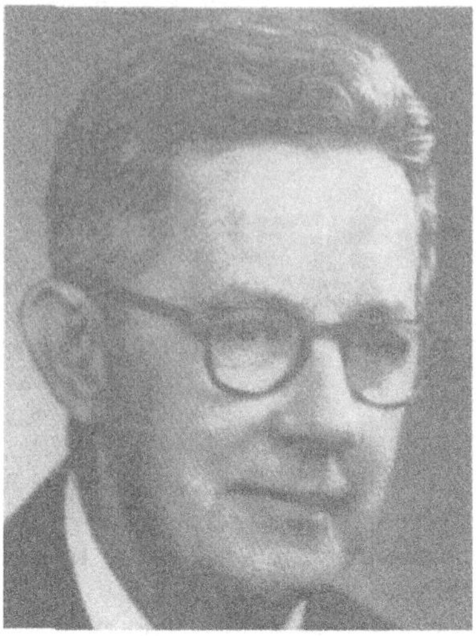

FIGURE 3.7. Alfred Blalock, renowned surgical investigator, teacher, and trainer of many academic surgeons.

prestigious academic chairs immediately following their completion of Halsted's training program at the Johns Hopkins Hospital[3] (Fig. 3.6). His astonishing success in the training of surgeons was later duplicated by such other notable figures as Blalock[4] (Fig. 3.7), Wangensteen[5] (Fig. 3.8), Ravdin (Fig. 3.9), and Rhoads (Fig. 3.10).

Halsted said "It was our intention originally to adopt as closely as feasible the German plan, which, in the main, is the same for all the principal clinics. . . ." He emphasized further: "Every facility and the greatest encouragement is [sic] given each member of the staff to do work in *research*." Halsted was deeply impressed by the contributions of those who involved themselves in original research, and he specifically cited the discoveries of Hunter, Pasteur, and Lister as being the foundation of modern surgical practice.

In his classic address, "The Training of a Surgeon," delivered at Yale in 1904, Halstead said:

The assistants are expected in addition to their ward and operating duties to prosecute original investigations and to keep in close touch with the work in surgical pathol-

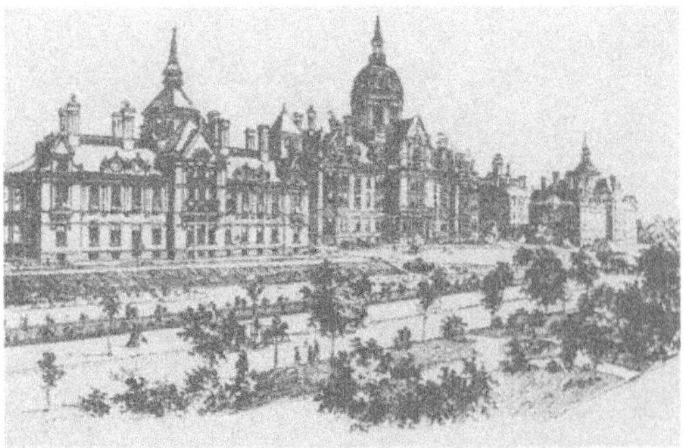

FIGURE 3.6. Johns Hopkins Hospital as it appeared when built in 1889 (from an original etching).

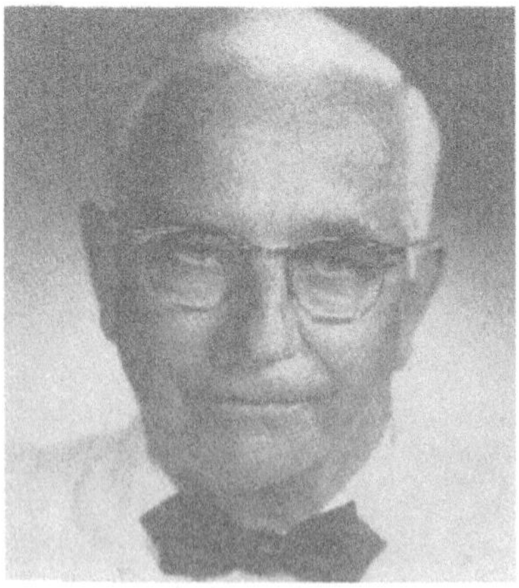

FIGURE 3.8. Owen H. Wangensteen, famed academic surgeon who trained many of the current leaders in surgery.

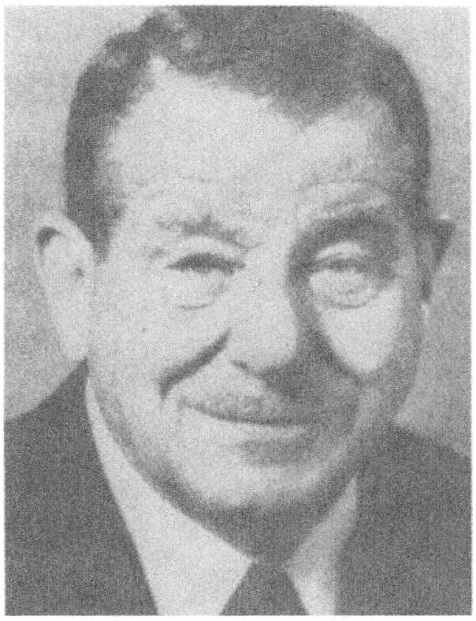

FIGURE 3.9. Isador S. Ravdin.

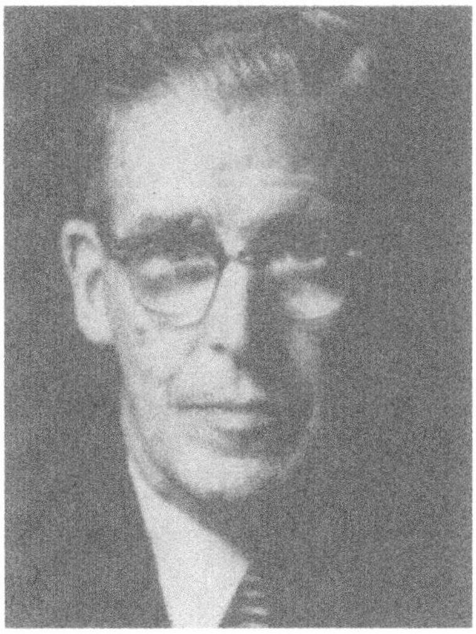

FIGURE 3.10. Jonathan E. Rhoads.

ogy, bacteriology, and so far as possible physiology. . . . Young men contemplating the study of surgery should early in life seek to acquire knowledge of the subjects fundamental to the study of their profession."[3]

"Halsted's men" were subsequently appointed to the most prestigious academic posts, and his concepts of surgical training with emphasis on clinical excellence, combined with research, spread rapidly and became widely adopted.[6]

In his frequently quoted presidential address to the American Surgical Association in 1956, Alfred Blalock said:

> The only way an interested person can determine whether or not he has aptitude in research is to give it a trial . . . My point is that he should not shy away from it because of a misconception and fear that he does not have originality. As a medical student, I felt pity for the investigator, but later this changed to admiration and envy.[7]

As his teacher Halstead had done decades earlier, Blalock realized achievements in clinical surgery, research, and the training of academic surgeons that elevated him to a towering position in the history of surgery.[4]

Responsibility for the training of surgical investigators is an obligation of surgical faculty members everywhere. More than two centuries ago, Samuel Johnson said:

> Every science has been advanced to a perfection by the diligence of *contemporary* students and the gradual discovery of one age improving on another, either truths, hitherto unknown, must be enforced by stronger evidence, facilitated by a clearer method, or more ably elucidated by brighter illustrations.

The distinguished Nobel laureate, Arthur Kornberg, in an essay entitled "Research–The Lifeline of Medicine," stated:

> Advances in medicine spring from discoveries in physics, chemistry, and biology. Among key contributions to the diagnosis, treatment and prevention of disease, an analysis has shown that two-thirds of these discoveries have originated with basic observations, rather than applied research. Without a firm foundation in basic scientific knowledge, innovations perceived as advances frequently prove hollow and collapse.

Surgical teachers are well advised to bear persistently in mind a comment of one of our greatest physiologists, Julius Comroe:

> I have always believed that a main responsibility of a faculty member is to be a talent source–to determine the special abilities of medical students in clinical care, in teaching, or in research and then to encourage them to do the very best they can in their field of unusual competence. One field, of course, is research. I see no way for faculty to determine this special talent of their students unless students have contact with research while they are still in medical school.

Quite clearly, it is highly desirable that students begin investigative work as soon as practicable.

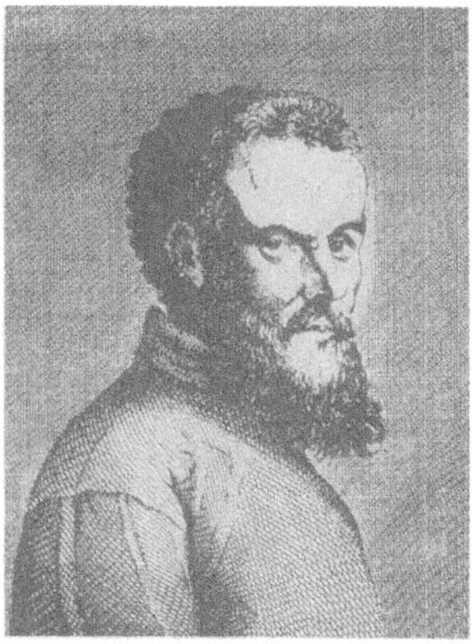

FIGURE 3.11. Andreas Vesalius, famed scientific anatomist.

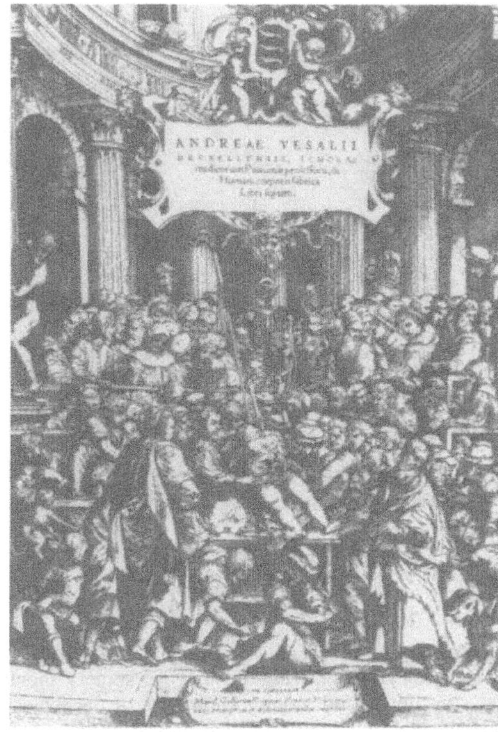

FIGURE 3.12. Frontispiece from Vesalius' *Fabrica*, published in 1543.

Research by Students

The major discoveries made by medical students are fascinating. Andreas Vesalius (Fig. 3.11) prepared his great anatomical text *De humani corporis fabrica* (Fig. 3.12) while a medical student and had it published four months after his graduation from the University of Padua as a doctor of medicine. The first microscopic observation of the function of the capillary circulation was made in 1665 by a medical student, Jan Swammerdam, who noted erythrocytes flowing through the capillary network. In 1799 Humphry Davy, a 19-year-old medical student, prepared and inhaled quantities of nitrous oxide, discovered its marked analgesic effect, and predicted that it would someday be used to prevent the pain associated with surgical operations. In 1846 another medical student, William T.G. Morton, administered ether as an anesthetic at the Massachusetts General Hospital. Paul Langerhans, a medical student working with Virchow in Berlin, first described the islets in the pancreas that now bear his name. Ivar Sandstrom, a medical student at the University of Uppsala in Sweden, discovered the parathyroid glands and wrote a monograph documenting his observations. In the team of Banting, Macleod, and Best, that pioneered the discovery of insulin, Best was a medical student, but only Banting and Macleod received the Nobel Prize. Jay MacLean was a second-year medical student working in the physiology laboratory of William H. Howell when he discovered heparin in 1916.

In 1929 Werner Forssmann became a superb example of a surgical intern, making a major discovery with great courage, by passing a ureteral catheter through a vein in his left arm into his own heart, after failing to convince a volunteer to undergo the experimental procedure. Once the catheter was in his heart, Forssmann pondered whether he would be believed unless he had objective proof of this daring human experiment. Consequently, he arose from the operating table, walked up several flights of stairs, had a chest radiograph (Fig. 3.13), and returned to remove the catheter. His forthright honesty is reflected in the last sentence of his report, in which he apologized to his readers because, when he removed the bandage from his forearm a week later, he had a superficial wound infection. He felt he must have inadvertently broken sterile technique during that historic procedure.[8]

Louis Pasteur made the famous statement, "Chance favors the prepared mind." Modern educational systems now approach complex sub-

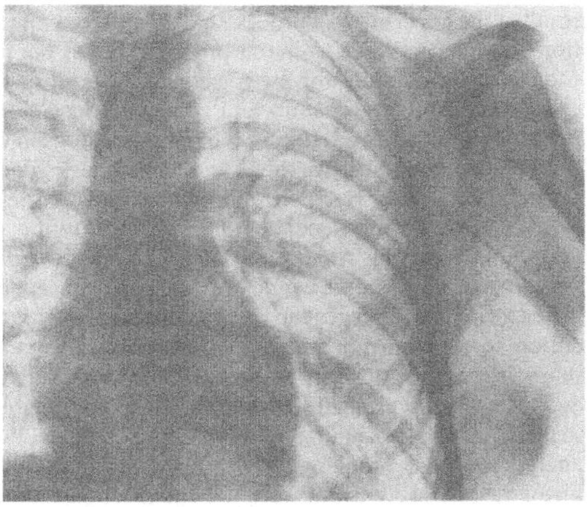

FIGURE 3.13. Chest film showing catheter self-inserted in the left antecubital vein and passed into the heart of Werner Forssmann.

jects much earlier in a student's life, and child prodigies are becoming much more frequent. Although such individuals account for a small percentage of those who become scientific investigators, stepwise progression of education remains the usual and most reliable means of nurturing productive investigators. Many medical students now begin original investigation while in college and continue in medical school. Although M.D.–Ph.D. programs have played an influential role in the training of medical investigators, research fellowships during surgical residency training have been of greater significance. Many residency training programs foster the concept of spending one or more years in research and, in many centers, most trainees obtain investigative experience. In the Duke program, nearly all surgical residents elect to spend two full-time years in basic research with a member of the faculty, a group of researchers or, occasionally, in a laboratory position, elsewhere (Fig. 3.14). Such programs have been the source of most recent academic surgical appointees in medical schools and centers. An academic appointment now generally depends on demonstrated competence in research, confirmed by significant publications.

The provision of stipends for young investigators is a matter of considerable importance. In the United States, the National Institutes of Health have traditionally been the primary sponsors of such awards (Fig. 3.15); other countries have similar sources of funding. Universities, private foundations, and industry have also provided financial support for traineeships. The results of research experience during residency programs is emphasized in a recent study. President Sanford of Duke University asked all departments in the School of Medicine to submit a summarized survey of the positions currently held by everyone who completed a residency training program at the Duke University Medical Center between 1970 and 1984. Of the 64 consecutive trainees who completed the chief residency in general and cardiothoracic surgery, 53 held full-time academic positions in departments of surgery throughout the country and 11 were in private surgical practice; that is, 82% entered full-time academic surgery and 18% became surgical practitioners. All residents, including those who did not elect to spend time in the laboratory, were sent a letter requesting their personal views on the role of research in the training of surgeons for

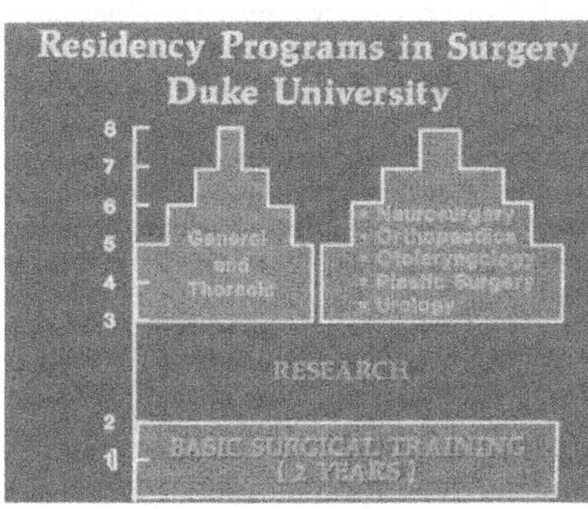

FIGURE 3.14. Residency Training Program at Duke University Medical Center; in the block labeled RESEARCH, the residents spend two or more years in basic scientific investigation full-time as research fellows.

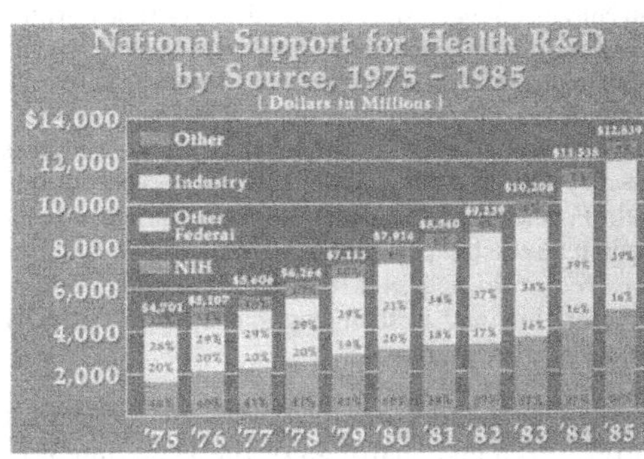

FIGURE 3.15. National support for health research and development by source, 1975–1985. (Source: National Institutes of Health Data Book, U.S. Department of Health and Human Services, 1985.)

careers in an academic setting *as well as* for those in surgical practice outside a teaching center. An update of the original report to 1990 shows a total of 93 chief residents (80%) in academic positions and 23 (20%) in surgical practice.

At Duke, the first two years of the residency training program are devoted to basic training in general surgery, with rotations in the surgical specialties. Residents then enter general or cardiothoracic surgery, or one of the surgical specialties, and continue there until completion of the "chief" year (Fig. 3.15). While it is *not* mandatory, most residents, particularly those in general and cardiothoracic surgery, spend two full-time years in basic research on surgically related problems. Most of these research fellows work with surgical faculty members who have qualifications permitting them to hold a second appointment in one of the basic science departments in the medical school. Several of the residents who completed the program elected not to take the full-time research experience and were under no obligation to do so; most agree it should be *elective*, since *required* time in the laboratory is generally unwise.

All the chief residents included in the study were asked to provide their views on the role of research in preparing surgeons for careers in academic settings, and for surgical practice outside a teaching center. A number of representative responses have been selected for direct quotation to reflect the views of the entire group. A distinct majority viewed research experience as being almost essential in the development of the complete surgeon for a career in academic surgery *or* clinical practice.

Dana K. Andersen, professor of Medicine and Surgery and vice chairman of the department at the State University of New York, Downstate Medical Center, said:

> I am convinced that a substantial period of time devoted to research is of considerable help to residents who intend to pursue clinical careers away from the academic setting. It is a rare surgical resident who, lacking investigative training, achieves the level of maturity that is shown by residents who pursue a research experience in depth. Furthermore, residents in surgical practice readily admit research experience has been not only valuable, but is specifically helpful in their efforts to evaluate clinical experience and in their ongoing need to critically evaluate the literature.

Robert W. Anderson, professor of surgery at Northwestern and chairman of the Department of Surgery at the Evanston Hospital responded:

> I believe that a period of research experience is valuable for anyone training to be a surgeon. Most of the significant advances that have been made in the field are the result of the experimental process and an orderly evaluation of results gathered from this progress. It may not be economically possible for every surgeon in training to spend time in the laboratory and conduct independent research, but I believe it is possible for every surgeon to become exposed to the methods and techniques of contemporary surgical research upon which their professional careers largely depend. It became clear to me as an examiner for the American Board of Thoracic Surgery that very few of the candidates have any concept of the experimental background that has provided the foundation for the current practice of cardiovascular and thoracic surgery. Although many were able to quote data and facts when presented with a problem, few were able to demonstrate a sound physiologic reasoning in the analysis of these problems. They appeared to lack any historical perspective and were, for the most part, both unfamiliar and disinterested with ongoing investigative efforts that may completely alter the current practice of surgery in certain areas within the foreseeable future. I think that by preparing the minds of *all* surgical trainees by exposing them to a research experience, we would not only make their own lives more interesting and productive, but would improve the overall state of medicine.

William A. Gay, professor of surgery and chairman of the Department of Surgery at the University of Utah, wrote:

> The practicing surgeon, as well as the surgeon who finds himself in a purely academic atmosphere, will find a research experience beneficial. In addition to the traditional concept of being able to better appreciate the research-oriented surgical paper more critically, it is my strong belief that the experience in basic research allows the individual to develop what I call scientific maturity.

Walter D. Holder, Jr., associate professor of surgery at Stanford University, holds the intermediate view:

> For those who follow the full-time practice of clinical surgery, I feel that residency research experience is very helpful in some circumstances and is generally positive. But for the majority, it does not contribute substantially to them in their eventual practice. In view of my current professional activities, I have found my research training experience to be invaluable. Without that experience I am certain that I could not have attained the position I now have nor could I be doing the many activities that I now enjoy.

Kent W. Jones, in surgical practice in Salt Lake City with a clinical appointment at the University of Utah Medical School, wrote: "Research training taught me the importance of precise technics, and the accurate results that this precision provides, not only in obtaining evidence on an experimental basis, but also in assessing clinical results."

William C. Meyers, associate professor of surgery at Duke, responded:

When I entered the program I had very little interest in spending time in the laboratory. This was primarily due to the fact that I had never spent such time before and due to the emphasis on pure clinical training at my medical school. However, I did have an important desire to be "the best" and this meant training in an academic environment, at least initially. I think that only with research experience can a clinician properly place into perspective his own personal experience and not spring to conclusions on the basis of a small experience or little data.

Kenneth P. Ramming, professor of surgery at the University of California at Los Angeles, who has special interest in the field of surgical oncology, wrote:

In any endeavor such as medicine, and particularly surgery, one cannot compete either in the marketplace or in the academic area without knowing at least the techniques and implications of disciplined scientific thought and the scientific method. Research experience is a requisite for the complete physician, and particularly for the complete surgeon. It forces him, sometimes reluctantly, into areas in which he may not feel initially comfortable. Accomplishment in such areas develops a whole new level of confidence, which is so important to successful surgical endeavor.

Andrew S. Wechsler, the Hunter McGuire Professor of Surgery and chairman of the Department of Surgery at the Medical College of Virginia, wrote:

The laboratory is an intellectually enriching experience. It teaches one to develop disciplines that are readily applicable to clinical surgery in the manner of requiring scientific data prior to making conclusions, to learning before making such decisions and in becoming aware of one's own cognitive processes. I do not think that a surgeon who has spent a couple of years in the laboratory approaches clinical decision-making in the same manner as one who acts on a purely pragmatic basis. For those who invest time in investigational areas in the laboratory, it is likely they will approach clinical problems with a new and fresh outlook.

Samuel A. Wells, Jr., Bixby Professor of Surgery and chairman of the Department of Surgery at Washington University–Barnes Hospital in St. Louis, said:

An experience in the laboratory is helpful for anyone interested in a career in clinical medicine. I do not think, however, that it is a necessity. I do feel that the best surgeons are those who have spent time in the laboratory, and from personal experience, I feel that the care of my patients is better because of the research experience that I have had. Had I not spent time in the laboratory, I doubt that I would have pursued a career in academic surgery. My concerns in earlier years were whether or not to spend a career in investigative laboratory work or to pursue a clinical career. Fortunately, I was able to balance these to some degree but consider myself more of a clinician than a laboratory investigator.

The young surgeon planning a career in academic surgery is wise to reflect upon the present fabric of the field and recognize that the *biological* basis of modern surgical practice grows increasingly significant. Depth of knowledge is particularly important in the fields of physiology, pathology, biochemistry, immunology, pharmacology, biostatistics, genetics, and other emerging areas of research. It is difficult to make significant surgical advances without such a knowledge of one or more of these disciplines and the ability to perform and utilize the associated laboratory techniques. Close association with a recognized investigator or team over a significant period of time merits considerable emphasis and should be thoughtfully planned in advance, in consultation with acknowledged contributors in the field and the director of the surgical residency training program.

A career in academic surgery is demanding but is also the source of much excitement and many pleasures. Alfred Blalock stated this very well:

No satisfaction is quite like that which accompanies productive investigation, particularly if it leads to better treatment of the sick. The important discoveries in medicine are generally simple, and one is apt to wonder why they were not made earlier. I believe that they are made usually by a dedicated person who is willing to work and to cultivate his power of observation rather than by the so-called intellectual genius. Discoveries may be made by the individual worker as opposed to the current practice of a large research team. Simple apparatus may suffice; all the analyses need not be performed by technicians; large sums of money are not always necessary. Important basic ideas will probably continue to come from the individual. Whether by accident, design or hunch, the diligent investigator has a fair chance of making an important discovery. If he is unwilling to take his chance, he should avoid this type of work.[4]

Finally, all those planning to enter investigative surgery should be continuously aware of the words of William Osler (Fig. 3.16), generally regarded as the greatest physician, worldwide, in the first half of this century; his astonishing career was characterized by tremendous happiness as well as achievement. While in his thirties, he became professor and Chief of the Department of Medicine at McGill University and the Montreal General Hospital in Montreal. Shortly thereafter, he was offered and accepted what was then the leading post in medicine in the United States at the University of Pennsylvania. Several years later, in 1889, he was offered the position of physician-in-chief and professor of medicine at the newly formed

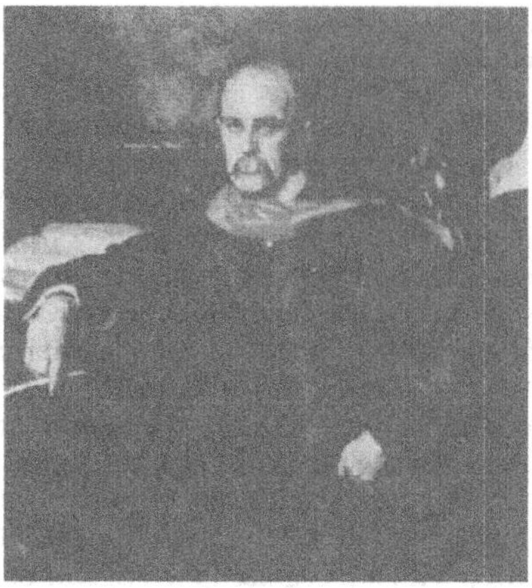

FIGURE 3.16. Sir William Osler, 1849–1919, Regius Professor of Medicine at the University of Oxford, England.

Johns Hopkins Hospital and Medical School, with a large number of beds and laboratories completely under his control. Since these beds were endowed and could be occupied by patients of any economic group, selected by the physician-in-chief, Osler was able to introduce medical students to the wards and to allow them *to perform* clinical examinations on patients. He was also a distinguished medical scholar who edited an extraordinary textbook of medicine that remained in publication for half a century; he was a skilled diagnostician, a superb speaker, and a clinical scientist of great renown. In 1905 Osler was offered the most prestigious post in medicine of that day, the Regius Chair at the University of Oxford in England.

When asked why he had been so successful in his career and why he was well known, by his friends and colleagues, to be an exceedingly happy individual who thoroughly enjoyed all aspects of the medical profession, Osler simply said:

It seems a bounden duty on such an occasion to be honest and frank, so I propose to tell you the secret of life as I have seen the game played, and as I have tried to play it myself . . . This I propose to give you in the hope, yes, in the full assurance that some of you at least will lay hold upon it to your profit. Though a little one, the master-word looms large in meaning. –WORK– It is the open sesame to every portal, the great equalizer in the world, the true philosopher's stone, which transmutes all the base metal of humanity into gold. The stupid man among you, it will make bright, the bright man brilliant, and the brilliant student steady. With the magic word in your heart all things are possible, and without it all study is vanity and vexation. The miracles of life are with it . . . To the youth it brings hope, to the middle-aged confidence, and to the aged repose . . . It is directly responsible for all advances in medicine during the past twenty-five centuries."[9]

References

1. Gloyne SR. John Hunter. Edinburgh: E & S Livingstone, Ltd, 1950:60.
2. Garrison FH. History of Medicine. Philadelphia: W.B. Saunders, 1929.
3. Halsted WS. The training of the surgeon. In: Surgical Papers by William Stewart Halsted, Vol. II. Baltimore: The Johns Hopkins Press, 1924:512–531.
4. Sabiston DC, Jr. Presidential address: Alfred Blalock. Ann of Surg 1978;188:255.
5. Wangensteen, OH. Teacher's oath, J Med Educ 1978; 53(6):524.
6. Carter BN. The fruition of Halsted's concept of surgical training. Surgery 1952;32:518.
7. Blalock A. The nature of discovery, Ann Surg 1956; 144:289.
8. Forssmann W. Experiments on myself. Klin Wochenschr 1929;8:2085.
9. Osler, Sir William. Aquanimitas with Other Addresses. Philadelphia: P. Blakiston's Son, 1932.

4

The Academic Surgeon

C.M. Balch, M.F. McKneally, B. McPeek, D.S. Mulder, W.O. Spitzer, H. Troidl, and A.S. Wechsler

The art and practice of academic surgery are mastered by defining and learning the pertinent basic principles and skills, and by practicing them under an experienced mentor. This requires a delineation of the personal qualities and professional skills needed to integrate surgical practice and investigation, and their attainment through an appropriately structured training program. This chapter discusses these qualities and skills, and the unique aspects of training that must be addressed by the academic surgical trainee in collaboration with his or her surgical program director.

The academic surgeon must:

1. Be an excellent clinical surgeon.
2. Be willing to initiate and test clinically relevant ideas.
3. Be a good communicator who willingly passes knowledge to others in an understandable way.
4. Be highly organized and able to maintain an appropriate balance among professional and personal objectives.
5. Have excellent interactive skills to facilitate research collaboration and fulfillment of administrative duties.

Many have discussed the dilemmas faced by a surgeon in the university setting who attempts to acquire all these traits and to master all these skills. In the words of William P. Longmire, "developing and maintaining the technical skills that will identify an individual as a well trained surgeon and at the same time qualify him or her as a scientist poses a greater challenge to surgery than to any other field of medicine."[1]

The diversity and multiplicity of challenges confronting the academic surgeon have become so great that the editors consider the pentathlete an illustrative analogy.

The Pentathlon Analogy

The modern pentathlon, an Olympic event, requires an individual athlete to be outstanding in five diverse athletic events: swimming, fencing, shooting, running, and riding—based on the skills required to qualify as a battlefield messenger in Napoleon's army. The critical characteristics of the pentathlete are personal strength, stamina, and commitment to excellence. The pentathlete is competitive in multiple areas but is not a record holder in events that are the single focus of other athletes.

Most successful pentathletes begin with a strong background in swimming and develop other athletic skills around it. In a similar way, academic surgeons build their careers around clinical skills. To achieve the level of excellence attained by someone who has chosen to focus on clinical surgery or laboratory research, the academic surgeon must be willing to spend extra time in training and additional working hours as a faculty surgeon.

Athletes competing in the pentathlon have unique individual combinations of relative strengths, but their training and prowess must encompass all five arenas of competition. Their real field of competition lies in their versatility and ability to build a combination of strengths to a competitive level of performance in multiple areas.

The analogy is that each aspiring academic surgeon must follow a training program specifically designed to expand his or her unique combination of talents, interests, and developed skills. The effort and dedication required of each individual presupposes an honest self-assessment of relative personal strengths and weaknesses, and a willingness to develop a diverse set of skills with a high degree of initiative and self-determination. There is no stereotyped or uniform approach to becoming an effective and productive academic surgeon.

The pentathlon analogy is not perfect. Only a few can win the pentathlon, but most academic surgeons can be effective and productive in a personally rewarding way, if they prepare themselves well for the challenges and take full advantage of the opportunities around them. Those who train well and meet the challenges are all winners.

As discussed in the remainder of this chapter, several areas of professional and personal skill must be developed, perfected, and maintained to have a successful and rewarding career in academic surgery.

The Academic Surgeon as a Clinical Surgeon

Academic surgeons must, first and foremost, be excellent clinical surgeons, even though they cannot devote their time solely to clinical surgery. Because they are role models for surgical residents and medical students, they must not only display superb operative skills and techniques, they must also be compassionate and respectful in their interactions with other people.

Although excellence in clinical surgery is an essential prerequisite for success as an effective academic surgeon, we will not dwell on the training of a clinical surgeon, since the purpose of this chapter is to describe the special features of training in other areas.

Willingness to Initiate and Test New Ideas

Ability to generate new knowledge relevant to surgical science and patient care is one of the most distinctive traits of an academic surgeon. It may be expressed through laboratory or clinical research, or a combination of the two.

Many surgical training programs emphasize scholarly acquisition of knowledge and skills, but surgical investigative trainees must also learn to be "constructive skeptics" about current scientific knowledge and standard surgical practice if they are to identify where opportunities for improvements and advances lie. They must be able to think "nontraditionally" and to channel ideas with clinical relevance into a series of formal investigations that will test them in a quantitative, analytical, and deductive manner.

Training To Be an Investigator

Because scientific methodology is the basis of evaluation and the medium of exchange of new ideas, it should be the centerpiece in the training of surgical investigators. The training program should focus on developing the ability to channel ideas into a formal, systematic scientific inquiry based on a hypothesis, a set of scientific objectives, and accepted and effective methodology for achieving the study's objectives.

What should trainees for academic surgical careers do to prepare themselves specifically for the unique challenges of their chosen careers?

A variety of pathways can lead to successful preparation for a career in academic surgery; many interesting options will suit some trainees better than others. Several programs proposed by the American College of Surgeons Conjoint Council on Surgical Research are outlined in Table 4.1.

A few core curricular requirements or fundamental courses essential to a scientific career should be incorporated in the formal/informal period of training in scientific methodology; biostatistics and computer methodology are two of them, as indicated in the following list.

1. Statistics.
2. Scientific writing.
3. Physiology.
4. Laboratory methodology.
5. Use of computers.
6. Research seminars.
7. Public speaking as applied to scientific presentations.
8. Grant writing.
9. Biomechanics.
10. Scientific instrumentation.
11. Teaching methods.

For surgical scientists whose primary language is not English, developing a command of the English language is highly desirable for international exchange. For English-speaking scientists, development of one or more additional languages will facilitate and enrich their scientific communication skills. An adequate understanding of the language of computers and statistics is an absolute requirement for success in surgical science.

When should the trainee learn scientific methodology? Ideally, an aspiring academic surgeon should embark on learning the experimental method as an undergraduate or medical student and expand this work during residency training. For those who have not had an earlier opportunity to gain experience in research in a scientific setting, the period of research immersion should occur, ideally, upon completion of the first two or three years of surgical training. It is important to know whether an individual can perform

TABLE 4.1. Examples of proposed programs for training in surgical research (Conjoint Council on Surgical Research).

I	II	III	IV	V
PG1[a]	PG1	PG1	PG1	PG1
PG2	PG2	PG2	PG2	PG2
Research 1	PG3	Research 1	Research 1	Research 1/PG3
Research 2	PG4	Research 2	Research 2/PG3	PG4
PG3	PG5	PG3	PG4	PG5
PG4	Research 1	PG4	PG5	Research 2
PG5	Research 2	PG5	PG5	Research2
Research 3	Clinical research	Research 3	Research 3	Research 3
Research 4		Research 4	Research 4	
Clinical research				

Post graduate year (PG)	Status
0	M.D. degree
1	Internship
2	Surgical resident
3	Surgical resident
4	Research
5	Research[a]
6	Surgical resident
7	Surgical resident (chief)
8	Basic/clinical research fellowship
9	Basic/clinical research fellowship
10	Basic/clinical research fellowship

[a] Board requirements met at end of PG5 year.

proficiently in the clinical surgeon's role before committing resources, time, and energy to his or her training as a surgical investigator. This subject is also discussed in the chapter on surgical research training in Sweden (Section V, Chapter 60).

At the end of the second or third year of surgical training, the trainee is sufficiently flexible to derive maximum benefit from new experiences; subsequent surgical training will be enriched by the principles learned and the habits and attitudes developed in the laboratory. While flexibility and diversity are to be encouraged, deferring the period of scientific training until the end of surgical residency is not as desirable, particularly if the laboratory experience is to be divorced from hands-on surgical experience.

Where should training in scientific methodology be obtained? The most significant requirement is that the period of training in scientific methodology be an immersion in a milieu so organized that the scientific method is the dominant cultural and educational experience. The academic discipline and setting should be appropriate to the trainee's interests—a strictly surgical laboratory, or such other departments as biostatistics, epidemiology, anesthesiology, immunology, anatomy, biochemistry, physiology, economics, or social science. Provided the standards of observation, hypothesis formulation and testing, analysis, critical review, and communication are high, the discipline is best chosen according to the interest and needs of the investigative trainee and the objective advice of his or her department chief or mentor.

Exposure to investigators who have different opinions and different approaches to solving problems in a given area of scientific inquiry is an important component of the surgical research training experience. *Visiting other institutions and laboratories, and meeting with visiting professors to discuss their distinctive perspectives on a problem of common interest are broadening experiences.* You will be surprised to learn how many different ways a given problem can be tackled.

Should the academic surgical trainee pursue a Ph.D. degree in basic science? Some trainees will find a Ph.D. program a sensible, enjoyable way to develop fundamental skills in scientific method. If you are facile at course work, enjoy examinations, are not deterred by thesis writing, and have an enthusiastic interest in the research and course work required for a doctorate in a given science, a Ph.D. program is an excellent route to developing a sound knowledge of scientific methodology. On the other hand, many highly successful surgical scientists and major contributors to fundamental science know that time at the laboratory bench, under the influence of an excellent scientist, can provide equal or possibly more appropriate preparation.

How do I support myself while I am learning scientific methodology? A variety of scholarships and research training fellowships are available through the National Institutes of Health in the United States, the Medical Research Council of Canada, and a variety of surgical organizations. They provide stipends to cover the trainee's living expenses and usually a small supplemental sum to the department for the support of the surgical research. They are generally available through such surgical organizations as the American College of Surgeons, the American Surgical Association, and others listed in Section V, Chapter 63. If the surgical scholar seeks out a department that fosters training in scientific methodology, departmental funds are often available to support appropriate candidates during prolonged periods of training in science.

The Academic Surgeon as a Communicator

The mere acquisition of knowledge is not sufficient: the knowledge must be communicated to the surgical and scientific community in an understandable way. Doing this requires oral and written skills, especially in English, which is now the primary scientific language.

The effective surgical investigator must know how to communicate with specific audiences in such varied settings as scientific and surgical meetings, seminars, and rounds. The role of educator requires the ability to communicate enthusiasm as well as knowledge. The dedicated surgical educator tries to arouse an interest in surgery in every student and then chooses those best suited to become surgeons.

Because the ability to assimilate meaningful information is an essential component of being a good communicator, the academic surgeon must have well-developed reading skills and be able to extract important conclusions from a wide array of frequently contradictory reports. The academic surgeon's skill in interpreting data and resolving major issues must be sufficiently sophisticated to allow the development of soundly based convictions and their courageous defense against opposition from any source.

Training To Be a Communicator

Writing and public speaking skills may come more easily to some than to others, but for most people they are the result of considerable effort. The rewards of such efforts are significant and will be garnered at scientific meetings and through published reports in the form of lucid, interesting and effective communication with other surgical investigators. To develop skill in talking about scientific topics, start by speaking to small groups, informally; master the content and delivery of your talk before speaking to larger groups. Most of the authors of this chapter regard enthusiastic critiquing by their colleagues and mentors, in small groups, as the best preparation they ever had for the academic surgical life.

To learn scientific writing, begin with a relatively simple, straightforward clinical or scientific paper before attempting to write a complex scientific manuscript. In addition to language and writing skills, trainees must learn to use the formats required for abstracts and for scientific manuscripts destined for publication; the successful surgical investigator communicates effectively through surgical and other scientific journals. Whether you are choosing a journal or a meeting, think about the audience you wish to address. Select the audience that is not only the largest with an interest in your report but also the most creditable and respectable forum to which you can convey your new finding.

We recommend participation in courses in scientific writing and public speaking. Some surgical trainees have found that Toastmasters International, an organization that meets in most major cities throughout the world for the purpose of enhancing effective public speaking, provides a good learning experience.

The Academic Surgeon Must Be Highly Organized

Academic surgeons must be highly organized to fulfill their responsibilities for multiple simultaneous professional activities. Maintaining an appropriate balance among competing priorities requires emotional maturity and stability, and the ability to keep a clear set of goals and objectives in focus. To master the juggler's art of "keeping all the balls in the air," you must become and remain adept at setting priorities and delegating responsibilities.

A perspective derived from the frequent review of responsibilities and objectives must be the basis for setting and balancing priorities. You must weigh and take account of clinical versus scientific, institutional versus national, and professional versus personal responsibilities. Development of the ability to use time effectively and wisely and to sort the urgent from the important, to prevent the former preempting the latter, is essential.

The following points will help you to learn how to be organized.

1. Look for role models. Analyze how busy, effective people organize their time.
2. Know your own strengths, weaknesses, and limitations. Have realistic expectations of yourself and others.
3. Have long- and short-range plans for all aspects of your professional activities.
4. Make your time meaningful by (a) identifying areas of wasted time, through time–motion studies if necessary, (b) developing the ability to dictate your thoughts clearly, (c) attending speed reading courses, etc.
5. Write things down. Most of us keep a "do list" in our pocket or briefcase, on an index card, a sheet of paper, or on a tape in a pocket-sized dictating machine. One of these should never be far away, day or night, so that thoughts can be captured as they come and before they evaporate.
6. Think constantly about priorities and delegations.
7. Maintain an appropriate balance between professional and personal life. Family and personal commitments are critically important. Develop areas and times for relaxation, such as hobbies, sports, and cultural and community activities.
8. Consider professional training in organizational and management skills.

We believe that family and personal commitments, including at least one relationship or friendship that is close and trusting enough to allow unburdening and sharing of very personal anxieties and aspirations, rank first among the important values to be maintained. "Burnout" is a not uncommon tragedy when rapidly rising successful young academic surgeons fail to maintain a balance in their personal lives, leading to turbulent periods of emotional instability or family disruption that undermine an individual's effectiveness in all areas.

The Academic Surgeon Must Have Interactive Skills

Multiple part-time responsibilities to collaborate in various clinical and scholarly activities demand significant interactive skills on the part of the academic surgeon. Success depends on maturity, humility, and the ability to delegate effectively. Learning to delegate is a form of training. You should arrive at an early appreciation of how to be an effective part-time, but wholehearted, coworker and learn how to establish effective, mutually beneficial partnerships in various areas of your professional life. In research, this usually means collaborating with full-time investigators within their departments or in basic science departments.

Think about the impact your activity will have on the discretionary time of the investigator and about the cost, to others, of the requests you make. Inspiring people to want to work with you requires a "give and take" personality. The successful academic surgeon strives to create "win–win" situations for all collaborators.

Learn to frame suggestions and delegations tactfully, positively, and constructively; cutting comments entail a cost! You must also learn how to challenge and criticize at the right time, in the right place, with the right approach. Insensitivity to the needs and feelings of others, or destructive public criticism, is especially counterproductive. Productive interaction presupposes a well-developed capacity for self-criticism and acceptance of constructive criticism by others. Learning interactive skills is a lifetime task in self-development.

Many of the topics just discussed are the subject matter of various books on managerial and leadership skills, but careful observation and consideration of how others work with and manage people, either well or badly, will make major contributions to your acquisition of their most desirable characteristics. Try to see yourself as others do and listen to criticism given to or by others.

Character Traits of the Academic Surgeon

We are convinced that the skills of the academic surgeon must be developed in candidates who have basic character traits appropriate to this choice of career. *The effective academic surgeon must be intellectually honest, with deep personal integrity, as well as generosity in the art of helping others.*

1. Commitment to excellence—be willing to put forth extra effort. This requires extra stamina and dedication to follow through and complete all responsibilities, even at the end of a long day.
2. Determination and initiative—these qualities may be more important than intellectual brilliance.
3. Integrity and honesty.
4. Judgment and intuition.
5. Creativity (i.e., nontraditional and innovative thinking).
6. Analytical, quantitative, deductive thinking.
7. Curiosity.

8. Humility and grace, particularly in giving credit to others.
9. Emotional stability and maturity.
10. A compulsive attitude toward getting things done right, coupled with flexibility about the methods of implementation.
11. Patience and tolerance toward the imperfections and shortcomings of others, and yourself.
12. Willingness to make financial sacrifices—in exchange for intellectual and personal rewards.
13. Consistency.
14. Courage.

Conclusion

To achieve a unique composite of special skills, the pentathlete lives with the frustration of not being the best in any one athletic field. Becoming and remaining competitive as a pentathlete demands dedication to working on areas of least skill to achieve overall excellence. Most pentathletes find their athletic careers amply rewarding.

Those who have chosen academic surgery as a lifetime career are similarly content. The breadth of the experience and the diversity of the challenges combine to create an exciting, stimulating, and rewarding professional and personal life.

References

1. Longmire WP—Conjoint Council on Surgical Research. Reports of the Committees of Special Interest, 1986. Published by the American College of Surgeons, Chicago, Ill., USA.

5

Strengthening the Research Environment

A.S. Wechsler, M.F. McKneally, C.M. Balch, F. Mosteller, B. McPeek, and D.S. Mulder

Sir William Osler, the legendary clinician-scholar-teacher, identified patient care, teaching, and research as the three traditional functions of an academic clinical unit. He noted that scientific investigation, the most recent of the three, was often the first to suffer when resources were strained.[1] Academicians everywhere find that their demanding roles as leaders in clinical care, teaching, and administration constantly encroach on whatever time is available for investigation.

Surgical research seeks an understanding of the factors influencing the pathophysiology of a disease and how a particular surgical approach modifies it. The environment in which the research is pursued exerts a decisive influence on how readily clinical problems will be scientifically examined, how significant the results of such investigation will be, and the extent to which research will become an integral part of a surgical unit's activities. Whether every surgical unit should do research is controversial; that not every surgical unit does research is factual. Some clinical units are committed to the investigative route to advanced knowledge, enhanced training, and improved surgical care. They are most effective when their organization, objectives, and commitment are the result of thoughtful and intensive planning. The addition of an investigative component to a strong clinical unit enhances all the endeavors of both; isolated surgical investigative units are anachronistic.

The Academic Department of Surgery

The academic department of surgery—in a university, hospital, or clinic—defines its goals within the surgical community and, in the course of achieving them, provides guidance to its members and its parent institution. If the departmental surgeons, physicians in other departments, and hospital and university administrators subscribe to the same or very compatible goals, success is likely; if they do not, the effort will fail.

However large or small the unit is, the research process begins in the pragmatic and philosophical commitment to investigation of its leader, generally the departmental chairman. The head of an academic department creates an environment that fosters collaborative clinical and laboratory investigation as the basis for successful research. The leader places *high priority on academic productivity*, sets a *personal example* of encouragement for scholarly research, protects time for investigators, provides appropriate clinical and research facilities, and develops suitable financial and collaborative support.

To accomplish this, chairmen use the weight of their influence in the hospital and university to obtain the necessary salaries, protected time, space, facilities, and support personnel. Since some trainees may not have a primary interest in investigation and some faculty members may find it a serious distraction from their clinical responsibilities, the unit's research and clinical missions must be constantly treated and reinforced as being indistinguishable.

Designating specific conferences for the presentation of ongoing investigations and requiring the same attendance at them as at clinical conferences are good starting points. Alternatively, the available time for each conference may be apportioned between presentations of clinical and investigative work. According the same status and importance to a research presentation as to the most recent series or isolated clinical operation is mandatory.

No national presentation should be made before it has been aired for "peer" review by the members of the department. This focuses the attention of the entire unit on the research project and draws individuals who have little research capability or interest into the process. Acceptance of papers for inclusion in the programs of national meetings, acquisition of research grants, recent publications, and other scientific contributions must be widely publicized within the department.

Individuals achieving such recognition deserve recognition at department-wide conferences, in their promotion packages, and in their financial reimbursement. The department's compensation plan must ensure that the incentives for research are not overshadowed by excessive financial rewards for clinical practice.

A research grand rounds draws the attention of all departmental members to the importance of research in relation to their day-to-day practice. On these occasions, and in other ways, the chief can tell those who augment the research effort by devoting time to committee work, teaching, and patient care that the department recognizes the importance of their contributions to the department's scholarly academic achievement in research. Special praise should be given publicly, and often, to residents who are engaged in or have completed research projects.

The chairman's message is that research is important, is rewarded, and is vital to the fulfillment of the role of the unit producing it. Although the demands on the departmental chairman's time and energy frequently preclude continuation of his or her own active research program, the chairman's abiding commitment to research must be obvious to everyone in the department, the hospital, and the university. The commitment and rapid ascension of those who are highly successful in research endeavors should be apparent to faculty members and should serve as a stimulus to similar endeavors on their part.

How to organize and integrate the research unit into the clinical program raises some difficult questions. It is not likely that every member of a clinical department of surgery can or should be a highly productive investigator. One approach to organization follows the natural departmental division into specific units of clinical expertise; it may be reasonable to have a strong research presence in each division, clinical unit, or clinical focal point. An appreciation within each division of the important rewards to be gained facilitates this arrangement. Individuals within the division should be given research time by transferring their responsibilities to members of the division who are less inclined toward research or less productive in it. Credit for successful research or grant acquisition should be accorded to all the members of the unit who contribute to making such investigative work possible.

Whenever possible, clinical investigative projects should recruit all the members of a unit and should gain their mutual agreement on the standards to be upheld in its execution. Research productivity should be viewed as a divisional responsibility and the accomplishment of very fundamental research as a divisional achievement.

If good intentions were enough, research could occur as a spiritual experience; unfortunately, they are not. The features and attributes that decisively influence a department or unit's research accomplishment are:

The physical environment.
The intellectual environment.
Personnel organization.
The reward system.
Collaboration.

The Physical Environment

Units do not always have the opportunity to determine their physical environment. Thought should be given to the physical setting of the research component in relation to the clinical activities of a unit at its inception, when physical moves are made for other reasons, or whenever an opportunity for restructuring arises. Physical proximity of the research and clinical practice areas is a great benefit to clinicians with combined clinical and investigative skills. The continuing, albeit intermittent, presence in the laboratory of the surgeon–investigator is important; movement of office space from one floor to another to achieve proximity to the laboratory will enhance productivity. Some institutions are able to collocate research laboratories and physicians' offices, or to connect the laboratory, the office, and the hospital area, structurally.

The McGill University Research Laboratory, for example, is an integral part of the Montreal General Hospital immediately adjacent to the surgical floors (Fig. 5.1). The research unit contains animal care facilities, an animal operating suite, and appropriate preparation space. The animal facility is separated from the patient care area by laboratory research offices, the research library, and the "dry labs" used for performing blood chemical determinations and other studies not requiring the physical presence of, or direct contact with, animals. A shared clinical and research conference room was built with the primary goal of situating

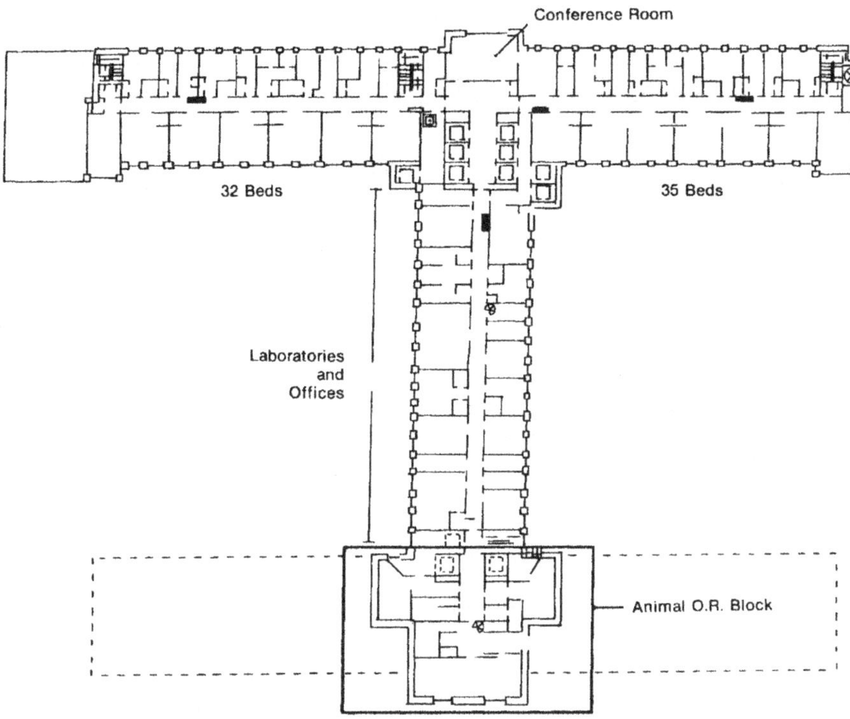

FIGURE 5.1. The McGill University Research Laboratory is an integral part of the Montreal General Hospital immediately adjacent to the surgical floors.

clinical teaching units in close proximity to basic laboratory space.

Three fully equipped animal operating rooms are located at the distal end of the research unit's corridor; with anesthesia machines, monitoring equipment, and a heart-lung machine, they can cater to virtually any operative procedure. Supervision of postoperative recovery and long-term care is provided by a veterinary surgeon. Office, laboratory and conference rooms are made available to investigators, residents, and students in the department of surgery under the director of research, who is a highly respected clinician and laboratory research scientist. All the residents and the chief of the division attend weekly rounds in the research unit, coordinated by the director.

The proximity of research and clinical teaching units promotes regular interaction between the residents and surgeons working on the clinical service and everyone currently involved in a research project. The importance of research in the activities of this surgical department is overtly acknowledged by the immediate physical presence of the research laboratory.

A similar spatial arrangement exists at the Marburg University Hospital, where the research team is located immediately adjacent to the departments of surgery and anesthesiology (Figure 5.2).

Access to the research laboratory should be as convenient and easy as possible. Locating research facilities in buildings not connected to the office, clinic, and hospital areas is a strong disincentive to spending time in the laboratory. The research "laboratories" should include operating rooms, critical care areas, ward units, and outpatient facilities.

The Operating Room

A surgical operation, like a scientific experiment, requires a carefully organized team of surgeons, anesthesiologists, nurses, perfusionists, and other specialized assistants. The team recognizes that its responsibility extends beyond providing outstanding care for today's patients to advancing knowledge and improving care for tomorrow's patients. Surgeons appreciate the importance of teamwork based on shared objectives and respect for the role played by each team member. Close understanding, cooperation, and personal interest are as important to patient care as they are to research. They are fostered by full discussion of research

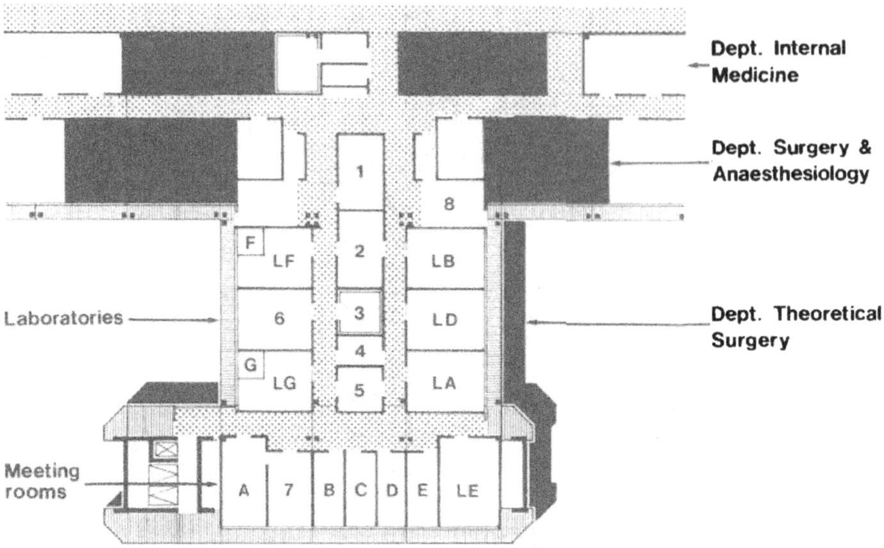

FIGURE 5.2. At the Marburg General Hospital the research team is located immediately adjacent to the departments of surgery and anesthesiology.

hypotheses and timely updates on both clinical and research progress (see Section III, Chapter 26).

Such simple steps as posting on the wall of the operating room the outline of a research protocol or data collection methods may enable research to proceed unobtrusively. For example, Naruke's maps of the mediastinal lymph nodes and the node station sampling required for inclusion of patients in Lung Cancer Study Group protocols were posted in thoracic surgical operating rooms in all the participating hospitals. This facilitated the collection of uniform data about each patient and the use of standard international nomenclature.[2] A full discussion of the scientific questions asked in the operative and perioperative research protocols brought a feeling of great satisfaction to the participating operating room personnel.

Anesthesiologists can ensure timely and complete collection and recording of specimens, data, and observations because they are not confined to the sterile operating field. The anesthesia department of the Massachusetts General Hospital has set a notable example of the value of interdepartmental collaboration in scientific analysis of pharmacologic interventions in hemodynamic problems encountered during cardiac surgery.[3] Such personnel as residents in surgery and anesthesia derive added satisfaction from their day-to-day work when they see it as part of a quest for a solution to a larger problem. Juniors watch their seniors, note their habits of observation and scholarly inquiry, and learn how to provide both clinical and research leadership. In the process of preparing for their own clinical and academic careers, they contribute greatly to the research effort. Surgical or anesthesia residents on full-time research rotations sometimes act as data managers in the operating room as part of their scientific experience.

Perfusionists can collect research data in the cardiac operating room, because they are familiar with the details of the surgical procedure and have well-established roles in recording the details of cardiopulmonary bypass. They contribute significantly to the randomized trials of coronary artery surgery conducted by the U.S. National Heart, Lung and Blood Institute by recording the data.[4]

Much good research originates in intensive care units and recovery rooms, where data can be collected on patients whose physiologic status is being actively monitored with invasive recording equipment. Some projects focus on the intensive care interventions; others use the intensive care data as short-term outcome measures for operating room interventions. For extraordinary examples of the effectiveness of clinical research in intensive care settings, see the work of Cerra,[5] at the University of Minnesota, and Civeta,[6] in Miami, in the recording of data in complex metabolic, pulmonary, economic, and ethical problems. (See also Section III, Chapter 27.)

Inpatient floors, outpatient clinics, and private offices can play important roles in the collection of follow-up data and the generation of new hypotheses for testing in the research protocols of scientific studies of patients. Clinicians encounter an abundance of unsolved patient care problems in the course of their daily rounds. Academicians perceive such problems as challenges to formulate researchable hypotheses as the first step toward finding solutions. Comparisons of postoperative analgesic regimens, postoperative anticoagulants in the prevention of pulmonary embolization, the efficacy and cost of preventive perioperative antibiotic treatment, early discharge and home care programs, and enteral versus parenteral nutrition are a few examples of productive research performed in surgical units. The results produce better care for tomorrow's patients, and the process of gathering and analyzing the data is an enriching experience for all those working in the participating units.

Residents, nurses, ward clerks, technical personnel from the laboratory, and members of the pump team participate in data collection for clinical research. A modest salary supplement for assisting in research can convert a nurse or a technician into a colleague who collects clinical information with faithful attention to the research protocol. This inexpensive and productive technique can eliminate the need to hire full-time data collection personnel and can have a galvanizing effect on the participants by endowing their daily work with a broader scientific purpose. A $1000-a-year salary supplement from research funds can turn a nurse in an intensive care unit into an on-site scientific colleague equipped to collect patient-related data. Participation in the scientific analysis of a patient care problem (e.g., decubiti, infected central line sites, the timing of a tracheostomy) helps to prevent "burnout" in nurses and other care givers by expanding their horizon; promoting their active personal involvement in scientific meetings has a further enhancing effect on their understanding and enthusiasm.

The Intellectual Environment

Although creating the appropriate intellectual environment need not require the bricks and mortar that may be necessary to establish physical proximity, it must be carefully planned. Centralization of certain facilities within a clinical unit can be cost effective, bring together investigators from multiple disciplines, and reducing personnel and space requirements. Polling of the research staff can identify which facilities and services are best centralized to form "core" resources that can be cost accounted back to individual investigators when central departmental funds are inadequate to support them. Glassware, supply room services, media preparation, high performance liquid chromatography, radioactive counters, cold rooms, ultracentrifuges, ultra-low-temperature freezers, atomic absorption instrumentation, spectroscopy instrumentation, and reagent pools are a few examples of such core services.

A conference area promotes the easy exchange of ideas and may serve as a central repository for grant information, meeting dates, and abstract deadlines. Similar centralization can be used for word processing, library services, and access to higher levels of computer power by linking personal microcomputers with mainframe computers (see Chapter 21, below).

The direction of the research effort may be difficult to define, but several models exist.

Investigator experience is the basis of one model. A highly talented investigator brings his or her expertise, frequently accompanied by appropriate personnel and equipment, to a unit that may never have done research related to the newcomer's field. A new area of investigation is introduced. Such ventures can be costly, but they certainly expand the breadth of the unit and are usually designed to fill a specific need. This approach, however, occasionally isolates the new investigator.

Clinical density, or a clinical-opportunity-based investigative program, gives rise to another model that "deals to" the established strengths of a unit. A unit with a very high incidence of trauma and a very low incidence of elective gastrectomies would be unwise to initiate research protocols requiring large numbers of patients needing gastrectomy. This is self-evident, but less obvious examples frequently occur, with consequent failure.

Capitalizing on clinical strengths has many advantages. A trained and active faculty is generally in place, patient enrollment is not a problem, and the research effort is constantly reinforced by reminders of the importance of the problem. Translation to the clinical setting of laboratory-defined opportunities becomes easy, and the need for extensive interinstitutional arrangements for initial trials is eliminated. The research team doing very fundamental work is bonded to the clinical activities of the unit by virtue of their common interest; research and clinical presentations receive an attentive hearing as the research and clinical teams naturally fuse. This may be a highly attractive model for departments initiating research programs.

Integrating Clinical Research into Patient Care Activities

In the Department of Surgery of the M.D. Anderson Cancer Center, a protocol-based clinical research program evolved over the past 5 years and now includes 27 prospective protocols that take in more than 350 patients per year. The research activities have produced a substantial increase in the number of scientific publications and an increased referral by community physicians of patients specifically for entry into clinical trials.

This approach to clinical research has a number of identifiable components. The first is a set of *protocols* approved by the entire general surgery faculty. At first, the faculty selected clinical protocols that were easy to incorporate into patient care routines (e.g., margins of excision for melanoma surgery, timing of drain removal after axillary lymph node dissection, antibiotic trials). During the ensuing years, faculty members, trainees, and research personnel learned to work as an increasingly sophisticated team capable of implementing complicated treatment protocols (e.g., investigation of drugs or biological agents, before or after surgery; intraoperative laser surgery versus radiation therapy; regional chemotherapy to the liver and extremities). The latter trials required a more elaborate system for accurate implementation and data management because they could induce serious morbidity if not performed correctly, or because if the research data were flawed, loss of access to investigational agents might result.

Members of the surgical faculty had to change their attitude toward and approach to patient care, because adherence to protocols required everyone to "think protocols" and to spend additional time in the clinics. Appropriate salary adjustments and promotion criteria were instituted as incentives for participation in clinical trials and research. Surgical trainees (residents and fellows) had to be trained in the design of clinical research protocols and were expected to participate actively in their implementation, because failure of such personnel to comprehend the importance of strict adherence to protocol requirements could cause violations. For example, a quality control audit revealed that before the residents were fully oriented to a breast drain protocol, they had been given prophylactic antibiotics, which produced inevaluable patients. A clinical research infrastructure had to be created to conduct the clinical trials.

Affinity groups, called sections, were created around different types of cancer (e.g., Breast Section, GI Section) so that faculty and research personnel with specific interests in these areas could provide intellectual leadership for the entire faculty in generating protocols and in monitoring their implementation. A clinical research committee was formed to supervise the protocol review system and the clinical research personnel.

Courses and seminars on such subjects as "How to Write Protocols" and "How to Use Computers for Clinical Research," and a 13-week symposium on clinical biostatistics, were added to the clinical research program. A weekly clinical research conference was instituted to involve the entire department—residents, students, fellows, and clinical research personnel—in research discussions.

The patient care system was altered to facilitate the entry of patients into clinical protocols. Reminders are distributed everywhere (e.g., protocol books in the clinic, a pocket guide of current protocols for every trainee), and the protocols are discussed in the weekly surgical conference. The research nurse flags the charts of eligible patients for protocols and assists the surgeon in determining eligibility and counseling patients about the merits of participating in a clinical trial.

A protocol-based clinical research system can address significant questions about patient care, offer the best patient care available, and delineate the benefits of new treatments or diagnostic approaches in an accurate and reproducible manner.

Collaboration

When Warren, Bigelow, and Morton demonstrated the efficacy of general anesthesia in 1846, they needed no clinical trial and no statistical analysis to convince the world of the importance of the discovery of anesthesia.[7] Although important innovations may have a profound impact on outcome in terms of death, disability, and discomfort, they are not so immediately striking, hence require the collaboration of a biostatistical colleague in the design and analysis of studies to demonstrate their value. The biostatistical colleague should be a full-scale partner in the research endeavor, beginning with the formulation of the hypothesis to be tested and moving on to the careful cooperative planning of the experimental design. A joint grant application is frequently the result. Continuing collaboration by the biostatistical partner will help to solve problems in data collection and to ensure that the chosen analytical methods extract accurately and efficiently all the information embedded in the data.

Clinicians who have received some training in statistics must realize that, valuable as this experience may be in developing a certain level of insight, it may be analogous to spending a single year as a resident in surgery or internal medicine. It is not a sufficient qualification to permit the giving of professional advice in biostatistics on which clinicians and their colleagues can depend. Statistics is a professional field; a half-trained statistician may be only slightly less dangerous than a half-trained surgeon. A growing number of statisticians who are experienced in medical science and a smaller number of clinicians who are well trained in biostatistics and epidemiology have made significant contributions to bridging the gap between the two fields.

Statisticians who are well adapted to collaborative research intuitively start with questions about patient referral patterns and the probability that patients and their physicians will accept proposed treatment alternatives. The first thought of surgeons who have become full partners with biostatisticians in design and analysis is to meet with their statistical colleagues to "brainstorm" about a project. They realize that the scientific methodologist is uniquely adept at formulating answerable questions from the presentation of clinical problems. Problems in experimental design and analysis are more easily prevented at the time of protocol writing than resolved after the control errors have been committed. When the clinician hears the biostatistician referring to "our patients" and "our treatments," he can be certain that the partnership has been established. The role of collaborators as true partners is clearly recognized by their status as coinvestigators on grants and as coauthors of published papers.

Physiologists, pharmacologists, biochemists, or other basic scientists may join, like biostatisticians, with clinicians in joint endeavors. Productive interactions require an investment of time and effort by all parties to the collaboration. Clinical investigators need to be aware of the costs of collaboration in terms of creative time and energy. Clinicians sometimes feel that the small amount of time they ask a basic science collaborator to devote to a research project is a relatively trivial claim to make on the coinvestigator. They may forget that all able people are very busy, and most are overcommitted. Teaching, administration, and other projects already in progress leave many basic scientists with only 10% of their time for their own creative work. Asking that half or all of this creative time be devoted to a new project takes on fresh meaning when viewed in this context.

Perhaps the most difficult issue to deal with in strengthening the research environment relates to the manner in which individuals with research, but not clinical, expertise should be employed—or deployed. The role in clinical departments of the fundamental scientist, usually a Ph.D. in a basic science, continues to undergo definition and is rarely consistent between institutions. During the past decade, as many basic scientists at the doctoral level have been appointed to clinical departments in the United States as have entered basic science departments in American medical schools.[8] Ideally, such individuals perceive clinical investigative opportunities as a chance to expand their own horizons, to extend their research into broader areas than were offered during their training, and to use such research accomplishments as a launching point for independently successful careers. In turn, the clinical members of the department learn from the basic science or biostatistical investigators, expand their own potential, and become part of a combination that is far more powerful, scientifically, than the sum of its parts.

In the worst scenario, basic scientists become pawns of clinical departments and "token investigators." They conduct projects identified by the clinical faculties—frequently without the understanding necessary to capitalize fully on them. In such settings, the basic scientists are truly "fish out of water," and they lose their identification with their basic disciplines. After several years, their ability to conduct contemporary research in their own disciplines wanes, their credibility among their scientific peers diminishes and, ultimately, their usefulness to the clinical units disappears. Everyone loses.

Careful thought is mandatory before a basic scientist is recruited. Whenever possible, dual appointments should be obtained in the clinical and basic science departments. These should not be "token" appointments. Whenever possible, a teaching responsibility should accompany them, and attendance at the basic science department's meetings and seminars should be encouraged. Some suggest that to maintain scientific credibility, a predesignated 25% of the scientist's time be allocated to work in the appropriate basic science department and attendance at meetings unrelated to the clinical discipline.

Some research scientists have been hired, assimilated, and inextricably linked to departments of surgery. These individuals—with their strong knowledge of the basic scientific process, heightened awareness of experimental techniques and greater knowledge of protocol development—serve as the focal point for departmental investigation. In Cologne, investigative science and clinical practice are so closely linked, and the careers of the trainees so thoughtfully planned, that clinical rotations are jointly determined by the chairman of the department and the head of departmental research.

This theoretical surgeon, as defined in Chapter 6, is responsible for organizing data processing, coordinating scientific and clinical meetings, helping to focus clinical training according to the ultimate investigative interests of the trainees, and devoting much time to the scientific training of "residents." Figure 5.3 depicts this relationship. This basic scientist is truly a member of the department who shares practice (research), teaching, and administrative responsibilities with the chairman.

This model may not work everywhere, but more institutions may wish to consider the development of specialized curricula for trainees, provided basic requirements for broad clinical training are fulfilled. In some institutions, new training programs are evolving for basic scientists to ensure that they are better equipped to make extended application of basic science to the human model. In particular, a degree in human biology combining basic science and fundamental medical curricula, without clinical experience, is one way to bridge the gap between disciplines and to relieve the tension that frequently develops when coverage of a broad spectrum of disciplines and concepts is attempted.

If a laboratory or research component is judged to be an important part of a clinical department, attempts should be made to organize and provide a relatively consistent basic curriculum for trainees and junior members of the faculty. The curriculum might include literature searching, use of personal computers, biostatistics, epidemiology, and the design of clinical investigations, as well as broadening the cognitive processes, vocabulary, and universe of the clinician. Investigators within a department should meet frequently to present their work, expose new technology and thought, and permit peer review. Basic scientists and clinical investigators must intermingle freely at such sessions. The traditional "visiting professor" program should be expanded to include role models who are successful investigators as well as brilliant clinicians. Participation in departmental conferences should be encouraged in such a way that those involved primarily in investigation attend clinical sessions and those primarily involved in clinical work attend research sessions.

Science and clinical practice must be so intermingled that they are conceptually inseparable. It would be interesting to know how frequently a basic scientist has been invited to be the visiting professor at a clinical conference. How often is a biostatistician or epidemiologist the visiting professor in a clinical department? Might exciting new ideas evolve from an awareness of how these disciplines could be applied to clinical problems?

Long-Term Stable Relationships Between Basic Science and Surgery

The "Marburg Experiment" (Chapter 6), is a classic example of highly productive, long-term, collaborative research involving committed clinicians and scientists. In Marburg, Germany, two scholars are linked together on a continuing basis to undertake joint exploration of scientific and clinical problems. Through constant review and direct personal exposure to the other's techniques and problems, each partner develops insight, asks new questions, and contributes a sympathetic but critical review of research procedures and results. This approach recognizes how difficult, or impossible, it is for surgeons to maintain expertise even in a basic science to which they have dedicated several years of full-time training and research. The Marburg model has been adopted by a number of centers and has produced excellent results.

Resident Experience in Research

Many academic programs require all, or selected, residents to have 1 or 2 years of exposure to the scientific discipline of research and scholarship. This experience enriches the education of clinicians, whether they intend to continue in research or to support it by providing clinical leadership.

At McGill University, every surgical resident devotes a minimum of one year to clinical or basic surgical research in the University Surgical Unit or in another department, such as pathology, anatomy, physiology, or immunology. This year of surgical scholarship follows the completion of a 2-year core clinical training program and precedes the senior clinical years of a general surgical residency. During this year away from clinical responsibilities, surgical residents work with a surgeon or a basic scientist on a project suited to their ability and interest. They review the literature and formulate a study program or experiment related to their mentor's ongoing research. The resident who attends formal lectures in biostatistics, anatomy, physiology, and pharmacology, and successfully completes a good research project and thesis is awarded the degree of master of science in experimental surgery. Residents with a special talent for research frequently decide, during this year, to enter academic surgery as a career. Appropriate candidates continue their research training for as long as 3 years, obtain the degree of doctor of philosophy in experimental surgery, and return to complete their two senior years in the clinical

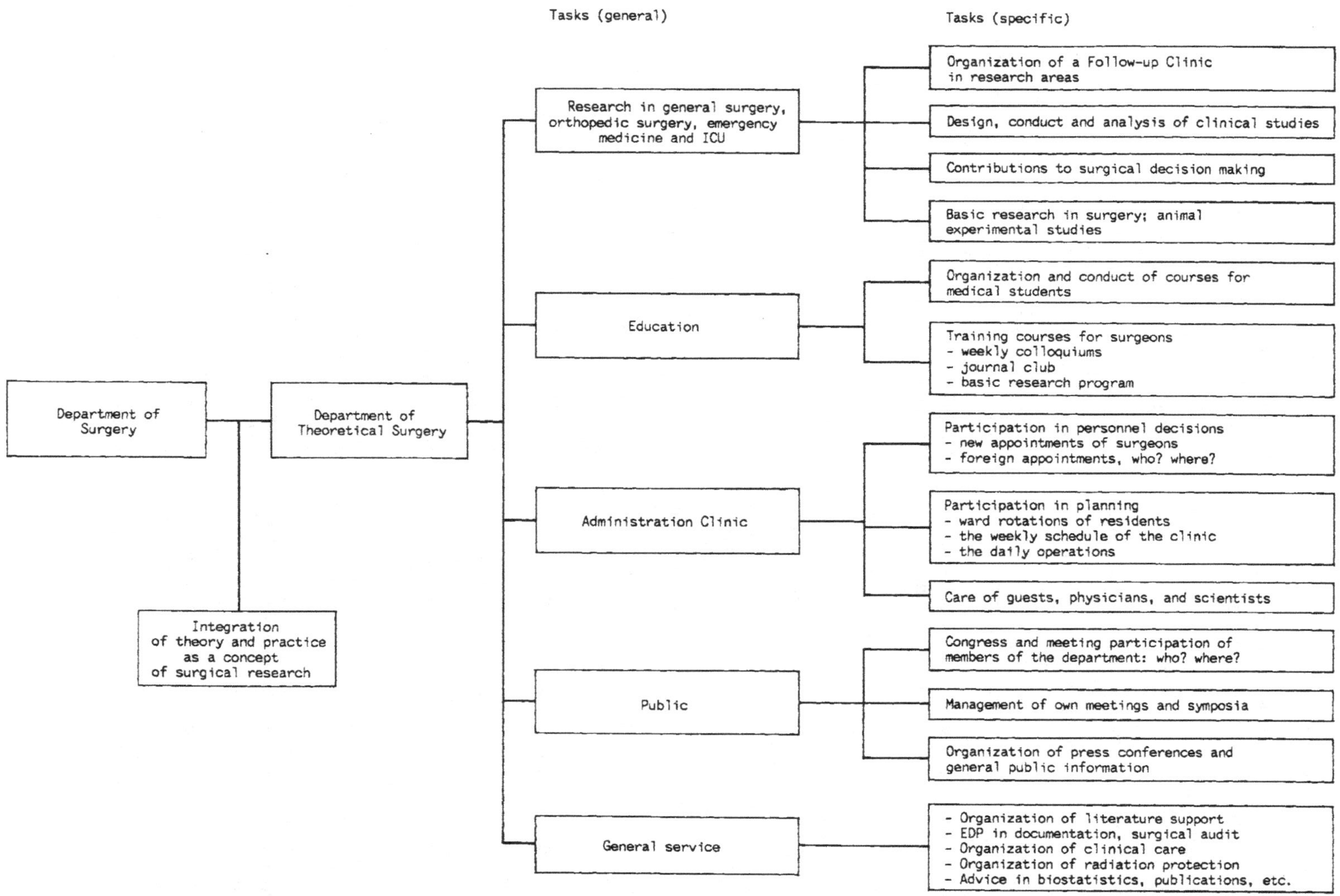

FIGURE 5.3. The relationship of the Department of Theoretical Surgery to such tasks as organizing data processing, coordinating scientific and clinical meetings, helping to focus clinical training according to the ultimate investigative interests of the trainees and devoting much time to the scientific training of "residents." An example from Cologne-Merheim.

surgery program. Ordinarily, they then assume academic positions with a major commitment to surgical research.

Every surgical resident in the training program of the Montreal General Hospital is encouraged to carry out a clinical research review with a member of the faculty during each academic year. Each resident, therefore, approaches clinical problems under the supervision of an experienced surgical teacher. The results of these clinical reviews, or of laboratory research by other residents, are presented each year at a special convocation. All residents are encouraged to submit their work to national and international meetings and are given financial support to attend them if their papers are accepted for presentation.

Medical and graduate students often impart a special stimulus to a research program by emphasizing and expanding the basic science aspects of a project. Their presence in clinics and laboratories heightens the atmosphere of academic inquiry, enhances their own education, and has a marvelously stimulating effect on the curiosity of their teachers. Research seminars expose students to clinical scholars, basic scientists, exciting investigations, and residents striving to advance their level of surgical knowledge. Student research fellowships during the summer months allow selected students to expand their exposure to research and to awaken a latent interest that eventually leads some into a lifetime commitment to surgical science.

Interinstitutional Research

Research collaboration between clinical units, or between research teams from different institutions, is especially effective in solving certain clinical problems. The interinstitutional collaborative projects of the National Surgical Adjuvant Breast Project (Section III, Chapter 29), are the Randomized Coronary Artery Surgical Study, and the Lung Cancer Study Group are notable examples of such collaboration.

These programs have drawn together surgeons, anesthesiologists, statisticians, internists, radiologists, pathologists, and other scientific personnel to formulate focused questions and to provide documented answers to problems that could not be resolved in any one institution. By developing, refining, and following joint protocols, the investigators have made significant advances in the definition of disease, standardization of optimal care, establishment of minimal criteria for reporting, and elimination of inappropriate use of surgical or adjuvant remedies.

The challenge of complex problems and the fun of working with friends motivate collaboration in research: synergism among partners is powerfully stimulating to investigators who might be frustrated in isolated attempts to find solutions.

Although we have discussed some of the special arrangements that have proven effective in some great academic centers, some of the most important and significant clinical research is performed by scholars working quietly in small departments or small clinics – sometimes alone, but more often in partnership with interested colleagues from other fields.

An inquiring mind that looks at problems in terms of potential solutions, and a spirit determined that tomorrow's patients will receive better care than today's, are much more important than great financial or technical resources.

References

1. Osler, Sir William. *The Collective Essays of Sir William Osler. The Classics of Medicine.* Birmingham, AL: The Medical Library, 1985.
2. Naruke T, Suemasu K, Ishikawa S. Lymph node mapping and curability at various levels of metastasis in resected lung cancer. *J Thorac Cardiovasc Surg* 1978; 76:832–39.
3. McIlduff JB, Daggett WM, Buckley MJ, et al. Systemic and pulmonary hemodynamic changes immediately following mitral valve replacement in man. *Cardiovasc Surg* 1980;21:261–66.
4. The Principal Investigators of CASS and Their Associates. The National Heart, Lung, and Blood Institute Coronary Artery Surgery Study (CASS). *Circulation* 1981;63(Suppl I).
5. Cerra FB, Mazuski J, Tusly K, et al. Nitrogen retention in critically ill patients is proportional to the branched chain amino acid load. *Crit Care Med* 1983; 11(10):775–78.
6. Civeta JM, Hudson-Civetta JA. Maintaining quality of care while reducing charges in the I.C.U.: ten ways. *Ann Surg* 1985;202:524–32.
7. Bigelow HJ. Insensitivity during surgical operations produced by inhalation. *Boston Med Surg J* 1846;35: 309–17.
8. Fishman AP, Jolly P. Ph.D.s in clinical departments. In: *Career Opportunities in Physiology*, Ramsay DJ, ed. Bethesda, MD: American Physiology Society, 9–12.

6

The Marburg Experiment: Developing the New Specialty of Theoretical Surgery

W. Lorenz, H. Troidl, and M. Rothmund

Most scientific endeavor now requires the active collaboration of scholars from a variety of disciplines.

Theoretical surgery started in response to the requests of clinical surgeons and anesthetists in Munich for help with research on practical problems. In 1968 two small permanent working teams of clinicians and biochemists were formed. A few years later, a system to promote surgical research in a nondepartmentalized university clinic was organized, in Marburg. This effort, known as the Marburg Experiment,[1] has grown over the past 20 years, but it continues to demonstrate one way of achieving close interaction between clinical surgery, basic sciences, and the care of surgical patients.

What is Theoretical Surgery?

Theoretical surgery is an integrated basic and clinical research system to support the scientific work of an academic department of surgery. It differs from traditional experimental surgical units in scope because it is not limited to laboratory studies. Unlike most basic scientists who work in clinical departments, theoretical surgeons are extensively trained in clinical research methodology, biostatistics, and human medicine. Their scientific interests are not limited to one or several projects within the department. They take responsibility for the scientific coordination of all of the work of the surgery department. Theoretical surgeons are distinguished by their willingness as well as their ability to put questions which arise in the clinic into terms amenable to solutions by the scientific method (see Figure 5.3, page 39).

Academic surgeons, who must devote much of their time and energy to patient care, teaching, and administrative duties, are frequently overwhelmed by the complexity of existing information channels and the problems of communicating with biostatisticians, pharmacologists, physiologists, biochemists, social scientists, and other basic research colleagues. If they choose to make major efforts in research, they risk isolation and eventual loss of some credibility as clinical surgeons.

The key to the success of the Marburg Experiment is integration—not just the frequently intended but rarely achieved cooperation. An academic clinician joins with a personal, permanent partner from the basic sciences for a long-term collaborative relationship. If biomedical research is to be responsive to the clinically relevant needs of patients, clinicians must play an active leadership role. We believe that the design and execution of original, methodologically reliable, and clinically relevant studies require close and continuing partnerships between skilful clinicians and experienced research workers. Interaction between these two groups must be characterized by complete and open communication if it is to result, at least, in better outcomes than either could achieve working separately. At best, it results in research incorporating the most sophisticated strategies, basic scientific techniques, and refined approaches to clinical practice.

Training of Theoretical Surgeons

As the Marburg Experiment continued,[2,3] it was found that a new type of problem-oriented (versus patient-oriented) research scientist was needed. We needed basic scientists who were truly comfortable with the ideas and concepts of clinical medicine. Gradually, a career training pattern for

TABLE 6.1. Organization of permanent working teams in theoretical surgery.

Principle	Integration of decision analysis with clinical and basic research among surgeons and theoretical surgeons in a practical, long-lasting arrangement
Composition	1 senior and 1 junior surgeon 1 basic scientist 1 or 2 technicians (electronic data processing and biomedical assistant) 1 or 2 students (medicine, biology, or chemistry)
Functions	Decision analysis and research in a defined part of the clinical and research program of the two departments Communicating at least once a week in a fixed meeting of about 2 hours Applying methods of decision making to current problems Designing and conducting clinical trials and animal experiments Running a systematic follow-up Documenting records, experimental data sets, and literature in the specific field
Rooms and equipment	1 room for meetings, for storing hard copies of records and data sets and files 1 laboratory with a microcomputer (LAN) and other (mostly biochemical) equipment Rooms provided by the theoretical surgeon with access to all apparatus of both departments

Modified with permission from Lorenz W, Hamelmann H, Troidl H[1] (1976). Other sources: Röher HD,[2] Lorenz W, Rothmund M[3] (1989).

those who would specialize in theoretical surgery was developed.

We recruited young scientists, fully qualified (Ph.D.) in one specialty of basic research (e.g., mathematics, pharmacology, biochemistry) and then sought to facilitate their acquisition of broad knowledge in surgical science and management. They tried to learn as much as they could about clinical and laboratory surgery under the leadership of practicing academic surgeons, and to acquire basic knowledge in a variety of scientific disciplines. They did not attempt to become professional practitioners of these other disciplines, but rather to become sufficiently knowledgeable to act as bridges or links between clinicians and basic scientists, and between the basic scientists, themselves. After about 6 to 8 years, this theoretical surgeon is qualified by habilitation (i.e., formal permission to act as an academic lecturer), a step similar to becoming an assistant professor in a faculty of medicine in North America. This usually happens at about age 35 to 38 years.

Organizing Collaborative Research

The aim of the Marburg Experiment is to create organizational structures that simultaneously foster enthusiasm and ability in integrating research across disciplines. Small working teams were assembled as permanent units that interwove the staffs of both the clinical and theoretical departments. The organization of these small working teams can be found in Table 6.1.

Decision Analysis

Nonoperative decision analysis is a continuing interest of theoretical surgery. In weekly joint meetings of the permanent working teams, decision trees for analyzing such clinical problems as duodenal ulcer are created and then tested by the clinicians; actions and strategies selected in upper gastrointestinal bleeding are other examples. These analyses use sophisticated computer hardware and software, select statistical models (Bayes theorem, cluster analysis, logistic regression), and create programs for measuring the performance characteristics of various diagnostic tests; the accurate quantification of perioperative risks has been a major thrust.

Contributions to Clinical Trials

The Institute of Theoretical Surgery has been instrumental in designing and supervising a number of controlled clinical trials. Some of the trials were generated to fill perceived gaps in decision-making algorithms dealing with such problems as stress ulcer prophylaxis in polytrauma, or preanesthetic administration of histamine receptor blockers.

Basic Research in Surgery

The research in biochemistry and pharmacology performed in the permanent working teams is applied and always has the aim of being immediately useful for clinical care.

Meta-analysis and Metasurgery

Meta-analysis comprises a group of new techniques by which clinical problems can be solved by analyzing data from patients, animals, cells, and other sources garnered from a series of published studies. A study design is developed with specific rules (e.g., a decision tree) for collecting individual trials from huge data bases, analyzing individual studies in detail, and submitting the whole body of trials to descriptive and very sophisticated inferential statistics.

Metasurgery comprises all systematic studies on the philosophy, epistemology, ethics, and social and psychometric aspects of surgery. The recent and increasing emphasis on consideration of such problems in surgical decision making has created a new demand for more solid data bases and the use of techniques already available in the social and behavioral sciences, and in the arts and humanities. This is been actively pursued by a permanent working team on metasurgery.

Advice

The Theoretical Surgery Department supports clinical trials, participates in local ethics committee deliberations, recommends the purchase and maintenance of special biochemical and electronic data processing equipment and software, and coordinates the various departmental activities in a central data processing unit.

Service Functions

The Department of Theoretical Surgery gathers information for clinicians by using retrieval systems with access to existing departmental and local data banks, as well as such international systems as MEDLARS. The permanent working team on metasurgery employs a trained librarian, complete hard disk facilities, and an assistant who is available for all technical and operational information transfer functions, including photocopying and duplicating services.

Surveillance Functions

The Department of Theoretical Surgery maintains surveillance over radiation, data, and animal protection. By creating a computerized system for medical decision making, theoretical surgery made a 10-fold reduction in the number of studies based on animal experiments, without diminishing the research productivity of the program. Such effectiveness is a potent argument for promoting this approach to medical decision making.

TABLE 6.2. Rules for theoretical surgeons and surgeons to achieve successful communication and progress of work in the permanent working teams.

Category	Specification
Psychological	Intention and sense of duty to communicate and work in a team
	Acceptance of different roles in treating patients: the surgeon is the king; the theoretical surgeon is the Brahman
	Fairness in authorship
Scientific	Careful selection of persons for the specific topic of the team
	Finding a common terminology between the clinician and the basic scientist by subtle exchange of information
	Mutual training in clinical science and basic research
	Combining special objectives with general methodological framework in selecting research fields to avoid superspecialization
	Flexibility in research fields to cope with unavoidable changes in hospital staff
	Patience of the theoretical surgeon in achieving harmonious discussion after an exchange of staff: the surgeon must treat the patients on the first day of starting work in the new hospital
Practical	Selection of an appropriate date for the weekly meeting—testing and retesting until it works
	Insistence by the theoretical surgeon that the meetings continue—even if the surgeon is tired
	Careful preparation of the weekly meeting agenda
	Theoretical surgeon: always approach the surgeon! Don't wait for the surgeon, the surgeon is always busy!

Reprinted with permission from Lorenz W, Rothmund M[3] (1989).

Interdepartmental Structure

Theoretical surgery is based, operationally, on an interdepartmental structure and permanent working teams that provide sustained development of an investigative approach. The teams are kept small (four to eight members) to foster easy communication, stimulate individual effort, and simplify cooperative efforts with others outside the team.

Some of the conclusions we have reached as a result of this 20-year experience are listed in Table 6.2. In a multidisciplinary effort, *communication is essential*. Meetings of the teams are held on Monday, Wednesday or Thursday evening, and on Saturday mornings, about 25 to 35 times per year. The benefit to participants is illustrated by the fact that this demanding schedule has endured for 20 years!

TABLE 6.3. Impact of theoretical surgery on efficacy in clinical care and decision analysis, in clinical research, and basic research in surgery.

Level of efficacy	Clinical care and decision analysis	Functions in academic surgery: Clinical research	Functions in academic surgery: Basic research
Performance	Development of safer anesthesia Perioperative, quantitative risk assessment by surgeons and anesthetists Argumentation in clinical decisions with quantities Defined strategies for peptic ulcer upper gastrointestinal bleeding Monitoring steroid levels administered in septic shock	First prospective clinical trial in German surgery, 1973 More than 30 randomized trials in anesthesia, intensive care, and surgery Cohort studies with simultaneous controls in peptic ulcer pathogenesis and surgery and on perioperative risk	Publishing articles in basic research journals with high impact Publishing articles on metasurgery in *The Lancet*
Changing strategies	Indication for operative treatment of peptic ulcer Indication for immediate operation in bleeding ulcer Stress ulcer prophylaxis Histamine H_1 − + H_2-antagonists in mesenteric infarction	Tremendous reduction in old-fashioned retrospective surveys without controls Publication of studies, mostly in English journals Spending much more time in planning clinical trials before conducting them and performing rotten statistics	Surgeons are *first* authors of articles in basic research Surgeons report at pharmacology meetings Animal models in basic research are changed by clinical considerations
Outcome	Decrease in lethality in upper gastrointestinal bleeding (15% → 6%)	Highly cited publications, including citation classics Editorials, invited lectures, and reviews in standard textbooks as parameters of common interest Promotion of careers for surgeons and theoretical surgeons Receiving considerable amounts of money in grants	Reduction of the gap between basic research and clinical science: man is an animal species Improved designs of studies in basic research: randomized trials More sound statistics in basic research (protection from the α-error)

Reprinted with permission from Lorenz W, Rothmund M[3] (1989).

Accomplishments of Theoretical Surgery

Quantifying the accomplishments of the Marburg Experiment during the past 20 years is difficult, but its impact on efficacy in clinical care and surgical research is currently being assessed by a technique using three levels developed by Loop and Lusted[4] (see Table 6.3). Its influence on existing surgical societies is just being felt. In 1980 the German Society of Surgery established a Permanent Working Party on Clinical Trials that distributes the concepts of theoretical surgery among its 200 members. In 1986 J.H. Baron of London helped us start the journal *Theoretical Surgery*. Several other universities (e.g., Cologne, Dusseldorf, and Innsbruck) now follow this approach to surgical research. For the Cologne organization see Chapter 5, on strengthening the research environment.

The role of theoretical surgery in furthering the progress of clinical practice is more subtle. Perhaps the major accomplishment has been impressing the reflexively critical approach to clinical decision making on our doctors and students, at all levels of expertise. Methodological rules were developed to approach various problems in surgery and to develop both heuristic and formal problem solving strategies.[5] The results of these studies were cited frequently in the literature including several citation classics.[3]

Acknowledgment. In preparing this chapter we have drawn on some of our previous work. In particular we cite references 1, 2, and 3.

References

1. Lorenz W, Hamelmann H, Troidl H. The Marburg experiment on surgical research: a five-year experience on the cooperation between clinical and theoretical surgeons. Klin Wochenschr 1976;54:927.
2. Lorenz W, Röher HD. Fifteen years of the Marburg experiment on surgical research. Part 1: Change from experimental to theoretical surgery. Theor Surg 1986; 1:21.

3. Lorenz W, Rothmund M. Theoretical research: a new specialty in operative medicine. World J Surg 1989; 13:292–99.
4. Loop JW, Lusted LB. American College of Radiology diagnostic efficacy studies. Am J Roentgenol 1978; 131:173.
5. Gross R, Lorenz W. Intuition in surgery as a strategy of medical decision making: its potency and limitations. Theor Surg 1990;5:54.

Further Reading

Interested readers will want to see the journal *Theoretical Surgery*, published by Springer-Verlag, New York.

Section II

Starting the Research Process

Good research ideas are rare and priceless treasures. Even when one lies glowing in your mind, translating it into the reality of a feasible research project often seems an insurmountable challenge. Before you can go very far with even an initial research plan, you must learn what your predecessors have done.

Reviewing the literature requires thoughtful effort to search, collate, classify, and assess material. We each want to be novel, we don't want to repeat work already done, and especially not the mistakes others have already made.

Orienting and reformulating an idea into a researchable question requires an understanding of feasible design strategies that will satisfy appropriate criteria of scientific rigor. The investigator must think through issues such as the nature of the interventions to be studied, the target endpoints, confounding variables, and the length of follow-up within a context of biological and clinical reality.

Ethical principles guide every aspect of research. Those who overlook such methodologic considerations as measurement, sample size, analytic approach, diagnosis, clinical significance, and probabilities do so at their peril.

Most large projects require resources that will be granted only after written documentation of a viable and promising research proposal. Thus before embarking on any but the smallest project, you must formulate and write, first, an initial plan; second, a detailed protocol; and finally, a formal research grant application.

Even if you are a newcomer to research, do not be discouraged by the steps you must take to achieve reliable results. In this section, we offer help as you take each successive step.

7

Taming the Literature

P. Hewitt

Computerized systems have not only taken much of the drudgery out of literature searches, but have also made them faster and more efficient. Computerization of indexes and abstracts enables you to search by any meaningful word in the article title, journal title, author's name, designated key words, and sometimes an abstract. The principles of organized literature searching apply whether your search is computerized or noncomputerized, but online searching is faster, more comprehensive, and more fun.

Getting Started

Once you have formulated a researchable question (see Chapter 11, below), you can embark on a literature search to determine what has been studied, what research designs have been employed, what controversies exist, and where your question fits into the field. Whether you use a computer or not, keep careful notes on what databases, indexes, and book collections you consult.

Ascertaining the content of online databases will let you know what other materials you need to investigate to make your review comprehensive; for example, are book chapters included in the database? Fortunately, most medical research is published in journals and MEDLINE and its printed form, *Index Medicus*, cover it well. This means that MEDLINE is a good place to begin.

MEDLINE/*Index Medicus* is 100% journal literature and covers approximately 3500 journals (2500 are *Index Medicus* journals and about 1,000 are "special list" journals, mainly in dentistry and nursing). EMBASE/*Excerpta Medica* covers other journals and has about a 35% overlap in coverage with MEDLINE. *Science Citation Index*/SCISEARCH covers a broad spectrum of scientific journals and some book chapters and meeting abstracts. Although each of the three has a printed counterpart, the online files are more flexible and may vary in content from printed versions (i.e., more online citations in MEDLINE and EMBASE than in the printed versions). None gives comprehensive coverage of books, book chapters, statistical sources, government reports, or meeting abstracts and proceedings. Other, specialized indexes afford access to some of this information.

Planning a Search

When planning a bibliographic search, you will need to ask some of the following questions.

1. Are there recent articles that I can use to formulate a subject search strategy?
2. What other subject terms should I search in indexes and other catalogs?
3. Is the journal literature the best place to find the information I need?
4. Are government reports and statistics, books, or meeting proceedings and abstracts a significant source of information on the topic of my search?
5. What time period should I cover?

Planning a research-level search will take about 45 minutes, but many searches (e.g., verification of a citation) require no planning. Author searching is easy, and compiling a bibliography of a specific person's work merely requires a standard format to produce comprehensive results. Most subject searches and all research-level literature searches, however, do require planning.

"Interviewing yourself" is a good technique for defining the question in MEDLINE/*Index Medicus*, EMBASE/*Excerpta Medica*, or other index terms. Libraries and online search centers ask clients to fill out a form to start the planning process;

you can use a similar technique to define and limit a search. The best request forms ask you to state the question in three different ways (i.e., three approaches to searching the index). Refining the question by using this interviewing process will remind you that (a) searches can be limited by human or animal studies, language, sex and age of patients, and geographic parameters; and (b) specific information is needed to achieve the purpose of your search (e.g., patient care, paper/article, research project, book/dissertation/grant proposal), helping to define how much information is necessary.

Pre-searching

One good strategy for choosing subject terms is to begin with a study that you have already identified as pertinent to your topic. It should be more than 3 weeks old – older if the vendor leases MEDLINE tapes from the National Library of Medicine or if the article is nonclinical – but not more than a few years old. Once you have selected the appropriate MEDLINE file, you can search by the author's name and look at the indexing of his or her study. The standard format for author searching in MEDLINE, on the National Library of Medicine's MEDLARS system, is

LASTNAME [space] INITIALINITIAL [space] (AU)

for example, Spitzer WO (AU)

Both *Index Medicus* and MEDLINE use this format, but MEDLINE offers an additional option. You may wish to include a truncated version of the name, for completeness or because you know only part of the name. The truncation symbol varies from vendor to vendor, but in MEDLARS it is : (colon).

For example,

Troidl H: (AU) (has he ever published with a middle initial?);

McPeek: (AU) (to find any McPeeks publishing in medical journals)

Wood: S: (AU) (to find authors Wood, Woodman, Woodle, Woodward, Wood-Dauphinée who have a first initial S).

The truncation symbol indicates that anything after it is acceptable. In the first example, any second initial is acceptable; in the second, any two initials; and in the third, any last name beginning with the root Wood and any initials beginning with S. You can use the truncation symbol with subjects, but avoid using it with common names and root words that will produce huge numbers of articles, [for example, cat: and Jones : (AU)].

When the pertinent article is located in MEDLINE, the PRINT FULL format will reveal its *Medical Subject Headings List* (MeSH) indexing. Table 7.1 is a FULL MEDLINE record. The MeSH headings indicate the article's major topics with an * (asterisk) and with subheadings that define the topic further. With one FULL record, you can proceed to an online search or an *Index Medicus* search in the library. Many searchers use two or three pertinent articles, log off the system, and formulate a complete search strategy using MeSH and the clues given by the pertinent articles. Select only the two or three MeSH terms that are most specific and most relevant to your search; too many terms will limit retrieval and lose good studies; too few will broaden retrieval and force you to sort through many irrelevant articles.

The Boolean operators *and*, *or*, and *not*; MeSH headings; authors' names; multiple author combinations; text words from the titles and the author-produced abstracts; and journal titles can be combined to tailor each online search to your specific question. The *and* of online searching is exclusive. GALLBLADDER/SURGERY *and* AGED, 80 AND OVER will not ask the reader to look at a thousand articles listed under GALLBLADDER/SURGERY and all the items indexed under AGED, 80 AND OVER; it will give only the number of articles indexed to both. You will always get fewer articles when you employ the *and* command. *Or* is inclusive; it will always get more articles. If you want all articles on gallbladder surgery, select GALLBLADDER/SURGERY *or* CHOLECYSTECTOMY to get a complete set of articles on the surgical aspect of the search before limiting it by some other factor using the *and* command (see Fig. 7.1).

Experienced online searchers use the *not* command, with caution. You can use it to "*not*" sets of online article citations you have already examined. For example, you could examine GALLBLADDER/SURGERY first, then realize that CHOLECYSTECTOMY may offer more citations to examine; using the *not* command, you would request CHOLECYSTECTOMY *and not* GALLBLADDER/SURGERY to eliminate duplication.

About 75% of the time you spend on a search should be devoted to planning its online portion. This saves money and gives you a fallback plan if your search yields far too much or too little. The online search planning form in Figure 7.2 is useful if you are doing a literature search yourself or with an intermediary librarian or research assistant. Write your question in sentences to put the medical

TABLE 7.1. FULL MeSH record on the MEDLARS system.

UNIQUE IDENTIFIER	89176368
AUTHOR	Wallace RJ Jr
AUTHOR	Musser JM
AUTHOR	Hull SI
AUTHOR	Silcox VA
AUTHOR	Steele LC
AUTHOR	Forrester GD
AUTHOR	Labidi A
AUTHOR	Selander RK
TITLE	Diversity and sources of rapidly growing mycobacteria associated with infections following cardiac surgery.
LANGUAGE	Eng
MESH HEADING	*Cardiopulmonary Bypass
MESH HEADING	Comparative Study
MESH HEADING	Cross Infection/EPIDEMIOLOGY/*MICROBIOLOGY
MESH HEADING	Disease Outbreaks
MESH HEADING	Drug Resistance, Microbial
MESH HEADING	DNA, Bacterial/ANALYSIS
MESH HEADING	Electrophoresis, Agar Gel
MESH HEADING	Endocarditis, Bacterial/MICROBIOLOGY
MESH HEADING	Human
MESH HEADING	Metals/PHARMACOLOGY
MESH HEADING	Mycobacterium/CLASSIFICATION
MESH HEADING	Mycobacterium Infections/*MICROBIOLOGY
MESH HEADING	Mycobacterium Infections, Atypical/EPIDEMIOLOGY/*MICROBIOLOGY
MESH HEADING	Mycobacterium, Atypical/*CLASSIFICATION/ DRUG EFFECTS/GROWTH & DEVELOPMENT/ GENETICS
MESH HEADING	Operating Rooms
MESH HEADING	Plasmids
MESH HEADING	*Postoperative Complications
MESH HEADING	Sternum
MESH HEADING	Support, U.S. Gov't, P.H.S.
MESH HEADING	Surgical Wound Infection/MICROBIOLOGY
ABSTRACT	Eighty-nine isolates of rapidly growing mycobacteria associated with cardiac bypass-related infections were characterized. Isolates from sporadic infections belonged to eight taxonomic groups and displayed numerous multilocus enzyme genotypes, plasmid profiles, and heavy metal and antibiotic resistance patterns. Compared with 449 noncardiac wound isolates, 45 sporadic cardiac isolates were more likely to be Mycobacterium fortuitum and M. smegmatis and less likely to be M. chelonae. About 80% of cardiac and noncardiac isolates were from southern coastal states. Eight outbreaks of cardiac bypass-related infections were identified. Strains from each outbreak were genotypically distinctive and five outbreaks involved more than one strain. In two outbreaks, isolates from environmental sources and noncardiac infections were similar or identical to isolates from sternal wound infections. The heterogeneity of these isolates suggests that most isolates are unrelated and are derived from local environmental sources rather than from contaminated commercial surgical materials or devices.
SOURCE	J Infect Dis 1989 Apr;159(4):708-16

terms in context. The literature search is divided into components using the standardized language of MeSH (or whatever thesaurus). There is a space for the relevant references you already know about; they can be searched by author and their indexing can be used to search for other relevant citations. You can be your own intermediary by using the form to begin to the refining of your question according to organization of the *Index Medicus*, *Excerpta Medica*, or another index.

More comprehensive and more specific citations for a literature review can be obtained if you understand the index and computer system. MEDLINE/*Index Medicus*, produced by the U.S. National Library of Medicine in Bethesda, Maryland, is a good example of an index available in printed (hard copy) and online form, in most medical libraries. MEDLINE is available internationally, through various vendors, for use on home or office computers. MEDLINE/*Index Medicus* will serve as an example, but the same principles of organized literature searching are applicable to any index. Other, complementary indexes will be discussed later.

The current MEDLINE file is 1988+, with backfiles to 1966. Is your search to be limited by time? Which backfiles will be searched? Because

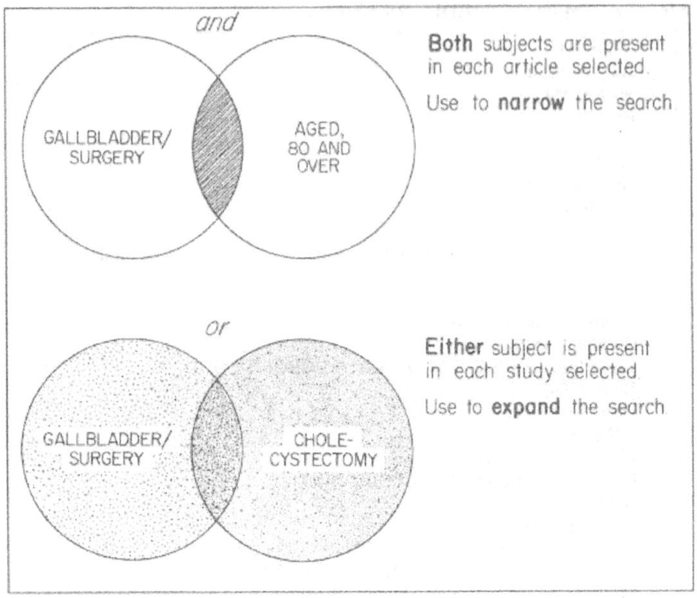

FIGURE 7.1. Boolean logical operators *and* and *or*.

1. Please write the question IN A SENTENCE or sentences.

____

____

2. Do you have a good article already? Please cite here.

____

____

3. TO NARROW THE SEARCH: Dates to cover ____________ Human/Animal? ____________

Language(s) ________________________ Age of patients ____________

AND	AND	AND	AND
OR			
OR			
OR			
OR			

FIGURE 7.2. Online search planning form.

TABLE 7.2. MeSH volumes.

Publication	Issued by	Publication number
Medical Subject Headings Annotated Alphabetic List, 1990	Bethesda, MD: U.S. National Library of Medicine, 1989	(PB90-180009)
Medical Subject Headings—Tree Structures, 1990	Bethesda, MD: U.S. National Library of Medicine, 1989	(PB90-1000007)
Permuted Medical Subject Headings 1990	Bethesda, MD: U.S. National Library of Medicine, 1989	(PB90-1000025)
List of Serials Indexed for Online Users—1990	Bethesda, MD: U.S. National Library of Medicine, 1989	(PB90-109851)

The publications listed above are available from:
National Technical Information Service (N.T.I.S.)
U.S. Department of Commerce
5285 Port Royal Road
Springfield, Virginia 22161, U.S.A.
These publications are revised with new subject headings each summer, and are available in September or October. In addition, each vendor will have a manual for the system and special instructions concerning MEDLINE and other individual databases.

different vendors of MEDLINE (for example, DIALOG, BRS, DATASTAR, DIMDI, and the National Library of Medicine's MEDLARS) have differently configured backfiles on their copies of the MEDLINE tapes, you will need to consult the system manuals in planning the dates to be covered in your search. Planning is easier if you use the printed version of *Index Medicus*—it is issued monthly, and cumulated yearly and every 5 years.

Indexing Organization

MEDLINE/*Index Medicus* uses the principle of bringing like subjects together. To do this, a preferred term is selected. Whenever synonyms occur in the literature, all relevant studies are indexed under that term. The terms are selected according to their frequency in the literature (i.e., "preferred" by authors in the field), and are published in lists that are updated yearly; sometimes more often. As indicated previously, the list of terms for MEDLINE/*Index Medicus* is called the *Medical Subject Headings List* (MeSH); it comprises three volumes and is available online as a separate database in the National Library of Medicine's MEDLARS system. In most medical libraries in the United States, MeSH is also used to classify books. Understanding MeSH organization will aid you in precision (retrieval of relevant articles) and recall (retrieval of all the articles on the topic).

Selecting MeSH Terms

The most serious error in using MeSH terms is choosing terms that are too broad. In MEDLINE/*Index Medicus*, specificity of indexing is the rule; articles are indexed under the most specific term possible. Failure to grasp this concept will cause you to miss more relevant articles than any other reason, including fatigue. Articles about AORTOCORONARY BYPASS will not be found under MYOCARDIAL REVASCULARIZATION (more general), HEART SURGERY (more general still), or THORACIC SURGERY unless the article is general and covers several types of surgery.

Where Are the MeSH Terms Listed?

The FULL format will give the MeSH terms for any citations in MEDLINE. The remaining MeSH terms are provided in the three volumes of the *Medical Subject Headings List*. (Table 7.2 lists the MeSH tools for 1990.) These volumes are updated yearly; you must use the latest MeSH, since terms are added, deleted, and rearranged each year. Volume I of MeSH, *Medical Subject Headings Annotated Alphabetic List, 1990*, is organized alphabetically; it has annotations for indexers (and searchers) and special notes about some terms. Under the MeSH term is noted the date it entered the list and cross references to related and more specific terms. A MeSH tree number, under the term, refers to the second volume of MeSH, *Medical Subject Headings—Tree Structures, 1990*. The trees rearrange the MeSH terms into a hierarchic structure and show the context of the term, as well as more specific and more general terms. CODEINE appears in three trees.

D3 - CHEMICALS — ORGANIC, HETEROCYCLIC COMPOUNDS
D14 - CHEMICALS AND DRUGS — NERVOUS SYSTEM DEPRESSANTS
D23 - CHEMICALS AND DRUGS — NEUROREGULATOR AND AUTACOID BLOCKADERS

E4 - PROCEDURES AND TECHNICS-SURGICAL

SURGERY, OPERATIVE
SURGERY, PLASTIC
LIPECTOMY

LIPECTOMY	E4.860.552			
RHINOPLASTY	E4.860.732	E4.847.677		
RHYTIDOPLASTY	E4.860.760			
SURGICAL FLAPS	E4.860.887	E4.936.664.		
TISSUE EXPANSION	E4.860.920			
SURGERY, UROGENITAL (NON MESH)	E4.887			
CASTRATION	E4.887.165	E4.779.282		
ORCHIECTOMY	E4.887.165.679	E4.779.282.	E4.887.774.	
OVARIECTOMY	E4.887.165.685	E4.779.282.	E4.819.608.	E4.887.690.
STERILIZATION, SEXUAL	E4.887.599			
STERILIZATION, INVOLUNTARY •	E4.887.599.450			
STERILIZATION REVERSAL	E4.887.599.500			
STERILIZATION, TUBAL	E4.887.599.683	E4.819.608.	E4.887.690.	
VASECTOMY	E4.887.599.900	E4.887.774.		
SURGERY, GYNECOLOGIC (NON MESH)	E4.887.690	E4.819.608		
HYSTERECTOMY	E4.887.690.399	E4.819.608.		
OVARIECTOMY	E4.887.690.680	E4.779.282.	E4.819.608.	E4.887.165.
SALPINGOSTOMY	E4.887.690.750	E4.35.832	E4.819.608.	
STERILIZATION, TUBAL	E4.887.690.766	E4.819.608.	E4.887.599.	
SURGERY, UROLOGIC (NON MESH)	E4.887.774			
CYSTECTOMY	E4.887.774.150			
KIDNEY TRANSPLANTATION	E4.887.774.175	E4.936.125		
NEPHRECTOMY	E4.887.774.435			
SURGERY, UROLOGIC, MALE (NON MESH)	E4.887.774.692			
CIRCUMCISION	E4.887.774.692.226			
ORCHIECTOMY	E4.887.774.692.618	E4.779.282.	E4.887.165.	
PENILE PROSTHESIS	E4.887.774.692.621	E4.659.762	E7.450.763	E7.858.565.
PROSTATECTOMY	E4.887.774.692.625			
VASECTOMY	E4.887.774.692.856	E4.887.599.		
VASOVASOSTOMY	E4.887.774.692.956	E4.35.956		
URINARY DIVERSION	E4.887.774.852			
CYSTOSTOMY	E4.887.774.852.240	E4.579.240		
NEPHROSTOMY, PERCUTANEOUS	E4.887.774.852.642	E1.341.642		
URETEROSTOMY	E4.887.774.852.947	E4.579.947		
SUTURE TECHNICS	E4.901			
SYMPHYSIOTOMY	E4.910			
THORACIC SURGERY	E4.920	G2.403.810.		
HEART SURGERY	E4.920.490	E4.752.376		
HEART ARREST, INDUCED	E4.920.490.460	E4.752.376.		
HEART MASSAGE	E4.920.490.490	E2.365.647.	E4.752.376.	
HEART TRANSPLANTATION	E4.920.490.505	E4.752.376.	E4.936.80	
HEART-LUNG TRANSPLANTATION	E4.920.490.505.450	E4.752.376. E4.936.162.	E4.920.800.	E4.936.80.
HEART VALVE PROSTHESIS	E4.920.490.520	E4.659.459	E7.450.500	E7.858.565.
MYOCARDIAL REVASCULARIZATION	E4.920.490.630	E4.752.376.		
ANGIOPLASTY, TRANSLUMINAL, PERCUTANEOUS CORONARY	E4.920.490.630.50	E2.148.102.	E4.752.376.	E4.752.814.
CORONARY ARTERY BYPASS	E4.920.490.630.280	E4.752.376.		
INTERNAL MAMMARY ARTERY IMPLANTATION •	E4.920.490.630.510	E4.752.376.		
INTERNAL MAMMARY-CORONARY ARTERY ANASTOMOSIS	E4.920.490.630.540	E4.752.376.		
PERICARDIAL WINDOW TECHNICS	E4.920.490.705	E4.35.720	E4.752.376.	
PERICARDIECTOMY	E4.920.490.720	E4.752.376.		
SURGERY, LUNG (NON MESH)	E4.920.800			
COLLAPSE THERAPY	E4.920.800.250			
PNEUMOTHORAX, ARTIFICIAL	E4.920.800.250.790			
LUNG TRANSPLANTATION	E4.920.800.495	E4.936.162		
HEART-LUNG TRANSPLANTATION	E4.920.800.495.450	E4.752.376. E4.936.162.	E4.920.490.	E4.936.80.
PNEUMONECTOMY	E4.920.800.780			
PNEUMONOLYSIS	E4.920.800.810			
THORACOPLASTY	E4.920.910			
THORACOSTOMY	E4.920.918	E4.579.918		

• INDICATES MINOR DESCRIPTOR

FIGURE 7.3. Example of MeSH tree structures.

CODEINE has one subset (more specific term) in the D23.338+ ANTITUSSIVE AGENTS category, and two subsets in each of the other categories. The second, OXYCODONE, may interest you if you are seeking information on pain relieving agents. The D3 and D14 trees indicate that codeine is a subset of opium and lists other more specific terms under opium. The terms ANESTHESIA AND ANALGESIA, which have their own tree, refer exclusively to types of anesthesia (for example, ANESTHESIA, INHALATION; NERVE BLOCK), not to anesthetic agents. A sample of the trees appears in Figure 7.3.

In the third volume, *Permuted Medical Subject Headings, 1990*, the MeSH terms appearing in *Alphabetic Annotated MeSH* and *Tree Structures* are sorted again, by each meaningful word. OSSICULAR REPLACEMENT PROSTHESIS is listed under the words OSSICULAR, REPLACEMENT, and PROSTHESIS. The term PROSTHESIS illustrates why *Permuted MeSH* is useful. Because it is

FIGURE 7.4. Example of permuted MeSH.

STRESS
DENTAL STRESS ANALYSIS
EMOTIONAL STRESS see STRESS, PSYCHOLOGICAL
FRACTURES, STRESS
POST-TRAUMATIC STRESS DISORDERS see STRESS DISORDERS, POST-TRAUMATIC
STRESS
STRESS DISORDERS, POST-TRAUMATIC
STRESS FRACTURES see FRACTURES, STRESS
STRESS, MECHANICAL
STRESS PROTEINS see HEAT-SHOCK PROTEINS
STRESS, PSYCHOLOGICAL
URINARY INCONTINENCE, STRESS

seldom the first word in a MeSH term, it is impossible to find in the other MeSH volumes. *Permuted MeSH* is the only place to go if you want to know all the terms containing the word PROSTHESIS. Figure 7.4 is an example of *Permuted MeSH.*

Why Use MeSH?

The National Library of Medicine's Unified Medical Language System (UMLS) will eventually link MeSH, ICD, SNOMED, and other methods of organizing information, so that any term typed into the system will offer the online user citations to articles on the topic. A "black box" will translate the query into appropriate terminology for the system. A metathesaurus will contain all the terms and map them to concepts to aid the searcher. To illustrate this: a disorder term will be linked to all its synonyms and variant spellings, and to treatments for that disorder. The information resources map will offer the user an array of terms from the metathesaurus and such other appropriate information sources as agencies producing categories of statistics or historical materials.

Until the more sophisticated computer systems are in place (work begins sometime after mid-1990), knowing how the system is organized will help you formulate more effective searches. All the online systems allow searching for title and abstract words, but indexing terms bring together like subjects and help to eliminate extraneous jargon. The concept "HUMAN" demands the following strategy in free-text databases (they do exist): WOMAN or WOMEN or MAN or MEN or CHILD or CHILDREN or INFANT or BABY or NEWBORN or TEEN or HUMAN or any other terms that the searcher can imagine; plurals and variant spellings must also be considered. A few techniques can make this cumbersome process easier, but the easiest way is to use the MeSH term HUMAN.

Search Helpers

Some online systems will help you to plan a search. Grateful Med software, installed in an individual microcomputer, will connect you to the National Library of Medicine's MEDLARS system. Grateful Med offers an input form screen and a MeSH component from which you can select terms that then move to the input form screen, before you connect to the National Library of Medicine computers; online charges do not begin until you are connected. Outside the United States, Grateful Med is currently available in Canada and Australia, and is planned for Great Britain.

PRO-SEARCH is another type of helper—a generic tool, not specific to MEDLINE or to medical databases in general. When it is installed in an individual microcomputer you can type in a search strategy before logging on to the system and it will help you with a series of menu screens. This is useful for new searchers, infrequent searchers, and slow typists since it offers easy login to two commercial vendors of MEDLINE; BRS and DIALOG. Grateful Med and PRO-SEARCH are purchased separately from any services of the National Library of Medicine, BRS, or DIALOG.

PaperChase and BRS COLLEAGUE are slightly different helper systems. Both lease the MEDLINE tapes. They are installed in the host computer, not in individual microcomputers. Both have menus to aid you by asking questions about your search requirements. PaperChase maps terms you type in, offers citations to articles with those words in the titles, and maps to the preferred MeSH term. If you type in CAT scan, the system will produce citations indexed under the MeSH term TOMOGRAPHY, X-RAY COMPUTED. The system then offers you the preferred MeSH term and additional terms to search for more citations on the topic. This is a step toward the Unified Medical Language concept, but PaperChase is geared to clinical use

TABLE 7.3. Sample MEDLINE search on MEDLARS.

```
NLM TIME 11:12:03 DATE 89:195 LINE 06C GM#040

WELCOME TO THE NATIONAL LIBRARY OF MEDI-
CINE'S ELHILL RETRIEVAL SYSTEM.
YOU ARE NOT CONNECTED TO THE MEDLINE
(1988-89) FILE.

SS 1 /C?
USER:
hip prosthesis

PROG:
SS (1) PSTG (630)

SS 2 /C?
USER:
Length of stay

PROG:
SS (2) PSTG (746)

SS 3 /C?
USER:
1 and 2

PROG:
SS (3) PSTG (5)

SS 4 /C?
USER:
prt

PROG:

1
UI - 89229552
AU - Dreghorn CR
AU - Hamblen DL
TI - Revision arthroplasty: a high price to pay.
SO - BMJ 1989 Mar 11;298(6674) :648-9

2
UI - 89083250
AU - Scalley RD
AU - Berquist KD
AU - Cochran RS
TI - Patient-controlled analgesia in orthopedic procedures.
SO - Orthop Rev 1988 Nov;17(11):1106-13

3
UI - 89044133
AU - Cushner F
AU - Friedman RJ
TI - Economic impact of total hip arthroplasty.
RF - REVIEW ARTICLE: 12 REFS
SO - South Med J 1988 Nov;81(11):1379-81

4
UI - 89032823
AU - Victor CR
TI - Rehabilitation after hip replacement: a one year
     follow up.
SO - Int J Rehabil Res 1987;10(4 Suppl 5):162-7

5
UI - 89016078
AU - Mallory TH
AU - Vaughn BK
AU - Lombardi AV Jr
AU - Kraus TJ
TI - Prophylactic use of a hip cast-brace following primary
     and revision total hip arthroplasty.
SO - Orthop Rev 1988 Feb;17(2):178-83

SS 4 /C?
USER:
stop y

TIME 0:01:59   NLM TIME 11:14:03
...

PROG:

GOOD-BYE!
THE ESTIMATED TOTAL ONLINE COST FOR THIS 2
MINUTE TERMINAL SESSION IS $
0.83.

*** END OF SESSION ***
```

and you cannot use some of the commands available in the MEDLINE tapes mounted on other systems, that are meant to help produce comprehensive searches.

BRS COLLEAGUE offers a variety of databases in addition to MEDLINE (*International Pharmaceutical Abstracts*, *Current Contents: Clinical Medicine*, and EMBASE/*Excerpta Medica*, and the full text of about 100 books and journals, including *New England Journal of Surgery*, *Gray's Anatomy*, and *The Merck Manual*). Investigators without access to libraries can get the text portion of all these documents, although technology does not yet allow transmission of illustrations, figures, or tables. As with PaperChase, this user-friendly system works best with simple searches; it cannot take advantage of some of the sophisticated features that professional online searchers use.

MEDLINE on CD-ROM (Compact Disk—Read Only Memory) is the newest way to access MEDLINE. Although a CD-ROM player is required in addition to a microcomputer and the disks are not inexpensive, for international users MEDLINE on CD-ROM may make economic sense. Telecommunications can be a problem for international users of online databases. Cost and quality of local telephone systems have mitigated against full use of online systems by medical professionals outside the United States. The advantage to CD-ROM databases is that there is no direct telephone communication and no per-use charge. The CDs are paid for and arrive by subscription. Most vendors of MEDLINE CD-ROM versions update them quarterly, some monthly. Several offer MeSH access on the CD-ROM disk. All have similar but slightly different commands and manipulation capabilities.

TABLE 7.4. Main offices of three major vendors of MEDLINE.[a]

Address	Telephone, fax, telex
U.S. National Library of Medicine MEDLARS Management Section 8600 Rockville Pike Bethesda, Maryland 20894 U.S.A.	Tel: (301)496-6193; (toll free) (800)638-8480
BRS Information Technologies Division Att: Vivian Daukysys MAXWELL ONLINE, INC. 000 Westpark Drive McLean, Virginia 22102 U.S.A.	Tel: (703)442-0900; (toll free) (800)955-0906 Fax: (703)893-4632
DIALOG Information Services, Inc. Marketing Department Hillview Avenue Palo Alto, California 94304 U.S.A.	Tel: (415)858-3810; (toll free) (800)334-2564 Fax: (415)858-7069 TWX: (901)339-9221 Telex: 334499 (DIALOG)

[a] For international offices of these vendors see Tables 7.5, 7.6, and 7.7. For countries not listed there, contact the U.S. office for the address of local data base agents.

Each of the various ways to access MEDLINE has different strengths and weaknesses. New software and systems will be available by the time this book is printed. The search plan aspect of the "user friendly" systems may interest you if you want to do your own online searching. A sample of a MEDLINE subject search is given in Table 7.3.

Major Medical Indexes

Of the 20 or so indexes of interest to medical professionals, three are primary tools for researchers: MEDLINE/*Index Medicus*, EMBASE/*Excerpta Medica*, and SCISEARCH/*Science Citation Index*. They cover different materials and they overlap.

MEDLINE indexes about 3500 journals and *Index Medicus* 2500, cover-to-cover, with up to 15 index (MeSH) terms per article, for both major and secondary topics. The major topics (5, at most) are the *Index Medicus* access points. Secondary topics are available in MEDLINE (for example, HUMAN, MALE, FEMALE, methodology terms, geographic terms, and other secondary points). *Index Medicus* is published monthly; MEDLINE is loaded twice a month. *Index Medicus* is cumulated yearly and every 5 years. MEDLINE is continuously cumulative—the latest citations appear first in any search. Backfiles are available to 1966, and the printed index goes back to 1879, in various forms. Abstracts, direct from the journals, are available for about 55% of the items in MEDLINE. *Index Medicus* contains the citations included in MEDLINE. Two special journal lists, *Index to Dental Literature* and *International Nursing Index* are available online but not in *Index Medicus*.

EMBASE/*Excerpta Medica* is available online and in print, but more articles are in the online file than ever appear in print. *Excerpta Medica* is not one large printed index, but 46 printed abstract bulletins and two printed drug literature bibliographies. Abstracts, created by *Excerpta Medica*, are available for 60% of citations. The controlled vocabulary called MALIMET differs from MeSH, but there are some organizational elements in common. 3500 primary journals are covered, and 1000 additional journals are scanned and indexed selectively. Based in Europe, *Excerpta Medica* covers journals not included in MEDLINE/*Index Medicus*. Its online files go back to June 1974 and its printed files to 1946.

Science Citation Index/SCISEARCH is available in print and online. It differs from MEDLINE and EMBASE. *Science Citation Index* has an author index (the *Source Index*), a subject index, a corporate index, and a unique feature, the *Citation Index*. The subject index uses text words from titles, with some augmentation, as "a key word in context" (KWIC) index. In contrast, MeSH and MALIMET are controlled vocabularies. The corporate index lists studies done by various corporate bodies, both commercial and academic. The *Citation Index* is useful if you have a good citation in hand. If the citation is about 2 years old or more, newer papers will have begun to cite it. You can use this index to find more recent papers citing key studies. SCISEARCH/*Science Citation Index* does not have subject headings lists or abstracts. It is produced monthly, and is cumulated yearly and every 5 years. Every online record is also available in the printed index. SCISEARCH covers journals in science, selected book chapters, and meeting

TABLE 7.5. International MEDLARS centers.

Australia
OZLINE National Library of Australia
Canberra A.C.T. 2600
Australia

Canada
Health Sciences Resource Center
Canada Institute for Scientific and Technical Information
National Research Council
Ottawa, Canada K1A 0S2

China
Institute of Medical Information
Chinese Academy of Medical Sciences
3 Yabao Road, Chaoyang District
Beijing, China

Colombia
Panamerican Federation of Associations of Medical Schools
Calle 123, No. 8-20
Bogota D.E., Colombia

Egypt
Centre for Educational Technology
21, Abdel Aziz Al Seoud Street
El Rhoda
Cairo, Egypt

France
Information Médicale Automatisée
Centre de Documentation de L'INSERM
78 rue du Général Leclerc
94270 Le Kremlin-Bicêtre, France

Germany (FRG)
German Institute for Medical Documentation and Information
5000 Köln 41, Postfach 420580
West Germany

Italy
Istituto Superiore di Sanita
Viale Regina Elena 299
00161 Rome, Italy

Japan
The Japan Information Center of Science and Technology
5-2 Nagatacho 2 Chome
Chiyoda-ku, Tokyo, C.P.O. Box 1478
Tokyo, Japan

Kuwait
Arab Centre for Medical Literature
P.O. Box 5225
Safat, Kuwait

Mexico
Centro Nacional de Informacion y Documentacion in Salud
Avda. INSURGENTESSUR #1397 2 Piso
Col. Mixcoac Insurgentes
CP. 03920 México D.F., México

South Africa
Institute for Biomedical Communication
South African Medical Research Council
P.O. Box 70
Tygerberg 7505, South Africa

Sweden
Medical Information Center
Karolinska Institute
Box 60201
S-104 01 Stockholm, Sweden

United Kingdom
Bibliographic Services Division
The British Library
2 Sheraton Street
London W1V 4BH, United Kingdom

Intergovernmental Health Organization
Pan American Health Organization
525 Twenty-third Street N.W.
Washington, D.C. 20037, U.S.A.

abstracts. The online files go back to 1974, and the printed index has been retrospectively created back to 1945. The 1945–1954 cumulation does not have a subject index.

These three indexes are the most general tools for bibliographic searching and are a good first stop. Such specialized tools as *INPHARMA*, *Biological Abstracts*, *Index to International Statistics*, and BIOETHICS can provide additional depth. There are about 20 databases of interest to medical professionals and nearly 3,000 publicly available databases on all topics. For information about contacting major vendors, in the United States and abroad, see Tables 7.4 to 7.7.

Evaluating Online Searches

The list of MeSH headings for each citation can be an important source of help to clinicians in the screening of articles. If the subject is MASTECTOMY, SEGMENTAL *and* PREANESTHETIC MEDICATION, these two terms will appear in the list, along with such other terms as HUMAN; ANIMAL; FEMALE; ADULT; AGED; AGED, 80 AND OVER; CHILD; INFANT; more specific infant terms, more specific animal terms, geographic areas, and other major and minor points of the article. The MeSH term CASE REPORT indicates a different sort of report from CLINICAL

TABLE 7.6. International BRS offices.

Address	Telephone, fax, telex
For Europe and Israel	
MAXWELL ONLINE, INC. Att: Claire Cree Achilles House Western Avenue London W3 OUA, England	Tel: (01) 992-3456 (01) 993-7334 Fax: (01) 993-7335 Telex: 8814614
Australia	
MAXWELL ONLINE, INC. Att: Russell Kendrick P.O. Box 544 Potts Point, NSW 2011, Australia	Tel: (02) 360-2691 (direct) (02) 331-5211 (switchboard) (008) 22-6474 (toll-free) Fax: (02) 332-2304 Telex: AA27458
Japan	
USACO Corporation 13-12 Shinbashi 1-Chrome Minatoku, Tokyo, 105 Japan	Tel: (03) 502-6471 Fax: (03) 593-2709 Telex: J26274 USACO TOKYO
Korea	
Samsung Co., Ltd. Business Development Dept. (SELPH) Taepyong-no. 2-GA, Chung-gu Seoul, Korea 100-742	Tel: (02) 751-2542 Fax: (02) 751-2776 Telex: STARS 3657, K22302

TRIALS or META-ANALYSIS. Printing the MeSH terms for each citation will also identify terms that did not occur to the planners of the online search and may suggest other search strategies. It is useful to begin the online search by examining the MeSH terms for a study the clinician knows as a good one; similar studies can probably be found by combining the MeSH terms assigned to it. Finally, the MeSH terms can be used to complement an abstract, or in lieu of one. The abstracts in MEDLINE are taken directly from the journal and reflect the bias of the author and the journal.

MeSH headings are assigned by professional indexers. While they do reflect the emphasis of the author, they place a study in the overall scheme of the medical literature. If the title a researcher gives to a paper does not mention "randomized control trial (RCT)", but the methods section does, there is a good chance the study will be indexed under CLINICAL TRIALS, and RANDOM ALLOCATION. Indexers do not "diagnose"—the author must discuss a subject in a substantive manner for it to be indexed—but they do try to index the primary and secondary points of all articles as emphasized by the author.

Too Little Information

If a search does not retrieve as many citations as you expected, it may be too narrow (i.e., it may be limited by age of the patient, date of publication, or other factors peripheral to the subject itself). Structure a new search with the essential items—two or three terms are often sufficient—and begin with the MeSH headings most frequently used for the articles you did retrieve. Other ways to enhance search retrieval are as follows.

1. Search retrospectively: MEDLINE backfiles go back to 1966.
2. Broaden the search strategy. If you have executed an online search on LIVER CIRRHOSIS, BILIARY (a very specific term), and retrieved too little, try CHOLESTASIS, INTRAHEPATIC, (a more general term). Consider synonyms. MEDLINE allows examination of the text words (title and abstract as opposed to the MeSH headings) for concepts that are very new or more specific than MeSH.
3. Reconsider the question. There probably is no literature on how many people experience headache in a general population, but there may be a survey of one specific population.

TABLE 7.7. International DIALOG offices.

Australia and New Zealand
Insearch Limited/Dialog
P.O. Box K16
Haymarket
Sydney, NSW 2000
Telephone: (02) 212-2867
Telex: AA127091

Brazil
PTI/Dialog
Publicações Técnicas Internacionais Ltda.
Rua Peixoto Gomide 209
01409 São Paulo SP
Telephone: (55-11) 257-2157
Telex: 1135844 (APTI BR)

Canada
Micromedia Ltd./Dialog
158 Pearl Street
Toronto, Ontario M5H 1L3
Telephone: 800/387-2689
416/593-5211
Telex: 065-24668

Denmark
Dialog/Denmark
DataArkiv
Glentevej 65
DK-2400 Copenhagen NV
Telephone: (45) 38-33-52-10

England
Learned Information Ltd./Dialog
P.O. Box 188
Oxford OX1 5AX
Telephone: (0865) 730275
Outside U.K.: (44-865) 730275
Telex: 837704 (INFORM G)

Egypt
Dialog/Egypt
MarketLink
Corniche El Nil
P.O. Box 533
Maadi
Cairo
Telephone: +20 2 363 8921

Finland
Dialog/Finland
Esselte InfoService
Box 112
00211 Helsinki
Telephone: (358-0) 692 6419

France
Dialog/France
75 avenue Parmentier
75011 Paris
Telephone: (33-1) 40-21-24-24
Telex: 211303 (CLIPSA F)

Mexico
AEID/Dialog
2a Cerrada de Romero de Terreros, 49A
Colonia del Valle
03100 México D.F.
Telephone: (52-5) 543-7207

Norway
Dialog/Norway
Axess A/S
P.O. Box 6753
St. Olavsplass
0130 Oslo 1
Telephone: (47-2) 20-91-30

Sweden
Dialog/Sweden
DataArkiv
Box 1502
S-171 29 Solna
Telephone: (46-8) 705-1300

West Germany
Dialog/Germany
EXIT Datenbankdienste
Graf-von-Stauffenbergstrasse 19
D-4800 Bielefeld 1
Telephone: (49-521) 16-10-21

4. Consider whether a database is the best source of information. For the headache question, MEDLINE may not be the best resource; a statistical database or printed index may be better. Some topics are textbook, rather than journal, material.

Too Many Citations

Too broad a question may result in too many citations. Retrieval can be limited by the age of the patient, type of treatment, years of publication, type of study, and more specific MeSH terms. Instead of a general look at HEART SURGERY, a search that combines CLINICAL TRIALS or PROSPECTIVE STUDIES or RANDOM ALLOCATION or DOUBLE-BLIND METHOD or META-ANALYSIS with the command EXPLODE HEART SURGERY will yield substantive studies on the 10 more specific HEART SURGERY MeSH terms, as well as on the general term HEART SURGERY. To limit by type of study, EPIDEMIOLOGIC METHODS (including more specific terms such as PROSPECTIVE STUDY), RESEARCH DESIGN, and COMPARATIVE STUDY are available. Limiting searches by study type can only be done online, as the printed *Index Medicus* does not have the cross-referencing capacity of a computerized system.

Critical Papers Not Found

First, check the citations of the papers to be sure they are within the MEDLINE years (1966 +), are in journals included in MEDLINE, and are *not* abstracts, government reports, or book chapters. These are not within the scope of MEDLINE. If the citations are within the scope, log on to the correct online file (which may vary with the online vendor), and request the article by author. You can analyze the MeSH headings to see how the indexers saw the emphasis of the study you have identified as "key." Whether you agree with the indexing or not, indexing analysis of key papers can help you identify all the studies needed. MeSH is revised each year, and the indexing for older files may not apply to newer files – new terms may have been added, and the *Tree Structures* may be rearranged. The newer the "key" paper is, the better your chances of finding more new papers under the same headings.

Online searching differs from other computerized tools. The user's sophistication determines the end product in a spreadsheet or in word processing, because these tools are not interactive and await the creative ideas of the user. The computerized online index is organized to be interactive; the choice of a MeSH term or strategy, and the request to MEDLINE to search it, allows immediate interaction with the system to modify the search. To take full advantage of this interactive capacity you should know some things about the system's organization. For instance, in MEDLINE used on the U.S. National Library of Medicine's MEDLARS system, when you type in "blood," the system will search the subject field (MeSH) for citations indexed to BLOOD. If you want to search the title and abstract fields, you must so specify with the qualifier (TW) (text word). If you want the author, Peter Blood, you must indicate the author field [for example, Blood P or blood (AU)]. Other vendors of MEDLINE have defined other default parameters for the fields to be searched, and you need to know which fields have been searched and which remain to be searched. It is not always most economical to search all the fields at the same time.

Always have a primary, a broader, and a narrower strategy prepared before you log on to the system so that you can interact with unexpected search results. Be prepared to scrap all previous strategies if MeSH headings appear that are better than those in your original strategy. Be prepared to log off, evaluate the search in progress, and log on again with a new approach. Online searching is an interactive process that should not end when you log off. Analyze each literature search, computerized or not, to be sure that the citations retrieved are appropriate to the question and that another avenue of approach would not yield better results; this need not take long. Sometimes searches should be augmented or redone with a new strategy.

The Librarian as Colleague

Increasingly, professional online searchers and medical librarians are becoming integral members of the research team. Although medical professionals do a good deal of online searching on their own, the advice of a colleague who performs many searches and is familiar with the gamut of bibliographic resources is valuable. Such a colleague can help with strategy for entire bibliographic searches, or check for logic and MeSH vocabulary problems in a strategy devised by the medical professional. The medical librarian may recommend a better index for a specific question, as well as books, special reports, other materials, other libraries, strategies for access to off-site resources, from interlibrary loans to data tapes at national centers.

Befriend an experienced professional online searcher or medical reference librarian. The experienced professional can evaluate overall online strategy, look for logic errors, pinpoint MeSH vocabulary problems, and advise on particularly difficult questions. The medical reference librarian, whether an online searcher or not, probably knows *Index Medicus* well, can advise on MeSH strategy, and has a general knowledge of the medical literature.

Bibliography

Beatty WK. "Libraries and how to use them." In: Coping with the Biomedical Literature: A Primer for the Scientist and the Clinician, Warren KC, ed. New York: Praeger, 1981

Conroy C. Online lifeline. Online Today 1986; 5May(5):14.

DeNeff P. The comprehensiveness of computer-assisted searches of the medical literature. J Fam Pract 1988; 27(4):404–8.

DeTore AW. Medical informatics: an introduction to computer technology in medicine. Am J Med 1988; 85(Sep)(3):399–403.

Harman SE. Getting the best results from your literature search request. Md Med J 1986;35(May)(4):255–7.

Haynes RB, McKibbon KA, Fitzgerald D, Guyatt GH, Walker CJ, Sackett DL. How to keep up with the medical literature: V. Access by personal computer to the medical literature. Ann Intern Med 1986;105(Nov)(5):810–6.

Hewitt P. Access to the medical literature. In: Data Analysis for Clinical Medicine: The Quantitative Approach to Patient Care in Gastroenterology, Chalmers TC, ed. Rome: International University Press, 1988:91–100.

Hewitt P, Chalmers TC. Perusing the literature. Methods of accessing MEDLINE and related databases. Controlled Clin Trials 1985;6(Jun)(2):168–77.

Hewitt P, Chalmers TC. Using MEDLINE for perusing the literature: software and search interface of interest to the medical professional. Controlled Clin Trials 1985;6(Sep)(3):198–207.

Hewitt P, Chalmers TC. Using MEDLINE to peruse the literature. Controlled Clin Trials 1985; 6(Mar)(1):75–83.

Hunter JA. When your patrons want to search – the library as advisor to end users . . . A compendium of advice and tips. Online 1984;8(May)(3):36–41.

Kolner SJ. The IBM PC as an online search machine – Part 1: Anatomy for searchers. Online 1985;9Jan(1): 37–42.

Kolner SJ. The IBM PC as an online search machine – Part 2: Physiology for searchers. Online 1985;9March (2):39–46.

Kolner SJ. The IBM PC as an online search machine – Part 3: Introduction to software. Online 19859May (3):44–50.

Kolner SJ. The IBM PC as an online search machine – Part 4: Telecommunications and CROSSTALK XVI. Online 1985 9July:(4):27–34.

Oxman A. Science of reading. Pediatrics 1989;83 (Apr)(4):617–9.

Schwartz DG. Techniques for accessing the medical literature. J Allergy Clin Immunol 1988;82(Oct)(4): 544–50.

Searching MEDLINE. Lancet 2(8612):663–4.

Van Camp AJ. The many faces of MEDLINE. DATABASE 1988 Oct;11(5)101–7.

Van Camp AJ. EMBASE PLUS – a new look for Excerpta Medica. DATABASE 1989;12(Apr)(2):34–8.

Williams PA. Overview of online information data bases in orthopedics. Orthop Clin North Am 1986;17(Oct) (4):519–26.

8

How to Organize Your Reference Material

R. Lefering and E.A.M. Neugebauer

Imagine you are starting to work on a new topic, such as endoscopy. First, you will gather together all the literature you have collected about endoscopy. Second, you may carry out a systematic literature search with MEDLINE, or some other data base—as described in the preceding chapter—to get the most recent publications. You may also talk to appropriate specialists to get leads to some key papers or the most recent books on the topic.

All these papers and books contain references to further reports in the literature. A regular examination of the most important journals on your topic (e.g., *Endoscopy, Surgical Endoscopy*), will keep you up to date, but you should make copies of the interesting articles. Some of your colleagues will give you other papers they think may be of special interest to you. By this time, you will have a stack of literature on your desk—and it won't stop growing.

This chapter is a guide through the world of literature organizing systems—to help you make maximum use of them and avoid drowning in a flood of papers. Some discussion about organizing a departmental literature system and some criteria for selecting a computer program for literature administration will follow.

Individual Literature Organization

You will usually have to deal with a daily or weekly input of new papers and, depending on the time you have available, you will peruse them and gain a degree of insight into their contents. Whatever information you extract will usually be stored in your mind. But, what should you do with a paper after you have scanned it? Throw it away or store it?

The only reason for not throwing it away is that you may wish to retrieve the information later—you will never be able to keep all the information in the articles you have read in your mind. An efficient retrieval system will facilitate access to what you have read and help you concentrate on the essentials. Access to articles in your own literature collection will be needed if you decide to prepare a paper or lecture, and will usually have to be supplemented by an on-line search for the most recent publications. You may also want to be able to retrieve articles to help some of your colleagues if they seek your advice. With a retrieval system, you will be able to give them some useful publications, immediately. You will also have many occasions to refresh your own knowledge about something in an article you have already read.

How do you deal with the flood of new literature? You cannot read everything! The first step is to sort your incoming papers into two categories: important articles you will very likely want to read again, and unimportant, boring papers, far from the center of your interest and of no foreseeable use to you. *Declare the second category instant litter.*

If what remains of your incoming stack is still too large, select the areas you are really interested in and restrict your attention to them, instead of struggling to get a broad oversight. You will still have to organize the remaining stack, because the only reason for keeping it is retrieval. The effort you devote to storing papers must be related to the frequency and types of request you make to your stored literature, and the amount of time it takes to make a retrieval from your collection.

If you decide to use one of the systems described below, weigh the real number of your requests to such a system—not the possible ones—against the cost to you, especially in terms of the time needed to keep it working.

TABLE 8.1. Differences of literature organizing systems to meet certain retrieval requests.

Task	Type of system[a]			
	Paper-based	Card index	Computer-assisted, citation only	Computer-assisted citation + keywords
Retrieve a *certain* paper...				
with complete citation	+	+	+	+
with author known	+	+	+	+
with coauthor known	−	−	+	+
with title (word) known	−	−	+	+
about a certain topic	−	±(1)	−	+
other (year, journal, ...)	−	±(1)	+	+
Retrieve *all* papers...				
of a certain author	±(2)	±(1)	+	+
with a certain title word	−	−	+	+
about a certain topic	±(1)	±(1)	−	+
other (year, journal, ...)	−	±(1)	+	+

[a] + = easy to carry out, ± = performable with restrictions, depending on (1) the chosen classification and (2) the alphabetical order and number of fields; − = impossible or very time-consuming.

Stack

This system is listed only to familiarize you with a type of cost-benefit analysis for measuring the usefulness of a storage and retrieval system. The "cost" is the effort involved in adding each new paper to your collection. In this example, the cost is zero because putting a paper on top of a stack requires no work. The "benefit" can be measured by the system's ability to answer the different types of possible requests listed in Table 8.1. Retrieval operations could be divided into looking for a certain paper, probably with incomplete knowledge of the specific reference, and getting overviews of a certain scope. The possibility of executing these operations and the time they require determine the benefit of a literature storage and retrieval system, because retrieval is the only justification for its existence. A simple stack responds very poorly to any type of request.

Paper-Based Systems

The usual way to organize literature involves paper-based systems. Typically, you identify the different fields or topics that cover your domain of interest. If the number of articles in a certain field is small enough, you can organize them as a stack; when the number is large, alphabetic storage by the author's name is more appropriate. The common classification for medical literature is by organ systems or diseases, but other categories, (e.g., animal/human study; review; case; ... surgical techniques; x-ray; ultrasound; CT; ...) or statistical approaches may be more suitable for your interests.

Some people like to collect all material for specific papers or lectures—figures, slides, and bibliography—in files on the topics of the proposed manuscripts, but problems arise when papers could be filed in several fields. A paper comparing the diagnostic value of x-ray versus ultrasound for detecting gallstones could be stored under "x-ray," "ultrasound," or "gallbladder." You could file a copy under each heading (usually not done because it requires extra duplicating and storing), or you could store it under one field and face additional effort when the time comes to retrieve it. Another approach is to subdivide each field into secondary classifications, but this can be carried only so far before the resulting categories become too small. If your topics are too narrow, you will have classification problems; if they are too broad, increased retrieval time.

Paper-driven systems have clear advantages for those who are uncomfortable with computers, especially when no research support staff is available.

Card Index

As your literature collection grows, a system based on condensed information rather than original papers may be more appropriate. Such information, written on a card, could include your remarks as well as the usual particulars about an article. This approach requires considerably more effort than a simple filing system, but the improvement in retrievability is small (see Table 8.1). It is much easier, however, to handle a card file on your desk than a cumbersome collection of original papers.

Computer-Assisted Systems: Citation

During the past decade, computers have become smaller, quicker, and cheaper, and these trends continue. Many boring tasks are now assigned to computers, including time-consuming searches for specific articles—once read or only heard of. Early on, computerized literature systems were nothing more than electronic card indexes, but even low-cost systems now offer a wealth of features. The act of storing an article is comparable to filling out a filing card; but retrieving the information is remarkably easier, even if you store only the citation with no keywords or comments. All stored items, or any combinations thereof, can be used as search criteria. Such a system can immediately give you a list of all the papers by T.C. Chalmers with the word "meta-analysis" in their titles published in 1980, or later.

Computer-Assisted Systems: Citation + Keywords

The computer-assisted system just described can be used without knowing anything about a paper beyond its author(s) and title. This may be an advantage if you are short of time, but the retrieval possibilities are rather limited. Your list of papers dealing with "meta-analysis" will be incomplete, because many relevant articles will not contain your search word in their titles [e.g., "Why do we need systematic overviews of randomized trials" from Peto R. Stat Med. 1987;6:233–40.]

Methodology is rarely mentioned in a title. If you are looking for an example of the application of discriminant analysis, searching titles will not be very fruitful. A successful search for special topics requires a short examination of each paper to enable you to attach a few keywords covering the main issue(s) dealt with by the author. These keywords, and a certain amount of discipline in choosing them, will produce an effective retrieval. Some computer programs allow keywords to be arranged hierarchically; for example, a search for papers dealing with "bacteria" will also yield all entries with the keywords "E.coli," "Streptococcus," etc. This can be a powerful tool, if it is used carefully.

The addition of an abstract to the stored information takes a lot of time and is useful only if access to the original paper is difficult.

The card index and the two computer-assisted systems bring a new feature to organizing your literature collection namely splitting it into original papers and "references" (titles, authors, years, journals, etc.). The separation process requires additional time to keep your system up to date, and two things need to be clearly recognized:

1. You have to maintain two systems: the references and the originals. Changes in one require the same changes in the other, or retrieval operations will not be successful.
2. You have to establish a "procedure" that connects the two systems. Every entry in the reference system must contain a sign, number, or signature that gives immediate access to the original paper. One commonly used procedure is to number every paper and store the originals in sequence. This allows the quickest retrieval of the originals. Another procedure is a "signature" system; here the signature indicates a certain topic or file where the original is stored (e.g., "SEPS_1," "META," etc.). This can be helpful if you have already established a well-structured filing system for your papers and want to move to a computerized system. If you keep your originals in some logical order, you can have access, with or without any computer assistance.

To summarize:

Keep only the papers you will probably use in the future; throw the rest away, immediately.

Organize the remaining literature by different fields or topics.

When the time required for searching, or the number of unsuccessful searches become intolerable, change to a computer-assisted system. File cards produce poor results compared with these systems.

Compare the expense of summarizing the content of a paper, and assigning some keywords, with the benefit to be derived from a high quality search for important topics.

Now, consider Dr. Readsalot, who has collected his literature in files divided into many small fields. He chose this method because he didn't want to have to look through a large file if he needed a certain piece of information. Because many of his papers could be correctly classified in several fields, he always chose one field as the main topic. Gradually, he came to realize that his files on a specific topic did not include all the relevant literature he had stored, so he decided to switch to a computer-assisted system.

As a start, he prepared a checklist of his requirements and visited some of his colleagues who used computers to organize their literature.

When he had chosen an appropriate system, his next decision was whether to use keywords. He soon realized that attaching keywords retrospectively to all his old papers would consume an enormous amount of his time, even if the input of basic reference data could be done by someone else. Consequently, he decided to use keywords when he started a new field. Because he knew that working with keywords requires some discipline, he prepared a list of keywords that would cover the important aspects of his interests.

The usual procedure Dr. Readsalot follows is:

1. Scan the article and assign it to a field of interest.
2. Mark this field as a signature on the paper itself.
3. Tick off some of the keywords on the predefined list and attach it to the paper.
4. Add the paper to the stack of other papers awaiting registration.
5. When the information has been stored in the computer, by someone else, the paper is immediately filed in the place indicated by the signature.

When papers registered in the computer are filed with papers that are not, marking the articles available in the computer is useful. Note that the old filing structure did not have to be reorganized—a great advantage. Dr. Readsalot learned the search operations of his software, without much difficulty. He can now use his system whenever he needs to and feels pleased when he perceives the growing power of his data base.

A different approach is to dispense with paper systems (i.e., to work entirely with computerized systems). The library of your medical school can do a search each time you prepare a new lecture, write a paper, etc. Scholars have ready access to centralized libraries with computerized search facilities and the capacity to obtain immediately copies of articles from journals. Other methods will gradually fall into disuse, but remember that a computerized search will only retrieve about two-thirds of the available information (see Chapter 7, "Taming the Literature").

Departmental Literature Organization

A system for joint use by all collaborators in a unit has limited justification if there are only two or three colleagues; individual search requests will probably yield similar results and some helpful remarks and advice, in addition. If the unit is large, an enormous effort is required to keep a joint system up to date. Shared systems are generally more vulnerable to piracy and incompleteness than private systems, especially if access is not limited. Each member of the unit will give priority to keeping his or her own system current, which is quite understandable. A collaborative system will never replace, but may enhance individual effort.

What are the benefits of such a system, if it won't replace an individual system? First, it will provide complete documentation of the literature available within your department, save some trips to the university library, and speed up your work. Second, any of your colleagues who do not store their references in a computer, will gain the advantages of electronic searching if the central data base is computerized. Third, a central system will relieve everyone of a large number of papers classified somewhere between "important" and "of no interest." Knowing that these "perhaps" papers are still retrievable, if you need them, can help you to concentrate on more important things. Finally, if one of your colleagues leaves, his or her references will not be lost by the unit.

You have no illusions about the expense of such a system. Keeping it current requires some hours per week—preferably the responsibility of a special reference librarian or research secretary who facilitates access to the literature.

The system installed in our research department, comprising five collaborators working in related fields, will serve as an example. We have a huge data base about shock that is being extended to other topics and made accessible to each collaborator. Keeping all our original papers in our unit library makes quick retrieval easy, allows each collaborator to organize his literature in his own way, independently, and creates an enduringly consistent data base.

Imagine a small department with an office for each assistant and a departmental library equipped with a computer. Each team member has to scan every new article arriving on his desk. If he decides a publication is rubbish and of no use to anyone in our unit, he immediately drops it into the litterbox. If he has any doubt about doing this and believes a colleague might make a different decision, he sends it to him with a remark like "Rolf, please check." Papers he deems important will be sent for central registration. If an article is particularly interesting and he wants to keep it in his office, he makes a copy immediately; entry into the central data base and storage in the unit library is done later by an assistant.

Each collaborator in our department contributes to a classification process that yields a stack of important literature in the central library and a wealth of valuable references in the computer. The original papers are stored according to the numbers attached to them.

We find this an effective way to reduce the stacks of new literature on everyone's desk, but it requires staff time and consistent attention. A systematic, increasingly valuable data base will be the reward for our efforts.

Criteria for Choosing Literature Software

Many programs, from low-cost public domain software to systems for huge libraries, are available and more will be as continuous changes and improvements are made. We cannot provide a complete list of current programs, nor do we wish to favor particular products. Accordingly, we present some options to consider when you are making choices.

Fields

The different components of a reference are stored in "fields"—one field for the title, one for the author(s), etc. Write down a complete reference as you want to store it. Does the program you are considering provide fields that are adequate for your needs? The fields in some programs are fixed (i.e., their names and lengths cannot be changed); other programs allow adaptations to be made by the user.

Search

Before you test a program, define some typical patterns of searching you will want to use on your data base. Don't forget to ask about the program's ability to find a certain word within different fields.

Duplicates

Testing on duplicates is a very helpful tool for assisting data input, but if such a test recognizes only completely identical entries, it is worthless. As an example, the test on year, journal, and pages only is a very good tool.

Keywords

Storage of some keywords is offered by nearly every program, but if you really want to work with keywords, look for such facilities as a predefined catalog of keywords or a capacity to structure them hierarchically.

Output

Several output formats should be available for different purposes, and it is advantageous to have them adjustable to meet your requirements. Some programs have the feature of being able to create a reference list from the data base, which is very helpful when you are writing a paper. This list can be produced in the format required by the journal you have selected, or stored in a file that can be transferred to your word processing system.

Protection

If you have reason to fear abuse of your literature data bank, or if you want to restrict the use or manipulation of your data, choose a program with protection mechanisms, such as passwords.

Amount

Try to estimate how much data your system will have to handle. Will the performance of the system still be satisfactory a few years from now? Does it have enough storage capacity? How long does it take the program to perform an operation like doing a special search within a large data base?

Import

If you want to take over an existing data base, or insert data from other data bases (e.g., MEDLINE or "Current Contents on Diskette"), you have to look for a program with this capability. An additional module is often available.

Tasks

In addition to looking after your literature requirements, some programs can execute such other tasks as organizing your books, slides, and lectures. It is a distinct advantage when a system that is familiar to you is usable for other purposes.

Testing

The manufacturers of large software programs often distribute a low-cost test or demo version that may help you to decide how practical or valuable it would be in meeting your requirements. It is much better, if you have the opportunity, to watch a colleague work with the system and ask him for his evaluation of it.

Summary

The only reason to think about organizing your literature is retrieval. Any effort you devote to storing information must be measured against how frequent, how sophisticated, and how big your retrieval operations are. A paper-based filing system with a carefully chosen classification system is often sufficient. A computerized system with keywords provides nearly optimal retrieval results, but it requires even more time for storing each paper. If you switch to working with a computer, don't discard your old system; reorganizing an existing collection will devour a lot of time. Departmental literature systems should support, but not replace, individual or centralized unit systems. A special documentation assistant is needed to assume responsibility for the operation and maintenance of a departmental system.

Any system for organizing literature is only as good as its classification criteria. Carefully selected topics and key words usually produce a better result than you can achieve with highly sophisticated computerized methods.

9

Systematically Reviewing Previous Work

E.A.M. Neugebauer, B. McPeek, and S. Wood-Dauphinée

Many of us regard reviewing previous literature as an unexciting chore, perhaps because well-read laboratory chiefs appear to consider the research review as a low-priority activity to be delegated to a research assistant or the most junior member of the team. For many, the excitement lies in carrying out a new experiment to add more information to what already exists. They regard poring over old research reports as a boring or less creative step. This is a major error in thinking. The accumulation of evidence is an important goal underlying all scientific inquiry. This is as true of medicine and surgery as of theoretical physics. An individual study is seldom an isolated event, but rather part of a continuum in which each new endeavor builds on preceding work. New findings lose much of their value if they are not linked with the accumulated wisdom, both theoretical and empirical, of earlier reports.

Quite apart from any associated research findings, the methods used by previous scholars may suggest fresh ideas. Some may present approaches to problem solving that have not occurred to you. Attention to earlier design and analytic methods may help you to avoid difficulties that plagued earlier efforts.

On a practical level, a thorough critical appraisal of existing literature provides background information for developing a research proposal, a grant application, or a report for publication.

A research review will likely lead to one of four products.

1. It may bring together what is known about a specific research area and lead directly to new work designed to test a specific hypothesis or add to the knowledge base.
2. It may analyze data from previous studies in a new way to answer new research questions.
3. It may summarize what is known in an area, appearing in a journal in its own right as a "state of the art" paper. Such a review will not only be of interest to those working in the specific field, but will also be particularly helpful to other specialists who wish to bring themselves up to date, quickly.
4. It may inform clinical decisions made by individual clinicians about the care of patients, or by chiefs of units about policy matters.

Approaches to Reviewing the Literature

Traditional Reviews

Most literature reviews are unsystematic and largely narrative presentations of studies and their findings; the methods employed in the studies are discussed selectively and informally.

Equally able reviewers often disagree about basic issues and occasionally arrive at diametrically opposite conclusions. With little concern for scientific rigor, reviewers frequently turn to a mindless vote count. When some studies show a positive treatment effect, others no effect, and still others a negative effect, the reviewer counts the number supporting each result and selects the majority view. This procedure, also called box score analysis or the vote counting method,[1] ignores the size of the effect found and the strength of the research design. If the number of previous studies is large, the traditional reviewer easily gets lost.

Despite the subjectivity, questionable scientific validity, and inefficiency of the traditional narrative approach to reviewing the literature, most scholars in medicine and surgery still use this antiquated procedure.

Over the past 15 years, new methods have been developed. Although they are not widely known to clinical scientists, they are significant advances in the methodology of reviewing scientific literature that bring it into the mainstream of modern science.

Data Analysis

Gene V. Glass[2,3] has written about three levels of data analysis: primary analysis, secondary analysis, and meta-analysis.

Primary Analysis

Primary analysis is the original analysis of data from a research study. This is what most of us think of as research, and articles describing such work form the bulk of medical communications.

Secondary Analysis

Secondary analysis, as described by Glass, is the reanalysis of original data to bring current statistical methods to bear on them or to answer new questions. We can learn much from secondary analysis. Better ways of looking at the data gathered in a project may be suggested after they have been published. For example, a variety of useful secondary analyses of the data collected by the University Group Diabetes Project (UGDP study) in medicine[4] advanced our understanding of how diabetes should be treated. Similarly, new hypotheses can be tested by the imaginative reanalysis of data already collected for a similar or even an entirely different purpose. Secondary analysis can be particularly useful in dealing with volunteer case reports, where volunteer reporting bias may have produced an effect if the data were collected prospectively. McPeek and Gilbert[5] used secondary analysis of published data to disprove a new hypothesis concerning postoperative jaundice following repeated exposure to halothane.

Meta-Analysis

Like secondary analysis, *meta-analysis* uses existing data but it focuses on the quantitative integration of findings across a group of independent studies and provides a more scientific alternative to the traditional narrative method of literature review.

There is no question that meta-analysis is a major advance, but we must remember that it is a comparative observational study with all the strengths and weaknesses of observational studies. We celebrate the fact that we now have a way to review work systematically, but guard against trying to extend it too far.

In thinking about meta-analysis, we lean heavily on three principles. First, *develop a strategy.* Bear in mind that the most effective review strategies and analytic techniques arise from the answers to the specific questions that are leading you to make the review. What do you want from the review? Do you seek a broad exploration of available information on a subject, or do you want to test specific hypotheses? Is an overall answer desirable, or are you interested in identifying interactions between specific treatments, patient populations, or settings, like hospitals or clinics? Are you interested in the feasibility of implementing a new program locally? If the plan is for an exploratory review, you ask what is known about a particular area of research, a specific disease, a clinical problem, or a treatment, such as an operation or an element of pre- or postoperative care. Your strategy will be to include diverse studies to increase the chance of uncovering interesting findings that may lead to new directions for future research. Unless you know what you are doing at the start, you may finish with a simple recitation of previous findings that does to little advance research, contribute fresh insight, or inform decisions.

The second principle is that *conflicting results must be carefully investigated.* When we find dozens of previous studies, we hope that most of them will agree. If they do, a review is easy, but this rarely happens. Conflicting findings have several potential explanations. There may be substantial differences between operations with the same name. Follow-up care may be quite dissimilar. Perhaps the treatment works poorly for some kinds of patients and well for others, or is effective in certain hands or settings and not in others. These explanations can only be uncovered through the careful study of the narrative reports of patients, treatment descriptions and details of hospital, clinical or laboratory procedures. A letter or telephone call to the authors may uncover new postpublication information or insights that clarify the analysis.

The third principle is that *we often need formal, quantitative, analytic methods to identify small effects across studies* that are not apparent through simple inspection of the results of the studies individually.

Beware! Drawing inferences about findings uncovered from exploratory analyses can be risky. Searching among many research studies for factors significantly related to outcome will lead to some false positives—statistically significant relationships due only to chance. If you examine many separate relationships, each at the .05 level of significance, you should not be surprised to discover that 1 in 20 is significant due entirely to chance—a finding consistent with probability theory.

If several treatments are compared, sample variation alone may make some look better than others even when they are truly equivalent. Similarly, when institutions are compared for success with an operation, sampling variation will make some look much better than others even if they are equal in excellence. For example, in the United States National Halothane Study[6] 34 institutions were compared for standardized surgical mortality rates and they appeared to differ, initially, by a factor of 24; after allowance was made for sampling variation, the ratio between the highest and lowest was only 3:1.

One way to prevent a review from *over-capitalizing on chance* is to break the data into parts. Half of the studies can be used to generate hypotheses about effective treatments or to predict treatment success; the other half can be used to test the hypotheses so generated. If the entire set of studies has some systematic bias, this procedure cannot eliminate it. Regardless of how you perform the review, your inferences will only be as valid as the underlying studies.

If your review is aimed at testing a previously established hypothesis, you must specify the hypothesis precisely, before you start. This may lead you to an early decision as to whether your review should look across studies to aggregate treatments (like operations), to aggregate patients, or to aggregate settings (like clinics or hospitals).

We ordinarily view the outcome of a clinical research study as being the result of interactions between the treatment, the patient, and the setting, compounded by random error. Reviews can answer many diverse questions, but we commonly seek answers to three:

1. What is the *average effect* of the treatment?
2. Are there *particular* patient *groups* or settings where the treatment works especially well?
3. *Can we implement* it in our department?

To answer the first question, we compare patients who receive the treatment with similar people who do not.

The second question asks for interactions. Do particular combinations of treatments and patients work especially well or poorly? For example, suppose a surgeon believes that a particular operation is especially valuable for elderly men while any one of several operations is as effective in younger men. A single research design that crosses different operations with patients of various age groups can test this hypothesis. But what do you do if no study systematically considers all of the combinations of operations and patients that you wish to examine? For example, one study may have looked at large numbers of elderly men and other studies at large groups of younger men. Taken together, these studies may give the reviewer some information about whether or not interactions exist, i.e., a collection of studies can sometimes shed light on complex interactions when studies considered individually do not.

The third question concerns implementation. Strictly speaking, studies tell us only what happened to the patients or the participants in the investigation. We are ordinarly interested in generalizing these findings to similar patients under our care. If we know from the start that a review is to inform a local policy decision, the reviewer will look for studies that bear particularly on the local circumstances. Information can be sought that would help us to decide how an operation is likely to work in our hands, at our hospital, on our kinds of patients.

Both qualitative and quantitative conclusions from meta-analysis can be updated as new study results become available. A wide array of descriptive, etiological, intervention, clinical tool validation, or diagnostic method testing studies may be the subject of meta-analysis. The general objectives of meta-analysis are as follows.[7]

To confirm information (hypothesis, proof, initial findings).
To find errors.
To search for additional findings—to develop new ideas (hypotheses) for further research and future original studies.

Origin and Types of Meta-Analysis

It is only during the past 15 years that scholars, particularly in the social sciences, have developed the notion of quantitative meta-analysis in a robust way. After the first stimulating article on the subject by Light and Smith,[8] Glass put forward his first definitions of meta-analysis[2]: the "analysis of analyses," or better, "the statistical analysis of a large collection of analyses results from individual studies for the purpose of integration of the findings." Quantitative methods and techniques were further developed by Rosenthal,[9,10] Hedges,[11] and others. The 1983 annual review of *Evaluation Studies* edited by R. Light[12] brought together an important array of methodological articles and many important original studies. Basic methodological textbooks,[13-17]

TABLE 9.1. Formal approaches various authors have used and/or proposed for evaluating the clinical literature.

Authors	Year	Reference
1. Mahon and Daniel	1964	22
2. Lionel and Herxheimer	1970	23
3. Horwitz and Feinstein	1979	24
4. Levine	1980	25
5. Chalmers et al.	1981	26
6. University of Rochester Clinical Pharmacology Group (Weintraub)	1982	27
7. DerSimonian et al.	1982	28
8. Haynes et al.	1983	29
9. Bailar et al.	1984	30
10. Evans and Pollock	1985	31
11. Neugebauer et al.	1987	32

monographs dealing with statistical methods,[18] and computer software[19] soon followed.

The usual purpose of quantitative or "classical" meta-analysis was to assess effectiveness of treatments, programs, and interventions and, less often, to study pathogenesis. To obtain reliable answers, meta-analysts gathered as many published and unpublished studies as possible. They did not, however, give enough consideration to the *quality* of the studies and were subsequently criticized on that score.[14] Problems of heterogeneity, experimental design and execution—especially in fields like education and medicine—soon demanded a *quantitative* approach (classical meta-analysis) *and* a "*qualitative* meta-analysis".[7] The latter is not only a systematic accumulation of the information in and characteristics of different studies, but also an assessment of quality, uncertainty, missing data, random error, and bias across relevant studies. In medicine, the greatest challenge of meta-analysis lies in the integration of the qualitative and quantitative assessment of given information (e.g., scoring of quality, weighing of the effect size by quality score).

Qualitative Meta-Analysis

Qualitative meta-analysis, in medicine, has been defined as a "method of assessment of the importance and relevance of medical information coming from several independent sources through a general, systematic and uniform application of pre-established criteria of acceptability to original studies representing the body of knowledge of a given health problem or question."[20] The objectives of qualitative meta-analysis, according to Jenicek,[7] are as follows.

To determine the prevalence, homogeneity, and distribution of quality attributes.

To expand the knowledge of missing and/or imperfect "outlines" (e.g., observation beyond a customary range).

Almost any clinical question or controversy can be subjected to qualitative meta-analysis, but the objectives for each meta-analysis *must* be clearly formulated *before* analysis. As in any research endeavor, development of a working protocol will formalize the decisions made at the design stage, to achieve the objectives. For each general objective, investigators can also identify such secondary objectives as determining the age groups for which a treatment may be most effective.

A valid meta-analysis includes as many relevant studies as possible, but the authors should provide details of their search procedures. At present, sole reliance on computer searches of the literature is not sufficient because they may yield less than two thirds of the relevant studies.[21] Efforts to minimize this bias include working from references of published studies, searching data bases of unpublished material, and questioning experts in the particular field. The meta-analysis will be clear only if the studies are chosen according to predefined inclusion and exclusion criteria whose rationale is clearly stated. Each meta-analysis should list the studies analyzed, the studies excluded, and the reasons for exclusion.

Qualitative meta-analysis calls for an adequate dimensional assessment of the quality of studies. Several methods of assessment of the quality of original studies are available.

Table 9.1 lists selected authors who have proposed criteria checklists, or other methods, to evaluate different types or parts of clinical studies; space limitations restrict our comments to only a few of them.

Mahon and Daniel[22] proposed a four-step method to evaluate reports of drug studies. Their process consists of applying only four criteria:

1. Were adequate controls used?
2. Were treatments randomized?
3. Were drug effects measured objectively? (This usually involves double-blind techniques.)
4. Were results analyzed statistically?

In 1970 Lionel and Herxheimer[23] presented the checklist they used to evaluate 141 clinical studies in four medical journals. Their checklist constitutes a formal assessment of whether an article is definitely acceptable, probably acceptable, or unacceptable. In 1979 Horwitz and Feinstein[24] proposed a set of 12 standards to be applied to retro-

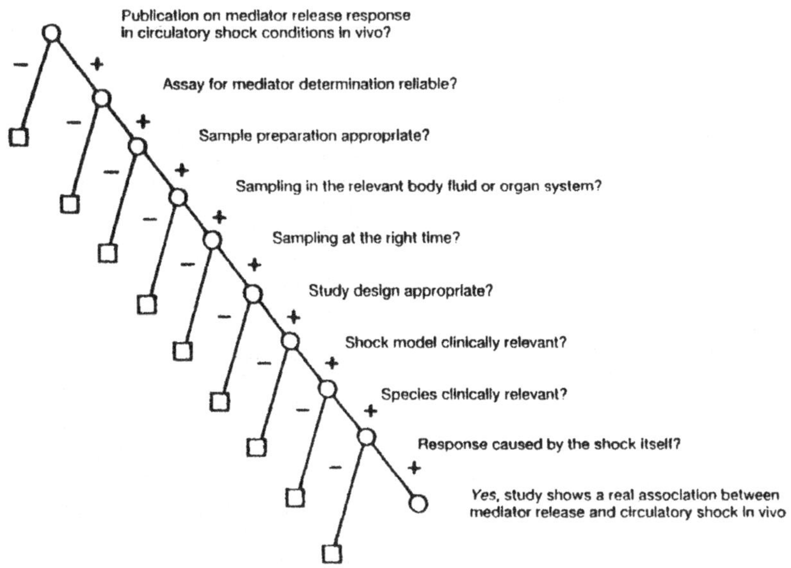

FIGURE 9.1. Decision tree for investigating a real, existing association between histamine release and septic/endotoxic shock under in vivo conditions. Reprinted with permission from Neugebauer E; Lorenz W.[58] (1989).

spective case-control research; the standards were successfully used in the evaluation of 85 studies.

There may be sound reasons for a study not having adequate external, or even internal, controls and having to rely on controls outside the study (e.g., historical controls). Bailar and colleagues[30] proposed a series of five questions for assessing the value (i.e., strength of evidence) of externally controlled studies and used them to evaluate a group of 20 publications in the *New England Journal of Medicine.*

Neugebauer and coworkers[32] used a decision tree (Figure 9.1) in their meta-analysis of the current status of histamine as a causal chemical factor in the pathogenesis of septic/endotoxic shock. All published studies investigating the presence of histamine release in septic/endotoxic shock, in vivo, and its absence in a state of health were evaluated by the criteria defined by the test nodes in the decision tree. All criteria and methodological standards at the test nodes were tabulated and set up in detail before the analysis was started. This meta-analysis suggested that, despite decades of histamine research, there is still no acceptable answer to the question of whether histamine plays a pathogenetic role in septic/endotoxin shock.[32]

In many cases, it may not be enough to list present or absent attributes of each study; these facts must have an appropriate dimension, where necessary. Scoring of quality is of particular interest. Evans and Pollock[31] proposed a qualitative assessment of clinical trials, based on the method of Chalmers and colleagues,[26] where—from a total score of 100—up to 50 points are given for the data base, design, and "protocol," with emphasis on blinding; up to 30 points for statistical analysis; and up to 20 points for the way the study is presented (Table 9.2). They used this method to rate 36 randomized controlled studies and found only 16 that scored more than 70 points. The same method was successfully used, recently, to answer the question: "Steroids in trauma patients—right or wrong?"[33]

The Trial Assessment Procedure Scale (TAPS) of Levine[25] is one of the most detailed trial assessment procedures with a scoring system. It involves an analysis of each report (e.g., trial protocol, completed study report, or journal article) in terms of attributes that reflect trial quality. The attributes are clustered into eight categories, each covering two to five related characteristics, to facilitate independent assessment of the quality of the various components of a trial—that is, to rate trial quality without regard to findings on treatment efficacy or safety. This form should be used only by very experienced raters.

The sequence followed in all the approaches above is qualitative assessment of studies, then

TABLE 9.2. Method of Evans and Pollock[31] for evaluating controlled clinical studies. Reprinted with permission from Evans M, Pollock AV[31] (1985).

Steps in evaluation	Yes	No
Design and conduct		
Is the sample defined?	2	0
Are exclusions specified?	2	0
Are known risk factors recorded?	3	0
Are therapeutic regimens defined?	5	0
Is the experimental regimen appropriate?	5	0
Is the control regimen appropriate?	5	0
Were appropriate investigations carried out?	2	0
Are endpoints defined?	5	0
Are endpoints appropriate?	5	0
Have numbers required been calculated?	2	0
Was patient consent sought?	1	0
Was the randomization blind?	3	0
Was the assessment blind?	4	0
Were additional treatments recorded?	4	0
Were side effects recorded?	2	0
Analysis		
Withdrawals:		
Are they listed?	3	0
Is their fate recorded?	4	0
Are there fewer than 10%?	4	0
Is there a compatibility table?	3	0
Are risk factors stratified?	3	0
Is the statistical analysis of proportions correct?	3	0
Is the statistical analysis of numbers correct?	3	0
Are confidence intervals reported?	2	0
Are values of both test statistics and probability given?	1	0
In negative trials, is the type II error considered?	4	0
Presentation		
Is the title accurate?	2	0
Is the abstract accurate and helpful?	3	0
Are the methods reproducible?	3	0
Are the sections clear-cut?	2	0
Can the raw data be discerned?	2	0
Are the results credible?	3	0
Do the results justify the conclusions?	3	0
Are the references correct?	2	0

selection of acceptable or best evidence, and finally quantitative meta-analysis of the latter. Frequently, quantitative meta-analysis is not needed because few studies fulfill the current standards of trial methodology[32] and survive the systematic qualitative assessment, or because the studies with acceptable quality are so heterogeneous (i.e., they used widely differing research designs, treatments, and target populations). Unacceptable studies must be rejected, for stated reasons, before quantitative meta-analysis is undertaken. Acceptable studies undergo quantitative meta-analysis according to the rules stated next.

Quantitative Meta-Analysis

In medicine, quantitative meta-analysis can be defined as a general, systematic, and uniform evaluation of dimensions across studies dealing with topics like the following:

The magnitude of a health problem.
The strength and specificity of a causal relationship in etiological research.
The strength and specificity of the impact of a preventive or therapeutic intervention.
The internal and external validity of clinical tools (e.g., diagnostic methods).
The costs and benefits of diagnostic methods and treatments.

The number of meta-analyses published in clinical journals increases each year. Some examples are as follows.

Evaluating the effect of weight loss treatment on essential hypertension.[34]
Assessing long-term beta-blocker treatment after myocardial infarction.[35]
Comparing the effects of intracoronary streptokinase and intracoronary nitroglycerin infusion for patients with acute myocardial infarction.[36]
Determining the effectiveness of antibiotic prophylaxis in colon surgery.[37]
Evaluating mortality, reinfarction, and side effects in patients with acute myocardial infarction given intravenous and intracoronary fibrinolytic therapy.[38]
Examining the effect of treatment with histamine H2-antagonists in acute upper gastrointestinal hemorrhage.[39]
Estimating the quality of life results in trials of coronary artery bypass surgery.[40]

Quantitative meta-analysis was developed to overcome the weakness of previous methods for research integration. Like any other scientific work, each meta-analysis should begin with a plan that clearly states the question to be answered and the methods to be employed, There is no single "correct" method for performing a meta-analysis, but several attempts have been made to define the basic methodological issues. The workshop on methodological issues in overviews of randomized clinical trials, sponsored by the National Heart, Lung and Blood Institute and the National Cancer Institute,[41] and the Versailles Meeting of the Meta-Analysis cooperative Group[42] were two recent examples. Sachs and colleagues[43] have evaluated the quality of 86 meta-analyses of randomized controlled trials, using a scoring method that considered the most important elements of meta-analysis (i.e., a meta-meta-analysis). The generally accepted issues in a quantitative meta-analysis are portrayed in Figure 9.2 and explained, briefly, in subsequent paragraphs.

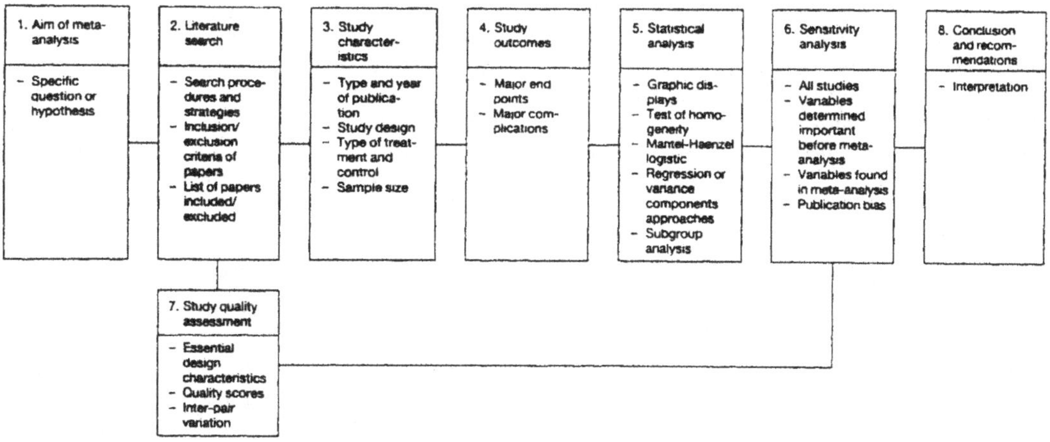

FIGURE 9.2. Methodological elements of a quantitative meta-analysis. Reprinted with permission from Neugebauer E, Lorenz W[58] (1989).

Methodological Elements of a Quantitative Meta-Analysis

Aim

A meta-analysis usually addresses sharper questions than a literature review, and seeks quantitative answers; thus its objectives must be clearly formulated before the study begins. A review of care for stoma patients might discuss treatment methods available, changing uses, and the pros and cons of different methods. A meta-analysis might take such a specific measure as the proportion of patients rehospitalized within one year of release under various conditions, combine the relevant evidence from several studies, and try to compare performance of different treatments. A distinction between two levels of questions leading to two different types of hypothesis can be made: (a) a search for tentative answers and their verification, and (b) verification or hypothesis testing.

Literature Search

As many relevant studies as possible should be included in a qualitative meta-analysis; details of the computerized and manual search procedures used to find them should be described. Computerized searches are not always straightforward and consistent, and several articles have examined this problem[44,45] (see Chapter 7). A professional librarian specialized in literature searches of clinical topics should be involved.

Literature searches will not find unpublished studies, and published studies may differ, systematically, from unpublished studies. Meta-analyses based on literature searches alone may display "publication bias."

Authors are more likely to submit, and editors are more likely to publish, work with statistically significant versus nonsignificant results. As a consequence, a reviewer who focuses on published studies will likely overstate treatment effects.

A computer search should be supplemented by consulting "Current Contents," reviews, textbooks, and people with relevant expertise, and by reviewing the references cited in the trials found.[43] Publication bias is one of the main criticisms leveled at meta-analysis, but sampling bias and data retrieval limitations are inherent in any literature review.

Selecting Studies for Inclusion

Studies for meta-analysis are chosen on the basis of inclusion and exclusion criteria. How you select studies for inclusion depends on the availability of research reports, the number and frequency of different designs, and the specific questions driving your analysis. Including everything you can find has the advantage of avoiding criticism for neglecting some work or including one study while excluding another, but it does present some problems. If you discover 1100 studies, such an embarrassment of riches will almost certainly sink your project and you must find some appropriate way of reducing the number. For example, you could draw a random sample of all the studies available and use the sample for your review.

It is important to include a wide variety of research designs and treatment variations, but if a particular study clearly has obvious, substantial, fundamental flaws, exclude it and state why. Wrong information is much worse than no information.

You may have trouble finding some studies; for example, it may be difficult to find a translator for a paper in a particular language, and certain monographs may be out of print. You may have to decide how much digging is warranted on the basis of a title or an abstract.

Another approach is to stratify your sample by dividing the available studies into categories for review. This procedure guarantees inclusion of each important type of study but only requires you to analyze in detail only the shorter list of selected studies.

Experimental design is often a strong predictor of research outcomes. In a review of almost 100 studies of portacaval shunt, Chalmers[46] found a clear negative relation between the degree of control in a research design and the level of success attributed to the surgical intervention; the higher the degree of control, the less enthusiastic the investigators were about an operation's effectiveness. Similar findings were reported by Gilbert, McPeek, and Mosteller[47,48] in a study of innovations in surgery and anesthesia. Such results support the "law" enunciated by the famous statistician Hugo Muench, that nothing improves the performance of an innovation more than the lack of controls.[49] Some papers suggest this rule is not universal,[50-52] but there is much evidence that it often applies in medicine and surgery.

Research design is not the only basis for stratification. You may wish to stratify by geography, treatment, type of operation, type of clinic or hospital, or the sociodemographic or clinical characteristics of patients.

In summary, we are not aware of standardized criteria for inclusion of studies in meta-analysis. Universal criteria are not appropriate, because meta-analysis can be applied to a broad spectrum of topics and criteria may need to vary for different objectives; disagreement on inclusion and exclusion criteria is to be expected among the readers of the published report of a particular meta-analysis. For this reason, *criteria and their rationale should be stated and all studies found, whether included or excluded, should be listed.*

Study Characteristics

After the studies have been collected and selected, it is helpful to record the key descriptive characteristics of each study on data abstract forms. The reader needs to be convinced that the results of separate trials have been meaningfully combined. Common methodological characteristics included in meta-analyses are type and year of publication; study design; type, dosage, route, frequency, and duration of treatment; control; sample size; and subject randomization and loss. Studies may differ in any of the foregoing characteristics. In general, the meta-analyst should note any differences between the primary studies and discuss how they affect the conclusions.

Study outcomes

Similar data abstract forms are useful for *study outcome characteristics*, because various endpoints or outcome variables are used to assess treatment effects. The outcome of interest may be measured by a continuous variable, such as blood pressure; by categorical variables, such as mortality or complication rates; by an ordinal variable such as tumor stage; or by time-related variables expressed in life tables. Meta-analysis has the advantage of being able to take several different dependent variables into account.[53] If you are reviewing the literature on the effects of selective vagotomy with antrectomy in patients with peptic ulcers, such outcome measures as mortality, recurrence, pain, or quality of life can be examined. When you are extracting data, record raw numbers rather than proportions, because the process is a potential source of bias. Control this type of bias by having the extracting done by more than one observer, by having each observer blinded to the various treatment groups through a coded photocopying process, and by measuring the interobserver agreement.[43]

Statistical Analysis

A major feature of meta-analysis is that the unit of analysis, when the results of many studies are being assessed, is not an individual patient or clinic, but a study. To compare studies, we must measure treatment impact for each study. Meta-analysis includes transformation of multiple study findings into a common matrix. The two most common measures are *statistical significance and effect size*.

Most research about the effectiveness of treatments asks the question: Do the differences between the treatment and the control groups exceed those we expect due to chance alone? If each of several studies compares treatment and control groups, we can take the p values as measures of statistical significance to interpret the effectiveness of treatment. This strategy has two problems. Many studies in medicine and surgery have rather few participants in each of the comparison groups. Small investigations have weak power because their ability to detect real differences between groups is low. If a weak study reports a difference, we can assume that the difference is substantial; if no significant difference was found, we can only wonder whether the findings indicate true absence of any important difference or only failure to detect a difference that does exist, because the study is too small. Consequently, relying on a *p* value may be misleading.

The sample size issue can cut the other way too. Occasionally, a study has very large sample sizes and tests of significance, like the *p* value, are heavily influenced by sample size. In a truly large study, very small or even trivial differences can be statistically significant. "Significant" does not mean "important"!

Effect sizes provide a simple estimate of how valuable a treatment is. Suppose we wish to compare the main results between the treatment group and the control group. If the information is reported in each of the individual studies, an average effect size for the entire group of studies can easily be calculated. For each study, we need to know the mean of the treatment, the mean of the control group, and the standard deviation of the control group. With an average size across a number of studies, we have a single summary value for the effectiveness of the treatment studies. In 1976 Glass and Smith[54] computed the average effect size for psychotherapy treatment across 400 separate studies to be .68. They concluded that an average patient receiving psychotherapy was approximately two-thirds of a standard deviation more improved than the average control group member.[3]

A comparison of proportions will give another measure of effect size. For example, one could compare the proportion of people who live longer than 5 years following different treatments for cancer. The effect size for proportions is calculated by simply subtracting the proportion surviving in the treatment group from that surviving in the control group.

Frequently, your chosen measure of effect size will depend on what numerical information is reported in the various studies. If the standard deviation of the control group, for example, is not reported or cannot be calculated, a mean-score effect size cannot be computed.

Another method of looking at the overall impact of treatment is to try to combine the significance tests from many separate studies into one comprehensive test of a null hypothesis for the studies as a whole. Rosenthal[9] has described nine ways to accomplish this. To illustrate one technique, consider the method of adding *Z*-scores (standard normal deviates). If each study has two comparison groups, there is a *Z*-score associated with each reported *p* value. The *Z*-scores from each individual study are simply added across studies. The sum of the *Z*-scores is divided by the square root of the number of studies. The probability associated with this total score gives an overall level of significance for the studies under review.

Combined significance tests are simple to compute and generally require only that we know the sample size and the probability level or the level of a test statistic, such as the value of *T*, *Z*, or *F*, for each individual study. The larger the overall sample size, the more likely it is that a given underlying effect size will be detected as statistically significant. For example, assume that patients with duodenal ulcer treated by vagotomy and antrectomy have slightly better results than those receiving vagotomy and pyloroplasty. If the two operations are repeatedly compared in very weak trials—small sample sizes for each group—many of the studies will not show statistically significant differences between the two operations, even if they exist. A traditional informal reviewer who did only a vote count would almost certainly fail to see the true effectiveness of vagotomy and antrectomy. A careful reviewer who combines the studies by adding *Z*-scores is much more likely to find that the overall statistical test is significant because the small numbers of patients in each weak study combine to become a much larger number of patients and produce a meta-analysis of greater power than any of the smaller studies taken individually.

Sensitivity Analysis

Because there will undoubtedly be differing opinions on the appropriate method for performing a particular meta-analysis, the investigator should always ask "How sensitive are the meta-analysis results to changes in the way the meta-analysis was done?" This process, called sensitivity analysis, is an important element in meta-analysis methodology[55] (Figure 9.2).

You may want to study how the pooled results change when randomized *and* nonrandomized studies, instead of randomized trials only, are included in a meta-analysis. This type of study simply involves the addition of a second analysis that includes data from the nonrandomized studies. A comparison of the results of the two meta-analyses will show that the type of study has little effect on the meta-analysis results and any disagreement about inclusion criteria is unimportant, or that the type of study is indeed an important factor in drawing conclusions from the analysis. Sensitivity analysis used as a tool within meta-analysis can help to resolve clinical controversies.

Factors influencing the sensitivity analysis can be discovered in the process of meta-analysis, such as differences between studies of young compared with old patients. By testing the effect of the more subjective elements of meta-analysis, such as the choice of inclusion and exclusion criteria, the conclusions drawn from a meta-analysis can be strengthened.

A related issue is the extent to which meta-analysis results are potentially distorted through publication bias. If one assumes that negative studies or studies showing no difference are less likely to be published than positive studies, this issue should be addressed if meta-analysis shows significant differences in outcome between treatment groups. Some published meta-analyses have estimated how many unpublished trials, showing no difference between treatments, would be required to convert a statistically significant pooled difference into an insignificant difference.[55-58] A carefully performed meta-analysis describes the different analyses used to strengthen the overall result obtained.

Study Quality Assessment

The scientific quality of the papers to be combined should be assessed and included in the sensitivity analysis. The resulting conclusion will be less reliable if the original trials were poor; see the earlier discussion of qualitative meta-analysis.

Conclusions and Recommendations

The extraction and pooling of data from published reports with the methodology of quantitative meta-analysis is time-consuming and tedious. At the end of the process the meta-analysis must put the results in perspective and, if the data are not decisive, should recommend appropriate future studies.

Presentation of Results

There are no hard and fast rules about the format for presenting the findings of a review employing meta-analysis. The format depends, to some extent, on the purpose of the final product and the organizational framework of the individual reviewer. Cooper[59] has suggested that such reviews follow an outline similar to the one used for primary research, that is:

1. An introduction defining the problem to be addressed and identifying the controversy in the literature.
2. A methods section describing how the articles were selected, the sources tapped, and the kind of information collected about each study.
3. A results section presenting the statistical procedures and findings.
4. A discussion section containing a summary of the findings, a comparison with other related work, and a statement of the direction future research might take.

Conclusion

A systematic synthesis of research results is needed to cope with the increasing number of published and unpublished studies. Meta-analysis can integrate research findings through an explicit approach that is more qualitatively and quantitatively rigorous than traditional methods. Although misuse of this powerful tool can produce misleading conclusions, it offers opportunities for analysis that are not possible by mere examination of co-variables, study design, and analysis. The methodology merits further testing and empirical evaluation in different fields of clinical and basic research.

References

1. Hedges LV, Olkin I. Vote-counting methods in research synthesis. Psychol Bull 1980;88:359–69.
2. Glass GV. Primary, secondary, and meta-analysis of research. Educ Res 1976;5:3–8.
3. Glass GV. Meta-analysis: an approach to the synthesis of research results. Res Sci Teach 1982;19:93–112.
4. University Group Diabetes Program (UGDP) Study. J Diabetes 1970;19(Suppl 2):740–850.
5. McPeek B, Gilbert JP. Onset of postoperative jaundice related to anesthetic history. Br Med J 1974; 3:615–17.
6. Moses LE, Mosteller F. Afterword for the study of death rates. In: The National Halothane Study; A study of the Possible Association Between Halothane Anesthesia and Postoperative Hepatic Necrosis, Bunker JP, Forrest WH Jr, Mosteller F, Vandam LD, eds. Washington, DC: Government Printing Office, 1969:395–408.
7. Jenicek M. Meta-analysis in medicine. Where we are and where we want to go. J Clin Epidemiol 1989; 42:35–44.
8. Light RJ, Smith PV. Accumulating evidence: procedures for resolving contradictions among different research studies. Harvard Educ Rev 1971;41: 429–71.
9. Rosenthal R. Combining results of independent studies. Psychol Bull 1978;85:185–93.
10. Rosenthal R. Assessing the statistical and social importance of effects of psychotherapy. J Consult Clin Psychol 1983;51:4–13.

11. Hedges LV. Statistical Methodology in Meta-Analysis. Princeton, NJ: ERIC Clearinghouse on Tests, Measurement and Evaluation, Educational Testing Service, 1982.
12. Evaluation Studies, Review Annual, Light RJ, ed. Beverly Hills, CA: Sage, 1983:8.
13. Glass GV, McGraw B, Smith ML. Meta-Analysis of Social Research. Beverly Hills, CA: Sage, 1981.
14. Hunter JE, Schmidt FL, Jackson GB. Meta-Analysis: Cumulating Research Findings Across Studies. Beverly Hills, CA: Sage, 1982.
15. Borg WR, Gall MD: Critical Evaluation of Research, Educational Research. An Introduction, 4th ed. New York: Longman, 1983.
16. Light JRJ, Pillemer DB. Summing-Up. The Science of Reviewing Research. Cambridge, MA: Harvard University Press, 1984.
17. Rosenthal R. Meta-analytic Procedures for Social Research. Beverly Hills, CA: Sage, 1984.
18. Hedges LV, Olkin I. Statistical Methods for Meta-Analysis. New York: Academic Press, 1985.
19. Mullen B, Rosenthal R. Basic Meta-Analysis: Procedures and Programs. Hillsdale, NJ: Erlbaum, 1985.
20. Jenicek M. Meta-analyse en medecine. Evaluation et synthése de l'information clinique et epidemiologique. St-Hyacinthe and Paris: EDISEM and Maloine, 1987.
21. Dickersin K, Hewitt P, Mutch I, et al. Perusing the literature: comparison of MEDLINE searching with a perinatal trials data base. Controlled Clin Trials 1985;6:306–17.
22. Mahon WA, Daniel EE. A method for the assessment of reports of drug trials. Can Med Assoc J 1964;90:565–69.
23. Lionel NDW, Herxheimer A. Assessing reports of therapeutic trials. Br Med J 1970;3:637–40.
24. Horwitz RI, Feinstein AR. Methodologic standards and contradictory results in case-control research. Am J Med 1979;66:556–64.
25. Levine J. Trial Assessment Procedure Scale (TAPS). Printed by U.S. Department of Health and Human Services, Public Health Service, Alcohol, Drug Abuse and Mental Health Administration, National Institute of Mental Health, Bethesda, MA, 1980. Available from Dr. Levine, University of Maryland, Maryland Psychiatric Research Center, P.O. Box 3235, Catonsville, MD 21228.
26. Chalmers TC, Smith H Jr, Blackburn B, et al. A method for assessing the quality of a randomized control trial. Controlled Clin Trials 1981;2:31–49.
27. Weintraub M. How to critically assess clinical drug trials. Drug Ther 1982;12:131–48.
28. DerSimonian R, Charette LJ, McPeek B, et al. Reporting on methods in clinical trials. N Engl J Med 1982;306:1332–37.
29. Haynes RB, Sackett DL, Tugwell P. Problems in the handling of clinical and research evidence by medical practitioners. Arch Intern Med 1983;143: 1971–75.
30. Bailar JC III., Louis TA, Lavori PW, et al. Studies without internal controls. N Engl J Med 1984;311: 156–62.
31. Evans M, Pollock AV. A score system for evaluating random control clinical trials of prophylaxis of abdominal surgical wound infection. Br J Surg 1985;72:256–60.
32. Neugebauer E, Lorenz W, Maroske D, et al. The role of mediators in septic/endotoxic shock. A meta-analysis evaluating the current status of histamine. Theor Surg 1987;2:1–28.
33. Neugebauer E, Dietrich A, Bouillon B, et al. Steroids in trauma patients – right or wrong? A qualitative meta-analysis of clinical studies. Theor Surg 1990;5:44–53.
34. Hovell MF. The experimental evidence for weight-loss treatment of essential hypertension: a critical review. Am J Public Health 1982;72:359–68.
35. Bassan MM, Shalev O, Eliakim A. Improved prognosis during long-term treatment with beta-blockers after myocardial infarction: analysis of randomized trials and pooling of results. Heart Lung 1984;13:164–68.
36. Rentrop KP, Feit F, Blanke H, et al. Effects of intracoronary streptokinase and intracoronary nitroglycerin infusion on coronary angiographic patterns and mortality in patients with acute myocardial infarction. N Engl J Med 1984;311:1457–63.
37. Baum ML, Anish DS, Chalmers TC, et al. A survey of clinical trials of antibiotic prophylaxis in colon surgery: evidence against further use of no-treatment controls. N Engl J Med 1981;305:795–99.
38. Yusuf S, Collins R, Peto R, et al. Intravenous and intracoronary fibrinolytic therapy in acute myocardial infarction: overview of results on mortality, reinfarction, and side-effects from 33 randomized controlled trials. Eur Heart J 1985;6:556–85.
39. Collins R, Langman M. Treatment with histamine H2 antagonists in acute upper gastrointestinal hemorrhage. N Engl J Med 1985;313:660–66.
40. Wortman PM, Yeaton WH. Cumulating quality of life results in controlled trials of coronary artery bypass graft surgery. Controlled Clin Trials 1985; 6:289–305.
41. Proceedings of "Methodological Issues in Overviews of Randomized Clinical Trials." Stat Med 1987;6:217–409.
42. Boissel JP, Perrieux JC, Panak E, et al. Guidelines for meta-analysis of clinical trials. 1989 (submitted for publication).
43. Sacks HS, Berrier J, Reitman D, et al. Meta-analyses of randomized controlled trials. N Engl J Med 1987; 316:450–55.
44. Hewett P, Chalmers TC. Using MEDLINE to peruse the literature. Controlled Clin Trials 1985;6:75–84.
45. Hewett P, Chalmers TC. Perusing the literature: methods of assessing MEDLINE and related databases. Controlled Clinical Trials 1985;6:168–78.
46. Chalmers TC. The randomized controlled trial as a basis for therapeutic decisions. In: The Randomized Clinical Trial and Therapeutic Decisions, Lachin J, Tygstrup N, Juhl E, eds. New York: Dekker, 1982, Chapter 2.

47. Gilbert JP, McPeek B, Mosteller F. Statistics and ethics in surgery and anesthesia. Science 1977;198: 684–99.
48. Gilbert JP, McPeek B, Mosteller F. Progress in surgery and anesthesia: benefits and risks of innovative therapy. In: Costs, Risks and Benefits of Surgery, Bunker JP, Barnes BA, and Mosteller F, eds. New York: Oxford University Press, 1977:124–69.
49. Bearman JB, Loewenson DB, Gullen WH. Muench's postulates, laws and corollaries. Biometrics Note 4. Bethesda, MD: Office of Biometry and Epidemiology, National Eye Institute, National Institutes of Health, 1974.
50. Stock WA, Okun M, Haring M, Witter R. Age difference in subjective well-being: a meta-analysis. In: Evaluation Studies Review Annual, vol. 8, Light RJ, ed. Beverly Hills, CA: Sage, 1983;8:279–302.
51. Straw RB. Deinstitutionalization in mental health: a meta-analysis. In: Evaluation Studies Review Annual, vol. 8, Light RJ, ed. Beverly Hills, CA: Sage, 1983:253–78.
52. Yin RK, Yates D. Street level governments: assessing decentralization and urban services. Los Angeles: Rand Corp., 1974.
53. Ottenbacher KJ, Peterson P. The efficacy of vestibular stimulating as a form of specific sensory enrichment. Clin Pediatr 1983;23:418–33.
54. Smith ML, Glass GV. Meta-analysis of psychotherapy outcome studies. Am Psychol 1976;32:752–60.
55. L'Abbe KA, Detsky AS, O'Rourke K. Meta-analysis in clinical research. Ann Intern Med 1987;107: 224–33.
56. Rosenthal R. The file drawer problem and tolerance for null results. Psychol Bull 1979;86:638–41.
57. Begg CB. A measure to aid the interpretation of published clinical trials. Stat Med 1985;4:1–9.
58. Neugebauer E, Lorenz W. Meta-analysis: from classical review to a new refined methodology. Introduction to the discussion forum about an example of meta-analysis in basic surgical research: the role of mediators in septic/endotoxic shock [Theor Surg (1987) 2:1–28]. Theor Surg 1989;4:79–85.
59. Cooper HM. Scientific guidelines for conducting integrative research reviews. Rev Educ Res 1982; 52:291–302.

10

Critical Appraisal of Published Research

M.T. Schechter, F.E. LeBlanc, and V.A. Lawrence

Every year thousands of articles appear in the surgical literature. While many present the results of careful investigations based on good methodology, many others report studies whose results are either invalid because of defects in their conduct or analysis, or ungeneralizable to other settings because of biases in the way they were executed. This chapter describes a framework within which the validity and generalizability of published research can be appraised and judged. We will examine two frequently published types of research, controlled trials of therapeutic interventions and review articles, according to six easily remembered appraisal criteria: WHY, HOW, WHO, WHAT, HOW MANY, and SO WHAT.

Controlled Trials

WHY: The Study Question

As a critical appraiser, you should always begin by considering the reasons for the study and determining whether sufficient evidence is presented to justify it. In the absence of clear statements of the purpose of the study and of the study hypothesis at the outset, you may well consider moving on to another article, because such statements are essential for two reasons. First, the design of the study, which includes the population to be studied, the variables to be considered, and the method of analysis to be utilized, depends very heavily on the purpose of the study. Second, you must be able to determine whether the hypothesis was specified in advance (i.e., a priori) or arose out of the data (i.e., a posteriori). The study hypothesis should also indicate whether the study is intended to be hypothesis-generating or hypothesis-testing.

Studies of therapeutic interventions should clearly state whether *efficacy* or *effectiveness* is being considered. Efficacy studies seek to determine whether an intervention results in a specific outcome under ideal circumstances, that is, in properly diagnosed and properly treated patients who are compliant. Effectiveness studies seek to determine whether an intervention does more good than harm in patients under normal clinical circumstances, that is, in patients who are diagnosed and treated, as in the community, and who may or may not comply, as in the community. In general, the outcome measures used in efficacy studies tend to be short-term and specific while those in effectiveness studies are longer term and more global. *Both types of study have their merits. Efficacy studies usually have their place in the early investigation of new therapies. It is the results of effectiveness studies that indicate whether a given intervention should be adopted.* Much of a study's methodology, especially the population to be studied and the outcome to be assessed, will be determined by which approach (i.e., efficacy or effectiveness) is chosen.

Consider a study investigating coronary artery bypass surgery as a treatment for coronary artery disease. To study the *efficacy* of this intervention, one would ideally utilize a treatment group consisting of patients with clearly documented coronary stenoses, all of whom undergo coronary artery bypass surgery. To test efficacy, one would consider short-term outcomes that this intervention is designed to produce, namely increased myocardial blood flow, relief of anginal symptoms, etc. In such a study, anyone who was allocated to receive the surgery but did not actually receive it, perhaps because of intervening illnesses, would not be included in the treatment group because any subsequent benefit could not be attributed to the efficacy of the intervention itself.

On the other hand, when one considers *effectiveness*, one is challenging not merely the intervention itself, but the *policy* of using this intervention in the study population. This is sometimes known as the "intent to treat" principle. A study of the effectiveness of coronary artery bypass surgery should consider a wider spectrum of outcomes, including long-term survival, quality of life, and level of function. In such studies, patients who are allocated to receive medical therapy but are given surgery at a later date should be analyzed within the medical group since it is the policies of initial treatment with medical versus surgical therapy that are being compared.

It is important to understand the difference between efficacy and effectiveness studies for two other reasons. Results of analyses from *both* perspectives often are reported and discussed in the same article; they may conflict and lead to different conclusions. Disagreement among colleagues may be due to interpretations from the differing perspectives of efficacy and effectiveness.

HOW: Study Methodology

You should next endeavor to determine the type of study methodology (see Chapter 16, below). The types of study design you are most likely to encounter, in relation to therapeutic interventions, include (a) *case studies*, which simply report the results of a series of cases treated with a given intervention, (b) *before–after studies*, which compare the patients' condition before and after the intervention, either in entire settings or within individuals, and (c) *controlled trials*, which compare the results in groups treated with experimental and standard therapies. In controlled trials, you should carefully assess how the patients were allocated to the experimental or the control group. Was the allocation truly randomized? If randomization was not employed, could any biases have occurred in the allocation of the patients? Be on the alert for *quasi-random allocation* in which patients are assigned on the basis of some seemingly random process, (birth date, chart number, day of week, etc.). Subtle biases can be introduced in such situations and there is no reason for not using a true randomization.

You should also attempt to determine what type of blindness was employed, and carefully assess whether any lack of blindness might have led to an expectation bias that distorted the results. *Single blindness* refers to studies in which only the patient does not know whether the experimental treatment or the "control" therapy was received. When *double blindness* is used, both the patients and the care providers are unaware of the allocation. In *triple blinded* studies the patients, the care providers, and those who assess the outcome, are all unaware of what treatment was given. In studies of surgical interventions, blinding of the patients and care providers is not always possible but, at the very least, those who perform the outcome assessment can be blinded to the treatment the patient received.

It is important to determine whether significant prognostic variables were equally allocated to the treatment and control groups. Although most prognostic variables will be equally distributed in large studies employing randomized allocation, maldistribution can occur in small studies. Consequently, it is wise for investigators to use *prognostic stratification*, a method in which patients are first stratified with regard to an important set of prognostic variables, then randomized from each stratum. This method usually guarantees equal distribution of the prognostic variables to the treatment and control groups.

Consider a clinical trial comparing two different treatments for astrocytomas. To make the comparison fair, the groups to which the respective treatments are applied should be comparable with regard to tumor grade, because histological grade is a very important predictor of prognosis in this disease. Since the number of available patients is likely to be small, a maldistribution could occur with simple randomization because an excess of patients with grades III and IV astrocytomas might be allocated, by chance, to one of the treatments. Prognostic stratification would avoid this; that is, patients entering the trial would first be stratified by the grade of their lesion and then randomized to treatment from within each grade. This would guarantee a more equitable distribution of the grades to the two treatment groups.

WHO: The Patient Population

Understanding the type of patient studied is one of the most important aspects of critical appraisal. You must determine whether the type of patient included in an investigation was sufficiently representative to allow the results to be applied to all patients in similar clinical situations or to your patients.

Representativeness can be assessed in a number of ways. Is the source population from which the study sample was drawn clearly described and suitably representative? Are demographic details of the catchment area provided? Was the study sample drawn from a primary, secondary, or tertiary referral center? Did the study sample represent the full spectrum of the disease, or only a small subsample?

Are clear and replicable inclusion and exclusion criteria specified, and do they match the goals of the study? If clear and replicable inclusion and exclusion criteria are not given, you cannot know exactly what type of patient was studied or to which of your patients the results can be applied. The inclusion and exclusion criteria should define a study population that matches the type of patient the investigators intend should benefit from the results. After the exclusion and inclusion criteria have been applied, compare the type of population that remains with the stated goals of the study, to see if they match.

Do the authors account for every patient eligible for the study who did not enter it? This is critically important. Typically, eligible patients (i.e., those meeting the inclusion criteria and not rejected by the exclusion criteria) are approached for informed consent and some decline. If the proportion of refusals is small (i.e., < 10%), it is of limited importance; but *volunteer bias* can occur if a significant proportion of eligible patients do not agree to participate. Participating patients tend to be more motivated, more compliant, and destined for better outcomes than those who decline. Investigators should recruit a minimum of 90% of all eligible patients, or provide evidence that those who declined had outcomes similar to those who volunteered; either approach provides some evidence that volunteer bias was not a significant factor.

Finally, determine whether the baseline comparability of the treatment and control groups has been documented. Although randomization of large numbers of patients should produce relatively equal distributions, maldistributions of important prognostic variables can still occur, especially with smaller sample sizes. The investigators should provide an assessment of the baseline comparability of the two groups; if any prognostic variable has been maldistributed, the analysis should take it into account.

WHAT: Intervention and Outcome Measures

This aspect of critical appraisal centers on two questions. What intervention is under study? What outcome measures are being assessed?

Investigators should provide a clear definition of the intervention; without one, you cannot really know what is being assessed. Some measure of *compliance* should also be included, even in trials of surgical interventions if such components of care beyond the surgical procedure as follow-up care, self-care, and adjunct medications require patients' compliance. Examine how noncompliers were analyzed. In effectiveness trials, noncompliers should be analyzed within the treatment arm to which they were randomized; in efficacy studies, it may sometimes be more appropriate to omit noncompliers from the analysis. Investigators should attempt to monitor *contamination* (patients assigned to the control arm who subsequently underwent the experimental intervention), *cointervention* (additional therapies were made available to patients in either arm of the trial), and all side effects.

All withdrawals (patients removed by the investigators) and dropouts (patients removed on their own volition) should be documented, along with the reasons for their departure. *Crossovers* occur when a patient in one arm of the trial receives the intervention assigned to another arm of the trial; for example, in studies of surgical versus medical treatment of coronary artery disease, patients originally assigned to medical therapy may deteriorate and subsequently undergo coronary artery bypass surgery. Determine whether withdrawals, dropouts, crossovers, and poor compilers were analyzed in accordance with the goals of the study. In an effectiveness study of coronary artery bypass surgery, patients initially assigned to medical therapy who cross over and receive the surgical intervention should be analyzed within the medical therapy arm to which they were originally randomized.

To critically appraise the outcome measures aspect of a study, determine whether all clinically relevant outcome measures were used and whether they matched the study's goals. A study comparing two interventions may focus on the subsequent 3-week mortality in the treatment and control groups, but an improvement in the three-week mortality with the intervention would not provide any reassurance about the long-term survival of patients. If you are deciding whether to use the intervention, you will want to know if the quality of life is improved for those undergoing the intervention. Was the measurement of the outcomes precise? This may not be an issue if the outcome was length of survival because the endpoint (death) is clear, but if the outcome measured was severity of pain, quality of life, improvement of clinical signs or symptoms, etc., you should determine whether a reliable and valid method was used to gather such information. Those who assess the outcome can usually be blinded to patients' allocations for the purpose of making unbiased assessments. Ascertain whether the process of observation required to assess the outcome could have influenced the outcome.

HOW MANY: Statistical Significance and Sample Size

Determine whether statistical significance was considered, whether the statistical tests used were applied appropriately (see Chapter 16), and whether the authors considered the methods of analysis and sample size requirements *prior* to initiating the study. The more analyses performed on a data set, the more likely it becomes that a significant result will be obtained by chance. Accordingly, a significant result obtained from a single prespecified analysis is much more meaningful than one derived from a series of analyses suggested by the data. Check for the possibility of the *multiple comparisons problem*, which occurs when investigators consider several different outcome variables and, by so doing, increase the likelihood of a significant result arising by chance. In such instances, the investigators should adjust their alpha level (see Chapter 16).

Where no statistically significant differences are found between the treatment and control groups, investigators must consider the possibility of a beta (i.e., type II) error and estimate the probability of its occurrence. If a type II error is not considered, you may well ask whether the study was large enough to detect important differences. All too often, investigators conclude that there is no difference between the experimental and control treatments when all they are justified in concluding is that their study failed to detect a difference.

Small sample size frequently leads to trials with weak power to detect important differences in outcome between treatment groups. Freiman and colleagues[1] found that in half the articles reporting no significant differences between the therapies studied, a 50% improvement in performance could easily have been missed. They concluded that type II errors and small sample sizes are ubiquitous in the medical literature. When no statistically significant difference was found, and you know the study was strong enough to have had a good chance of detecting a clinically important difference, you can conclude that the matter is fairly well settled. If the authors do not discuss the power of their trial, you have the right to suspect the study was not large enough to detect important differences.

SO WHAT: Clinical Significance

The heading "so what" reminds you to form some overall conclusion about the importance of the information provided in the article and its relevance to your own clinical practice.

If differences were detected, was their CLINICAL SIGNIFICANCE discussed? Clinical significance refers to the magnitude of the difference observed between treatment and control groups measured in clinical, rather than statistical, terms. If a statistically significant difference is also clinically significant, it implies that a change in clinical behavior is warranted. For example, a study may observe survival rates of 55% in the treatment group and 50% in the control group. If large numbers of patients are involved, this difference may be statistically significant. If the intervention is exceedingly expensive, however, or entails considerable morbidity, it may be hard to justify using it to obtain such a marginal gain in survival, that is, the difference is not clinically significant.

Were the patients included and analyzed in the study sufficiently representative to allow the results to be generalized to other patients? By considering the source population from which the study sample was obtained, the method by which patients were recruited, the inclusion and exclusion criteria, the possibility of volunteer bias, and the patients actually analyzed, you should be able to decide whether the type of patient studied was sufficiently similar to your patients to make the results applicable to them. A simple rule of thumb is: THE TYPE OF PATIENT INCLUDED AND ANALYZED IN ANY STUDY IS THE ONLY TYPE OF PATIENT TO WHICH ITS RESULTS CAN BE APPLIED.

Was the intervention as performed in the study sufficiently feasible that the results can be generalized to other settings? Is the intervention available in other settings? Were those who performed the intervention highly specialized? If the study involved highly motivated, highly trained, and compliant care providers, questions may arise as to how well the intervention will be performed on a community wide basis. This is particularly true in studies of surgical interventions performed in specialized settings by highly skilled surgeons, practiced in the technique under study, and supported by highly specialized adjunct care.

Are the outcomes assessed in the study adequate to establish which of the therapies under study does the most good? If 6-week mortality was the outcome variable of central interest, you may not consider that the results justify incorporating the intervention into your clinical practice; you may well prefer to await evidence that the benefit is not only a short-term reduction in mortality but also a long-term improvement in survival, morbidity, quality of life, level of function, etc.

In conclusion, the goals and hypotheses (the "why") on which a study is based are inexorably linked to several crucial methodological components of the study design, namely the source population to be sampled, the inclusion and exclusion criteria, allocation methods, appropriate handling of various events (withdrawals, crossovers, etc.), outcome assessment, methods of data analysis, and interpretation of clinical significance. A CLEAR UNDERSTANDING OF STUDY GOALS AND HYPOTHESES IS FUNDAMENTAL TO GOOD RESEARCH METHODOLOGY AND ASTUTE CRITICAL APPRAISAL.

Summary: Controlled Trials

WHY: The Study Question

Is sufficient evidence presented to justify the study?
Is the purpose of the study clearly stated?
Is the study hypothesis clearly stated?
Is it clearly outlined whether the study is considering EFFICACY or EFFECTIVENESS?

HOW: Study Methodology

What exactly is the study design?
If it is a controlled trial, is the allocation truly randomized?
If it is not a controlled trial, are there any biases in the allocation to treatment?
What type of blindness is employed (single, double, triple, etc.)?
Was prognostic stratification used?

WHO: The Patient Population

Is the population from which the study sample was drawn clearly described?
Are inclusion and exclusion criteria specified and replicable?
Do the criteria match the goals of the study?
Do the authors account for every eligible patient who did not enter the study?
Is the baseline comparability of the treatment and control groups documented?

WHAT: Intervention and Outcome Measures

What, exactly, was the intervention performed? Is it clearly defined and replicable?
Was compliance with the intervention(s) measured, and were noncompliers analyzed appropriately?
Were contamination and cointervention considered?
Were all patients who entered the study accounted for?
Were withdrawals, dropouts, crossovers, and poor compliers analyzed in accordance with the goals of the study?
What outcomes were assessed in the study?
Were all relevant outcomes utilized?
Could the process of observation have influenced the outcome?

HOW MANY: Statistical Significance and Sample Size

Was statistical significance considered in the study?
Were statistical tests applied appropriately?
Did the authors consider the methods of analysis and the sample size requirements prior to the study?
When no statistically significant differences were found, did the authors consider the possibility of a beta (type II) error and estimate its probability?
Was the study large enough to detect important differences?

SO WHAT: Clinical Significance

If differences were detected, was their clinical significance discussed? Were the patients entered and analyzed in the study sufficiently representative to allow the results to be generalized to other patients?
Was the intervention, as performed in the study, sufficiently representative to permit generalizing the results to other settings?
Do the outcomes assessed in the study provide an adequate basis for establishing which of the studied therapies does the greatest good?

Review Articles

A review article requires a special type of critical appraisal. Given the volume of medical literature, clinicians and researchers depend on review articles to keep them abreast of medical knowledge across specialty boundaries and within their own areas. The review article is a special type of study or research tool. It should synthesize or carefully evaluate a body of information. Its quality depends on the extent to which evidence is systematically and critically evaluated. You will want to judge the validity and generalizability of review articles carefully, to maximize your knowledge and efficiency in handling the literature. Assess a review article using the appraisal criteria described above.[2,3] (see Chapter 9).

WHY: The Study Question

The purpose or question being addressed by the review article should be clearly stated. You must have a clear statement of the question to give you a frame of reference for choosing types of investigation to review (e.g., using only data from controlled clinical trials for a review of a particular therapy).

HOW: Review Methodology

For a review, the data are published investigations. You should be given clear information on (a) how published studies were identified (personal knowledge or computerized literature data bases such as MEDLINE), (b) inclusion and exclusion criteria used in selecting articles for review, and (c) how methodological validity was assessed. Without this information, you cannot determine how representative the reviewed material is in relation to all the available literature, whether relevant material may have been excluded, or whether selection bias may have been present. In this setting, "selection bias" refers to the degree to which reviewers preferentially choose data that supported their own opinions. There should be explicit criteria with respect to how published studies, once identified, were included or excluded from review. Articles rejected from consideration should be logged, like patients excluded from a clinical trial. In addition, systematic appraisal of the quality of the studies covered by the review is necessary for accurate conclusions and to determine their generalizability to your own patients. If we are to depend on the reviewers' expertise and ability to read and appraise the literature for us, the review article must describe a systematic process and standardized criteria for judging articles.

WHO: The Patient Populations

The review should include information about the types of patient and clinical settings in the published investigations being reviewed. The range of patient characteristics and the spectrum of disease should be described. When such information is lacking, it is difficult to assess the quality of the original data, the reviewer's expertise in collation and integration of data, or the generalizability of the reviewer's conclusions to your clinical setting. If a quantitative assessment is to be carried out by pooling the data, the authors must establish that the populations are sufficiently homogeneous to make such a process valid.

WHAT: Interventions, Outcome Measures, and Synthesis

The interventions and outcome measures used in the individual studies covered by a review article are major factors in the synthesis of data to reach conclusions about a body of evidence. The review should provide adequate information about differences in patient populations among studies, specific interventions, and the limitations and inconsistencies in the data. You must have this information before you can place your confidence in the reviewer's ability to identify good quality data, integrate information from a variety of sources, and explain conflicting results among studies.

If a quantitative assessment is to be carried out by pooling data, the review's author(s) must also establish that the interventions, outcomes measured, and measurement techniques were sufficiently homogeneous to permit such pooling.

HOW MANY: Quantitative Review

Information synthesis may be qualitative (review article) or quantitative (meta-analysis). Critical assessment of both types of review article is similar up to this point. In qualitative reviews, the author(s) should weigh the value of each study according to the appropriateness of the statistical methods it used and its power to detect important differences. Meta-analysis adds an extra quantitative dimension by formally pooling data from several studies. In such analyses, the reviewer should use or derive a common unit of comparison and be able to assess statistical variance in every study used as a source of data for inclusion in the pooling process. The best overall estimate of the treatment effect is not obtained by simply averaging the individual estimates or by combining the number of treatment successes across the trials. Some form of pooling that takes account of individual variances in the estimates is preferable (e.g., the Mantel–Haenszel procedure or other methods of combining contingency tables).

An advantage of meta-analysis is its ability to identify small effects in subgroups that may be statistically undetectable in individual small studies. You should be wary, as usual, of the multiple-comparisons problem—that is, the likelihood of a false-positive result increases with the number of subgroups analyzed.

SO WHAT: Clinical Significance

When you read a review article, you should decide whether any summary differences found were clinically significant, whether the combined study patients were sufficiently similar to your own, whether the intervention was feasible and representative in your setting, and whether the outcomes establish the therapy that does the greatest good. In a review article, clinical significance rests not only on the validity, magnitude, and generalizability of the conclusions but also on the identification of unanswered questions. Conclusions are valid only when the review process has been scientific. A good review article directs our attention to a research agenda so that subsequent investigations will maximize methodological quality and will not be redundant or address unresolved issues. The overwhelming breadth of the medical literature compels us to rely on "ghost readers." If review articles are viewed as scientific endeavors in their own right and their quality withstands critical appraisal, we can be more confident that such ghosts are scientific spirits.

Summary: Review Articles

WHY: The Study Question

Is the purpose or question addressed by the review article clearly stated?

HOW: Review Methodology

Is the method used to select articles clearly described?
Are the inclusion and exclusion criteria for selecting articles clearly stated?
How was the quality of the studies under review evaluated?

WHO: The Patient Populations

Are the populations of patients clearly described?
If data have been pooled, did the author(s) establish the homogeneity of the patient populations?

WHAT: Interventions, Outcome Measures, and Synthesis

Is adequate information provided about differences in patient populations among studies, interventions used, and data limitations and inconsistencies?
If data have been pooled, did the author(s) establish the homogeneity of the interventions, outcomes, and methods of outcome assessment?

HOW MANY: Quantitative Review

In qualitative reviews, have the authors appraised the quantitative methods and the power of each study?
In pooled analyses, have the authors combined the results in a way that takes account of individual variances?
In subgroup analyses, have the authors taken account of the multiple comparisons problem?

SO WHAT: Clinical Significance

Are any detected overall differences clinically significant?
Were the combined study-patients sufficiently representative to permit generalization of the results?
Are the interventions reviewed sufficiently feasible and representative to permit generalization of the results to other settings?
Were the outcomes sufficient to establish the therapy that does the greatest good?
Did the authors identify key questions and outline a future research agenda that follows logically from the present state of knowledge?

References

1. Freiman JA, Chalmers TC, Smith H Jr, Keubler RR. The importance of beta, the type II error and sample size in the design and interpretation of the randomized control trial. Survey of 71 negative trials. N Engl J Med 1978;299:690–94.
2. Mulrow CD. The medical review article: state of the science. Ann Intern Med 1987;106:485–88.
3. Sacks HS, Berrier J, Reitman D, Ancona-Berk VA, Chalmers TC. Meta-analyses of randomized controlled trials. N Engl J Med 1987;316:450–55.

Additional Reading

Chalmers TC, Celano P, Sacks HS, Smith H Jr. Bias in treatment assignment in controlled clinical trials. N Engl J Med 1983;309:1358–61.
DerSimonian R, Charette LJ, McPeek B, Mosteller F. Reporting on methods in clinical trials. N Engl J Med 1982;306:1332–37.
Emerson JD, McPeek B, Mosteller F. Reporting clinical trials in general surgical journals. Surgery 1984;95:572–79.
Fletcher RH, Fletcher SW. Clinical research in medical journals. N Engl J Med 1979;301:1809–83.
Sackett DL, Tugwell PT. Deciding on the best therapy. In: Clinical Epidemiology: A Basic Science for Clinicians, Boston/Toronto: Little, Brown, 1985;171–97.
Sackett DL, Haynes RB, Tugwell PT. How to read a clinical journal. In: Clinical Epidemiology: A Basic Science for Clinicians, Boston/Toronto: Little, Brown, 1985;285–321.

11

Formulating an Initial Research Plan

R.E. Pollock, C.M. Balch, J. Roth, B. McPeek, and F. Mosteller

Much thought occurs before you are ready to formulate an initial research proposal. At the broadest level, a fertile mind must be receptive to fresh ideas, ready to nurture and support a nascent plan and, after a period of intellectual germination, able to formulate the idea into a written research proposal. The process, and this chapter, operates on two levels, one, broad, conceptual, and philosophical; the other, focused, structural, and expository.

Nurturing Scientific Creativity

Research aims at learning more about the world we live in. Ordinarily, we cannot study the world or nature without first simplifying it to make our learning assignment more manageable. We study nature by abstracting it so it becomes possible to handle, to describe, to measure in a controlled, systematic way. We try to take nature into our laboratory. We subject it to experimental manipulation using modern techniques of biology and chemistry, biostatistics and epidemiology, etc.

In theory, we first conceive a scientific topic or issue and then try to fashion a project we could do that would yield information on the issue. In an orderly world, one might first think about the issue, what is known about it, perhaps what's not known, and some scientists do work this way. More commonly, we conceive of a project and then realize it could produce information bearing on nature.

A variety of strategies help bring fresh insights. Ideas or techniques from one field can be applied to another, producing information that is novel and not yet available in the second field. If you hope to do scientific work, read widely. Discuss your research ideas with a variety of people who work in different scholarly areas. The literature in your own field may have a limited view of research or approaches to your topic or issue. Make a habit of browsing and reading widely in science. Remember that social scientists as well as natural scientists and clinical scholars have much to offer that is relevant to bedside medicine and surgery. Go to national scientific meetings, particularly meetings in fields other than your own.

Teaching students offers a frequent source of new ideas or insights. Students may be less constrained by the limits we see in our present knowledge and methodology. Students often ask "why?" They have mental flexibility and recent exposure to other fields.

You must have a skeptical attitude toward conventional wisdom. Do the explanations we offer about nature or about the problems we see in our clinic really make sense? Think about what is really known and how surely it is known. Most of us are far too confident of the state of our own knowledge.

Good Questions

What makes a good research question? A good question seems interesting; the more you think about it, the more interesting it appears. As you think about it and discuss it with your research team, you want to work on it. It sparks your curiosity and emphasizes your strengths and those of the team. Its solution seems important. You would feel rewarded for your effort.

Scientists seek questions that offer originality and answers that would aim toward the solution of a basic scientific problem or have clear clinical value. We don't always think enough about feasibility. Most of us are good at devising infeasible projects requiring the key to the national treasury, as well as collaborators, patient material, equipment, space, or knowledge that is not available.

This is not just an issue of a team's strengths and weaknesses (e.g., pediatric projects are difficult to run in a veterans' hospital). It is a more general problem. Inexperienced workers constantly find themselves asking too much of a research project. We forget that there is no scientific project that our own grandiose ideas cannot inflate to the point of infeasibility.

Build on Experience

As you start to develop your research project, take advantage of past experience, talk to your friends who work in the field. Seek the help of a senior scientific mentor if you are just starting out. Try to view your project as part of a continuing research program. This will serve to focus some of your interests and help you build on previous successes. It may subtly keep you from dissipating your efforts across too wide an area.

Team Work

As you develop a project, consider working with other people. Most of us find it is fun, and it is very productive. Different people have different strengths, different experiences, different insights. As you advance an idea, a whole new formulation may occur to your partner. When you plan a joint project, try to develop a series of short-term goals. They make definite what is needed or expected of individuals at a given time. They also subtly assign guilt for not having produced work ("subtly" is an important word because nothing will end a collaboration quicker than an atmosphere of blame). On the other hand, a tiny amount of self-felt guilt may advance a project as partners take their responsibilities more seriously. Regular meetings are vital for production because they provide definite expectations and deadlines.

Let us say you have an idea that seems promising and feasible, and you think it will be fun. An initial research proposal helps structure, focus, and communicate your ideas to others.

Writing a Research Proposal

A research proposal is an internal working document—not to be confused with a grant application—used by many investigators to formulate their ideas. It facilitates original and productive research by structuring intuitive intellectual processes into a carefully defined set of plans. These plans should delineate the hypothesis to be tested, appropriate controls, and an experimental design that will promote originality and clinical relevance.

In our laboratories, we continuously develop a variety of research proposals as a means of structuring, focusing, and communicating our ideas.

General Principles

1. The proposal should address one or more hypotheses to be tested. These hypotheses should be grounded firmly in underlying biological or physiological principles. Occasionally, the necessary experiments are observational (phenomenological), and a successful outcome depends on a positive result. The more incisive studies usually address hypotheses of significant scientific interest, whether the results are positive or negative.
2. Have a clear understanding of the potential clinical relevance of your proposal. Most surgical investigations are preclinical studies, in relevant animal or in vitro models, having ultimate applicability to the surgical patient, or clinical studies that use human materials in vitro or accompany clinical research protocols.
3. Use the proposal-drafting process to capture and focus your ideas. Drafts only 1 to 3 pages long provide good frameworks for organizing data and concepts as they mature over time; review and update them periodically. Circulate your drafts among laboratory workers or possible collaborators as a means of initiating later discussion.
4. Know and keep up with the literature in your field. The essence of good research is originality and significance; remaining abreast of the literature helps to ensure that your own work will maintain its originality. It also allows you to design experiments that permit comparisons with published results.
5. Establish research collaborations and mentorships wherever possible. A research proposal provides a good basis for discussion and delineation of responsibilities in a multifaceted and collaborative research effort.

Outline of a Research Proposal

The basic elements of a research proposal include title, investigators, hypothesis, objectives, research design, and budget.

Title

The title delineates the theme of the research proposal; it should be as concise and focused as possible.

List of Investigators

When multiple investigators are participating in collaborative research, it is especially important to name the principal investigators and to delineate their degrees of responsibility at the outset of a research proposal. Since the order of listing may well reflect the authorship sequence on subsequent manuscripts or abstracts, the hierarchy should be decided at the start, to avoid later conflicts about authorship.

Hypothesis

The hypothesis should be based on the specific questions to be asked. An effective hypothesis usually examines the biological or physiological mechanisms underlying an unexplained observation; it should not be global but should focus on the specific area of inquiry.

Research Objectives

No more than four or five concise, *specific* questions should be listed as objectives, and they should be compatible with the research theme reflected in the title and the hypothesis being tested.

Research Design

This section summarizes the overall strategy and specific tactics to be employed in testing the hypothesis and achieving the research objectives. It is an outline of the basic experimental design, including a delineation of the appropriate controls, sample size, and statistical methods to be used. It might also include a data flow sheet in a format suitable for automation and computerized statistical analysis.

Research Budget

Make a strenuous attempt to take specific account of all the costs of conducting the research project, to ensure the availability of sufficient funds to complete the study. Funding requirements for new supplies or equipment needed, or potentially needed, to conduct the research should be identified.

Summary

Preparing research proposals is an integral part of the effective functioning of any research laboratory, whether the research projects are large or small. The process engenders a rigorous and analytical focusing of research ideas and minimizes the risk of wasting time and resources associated with more casual or informal approaches to laboratory research. After preliminary data have been generated, a research proposal may become the basic framework for a formal research proposal and grant application.

12

Ethical Principles in Research

D.J. Roy, P.McL. Black, and B. McPeek

"The surgical act is just too powerful and too dangerous to be loosed on an unsuspecting public in the hands of a surgeon who uses only his cerebellum."
Judah Folkman, M.D.[1]

Research ethics is as integral a part of scientific judgment as clinical ethics is of clinical judgment.[2] Many ethical issues in research arise from a failure to think as rigorously about the conditions for ethical consistency as about those for scientific validity. The ethical principles governing all surgical, clinical, and biomedical research with human subjects are fundamentally the same. They have been listed and discussed in numerous documents and countless publications over the past 40 years.[3-10]

Although due regard must be maintained for the utility and necessity of institutional review boards, ethics committees, and public participation in the ethical evaluation of the protocols for research with human subjects, it is a mistake to view ethics as an external, authoritarian imposition of regulations or possibly arbitrary constraints on the process of clinical research. The design and the practice of research ethics should be primarily, though not exclusively, a matter of self-consistency and self-governance within clinical investigation.

Ethics and Research

Research ethics and scientific research pursue a common cognitive goal; to distinguish mere appearances from reality. Scientific research, using measurement as its cardinal procedure, seeks to ascertain the actual relationships between phenomena. Uncritical reliance on initial observations, potentially distorted by bias, can lead to a systematic divergence from the truth.[11] Rigorous research methods are devised precisely to counter the tendency to mistake a mere semblance of correlation for a judgment of fact.

Research ethics, a process of critical reflection and interdisciplinary collaboration, acts against the tendency to diverge systematically from what is right. As initial observations may fail to reveal true correlations, spontaneous desires or compulsions may not correspond with what we ought to do. What appears to be good in a limited perspective may contradict a greater and more commanding value. True values, like real correlations between phenomena, are not always immediately obvious. A spontaneous apparent good acquires the moral force of a value only after passing through a process of critical reflection in which proposed courses of action and possible objects of choice are subjected to a series of questions that result in value judgment. Value judgments, like judgments of fact and of truth, are governed by assent to sufficient evidence, not by submission to custom, convention, authority, brilliance, or emotion.

Working out the ethics of research requires the exercise of critical intelligence and judgment by a community of humans engaged in attentive and mutually corrective discourse rather than isolated monologues. Combining interdisciplinary dialogue with the study of specific cases, whether of clinical practice or clinical research, counteracts moral atomism, rampant relativism, and what Stephen Toulmin has called the tyranny of principles.[12] Principles, guidelines, and codes, alone, do not decide concrete cases. Principles will fail to reveal their meaning—what they command, permit, and prohibit—until they are interpreted in the light of specific research situations. This approach to ethics provides a basis for institutional review boards (IRBs) or research ethics committees without, necessarily, justifying their specific modes of operation. It must be emphasized, however, that ethical judgment is an integral component of clinical and scientific intelligence; clinical investigators are expected and entitled to perform as integrated humans and professionals.

Controlled Clinical Research: An Ethical Imperative

A physician's moral obligation to offer each patient the best available treatment cannot be separated from clinical imperatives to base any choice of treatment on the best accessible evidence. The tension between the interdependent responsibilities of giving care that is personal and compassionate, and treatment that is scientifically sound and validated, is intrinsic to the practice of medicine. This tension, which arises prior to and as a moral reality distinct from any conflict of interests, is a structural part of the medical profession's covenant with the human community, not merely the expression of an individual physician–investigator's disordered intentions.

Controlled clinical trials—randomized and multiply blinded (when these are feasible), ethically achievable, and scientifically appropriate—are an integral part of the ethical imperative that physicians and surgeons know what they are doing when they intervene into the bodies, psyches, and lives of vulnerable, suffering humans. The ethical requirement of precise and validated knowledge gathers force with the likelihood that clinical interventions will have decisive and irreversible impacts on patients' futures and on future patients. Future patients have faces; they cannot be lumped together as part of society and set in opposition to patients occupying hospital beds today.

The standards of good medicine, determined by professional consensus based on reliable methods of achieving validated knowledge, enter into the inner structure of the doctor–patient relationship. "What doctor and patient choose is not the untrammelled expression of the knowledge and values of each. It is limited by the professional norms that constrain the doctor's judgment and constrain it in the name of good medicine generally."[13] Something more, though, is required. If the achievement of good medicine is an ethical imperative, it must exert not only the *protective force* of a constraint on potential misguided judgment and choice, but also the *constructive force* of an invocation to comprehending and voluntary collaboration in constantly redesigning the standards of good medicine. Professionally validated knowledge, without the collaboration of individual physicians and patients, would remain a utopian dream.

When there is uncertainty or definite doubt about the safety or efficacy of an innovative or established treatment, this position supports the strong view that there *is*, not simply *may be*, "a higher moral obligation to test it critically than to prescribe it year-in, year-out with the support of custom or wishful thinking."[14] When large numbers of innovative treatments are being continuously introduced into clinical practice, rigorous testing is ethically mandatory for the protection of individual patients and the just use of limited resources. This holds true with even greater force in the light of evidence that many innovations show no advantage over existing treatments when they are subjected to properly controlled study.[15] They may even be less effective, or harmful.[16]

Conditions for the Ethical Conduct of Clinical Research

Conditional Ethics

If the practice of medicine is both morally mandatory and inherently experimental,[17] controlled clinical trials cannot be inherently unethical. Clinical trials, whatever the tactics used to control for bias, will be unethical only to the extent that they fail to meet a set of necessary and interrelated conditions. "Ethical justifiability" means consistency with the ethos and morality of the human community. Human communities vary from one culture and society to another, not only in their customs and art, but also in their governing perceptions and values regarding the body, health, disease, suffering, death, and a host of other realities affecting the practice of medicine. The conditions for ethically justifiable research with human subjects arise from the requirements for consistency along each of these dimensions.

These conditions are structured. They range from fundamental principles of science, medicine, and philosophy across more specific norms, procedures, and regulations to encompass the tailored ethical judgments required for the unique characteristics and designs of individual clinical trials. The ethics of clinical research is open-ended, cumulative, and unfinished. A continual process of feedback is at work between tailored ethical judgments on specific trials and the principles, norms, procedures and regulations requisite for the ethical conduct of clinical research. Our knowledge of right and wrong is as subject to the process of evolution and cumulative growth as our knowledge of fact and truth in science.

The concept of conditional ethics, so understood, implies that ethical justifiability is a graded, not a binary, characteristic of clinical trials. The rheostat rather than the on–off switch suggests an appropriate image.

Research Ethics and Cultural Diversity

Though science is largely transcultural, the human community has not yet developed a completely corresponding body of transcultural ethics. Differing views about what is normative in person–person, doctor–patient, and investigator–subject relationships may create the need for ethical compromise or accommodation in some multicenter trials, particularly when the collaborating centers are situated in different nations.

A Japanese physician–investigator may find it difficult to honor North American insistence on detailed disclosure to patients about the randomization process used to select treatment in a clinical trial for breast cancer or cancer of the prostate. In a culture that places great emphasis on trust in the physician as an integral part of the healing process, both physicians and patients may find an open admission of physician ignorance or uncertainty therapeutically damaging or even absurd.

North American culture emphasizes the value of individual autonomy; some Asian cultures, the value of the family and the community. The approaches to informed, comprehending, and voluntary consent may be quite different in these two cultures. In China the family and the community play a central role in resolving disputes and in obtaining a patient's consent in difficult situations.

> First, community social pressure is the first and usually very effective mode of obtaining agreement. Second, the family plays an important role in securing patient consent, even with adult patients. However, others, such as fellow-workers, are also involved.[18]

Sensitivity to the dominant values of other cultures should be an ethical requisite of international collaboration in multicenter trials. Accommodating cultural differences, even in ethnic groups within the pluralistic society of Western nations, will usually require a flexibility in procedures rather than the compromise of fundamental principles.

Scientific Adequacy

The Nuremberg Code and the Declaration of Helsinki state that research with human subjects must, as a general condition of ethical justifiability, conform to the canons of scientific methodology.[19,20] Both documents insist on respect for accepted scientific principles, knowledge of the natural history of the disease or problem under study, adequate preliminary laboratory and animal experimentation, and proper scientific and medical qualification of investigators. This emphasis, though covering the basic preconditions for a valid and credible clinical trial, may sound like a quaint overemphasis of the obvious. However, the attempt in the early 1980s to treat two β-thalassemic patients by modifying bone marrow with human β-globulin gene implants was widely criticized as premature and unethical, chiefly on two grounds. The treatment was tried without adequate preliminary experimentation with animal models of β-thalassemia or a solid foundation of adequate basic knowledge about the regulation of gene expression.[21-25]

David D. Rutstein's maxim—"A poorly or improperly designed study involving human subjects . . . is by definition unethical"[26]—directs attention to the general rule of proportionality ethics. Inviting human beings to submit themselves to possibly heightened risk of discomfort, inconvenience, harm, or death; consuming scarce precious resources; and raising hopes, particularly when hope is about all that patients have left, demand the balancing weight of a clinical trial that exhibits a high probability of achieving the three objectives identified by David L. Sackett. They are: "validity (the results are true), generalizability (the results are widely applicable), and efficiency (the trial is affordable and resources are left over for patient care and other health research)."[27]

Only reliable clinical knowledge merits widespread clinical application. The generalization of invalid clinical knowledge is inherently unethical and the extensive application of nonvalidated procedures is, at best, ethically dubious. In this context, randomization has gained wide recognition as one of the most effective tactics to control for selection bias—a major form of bias that leads to false conclusions about the safety, efficacy, or superiority of a given treatment.

Although the emphasis on randomization in scientific and ethical discussions of controlled clinical trials with human subjects has not been misplaced, a major shift of ethical attention is long overdue. The ethical difficulties raised by the randomization process may be less significant than the methodological confusion and deficiencies it contributes to the generation of randomized clinical trials that are humanly costly and resource intensive and whose results are clinically implemented only in very limited ways. The problem is not limited to the admitted need to translate the results of clinical trials into practice more effectively,[28] nor can it be solved by technique alone or by more intensive and restricted focus on the careful blueprinting of randomization designs.[29] Randomization, whatever its power, glorious achievements, limitations, or ethical challenges, is not the root of the basic problem of scientific adequacy as a condition for ethically justifiable clinical research with human subjects.

The problem is rooted in the current limitations of basic biomedical science. Meeting the demands of scientific adequacy, as a condition for the ethical justifiability of clinical research with human subjects, requires the development of what Alvan R. Feinstein has called "the basic science of clinical practice." This requirement, as yet unfulfilled, is based on the fact that "the experiments of the laboratory and the bedside have major differences in scientific orientation, motivation, hypotheses, and values."[30]

A continuing failure to implement the consequences of the differences will exacerbate the ethical problems of clinical research, however much greater the increases in the number of publications and conferences on the meaning of respect for human dignity and the specifications of informed consent. Feinstein's suggested additional basic science of clinical practice would aim to bring cogent human information, derived directly from the patient, back within the boundaries of science. The goal of this science would be to give physicians and patients power over medical science and technology "by expanding it to include human data, by aiming it at human goals, and by making it respond to human aspirations."[31]

Clinical Research: A Human Relationship

Research with human subjects is ethically unjustifiable to the extent that it fails to honor four fundamental characteristics of an authentically human relationship. Charles Fried[13] has identified these as humanity, autonomy, lucidity, and fidelity. These characteristics are essential qualifications of how physicians, clinical investigators, patients, and subjects should behave toward each other. Our attention, in this discussion, is understandably focused on the behavior of physicians and clinical investigators.

In a human relationship, a person is not treated simply as one of a class. The characteristic *humanity* stresses that each person is a unique individual with a correspondingly unique biology and individualized needs, weaknesses, strengths, and life plans. *Humanity* means attention to and respect for this "full human particularity."[13] Autonomy or self-determination implies the need and the capacity to deliberate about personal goals and the liberty to act accordingly. A relationship that fosters autonomy is notable for the absence of fraud, force, and the tendency to use another human being as a disposable resource.

Lucidity qualifies communication as honest, candid, and open to imparting all known information that is material to another's self-determination, deliberation, and choice of alternatives to realize individual life plans. This means sensitivity to another person's total life interests and capacities for comprehension. Lucidity is ill-served if clinical investigators look on "obtaining informed consent" as some kind of legally imposed ritual. Clinical investigators sometimes speak as though consent is something they need for their research. They fail to grasp the reality that adequate information is primarily a need of the patient and a moral requirement of integrity in a human relationship.

Fidelity means faithfulness in responding to justified expectations that are integral components of a relationship. These expectations will vary from one kind of relationship to another. Patients enter into relationships with doctors justifiably expecting, however implicitly, that their doctors are suitably qualified, are up to date with current standards of good medicine and skillful surgery, and are committed to restoring their patients to good health.

Informed, Comprehending, and Voluntary Consent

Physicians and clinical investigators have a primordial obligation to assure that their patients and volunteer subjects are adequately informed to be able to consent comprehendingly, and without coercion, to the research procedures and interventions they are being invited to undergo. This condition for ethically justifiable research with human subjects, clearly established in the Nuremberg Code,[19] has been subjected to relentless and detailed scrutiny over the past 30 years in more than 4000 publications.[32]

The ethical norm of informed, comprehending, and voluntary consent has its origin in the four characteristics of an authentic human relationship discussed earlier. Though each shapes the process of consent, humanity is the most difficult to respect. It is, nevertheless, singularly important in gauging the scope of disclosure of information in clinical practice and in clinical research.

The particularity of the patient's situation was a central issue in the Canadian Supreme Court case of *Reibl* versus *Hughes*. The court's decision clarifies that, of three possible standards for determining the kinds of information that must be disclosed (i.e., the professional, subjective patient, and objective patient standards) the latter is to be followed. If the professional standard would allow doctors and clinical investigators to set the threshold of disclosure "at a lower level than would serve the public interest and protection," the subjective patient standard would place physicians "at the mercy of the patient's bitter hindsight."[33]

The court clarified that the objective or reasonable patient standard implies the need to match information to a patient's reasonably based particular concerns and preferences.[34] This legally and ethically important case illustrates the essential moral difference between "obtaining" informed consent, as a ritual kind of act performed primarily to get treatment or research moving, and "educating" a patient or subject in an open, searching conversation, carried out primarily to assure that the patient knows and understands everything required to make a free and reasonable decision.

The Canadian case also emphasizes that "informed consent" is part of a two-way transaction.[33] The doctor also needs information if the patient is to be adequately informed. How can a physician or clinical investigator serve the life plans of a patient or subject if nothing is said about them in conversations about the treatment or research? Doctors and clinical investigators are as much in need of knowing every essential of the life plans, concerns, and bodily situation of patients and subjects as the latter are in need of knowing every essential of the preferred treatments and proposed research procedures.

Physicians and clinical investigators bear primary responsibility for organizing consent conversations and making certain that this mutually informing process really takes place. Insecure and vulnerable patients and subjects may easily be cowed into silence, or even acquiescence, by the awesome environment of the hospital and the authority-laden image of the doctor.[35] The hospital is the doctor's daily domain and home territory, which the patient enters as a frightened stranger. In these circumstances, voluntary consent doesn't come naturally. Sensitive perception and dedicated commitment are necessary if physicians and clinical investigators are to serve the needs and goals of those who come to them for care and cure.

Clinical Research: A Therapeutic Relationship

Henry K. Beecher's statement "Ordinary patients will not knowingly risk their health or their life for the sake of science"[36] is as true today as it was in 1966. Sick people come to doctors for care, relief, and cure. Though cure cannot be guaranteed and every intervention into the body carries its risk of harm, care encompasses the granting by patients, and the appropriating by doctors, "of some power over another so that the other will benefit."[37]

The expectation that doctors will help, and not harm, is the basis of the patient-doctor relationship, the primary content of the medical profession's societal mandate, and the guiding norm of one of medicine's most ancient ethical maxims.[37] Fidelity to this expectation is an essential condition for ethically acceptable clinical research.

Claude Bernard gave precision to the meaning of this fidelity in his statement of a principle of medical and surgical morality:

> It is our duty and our right to perform an experiment on man whenever it can save his life, cure him, or gain him some personal benefit. The principle of medical and surgical morality, therefore, consists in never performing an experiment which might be harmful to him to any extent, even though the result might be highly advantageous to science, that is, to the health of others."[17]

This principle sets a basic right of patients, and a corresponding fundamental duty of doctors, that takes precedence over any utilitarian calculus that would tolerate a sacrifice of the health or lives of individuals today for the putatively greater good of society or the patients of tomorrow.

This "Bernard" principle, though clearly essential for the ethical justifiability of clinical research with human subjects, is too pure and absolute in its original wording to be realistic. Medicine is inherently experimental. It is clearly impossible, either in uncontrolled clinical practice or in controlled clinical trials, to abstain totally from interventions that might be harmful "to any extent." The factors of uncertainty and risk of harm, attendant upon any clinical intervention into the body, must be taken into account in this principle of the primacy of the therapeutic obligation.

The therapeutic obligation in clinical practice, regardless of whether physician and patient are participants in a controlled clinical trial, has to be governed by proportionality ethics. Risks of harm or detriment have to be balanced by a probability of benefit for the patient that is weighty enough to compensate for any loss or injury that might occur. This principle complements the Nuremberg and Helsinki emphasis on the proportion to be maintained between the risks undertaken by subjects in clinical research and the scientific and humanitarian importance of the research objectives.[19,20]

Harms and benefits are not totally susceptible to objective, generalizable measurement. They comprise both "hard" and "soft" data. The ethical implication is that it is impossible to determine that a proportion between harms and benefits holds for particular patients, without giving due attention and weight to their personal interpretations of the total impact of a clinical intervention on their lives.

This is the target of Feinstein's justified criticism of attempts to balance harms and benefits, or to judge a treatment's efficacy, on the basis of a dehumanized array of data. Such attempts fall short of their objective because they fail to assess the "total spectrum of a treatment's impact."[38]

The Therapeutic Relationship in Randomized Clinical Trials

One of the strongest recurrent ethical criticisms of randomized clinical trials is that they sin against the therapeutic relationship. Physician-investigators participating in such studies, so the critique runs, abandon fully individualized care of their patients and even subject some patients, via the randomization process, to inferior treatment. One assumption behind this criticism is that equipoise regarding safety and efficacy rarely exists between alternative treatments at the initiation of a controlled trial. There is usually some indication that one treatment is better than another, even if the indication falls short of a statistically rigorous demonstration. Even if equipoise does seem to hold at the initiation of a trial, secrecy about interim results when these favor one treatment over another means that some randomized patients, including both early and newly entered patients, will receive inferior treatment.

How can randomizing patients to inferior treatment, or maintaining them on inferior treatment until the trial reaches a certain minimum probability of error, be squared with the demands of the therapeutic relationship? This bottom-line question gathers force when patients die or suffer serious deterioration of health as a consequence of the inferior treatment.

The foregoing criticism of randomized clinical trials does not reflect sufficient appreciation of the proliferation of innovations and the attendant pervasiveness of uncertainty in medicine, the associated danger of using invalidated procedures in clinical practice, and the intersection of goals in clinical therapy and interventional trials.

Surgical trials with human subjects are, with few exceptions, interventional rather than explicatory. Feinstein has identified the ethical significance of the differences between these two kinds of trial.[39] In an *interventional* trial, the goal of the treatments employed is to change a patient's clinical course, not in a passing way to study some physiological variable, but in an enduring way, and to enhance health and postpone death.

The goal of the therapeutic relationship—to care, relieve, and cure a suffering patient—is identical to the goal pursued by the physician-investigators in an interventional trial. The goal of the trial is to determine, reliably, whether the effects observed to follow upon a clinical intervention are due to treatment, or whether one treatment is safer or more effective than its alternatives.

When there is no uncertainty about the safety, efficacy, or comparative worth of treatments, there is no need for an interventional trial. To the extent that such uncertainty does hold sway, it is impertinent to ask whether physician-investigators in an interventional trial are withholding known effective treatments from patients or are consigning patients to inferior treatment. That is precisely what is unknown and can be reliably determined only by a properly designed trial. An interventional trial, assuming the fulfillment of essential scientific and ethical conditions, is more consistent with fidelity to the therapeutic relationship than unquestioning recommendation of one of several invalidated treatments whose comparative worth is in dispute.

This position does not reject the principle of conscience. A physician, convinced of the superiority of a given treatment on the basis of available evidence, would be acting against his or her personal and professional conscience in participating in a randomization of patients to an alternative treatment that causes higher mortality or morbidity in the physician's opinion. It must be realized, however, that evidence sufficiently strong to constitute ethical ground for an individual physician's refusal to participate in a randomized clinical trial may fall far short of a decisive argument against the ethical justifiability of the trial itself.

Clinical Trials and Surgical Research: Ethical Issues

To fit the reality of particular clinical trials, ethical decisions need two synchronized cutting edges: an upper blade of general ethical principles, and a continually reshaped lower blade of definite answers to specific questions.

The Ethical Use of Animals in Surgical Research

It is generally and correctly assumed that the ethical justifiability of research with human subjects depends on adequate prior experimentation with animals. This does not mean that the use of animals in research requires no further justification. However, a comprehensive response to the question about whether we are morally justified "in imposing suffering on or taking the lives of other species solely for our own benefit"[40] would require an analysis of the expanding and unfinished debate on these issues.[41-44] Since such an analysis would exceed the boundaries of this chapter, two major points have been selected for discussion.

First, differences between species do have moral significance. Ethical constraints on what we may impose on other animals to satisfy our own good and our own needs increase as the capacities and needs of the animals approach those of human beings. Second, the critical question is not whether, but under what conditions we may use animals in research.

Effective measures to assure the humane treatment of animals in research, and to protect animals against wanton disregard of their needs and welfare, are essential requirements of civilized scientific behavior. Fulfilling these requirements does not necessitate acceptance of any of the following positions.

Humans have no right to treat animals any differently from how they would treat any member of their own species.[45]
Animals should be used in research projects only when the results will directly benefit the animals themselves.[45]
There should be an immediate replacement of all animals used in experiments by alternative systems.[43]

Sensitivity to the needs of animals and to their differential capacities for suffering from pain, constriction, and deprivation does necessitate careful attention to Lane-Petter's five basic questions.

Is the animal the best experimental system for the problem?
Must the animal be conscious at any time during the experiment?
Can the pain and discomfort associated with the experiment be lessened or eliminated?
Can the number of animals involved be reduced?
Is the problem under study worth solving?[46,47]

Necessity of experiment, humaneness of design, and a standard of pre- and postoperative care at least as good as that required for acceptable clinical veterinary practice[48] summarize the conditions for the ethical justifiability of using animals in research.

Standards in Surgical Research

There is no controversy about the desirability of high standards of evidence in surgical research. The well known division of opinion is about the kinds of design that are practicable and effective in producing such evidence.[49-56] The rule governing such discussions should be: avoid fervent answers to global questions. Variations in the nature of the procedures under study, the clinical conditions to be treated, and different surgical specialties require differentiated judgments about the research design most appropriate for each research project.

The principle of differentiated judgment modifies, and is not a substitute for, the more general ethical rule: employ every possible tactic at the most opportune moment in the development of innovative surgical procedures to reduce the devastating effects of bias. Demanding that the standards of surgical research match the highest currently attainable in clinical investigation is not the same thing as insisting on identity of research design in surgical and medical trials. Methodological sophistication may indicate the need for research designs uniquely tailored for some surgical specialties.[51,56-58]

Ethics and the Design of Surgical Research

The methodologically rigorous design of surgical trials poses several distinct and widely recognized difficulties,[59-60] which have ethical implications.

First, it is generally impossible to achieve full blinding in surgical research. The extent of blinding achievable will vary according to the purpose of the trial, that is, whether an operation is being compared with nonsurgical treatment or with the comparative safety and efficacy of two operations. Though sham operations are ethically unjustifiable and would not be considered today, a measure of blinding may be possible when the physicians evaluating the patients' progress have not been involved in the trials.[50,60-62]

Second, surgery has a powerful placebo effect that may exist independently of an operation's genuine efficacy. This fact, for which internal mammary artery ligation for the relief of angina offers some evidence, underscores the importance of blinding as a tactic in a methodologically rigorous trial. It is difficult to ethically justify the continued use of surgical operations having little more than placebo efficacy.[60]

Third, Francis D. Moore has observed that "the most remarkable and effective extensions of surgery have often not required elaborate statistical analysis for their establishment."[63] Though "often" is not equal to "regularly" or "generally," this observation invites a flexible attitude toward what H.A.F. Dudley has called the central dogma, namely "the concept of overriding need to prosecute controlled clinical trials as the only way of ensuring reliable knowledge."[64]

Fourth, there are situations in which randomized clinical trials may be both impractical and ethically dubious. The advisability of a trial is open to serious questions when "thousands of patients must be treated to establish statistically significant, but very small, differences."[63]

Fifth, randomized clinical trials may be impossible when the course of treatment for a given condition is in a state of rapid evolution. For example, the arrival of coronary artery bypass grafting led to the abandonment of a randomized clinical trial of the Vineburg surgical procedure.[57] Randomized clinical trials are perilous and dubious undertakings when innovations are likely to be rapidly replaced by even better new procedures.

Sixth, the controversy over radial keratotomy, a surgical procedure to correct myopia, has emphasized once again how difficult it is to launch controlled studies of surgical innovations after they have become popular. The standard ethical objection to randomized trials in this situation is: How can one justify withholding a widely acclaimed procedure from a control group? The radial keratotomy controversy has added another objection: How can one justify withholding business from surgeons by concentrating use of the operation to those surgeons participating in a randomized clinical trial? The lawsuit launched in the United States against George O. Waring, an associate professor of ophthalmology, and against others involved in the "Prospective Evaluation of Radial Keratotomy" trial, has intensified and hardened divisions of opinion about how surgical innovations should be brought into the health care system.[65]

Although a judgment on the justification of this particular lawsuit must be withheld, the wisdom of charging clinical researchers with conspiracy to monopolize an operation and with violation of antitrust laws, when they undertake the evaluation of a new operation for safety and efficacy, must be vigorously questioned. The good conscience of individual surgeons will never be an adequate substitute for methodologically rigorous evaluations of surgical innovations. The prospective evaluation of radial keratotomy, the PERK study, indicates that this surgical operation tends to have unpredictable outcomes. The risks have to be balanced against the small gains.[66,67]

The goal of controlled clinical trials should not be confused with any set of methodological strategies or tactics. The goal is reliable knowledge. H.A.F. Dudley has emphasized that "there is a continuous rather than a discontinuous scale of reliability, not a quantum leap from none to near total reliability."[64] The role of randomized clinical trials should be gauged against that scale and in the light of the varying constraints of different clinical situations. We are coming to a more precise identification of the circumstances in which evaluations of efficacy cannot be made with randomized prospective studies.[51,57,68] However, the recent results of the extracranial–intracranial bypass study should exercise a braking restraint on any latent enthusiasm for liberation from the rigors of controlled clinical trials.[69]

Pre-Randomization Learning and Early Randomization

Thomas C. Chalmers has advanced methodological and ethical reasons for early randomization, indeed for the randomization of the first patient, in the evaluation of new medical treatments and surgical procedures.[50,70] Succinctly, his position is: "Randomization from the beginning, with truly informed consent, is the only ethical way to begin the exploration of new therapies."[50]

Attention should be given to two methodological considerations, one supportive, the other critical of early randomization, before analyzing the ethical issue raised in the Chalmers position.

Pilot studies and prerandomization learning periods, followed by positive observations reports, increase the likelihood that methodologically rigorous evaluations of new surgical procedures will be postponed unduly or never initiated. It becomes ethically difficult to randomize patients when one of the procedures under study has already won an enthusiastic constituency, however illusory the evidence for this enthusiasm may be.[71,72] Early randomization, if practicable and successful, counters this tendency.

Early randomization may, however, be impossible or methodologically dubious in some surgical trials. Experience, technical skill, and masterful craftsmanship have to be acquired through practice. They cannot be taught and learned before an operation is actually performed. A new operation has little chance of being judged on its own merits before the surgeons performing it in a trial have acquired sufficient mastery of the procedures to permit a sufficient degree of standardization. Short of this, the same operation in the hands of different surgeons possessing quite variable levels of skill may well have quite divergent results.[73] In such circumstances, a trial would more likely measure variances in surgical craftsmanship rather than the safety and effectiveness of the new operation. Indeed, with wide variations in surgical skill, the operation under study may not be the same. Moreover, potential promising new operations for which "it takes years to reach optimum low risk and clinical benefit"[53] could be rejected, not on the basis of their real therapeutic merit, but because of initial high mortality rates due to surgeons' inexperience.

Chalmers recognizes the force of the methodological objection to very early randomization of patients in the evaluation of surgical innovations, particularly of technically difficult new operations. He has stated that "from the scientific standpoint alone, the technique should be fully developed before the randomized trial is begun."[50] Consonant with this observation, William Van der Linden has proposed a pre-randomization practice period that "should last until the participants are fully conversant with every single detail of the new technique. It is not until then that a fair trial can be run."[62]

The Chalmers position holds that running a fair trial can be in conflict with running an ethical trial. Though prerandomization practice periods would set the stage for a more reliable comparison of a new against an established operation, Chalmers observes that patients honestly informed about the potentially higher initial mortality or morbidity rates, to be expected during this period, would likely refuse to enter this surgical novitiate and demand the established operation.[50] He argues that randomization from the beginning, with truly informed consent, is the only ethical way to evaluate new operations because patients are more likely to accept randomization if they are convinced that there is "an equal chance that the new operation might be better than the old from the beginning."[50]

The Chalmers exclusive position on the ethical superiority of very early randomization is not convincing. The fact that a new operation has a good chance of being superior to an older established surgical treatment must be modified by the word "eventually." The potential intrinsic merits of a new operation, once mastered, are not an antidote to the risks of potentially higher mortality or morbidity resulting from surgeons' underdeveloped skills in performing the new procedures. Lawrence Bonchek's observation and counterquestion are in order: "Randomization does not alter operative risk; it simply dictates that chance, not the patient, will determine exposure to the risk. Is such an arrangement more ethical?"[49] The real ethical issue is whether patients know about, and freely assume, the risks of new operations.

Informing Patients About Randomization: Conflicting Views

Do the ethical principles requiring informed, comprehending, and voluntary consent necessitate telling patients how their treatments are selected in randomized clinical trials?

The ethical justifiability of randomization does not hinge only on physician "indifference" to the treatments. Equipoise of outcome of different treatments, whether apparent only at the beginning of a trial or increasingly evident as the trial progresses, does not justify the inference that patients will be, or ought to be, "indifferent" about the treatment they will receive.[74] Physician–investigator uncertainty about the relative merits of alternative treatments does not mean that patient preference for one treatment over another is necessarily, or even generally, "capricious."[75] The treatments in a trial may exert significantly different impacts on patients' quality of life and life plans, whatever the initial state of knowledge or the eventual statistical results of the trial may be.

The management of breast cancer and cancer of the prostate are two clinical trial situations for which the following conclusion is entirely appropriate: "It is not enough for the physician to have no reason to prefer one treatment over the other, in addition, there must be no reason for the patient to prefer one treatment."[74]

The harm–benefit ratio is a resultant of balancing multiple factors that must include effects that patients consider personally important. Reducing the ratio to the "hard" variables the trial is designed to measure can easily amount to a disregard of a patient's particular situation. Physician–investigators are not ethically justified in perceiving and treating patients exclusively as representatives of a given disease category. It is methodologically and ethically important that surgeon–investigators pay close attention to patient–subjects' unique personal differences. Good ethics and good science demand precisely that everybody not be treated alike in consent negotiations.[77,78]

Lack of candor about randomization, and the associated additional concealments of information this would often entail, can constitute an act that bars patients from what they need to know to make the choices they consider to be the most important for their lives. This is ethically unjustifiable in a trial that would otherwise be ethically acceptable. As a rule, patients should be informed about randomization. Justifiable exceptions will have to be justified. A generalization of such exceptions could arise when the differential impact on patients' lives are perceived, by patients and surgeons alike, as being just as important as the treatments' initial putative equality of outcome. In such situations, surgeons may be no less deterred from enrolling otherwise eligible candidates into a trial than the patients themselves are from participating.

The National Surgical Adjuvant Project for Breast and Bowel Cancer (NSABP) trial to compare the relative effectiveness of total and segmental mastectomy, with and without radiation, presents a challenging illustration of these difficulties[79] (see Chapter 29).

Harmonizing a surgeon's responsibilities, as physician, with his or her duties as clinical investigator may be easier in word and in theory than it frequently is in act and practice. The U.K. Cancer Research Campaign Working Party in Breast Conservation has noted: "It is one thing to admit doubt among one's colleagues, quite another to have to admit it to a patient."[35] The need to confess to patients that chance, not their surgeon, is in charge of selecting their treatment is at least as difficult as admitting uncertainty or ignorance. These admissions do require "mental gymnastics beyond the abilities of many,"[80,81] surgeons as well as patients. Admittedly, this is not the way surgeons traditionally behave towards their patients in normal practice. Whether behavior in normal practice should be the norm for clinical research or vice versa is a question meriting its own discussion.

Enrolling patients into randomized surgical trials without their knowledge and consent is not an answer to these and other difficulties surgeons experience with the process of randomization. Randomizing patients to treatment groups before initiating consent negotiations seems to alleviate the difficulty surgeons have when asking patients to participate in a trial without being able to tell them what treatment they will receive. Prerandomization designs are less problematic ethically when all patient candidates, those assigned by chance to standard therapy and those similarly assigned to innovative therapy, are involved in consent negotiations. It is unethical to conduct a trial when some of the patient-subjects are totally unaware of the research process in which they have been enrolled and quite unaware of the alternative treatments they might have preferred.

Involving all patient-subjects in consent negotiations does not, however, directly guarantee that prerandomization designs are ethically innocuous. Even if patients are told that their treatment has been selected by chance—and they should be told—the way in which the advantages and drawbacks of the alternative treatments are presented can amount to tender but real coercion.[82] The voluntary, if not the informed, character of consent may be jeopardized by a linguistic tailoring of information that manipulates the patient's will without blinding the patient's intellect.

It should be emphasized that this danger is not peculiar to randomized clinical trials, whatever the randomization tactic may be. The danger is equal or greater when a surgeon, who is not participating in a trial, convincingly presents one of several alternative treatments under study in a trial, elsewhere, as the best "in my judgment." This situation is the target of the U.K. Working Party's fifth practical proposal:

> Those doctors who treat patients with cancer but do not participate in randomized clinical trials should realize that they too have an obligation to discuss alternative forms of treatment with their patients. In our view the fact that they are not formally randomizing their patients does not reduce their obligation in this respect."[35]

This proposal suggests a return to the point mentioned earlier about norms of surgeon behavior toward patients in routine practice as contrasted with randomized surgical trials. Some respondents to the investigation of surgeons' reasons for not enrolling patients into the NSABP trial of treatments for breast cancer "believed that participating in a clinical trial would necessitate a major change in the traditional physician-patient interaction."[79] Some changes in that relationship, motivated or necessitated by participation in randomized surgical trials, may be highly desirable, meriting introduction into routine surgical practice. Dropping the guise of sapiential authority, when the state of clinical knowledge offers no warrant for such an assumption of power, may advance the education of patient expectations, bolster patient autonomy, and, paradoxically, strengthen the trust of patients in their physicians.

Human Studies Permission: Some Practical Points

Perhaps the most important practical point for the potential surgical investigator is to take human studies permission seriously. The present climate, and the requirements for appropriate treatment of other human beings, make it mandatory that human studies forms be filled out honestly and accurately. For purposes of this discussion, the human studies form of the Brigham and Women's Hospital in Boston will be used as a guideline. At this hospital, all protocols involving human tissue or subjects are reviewed by a research committee that meets twice a month. Four categories of information are required:

1. General information, including the name of the investigator and the department, the date of beginning and ending the study, and the co-investigators.
2. Funding information, specifically whether there are costs not covered by outside research funds or third party payers.
3. Patient-subject information, including the total number of subjects, the facilities required (inpatient, outpatient, or clinical research center), potential use of special groups (children, newborns, fetuses, medical students, the mentally handicapped, pregnant women, prisoners, or adolescents), duration of study for individual subjects, remuneration, and the use of drugs, radioactive materials, medical devices, nursing services or dietetic services.
4. A description of the research and training project.

The fourth category probably has the greatest import because it essentially justifies the project for human studies. It begins with a statement of the general purpose of the research and the specific hypothesis to be tested. It moves then to the proposed experimental procedures, including background information, number of subjects to be involved in the study, procedures and methodologies to be used, names and details of medications, and the use of data to test the proposed hypotheses. The next section documents stresses or aggravation of "chemical, physical, biological, psychological, and other nature" and the investigators' experience in this kind of research. There follows a listing of possible benefits or advantages to the individual patient or society, and potential discomfort or risks. (A risk is defined here as exposure to "the possibility of any harm, physical, psychological, sociological or other as a consequence of any activity which goes beyond the application of those established and accepted methods necessary to meet the patient's needs.")

The application must describe the manner in which patients will be recruited and informed consent will be obtained, appropriate alternative procedures, provisions made to answer patient inquiries, measures taken to ensure that involved subjects will be free to omit specific procedures, and changes in experimental design that might be necessary to complete the formal information portion.

The informed consent form lies at the heart of the study. The consent form should have the following elements in it: the purpose of the study, procedures to be used, risks and discomfort, benefits, alternative procedures, standard release form, confidentiality of information, a compensational clause, and option to withdraw.

The study's goals should be clearly stated at the beginning. The section on procedures should include a description of how the proposed procedures differ from standard care, the duration of the subject's participation, the details of the procedure to be used, and any compensation for participation.

Risks, discomforts, and benefits should include direct benefits to the patient and any risks he or she might run. Alternative procedures should be discussed, and the availability of the physician in charge to answer inquiries should be emphasized. Assurance should be given that information will be kept confidential. It should be stated that the subject will not be compensated for injuries occurring and that he or she is free to withdraw at any time. Finally, there should be a statement that the procedure has been explained.

At our institution, the range of potential investigative procedures is rather wide. Blood drawing for purposes of doing blood testing; chart reviews; use of nursing services, women, prisoners, or adolescents; duration of study; and the use of discarded material are all part of human experimentation and must be proposed and justified. Special information is required for drug data, isotopes, and nursing services. Short forms, to expedite processing, are available for human discarded material and for record reviews.

These requirements may seem onerous, but they ensure that the patient is not abused.

Conclusion

The opening quotation was a surgeon's warning to fellow surgeons about the danger of acting without reflecting. A number of matters to which surgeon-investigators should give primary attention in planning and conducting clinical trials have been discussed, but there are many other issues that are just as important.

The most prominent of these issues might be: the just distribution of burdens and benefits in the selection of patients as candidates for clinical trials; compensation for subjects injured in clinical trials; the requirements of clinical investigators' collaboration with institutional review boards or research ethics committees; the ethical conditions for terminating a controlled study; and the ethical dilemma of releasing interim results during the course of a randomized clinical trial (see also Section I, Chapter 1). The discussion of these matters requires far more than the space that can be reasonably allocated to this chapter. The principle adopted was to offer in-depth discussion of the questions distinctively important for surgical trials rather than to attempt a more superficial treatment of many issues, however germane they may be to all clinical trials.

References

1. Folkman J. Surgical research: a contradiction in terms? J Surg Res 1984;36:298.
2. Pellegrino ED. The anatomy of clinical judgments; some notes on right reason and right action. In: Clinical Judgment: A Critical Appraisal, Engelhardt H, Tristram Jr, Spicker SF, Towers B, eds. Dordrecht-London-Boston: Reidel, 1979:169–195.
3. Bankowski Z, Howard-Jones N. Human Experimentation and Medical Ethics. Geneva: CIOMS, 1982.
4. Beecher HK. Research and the Individual. Boston: Little, Brown, 1970.
5. Freund PA, ed., Experimentation with Human Subjects. New York: Braziller, 1970.
6. Gray BH. Human Subjects in Medical Experimentation. New York: Wiley, 1975.
7. Katz J. Experimentation with Human Beings. New York: Russell Sage Foundation, 1972.
8. Levine R. Ethics and Regulation of Clinical Research. Baltimore–Munich: Urban & Schwarzenberg, 1981.
9. Shapiro SH, Louis TA, eds. Clinical Trials. New York: Dekker, 1983.
10. WHO and CIOMS. Proposed International Guidelines for Biomedical Research Involving Human Subjects. Geneva: CIOMS 1982.
11. Sackett DL. Bias in analytic research. J Chronic Dis 1979;32–60.
12. Toulmin S. How medicine saved the life of ethics. Perspect Biol Med 1982;25:736–50.
13. Fried C. Medical Experimentation. Amsterdam: North Holland, 1974;151:101–4.
14. Green FHK. Quoted by Jackson DM. Moral responsibility in clinical research. Lancet, 1958;1:903. This reference comes from Feinstein AR. Clinical biostatistics: XXV1. Medical ethics and the architecture of clinical research. Clin Pharmacol Ther 1974;15:320.
15. Gilbert JP, McPeek B, Mosteller F. Statistics and ethics in surgery and anesthesia. Science 1977;198: 684–89.
16. Silverman WA. The lesson of retrolental fibroplasia. Sci Am 1977;236:100–7.
17. Bernard C. An Introduction to the Study of Experimental Medicine, Greene HC, transl.:Henry Schuman, 1949:101–261.
18. Engelhardt HT Jr. Bioethics in the People's Republic of China. Hast Center Rept 1980;10:8.
19. The Nuremberg Code. Trials of war criminals before the Nuremberg military tribunals under control council law, no. 10, vol 2. Washington, DC: Government Printing Office, 1949;181–82. Reprinted as Appendix 3 in Ethics and Regulation of Clinical Research.[8]
20. World Medical Association Declaration of Helsinki: Recommendations guiding medical doctors in biomedical research involving human subjects. Reprinted as Appendix 4 in Ethics and Regulation of Clinical Research.[8]
21. Anderston WF, Fletcher JC. Gene therapy in human beings: when is it ethical to begin? N Engl J Med 1980;303:1293–97.
22. Cline MJ, Mercola KE. The potential of inserting new genetic information. N Engl J Med 1980;303: 1297–1300.
23. Editorial. Gene therapy: how ripe the time? Lancet 1981;1:196–97.
24. Grobstein C, Flower M. Gene therapy: proceed with caution. Hastings Center Rept 1984;14:13–17.
25. Wade N. UCLA. Gene therapy racked by friendly fire. Science 1980;210:509–11.
26. Rutstein DD. The ethical design of human experiments. In: Experimentation with human subjects, Freund A, ed. New York: Braziller, 1970:383–401.
27. Sackett DL. The competing objectives of randomized trials. N Engl J Med 1980;303:1059–60.
28. Frederickson DS. Welcoming remarks, national conferences in clinical trials methodology. Clin Pharmacol Ther 1979;25:630–31.
29. Zelen M. A new design for randomized clinical trials. N Engl J Med 1979;300:1242–45.
30. Feinstein AR. An additional basic science for clinical medicine: I. The constraining fundamental paradigms. Ann Intern Med 1983;99:393–97.
31. Feinstein AR. An additional basic science for clinical medicine: IV. The development of clinimetrics. Ann Intern Med 1983;99:843–48.
32. Woodward FP. Informed consent of volunteers: a direct measurement of comprehension and retention of information. Clin Res 1979;27:248–52.
33. Dickens BM. The modern law on informed consent. Mod Med Can 1982;37:706–10.
34. Reibl v. Hughes. 1980;2 S.C.R.:882.
35. Cancer Research Campaign Working Party on Breast Conservation. Informed consent: ethical, legal and medical implications for doctors and patients who participate in randomized clinical trials. Br Med J 1983;286:1117–21.
36. Beecher HK. Ethics and clinical research. N Engl J Med 1966;274:1354–60.
37. Jonsen AR. Do no harm. Ann Intern Med 1978;88: 827–32.
38. Feinstein AR. Clinical biostatics: XLI. Hard science, soft data, and the challenges of choosing clinical variables in research. Clin Pharmacol Ther 1977;22:485–98.
39. Feinstein AR. Clinical biostatistics: XXVI, Medical ethics and the architecture of clinical research. Clin Pharmacol Ther 1974;15:316–34.
40. Dresser R. Book reviews: In: Scientific Perspectives on Animal Welfare, Dodds WJ, Barbara F, Orlans, eds. 1982, New York: Academic Press, 1982. Also in J Med Philos 1984;9:423–25.

41. Naverson J. Animal Rights. Can J Phil 1977;vii: 161–78.
42. Regan T, Singer P. Animal Rights and Human Obligations. Englewood Cliffs, NJ: Prentice Hall, 1976.
43. Rowan AN, Rollin BE. Animal research—for and against; a philosophical, social, and historical perspective. Perspect Biol Med 1983;27:1–17.
44. Singer P. Animal Liberation. New York. Random House, 1975.
45. McIntosh A. Animal rights and medical research. Future Health, Winter 1985:10–11.
46. Editorial. Animal experiments. Br Med J 1982;284: 368–69.
47. Lane-Petter W. The place and importance of the experimental animal in research. Proc R Soc Med 1972;65:343–44.
48. Russell JC, Secord DC. Holy dogs and the laboratory; some Canadian experiences with animal research. Perspect Biol Med 1985;28:374–81.
49. Bonchek LI. Are randomized trials appropriate for evaluation new operations? N Engl J Med 1979; 301:44–45.
50. Chalmers TC. Randomized clinical trials in surgery. In: Controversy in Surgery, Varco RL, Delaney JP, eds. Philadelphia: Saunders, 1976:3–11.
51. Feinstein AR. The scientific and clinical tribulations of randomized clinical trials. Clin Res 1978; 26:241–44.
52. Haines SJ. Randomized clinical trials in the evaluation of surgical innovation. J Neurosurg 1979;51:5–11.
53. Loop FD. A surgeon's view of randomized prospective studies. J Thorac Cardiovasc Surg 1979;78:161–65.
54. Spodick DH. Randomized controlled clinical trials. The behavioral case. JAMA 1982;247:2258–60.
55. Spodick DH et al. Standards for surgical trials. Ann Thorac Surg 1979;27:284.
56. Van der Linden W. On the generalization of surgical trials results. Acta Chir Scand 1980;146:229–34.
57. Feinstein AR. An additional basic science for clinical medicine. II. The limitations of randomized trials. Ann Intern Med 1983;99:544–50.
58. Feinstein AR. An additional basic science for clinical medicine. III. The challenges of comparison and measurements. Ann Intern Med 1983;99:705–12.
59. Fisher LD, Kennedy JW. Randomized surgical clinical trials for treatment of coronary artery disease. Controlled Clin Trials 1982;3:235–58.
60. Merlo G. Surgical trial: possibilities and objections. Eur Surg Res 1984;16:1–4.
61. Editorial. Blindness in surgical trials. Lancet 1980; i:1229–30.
62. Van der Linden W. Pitfalls in randomized surgical trials. Surgery 1980;87:258–62.
63. Moore FD. Perspectives, surgery. Perspect Biol Med 1982;25:698–720.
64. Dudley HAF. The controlled clinical trial and the advance of reliable knowledge: an outsider looks in. Br Med J 1983;237:957–60.
65. Norman C. Clinical trial stirs legal battles. Science 1985;227:1316–18.
66. Waring GO, Lynn MJ, Fielding B, et al. Results of the prospective evaluation of radial keratotomy (PERK) Study 4 years after surgery for myopia. JAMA 1990;263:1083–91.
67. Editorial. Radial keratotomy. Lancet 1990;335: 1131–32.
68. Fyfe IM. The randomized clinical trial: panacea or placebo? Can Med Assoc J 1984;131:1336–39.
69. EC/IC Bypass Study Group. Failure of extracranial-intracranial arterial bypass to reduce the risk of ischemic stroke: results of an international randomized trial. N Engl J Med 1985;313:1191–1200.
70. Spodick DH. Randomize the first patient: scientific, ethical, and behavioral bases. Am J Cardiol 1983; 51:916–17.
71. Editorial. Managing severe head injury—doing more and faring worse? Lancet 1980:i:1229.
72. McKinlay JB. From promising report to standard procedure: seven stages in the career of a medical innovation. Milbank Mem 1981;59:374–411.
73. Feilding LP, et al. Surgeon-related variables and the clinical trial. Lancet 1978;ii:778–9.
74. Hill Sir Austin Bradford. Medical ethics and controlled trials. Br Med J 1963;I:1043–49.
75. Esenberg L. The social imperatives of medical research. Science 1977;198:1105–10.
76. Angell M. Patients' preference in randomized clinical trials. N Engl J Med 1984;310:1385–87.
77. Brewin TB. Consent to randomized treatment. Lancet 1982;ii:919–21.
78. Sade RM, Miller III, Clinton M. Letter. N Engl J Med 1983;308:344.
79. Taylor K, Margolese RG, Soskolne CL. Physicians' reasons for not entering eligible patients in a randomized clinical trial of adjuvant surgery for breast cancer. N Engl J Med 1984;310:1363–67.
80. Dudley HAF. Informed consent in surgical trials. Br Med J 1984;289:937–8.
81. Editorial. Consent: how informed? Lancet 1984;i: 1445–47.
82. Ellenberg SS. Randomization designs in comparative clinical trials. N Engl J Med 1984;310:1404–8.

13

Selected Nonexperimental Methods: An Orientation

W.O. Spitzer and S.M. Horwitz

Clinical investigators and members of interdisciplinary research teams may often find that they must employ nonexperimental strategies characteristically used by epidemiologists and biostatisticians, particularly when randomized controlled trials (RCTs) are not ethically or practically feasible. These designs are used less frequently than controlled trials in surgical and anesthesia research. This chapter is intended as an orientation for those who seek meaningful and knowledgeable partnership in clinical and epidemiologic research. The bibliography will assist those who wish to pursue an in-depth understanding of the strategies presented here.

Uncontrolled case studies and case series have been mentioned in this textbook. Such efforts are indispensable precursors to good clinical and epidemiological research. However, the role of such work should be restricted to *hypothesis generation*, except when findings are dramatic. The discovery that penicillin could cure hitherto consistently incurable disorders was so striking that controlled studies and inferential statistics became unnecessary. Such dramatic advances in any field of medicine are, however, the exception rather than the rule. Characteristically, advances in clinical science are small, and progress is incremental. Improvements can be so subtle that the changes must be demonstrated carefully with the best attainable rigor of design and the highest sophistication of appropriate statistics. Admissible rules of scientific logic must be followed.

One of the key rules is that research questions or hypotheses are tested only after they have been set forth in advance, not through fishing expeditions in existing data or even data-dredging of information we may have gathered ourselves. It is important to generate hypotheses, but it is essential to test them following an explicit protocol, written and evaluated according to principles that assess the extent to which the results support a causal association.

Association Is Not Necessarily Causation

All clinicians must constantly remind themselves that association does not mean causation. Ordinarily, we can develop truly convincing evidence for causation only through experimental approaches. The strongest and most reliable evidence for cause and effect is the randomized controlled trial. Without evidence from such trials, the determination of whether an association is a causal one becomes more problematic. Sir Austin Bradford Hill suggests the consideration of nine features in looking at associations between factors and outcomes when the evidence is derived from nonexperimental methods. If many of these features are present, we are more secure in postulating causation.

Hill put the *strength of the association* first on the list. If the exposed population shows the outcome variable in a very marked degree, we are much more comfortable in inferring causation. High odds or risk ratios mean a strong association. Of course, we are sometimes misled. A very strong association between two factors may be just that, a strong association and not cause and effect.

Next on Hill's list of features to be considered in attributing causation is *consistency* of the observed association. The connection between smoking and lung cancer has been repeatedly observed by different workers in different countries using quite different populations over many years. Hill places great weight on similar results reached from quite different designs. He finds this much more convincing than similar results from a collection of similarly designed studies. We know in medicine and surgery that very weakly designed studies all pointing in the same direction have led us to assume causation when, in fact, the consistency of association was merely the repetition of a mistake.

Hill's third characteristic is the *specificity of the association*. If the association is unusual, if it is limited to specifically exposed persons who develop unusual outcomes, this is a strong argument in favor of causation. The peculiar form of deformity in newborns produced by exposure of pregnant women to thalidomide and the association between acquired immune deficiency syndrome and very rare Kaposi sarcomas are recent examples of this characteristic.

The fourth factor Hill considers is the *temporal relationship of the observed association*. An inference of causation is severely undermined when the effect appears before the cause. In the epidemics of Minamata disease seen in several parts of the world a few years ago, the emission of organic mercury toxic wastes preceded the great increase of reported cases of the neurological disorder.

As a fifth factor, Hill looks for an association that reveals a *dose-response curve or a biological gradient*. For example, those who smoke more cigarettes have higher death rates from smoking than both nonsmokers and those who smoke but a few cigarettes. A reverse gradient, such as a decreasing incidence of cancer of the lung among former smokers, is particularly persuasive.

The sixth feature Hill looks for is *biological plausibility*. If the association seems to make no sense at all, as in a relationship between the number of Presbyterian ministers in Scotland and the increasing population of Chicago, Hill suggests that we should be cautious in inferring causation. However, as we learn more and more about biology, associations that once made no sense become biologically plausible. When Professor Oliver Wendell Holmes of the Harvard Medical School drew attention, in 1847, to the association between the hand-washing habits of obstetrical surgeons and the incidence of puerperal fever among the mothers they attended, no one paid much attention because people could see no biological plausibility in the association. Twenty years later, after the work of Pasteur and Lister, the association acquired biological plausibility.

Hill's seventh factor is *coherence of the evidence*. Hill says that a cause and effect interpretation of an association should not seriously conflict with the generally known facts of the natural history and biology of the disease studied. Hill points out that the association of lung cancer and cigarette smoking is coherent with the increase in smoking among men that took place between 1910 and 1920 and the later increase among women. The isolation of carcinogenic factors from cigarette smoke and the histopathologic evidence of irritation of the airway epithelium of heavy smokers lends further evidence of coherence.

For his eighth factor, Hill asks if the *trends are reversible*. When the government withdrew the suspect pharmaceutical from the market, did reported cases of phocomelia fall? When smokers stop using cigarettes, do the rates at which they develop lung cancer fall? We call this evidence of reversibility.

Finally, as a ninth factor, Hill suggests we look for *analogies*. After having discovered a drug effect of thalidomide on fetuses, we are readier to accept somewhat similar evidence that another drug might cause fetal defects.

None of the nine factors brings indisputable evidence for or against a cause and effect hypothesis. Nevertheless, they do, with greater or lesser strength, suggest instances when an association may be one of causation.

For causation we prefer to have the evidence of a soundly conceived and well-executed experiment—one that employs the strengthening factors of random allocation to treatment and appropriate varieties of blindness on the part of the experimenter, the patient, the evaluator of the outcome and, perhaps, the statistician who analyzes the data. Employing strengthening factors such as random allocation and blindness is no more an aspersion on the honesty of experimenters than requiring rubber gloves is a comment on the personal hygiene of surgeons.

Ascribing causation is serious business. The best advice about drawing conclusions on cause and effect from nonexperimental designs is to invoke Bradford Hill's criteria judiciously and to interpret the relationships carefully.

Experimental Versus Nonexperimental Designs

An experimental design is one in which one group of eligible subjects or patients exposed to an intervention or a maneuver is compared to one or more control groups comparable to the intervention groups in all respects, save for the intervention or maneuver of interest. *The first essential characteristic of an experiment is that the intervention or the maneuver is assigned by the investigator to the exposed group and that the comparison interventions or maneuvers (e.g., placebo or the best accepted current therapy) are also assigned by the investigator to the control group or control groups.*

To express it another way, the assignment of the *maneuvers is under the control of the investigator.*

The second essential characteristic of an experiment is that assignment of subjects to the control and experimental groups be done by systematic, prespecified means presumed to guarantee the assembly of two absolutely comparable groups except for the effects of the maneuver of interest. Generally, an investigator chooses to assign subjects to the intervention and control groups randomly, assuming that, with a large sample size, random assignment will evenly distribute unmeasured potential risk factors. However, experimental and control group assignment may be done in a systematic fashion by other preselected means, such as alternate assignment rules like odd–even hospital file numbers.

In our current understanding of clinical science, the experiment that is an RCT is the "gold standard" of research. In their chapter on clinical research, Walters and Sackett discuss the advantages of the randomized and controlled approach for the assessment of effectiveness (see Section III, Chapter 24). Yet no matter how well designed, these RCTs are not without problems due to human error, human folly, and chance. RCTs are difficult to carry out, must often sacrifice internal validity for generalizability, and evaluate clinical maneuvers only under optimal circumstances, as opposed to conditions approximating usual clinical care.

Designs belonging to a group in which random assignment of subjects is not possible, although investigator control over the assignment of the clinical maneuver is maintained, are called subexperimental (a term used by Walters and Sackett) or quasi-experimental (a term borrowed from the social sciences). These designs can employ one group or multiple groups. In the one-group design, the comparison of interest is the outcome variable before and after the application of the intervention. Consider all eligible drivers in the state of Victoria, Australia, as a group; for the intervention of interest, take the introduction of compulsory use of seatbelts while driving. Given that it is possible to determine the number of injuries entailing death or physical injury to drivers and passengers per 100,000 persons "exposed to automobile transport," you could conduct a "before and after study." You could determine the number of injuries in the exposed citizens of that state, within certain age groups, for the full year prior to the new law. With the same determinations for one full year after the law came into effect, you could see whether there was any difference in rates. If the change (presumably a drop) is truly dramatic, you may not need comparison cohorts or concurrent experimental trials of any kind.

When before and after studies must be done, the design is strengthened by having several sequential measurements before the event or "independent variable" of interest, and several measures after. In the seatbelt example, suppose you had taken measures for odd-numbered years for a decade *before* the introduction of the law, and suppose further that the rates of identically classified and measured injuries were stable. If you made the same ascertainments for a decade *after* the introduction of the new law in odd years, and there was a stable *sustained* new lower level, your conclusions about the relationship between the new law and the prevention of accidents and death would be greatly strengthened. If you are doing before and after studies, seek every opportunity to have at least two before measures and two after measures. A "step down" or "step up" of the measurement in the dependent variables coinciding with the "treatment" or exposure to the independent variable is a much stronger set of data on which to base conclusions on association.

If a "before and after" study does not give convincing evidence of change, you should be very cautious in interpreting the results, even if you have several before and after determinations. Other factors (confounders or effect modifiers) could have been operating at the same time. The price of gasoline might have changed, driving habits might have altered, or other laws setting lower speed limits might have affected the rate of accidents. It then becomes important to attempt additional before and after studies, historically or concurrently, in other jurisdictions (multiple group comparisons). The replications can be helpful in elucidating the confounding or effect-modifying impact of unrelated factors.

Designs that incorporate neither random allocation nor investigator assignment of the maneuver of interest are called observational or nonexperimental designs, even if two or more groups of study patients are compared. The balance of this chapter will introduce you to the major types of nonexperimental design, but our discussion of them will not be exhaustive. Many variations of these basic designs exist, and our brief orientation provides only a basic road map for this territory of research methodology. We have organized our discussion of nonexperimental designs according to the Canadian Task Force on the Periodic Health Examination[1] hierarchy of evidence: cohorts, case-control studies, cross-sectional research, and ecologic studies. Uncontrolled case studies and case reports will not be considered further.

Before detailing specific designs, we need to introduce a number of concepts that are important to keep in mind when digesting methodologic material. The first is the purpose of the study to be undertaken. Are we simply describing the state of affairs (i.e., a *descriptive* study) or are we generating information about the relationship of particular factors to a disease (i.e., an *analytic* study)? We generally undertake descriptive studies when we know little about the determinants of disease or its natural history. Descriptive studies provide us with basic information about the disease or condition of interest and help us generate specific hypotheses about possible etiologic agents.

The second issue is the direction of the study design with respect to the potentially related factor and the outcome of interest. Are we observing a group of individuals at a defined point in time, gathering detailed information on the etiologic agents of interest and following these individuals *forward* in time, concurrently, to determine disease status? Or, are we assembling a group of individuals with the disease of interest, a second group of individuals without the target disease, and pursuing the information backward with *backward* logic? Finally, are we measuring both etiologic agents and disease at the *same* point in time (cross-sectional)?

Another issue to consider is the unit of observation. Are we measuring our targeted features in individuals, in small groups (e.g., a family), or in larger groups (e.g., countries)? In most medical and surgical studies, the individual is the unit of observation. Further details for subsections of these observational designs can be found in Chapters 10, 15, 19, 24, and 29.

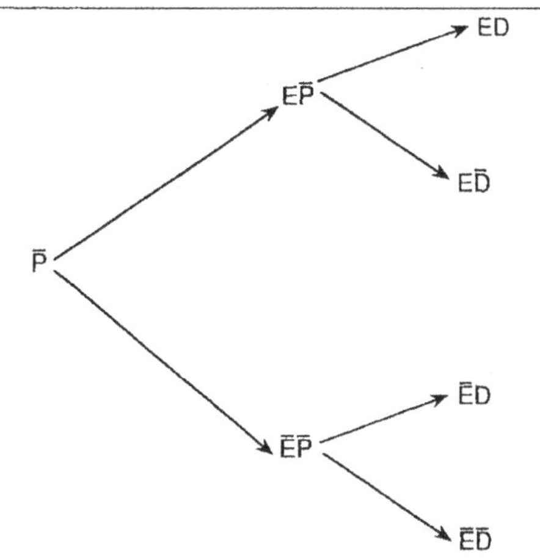

$\bar{P}$ = study population of interest, usually some group of individuals without the disease of interest, some proportion of whom will become exposed to the agent of interest.

E = exposed, $\bar{E}$ = not exposed

D = diseased, $\bar{D}$ = not diseased

FIGURE 13.1. A cohort study.

Cohorts

The Latin word *cohort* was a Roman military term. It referred to a group of soldiers of a certain category. It could have been 100 or 500 infantrymen, 500 cavalry warriors, etc. The first and most important use of "cohort" in clinical and epidemiologic research is to designate a number of persons (patients or healthy individuals) who share common attributes considered to be relevant to the research questions at issue. It could be 500 persons, 20–49 years old, experiencing a first incidence of low back pain, who have no clinically objective signs of neurological deficit. The cohort could be 10,000 diabetics 50–79 years old, eligible for inclusion by definite criteria and unaffected by peripheral vascular complications. It could be 25 one-week survivors of liver transplants, aged 13 to 60 months.

Sometimes the only intervention or maneuver of interest in studying a cohort is the passage of time. Thus, for the diabetics unaffected by peripheral vascular complications, one might wish to discover how many complications affect that *population* of diabetics over a 5-year period, stratified by age in half-decades. Or, a new drug to delay or prevent peripheral vascular complications may have been introduced into the market. A study might then determine the rate of development of such complications in a cohort of persons prone to peripheral vascular disorders and using the drug.

For any cohort, it is important to decide in advance what the dependent variable or the target outcome will be. The outcome events become the numerators for rates (such as incidence) calculated in cohort studies. For survivors of liver transplants, the dependent variable or target outcome might be death. For a cohort of patients with osteosarcoma, it might be length of disability-free survival. For a cohort of women with indwelling urinary catheters, it might be new infections in the postoperative period. The fundamental characteristic of the cohort is that the study subjects are identified and delineated by explicit criteria *before* the declared target outcome or dependent variable of interest is manifest among the same subjects. Cohorts are denominators for target outcomes. The target outcomes or dependent variables are the numerators. *In cohort studies, the denominators are always identified and delineated before the dependent variables are observed.* That is why cohort studies are sometimes called follow-up studies.

Cohorts may be followed in time as a single group without making any comparisons with any other group. Such work is referred to as descriptive. Figure 13.1 diagrams the basic structure of

TABLE 13.1. Data layout for a prospective cohort study.

		Disease status		
		D	$\bar{D}$	Totals
Exposure status	E	a	b	$a + b$
	$\bar{E}$	c	d	$c + d$
	Totals	$a + c$	$b + d$	$(a + b) + (c + d)$

disease among exposed = $a/(a + b)$
disease among unexposed = $c/(c + d)$

$$\text{relative risk} = \frac{a/(a + b)}{c/(c + d)}$$

a classical cohort design. Notice that the direction of the study is forward and the unit of analysis is the individual.

Table 13.1 shows the data layout for the analysis of a cohort. Individuals' exposure status is on the left-hand side and follow-up disease status is across the top of the table. To determine whether those exposed to the putative agent of interest—for instance, amount of caffeinated beverages consumed daily by a cohort of 40- to 60-year-old men and women, who develop the targeted outcome (gallbladder disease)—we use the ratio of those diseased among caffeine consumers $[a/(a + b)]$ divided by the ratio of those diseased among the nonconsumers $[c/(c + d)]$. The resulting measure, the *relative risk* or *risk ratio*, gives us an idea of the association of caffeinated beverages with gallbladder disease. If this ratio is greater than one, we usually say that the putative agent is associated with an increased risk of disease. If the ratio is less than one, we say it is associated with a decreased risk of disease or it is a protective factor. In Chapter 15 on clinical biostatistics, Kramer presents additional analytic methods appropriate for use with categorical outcome measures.

Sometimes it is possible to compare two or more cohorts and follow them simultaneously. For instance, it may be possible to assemble 20,000 men who become exposed to occupationally related radiation in nuclear plants starting in 1971, and continue to be exposed, and follow them to determine the total number of new cancers detected through 1995. This could be done at the same time as one follows another 20,000 men in other energy-related industries, similar in most respects to nuclear power generating plants, except for the exposure to measured levels of radiation in the workplace. This second cohort of 20,000 men assembled in 1971 would also be followed through 1995. Note why this is not an experimental design. The investigator did not assign the men to be or not to be exposed to radiation, or to be or not to be in one type of industry or another. *The men self-selected their own jobs*. However, it can and should be established that the two self-selected cohorts are sufficiently comparable to follow them forward in time and compare the rate of development of new cancers between two groups. With two or more groups, we have a cohort comparison study. It is worth emphasizing that all 40,000 men, the 20,000 exposed and the 20,000 not exposed, were free of the target outcome of interest (cancer) *at the time the cohort was assembled in 1971*.

One of the main disadvantages of cohort studies is that they generally require a very large number of subjects in the denominator so that meaningful numerators can emerge as dependent variables. That is not true in certain clinically oriented studies (e.g., liver transplant studies, where the outcomes of interest are not rare). The precision of the answers depends greatly on the size of the numerator. Also, cohort studies sometimes require long follow-up with all the consequent problems of logistics, the most important one being losses to follow-up.

One frequently used strategy in cohort studies, which gets around the disadvantage of many years of waiting to ascertain outcomes in cohorts assembled according to exposure criteria, is to do a historical cohort. An investigator studying cancers among cohorts of workers assembled in 1971, in conventional and nuclear plants, could have started the work in 1986. The pursuit of the data is *still forward*, from 1971 to 1995, but the investigator has gone backward in time for 15 of the 25 years. The method is partly historical and partly concurrent.

If the investigator had fielded this work in 1995, following the workers from 1971 through 1995, the entire project would have been a historical cohort study. We emphasize, however, that a historical cohort, even when implemented historically, is *prospective* in common terminology, because the pursuit of the data is forward. Other cohort studies that we designate concurrent also pursue the data forward but, from the present to the future. They are also classified as *prospective*, conventionally, but this use of the term "prospective" to qualify cohort studies is ambiguous and confusing. It is also not useful as a qualifier of randomized controlled trials. RCTs are always prospective.

Case-Referent or Case-Control Studies

The distinct feature of the case-referent or case-control study, as it is commonly called, is that the two groups compared, the group of *cases* and the *subjects from the referent group* (i.e., controls) are

FIGURE 13.2. The case-referent/case-control study.

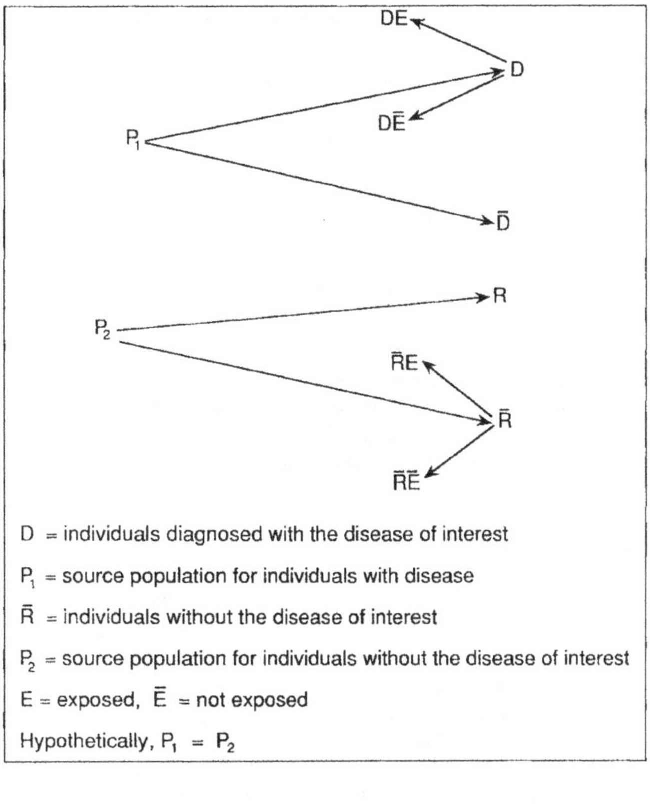

identified with reference to the presence or absence of the target outcome of interest, usually incident cases of disease. Characteristically, you obtain information on outcomes and exposure at the same time. You then determine, in each of the two groups of patients compared, how frequently a prior exposure of interest occurred.

You might, for instance, take 400 neonates with meningomyelocele from among a group of university childrens' hospitals and compare them to a second reference group of 400 very young children, matched by age, who were referred to the same hospitals for management of severe trauma.

The question of your project is whether exposure of the mother to a particular garden herbicide during pregnancy might be associated with development of meningomyelocele. You would interview the mothers of both groups of children to determine the proportion of exposure of each group during the corresponding pregnancies. Suppose that 32% of the mothers of children with meningomyelocele report being exposed to the chemical herbicide and only 8% of the mothers of children with multiple trauma report such exposure. You would conclude that mothers of children with meningomyelocele are four times more likely to have been exposed to the herbicide. Using these data to calculate an odds ratio, as the exposure ratio in the cases (32/68) divided the exposure ratio in the controls (8/92), you would say that the exposed mothers are approximately five times more likely to bear children with meningomyelocele.

Figure 13.2 shows the structure for a case-referent or case-control study. Notice that the cases and referents or controls are selected from two different populations and that the direction of the study is backward. Subjects are selected on the outcome of interest (disease or condition under study versus no disease) and the information on etiologic exposures is collected retrospectively. Table 13.2 shows the data layout for a case-referent study.

Continuing our caffeinated beverages example, we would gather cases of disease of interest—for instance, cancer of the pancreas—and compare them to a group of patients entering area hospitals for elective surgery with respect to the exposed factor of interest, caffeinated beverages. We would then compare the proportion of exposed among the cases $[a/(a + c)]$ to the proportion exposed among the controls $[b/(b + d)]$. The resulting measure, the odds ratio, gives us a sense of the degree of caffeinated beverage exposure among the cases

TABLE 13.2. Data layout for a case-referent/case-control study.

		Cases	Referents or controls
Exposure status	E	a	b
	$\bar{E}$	c	d
		$a + c$	$b + d$

exposure among the cases $= a/(a + c)$
exposure among the referents $= b/(b + d)$

$$\text{odds ratio} = \frac{a/(a + c) \div c/(a + c)}{b/(b + d) \div d/(b + d)} \text{ or } \frac{ad}{bc}$$

compared to the referent group. Again, when the odds ratio is more than one, or unity, we associate an increased risk of disease with exposure. When the disease under study is rare, as is usually the case when we use a case-referent design, the odds ratio comes close to the value of the risk ratio or the relative risk.

In case-referent research, if you obtain odds ratios that are high, like 6 or 11 or 20 (meaning that a target outcome is 6 or 11 or 20 times more likely to occur in the presence of a suspected risk factor as compared to the absence of the risk factor), you have evidence of *association* between the target outcome and the risk factor, and the strength of the association, as reflected in the high odds ratios, *would strongly suggest but does not prove causality* of the risk factor with respect to the target outcome. Findings from case-referent studies can seldom be taken as conclusive evidence of cause, no matter how high the odds ratios. Moreover, odds ratios from case-referent studies are weak, often only in the order of 1.3 or 1.8 or about 2. In such cases (assuming that statistical significance has been attained), the evidence of association can be invoked to draw causal inferences only at great peril. The previously discussed specific ground rules about diagnosing causality from association should be invoked when evaluating evidence from case-referent studies.

In recent years, Miettinen[2] developed the theory underlying case-referent studies that permitted substantial advances in the understanding of this strategy. He introduced the concept of *study base* as the hypothetical conceptual denominator of relevance for these types of studies. Clinicians participating with methodologists in case-referent studies should make a serious attempt to master both the theory and the logistical challenges of the case-referent approach. The theoretical and practical difficulties can be formidable despite the advantages of smaller sample sizes and much shorter study periods.

The key disadvantages to the case-referent method are vulnerability to bias[3] and the difficulty in judicious choice of reference groups for comparison. The advantages include smaller numbers of patients and shorter follow-up. In the case of a rare disease, the case-referent method is often the only feasible way of evaluating association between a risk factor and a clinical outcome.

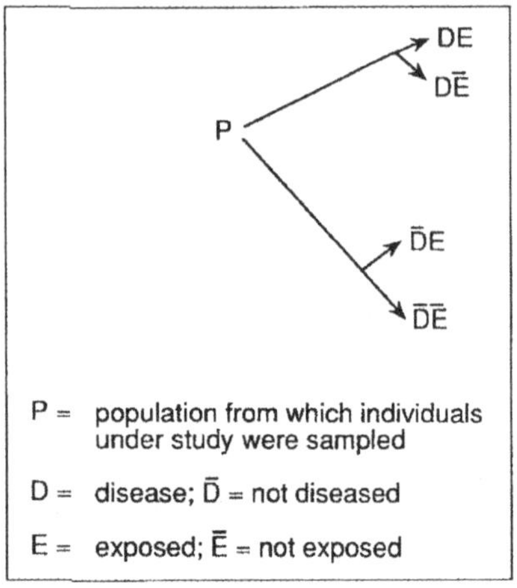

FIGURE 13.3. The cross-sectional study.

Cross-Sectional Designs

Cross-sectional designs are those in which denominators are delineated at the same time as the numerator events are measured. You might enumerate all victims of motorcycle accidents within a particular city of 500,000 persons and designate them as the denominator of interest; for the target outcome in the numerator, you might measure the extent of their resulting physical disabilities. This outcome will be established *at the same time* as the eligible study subjects are included in the denominator.

Figure 13.3 shows the structure of a cross-sectional study. The absence of lines indicating the passage of time shows that data on exposure status and the outcome of interest were collected at the same time. Unlike the case-referent study, in which exposure and outcome are also gathered at the same time, all individuals under study come from the same source population. If we did a cross-sectional study on the effects of caffeinated beverages, focusing on minor gastric disorders, we would choose a sample of individuals from a population of interest (e.g., community A) and interview them on their use of caffeinated beverages and their symptoms of gastric upset. The unit of analysis is the individual and the study is nondirectional.

Table 13.3 shows the data layout for a cross-sectional study. The comparison of interest is the ratio of the rate of disease among those with exposure to caffeinated beverages [a/b)] divided by the rate of disease among those without caffeinated beverage exposure [c/d)]. An elevated risk ratio or relative risk would suggest, but not prove, some association.

A more rigorous approach is a cross-sectional study that makes comparisons among groups of people. You might study all motorcycle victims in one city of 500,000 and compare them with motorcycle victims in another city of 500,000 in a neighboring state. The difference is that the use of helmets is not mandatory in the first city, but is in the second. You could make a quantitative assessment of the extent of disability among the victims in both cities, using a new "disability index" (0 = death, and 100 = freedom from disability). Suppose you measure an average "disability index" of 68 points in city A and 48 points in city B. You would tend to conclude that city B is better off than city A and to impute the benefit to the law on helmet use.

This example was chosen to show the pitfalls cross-sectional designs can harbor and to illustrate how cohort studies are superior, when feasible, because they are not as vulnerable to biases and misinterpretation. Community A could actually be better off than community B by virtue of having had lower mortality; community B may have had higher mortality with less disability among the surviving victims. If you had started with a cohort approach that identified all motorcycle *riders* in both communities before introduction of the law and followed both groups forward from a time close to the introduction of the new law in city B, there would be no confusion between survival and residual disability.

Budgetary limitations, unavailability of data, lack of time, or ethical constraints may often preclude a cohort study, however, and all we can do is a cross-sectional study. Remember that when your data emerge from cross-sectional studies only, you can reach only tentative conclusions that a particular exposure factor or a particular intervention is *associated* with a particular target outcome or dependent variable.

Cross-sectional designs do not provide reliable information on the temporal relation between suspected causal factors and the health outcomes of interest. Only cohort studies and controlled studies give such information.

Ecologic Studies

Ecologic studies, also called heterodemic, aggregate, or descriptive studies, use the group as the basic unit of analysis. Groups are commonly defined according to geographic, geopolitical, or time criteria. Although ecologic studies often use mortality data as the outcome of interest, they may use any such commonly collected types of data as rates of hospitalization for various conditions, numbers of cases of reported infectious diseases, or numbers of births. Beginning with Durkheim's analysis of the relation between the number of suicides in European countries and the proportions of Protestants in the regions under study, ecologic studies have been used to show relationships on the group rather than the individual level. Wennberg and Gettelsohn's study, showing the relation between rates of surgical procedures and the numbers of physicians performing surgery, is a more recently published example of this type of analysis.[4]

TABLE 13.3. Data layout for a cross-sectional study.

		Disease status		
		D	$\bar{D}$	Totals
Exposure status	E	a	b	$a + b$
	$\bar{E}$	c	d	$c + d$
	Totals	$a + c$	$b + d$	$(a + b) + (c + d)$

disease among exposed $= a/(a + b)$
disease among unexposed $= c/(c + d)$
prevalence odds ratio $= \dfrac{a/b}{c/d}$ or $\dfrac{ad}{bc}$

Figure 13.4 shows the basic structure of an ecologic study in which the joint distribution of exposure and disease is not known. We gather information on exposure or disease only, the information commonly found in the marginals of a standard data layout table (Table 13.4). In our illustrative study of caffeinated beverages, we might be interested in the relation between caffeinated beverage consumption and bleeding ulcers. An ecologic study might look at the association of caffeinated beverage sales with hospitalizations for bleeding ulcers in two demographically similar regions that differ in their use of caffeinated beverages. If such an association were found, it might encourage the interested investigator to pursue the possible causal relationship further.

Ecologic studies warrant much caution. They are attractive because they use existing data, and require less time and money, but they may be subject to a phenomenon known as the "ecologic fallacy." The data available in an ecologic study consist of the information portrayed in the marginals of a standard data layout table. If the grouping of the individuals studied distorts the effect of interest, *or* if certain factors related to the group are

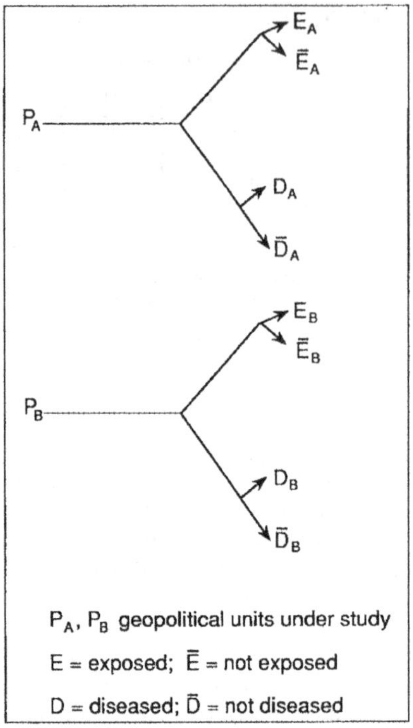

FIGURE 13.4. The ecological study.

TABLE 13.4. Data layout for an ecologic study.

Population$_i$ — Disease status

		Diseased	Not diseased	
Exposure status	Exposed	---	---	$a_i + b_i$
	Not exposed	---	---	$c_i + d_i$
		$a_i + c_i$	$b_i + d_i$	N_i

Population$_j$ — Disease status

		Diseased	Not diseased	
Exposure status	Exposed	---	---	$a_j + b_j$
	Not exposed	---	---	$c_j + d_j$
		$a_j + c_j$	$b_j + d_j$	N_j

comparison: $\frac{a_i + b_i}{N_i} > \frac{a_j + b_j}{N_j}$ and $\frac{a_i + c_i}{N_i} > \frac{a_j + c_j}{N_j}$

affecting the occurrence of the outcome of interest, an ecologic study will lead us to the wrong conclusion about the relationship under investigation. If we found a relationship in the caffeinated beverages study, we would have no way of determining whether the individuals who were hospitalized with bleeding ulcers were actually drinking caffeinated beverages.

Summary

The three broad purposes of clinical and epidemiologic investigation are (a) *describing what is*, (b) *predicting what could happen* in the future, and (c) *establishing cause and effect* in etiologic and therapeutic investigation.

The experiment is by far the strongest evidence that can be invoked to differentiate causality from association. It is the gold standard of clinical, epidemiologic, and health care research that should be used whenever ethically and practically feasible. In the history of medicine, nonexperimental studies have rarely led to firm conclusions about cause and effect.

If one cannot do an experiment, a series of nonexperimental strategies can be considered. To establish a causal significance from an association, the hierarchy of rigor of evidence gives highest weight to the cohort comparison study. The next levels, in order of descending rigor, are the well-designed case-referent study, the cross-sectional study and, finally, the ecologic association study. Only when striking findings show major changes should case studies be invoked to establish cause and effect relationships. Generally, unless it is an experiment, no single study should be used as conclusive evidence about any one question.

It is important to create a profile of several nonexperimental studies. If most of them tend to point in the same direction, especially if they were planned and designed by different investigators in different countries at different times, with complementary designs in different kinds of patients, causality may become a tenable verdict. Other important rules about the scientific admissibility of evidence were summarized earlier in this chapter in Bradford Hill's criteria.

Prediction of the future depends, in part, on how faithfully interventions—assessed through experimental, subexperimental, and nonexperimental methods—reflect current and future realities. There must be an adequate sense of all the circumstances surrounding an intervention, such as competing medical treatments, the milieu in which health service organizations operate in a particular country, and the conformity between the characteristics described and studied in a particular project and the basic nature of the population for which predictions are being made.

Mathematical modeling, based in part on empirical evidence gathered through experimental and nonexperimental studies, can play an important role in predicting the future. Although this chapter has not dealt with such modeling, nor has it presented laboratory simulation in detail, a balanced overview of selected strategies requires that they, at least, be mentioned.

Some investigators scorn the use of anything less than the gold standard of randomized controlled double-blind trials in clinical and epidemiologic research. While we believe that the highest feasible level of rigor in design should always be attempted, we also feel that it is usually better to have some data than none. When legitimate real-world constraints do not permit randomized controlled trials, every other avenue to new knowledge should be followed as far and as carefully as possible.

The substantial compromises in strategy that must be made in nonexperimental research require the exercise of even more care in the choice of all patients or study subjects, in the validity and reliability of data gathering, and in the selection of the best possible statistical techniques than in experimental trials.

References

1. The Canadian Task Force on the Periodic Health Examination: 1989 update. Can Med Assoc J 1989; 141:209–16.
2. Miettinen OS. Theoretical Epidemiology: Principles of Occurrence Research in Medicine. New York: Wiley, 1985.
3. Ibrahim M, Spitzer WO. The case-control study: consensus and controversy. J Chronic Dis 1979;32: 1–190.
4. Wennberg J, Gettelsohn A. Small area variations in health care delivery. Science 1972;182:1102–8.

Additional Reading

Bradford Hill A. Principles of Medical Statistics. 9th ed. New York: Oxford University Press, 1971, Chapter 24.

Campbell DT, Stanley JC. Experimental and Quasi-Experimental Designs for Research. Skokie, IL: Rand McNally, 1963.

Cook TD, Campbell DT. Quasi-Experimentation. Skokie, IL: Rand McNally, 1979.

Feinstein AR. Clinical Epidemiology: The Architecture of Clinical Research. Philadelphia: Saunders, 1985.

Fletcher RH, Fletcher SW, Wagner EH. Clinical Epidemiology: The Essentials. Baltimore: Williams & Wilkins, 1982.

Friedman GD. Primer of Epidemiology, 2nd ed. New York: McGraw-Hill, 1980.

Kelsey JL, Thompson WD, Evans AS. Methods in Observational Epidemiology. New York: Oxford University Press, 1986.

Kleinbaum DG, Kupper LL, Morgenstern H. Epidemiologic Research. Belmont, CA: Lifetime Learning Publications, 1982.

Lilienfeld AM, Lilienfeld DE. Foundations of Epidemiology, 2nd ed. Oxford: Oxford University Press, 1980.

Sackett DL, Haynes RB, Tugwell P. Clinical Epidemiology: A Basic Science for Clinical Medicine. Boston: Little, Brown, 1985.

Schlesselman JJ. Case-Control Studies. Oxford: Oxford University Press, 1982.

Swinscow, TDV. Statistics at Square One. London: British Medical Association, 1976.

14

Experimental Methods: Clinical Trials

B. McPeek, F. Mosteller, M.F. McKneally, and E.A.M. Neugebauer

We frequently do not know which is the best of several possible treatments. Worse yet, we may not know if any of them are better than what we are now doing, or better than providing only encouragement and sympathy.

We can think, compute, theorize, observe, or guess, but the answers to such questions, even approximate and uncertain answers, must finally be found by studying treatments in a controlled, practical tryout under field conditions. Our language reflects how well we know this: the proof of the pudding is in the eating. This chapter is about the practical evaluation of innovations in the field, using controlled trials.

Controlled Clinical Trials

In a controlled trial, the investigator imposes two (or more) different treatments on selected groups of individuals to see how well each treatment achieves a prestated goal. The results are usually also reviewed for effects not included in the original plan.

The Logic of Trials

A simplified version of the rationale of basing inferences on a comparative trial assumes that:

1. Initially, the individuals in each group receiving one treatment are similar to the individuals in the groups receiving the other treatment(s).
2. The difference in their treatments is the only factor affecting the outcomes in the different groups.
3. The individuals in the treated groups react to the treatments in the same way as the rest of the population would react.

We then conclude that because the only difference is in the treatment, it must have caused any differences in observed outcome, and because the individuals in the trial react like the rest of the population, applying a treatment to other members of the population will produce the same effect as it did on the individuals in the trial.

Strength of a Trial

Many simpler strategies provide information about what happens after a treatment is given; each is sometimes used to say something about the effectiveness of a treatment. They all lack the strength of a controlled trial because their designs are inherently weaker. They are frequently described as being "almost as good as" or "closely approaching," but it is never suggested that their weaker designs offer the strength of inference one can provide with a controlled trial. For this reason, the carefully executed controlled trial continues to supply our best evidence of cause and effect, and our best evidence of the effectiveness of diagnostic and therapeutic maneuvers.

The confidence we have in the results of a controlled trial lies, in large measure, in the strength of the control. Were the groups of individuals that received the different treatments truly initially similar? We are most likely to be convinced of this if the groups were selected from the same population and divided or allocated into groups by a reliably unbiased method.

The most convincing of such methods is randomization using a table of random numbers, giving each individual an equal chance to be assigned to each of the groups. Although "randomization" based on throwing dice, tossing coins, or drawing cards can seem to be reliable, it may have serious weaknesses. Such methods are more easily interfered with and cannot be checked if questions about them arise later.

Odd or even birthdays, patient identification numbers, or alternate arrival in the clinic are not proper bases for random allocation. They are systematic allocation procedures. They may appear to be unbiased, but such procedures have the weakness of tipping the patient assignment in advance so that someone who knows the procedure, perhaps a referring physician or clinic secretary, can allow personal prejudice to bias allocation by pushing forward or holding back otherwise eligible patients.

The use of concurrent control groups from the same population lends strength to our belief in the initial similarity of the treatment and control groups, but such confidence would quickly run down the drain if we thought the selection had been done in a biased fashion, resulting in sicker, younger, or wealthier patients being assigned in greater number to one group or the other.

Sometimes a controlled trial is designed to use nonconcurrent treatment groups. For example, treatment 1 may be applied in January and February, and then treatment 2 is applied to everyone in March and April. This strategy, at least, selects group members from the same population in the same institution, but we wonder what other changes may have occurred. Did the surgeons on the service change at the time the treatment change occurred? Were there more or fewer nurses in March than in January? The possibility for such differences increases if the groups are separated more widely in time. A design that compares one treatment given in the 1980s with another treatment administered in the 1990s raises real questions. Have our diagnostic criteria remained stable over time? Have other treatments been introduced, or other changes occurred in the patients or their environment?

Occasionally, a controlled trial in which the treatment group comes from one institution and the control group from another is attempted. It is always difficult to assure ourselves, let alone those who will later read the published reports of such a trial, that the treatment groups were indeed initially similar and that the only difference lies in the treatments being compared.

Sometimes trials attempt to draw a comparison group from patients previously reported in the literature. It is usually very difficult for such "control" groups to be convincing except perhaps in the special case of a known course of events, with the literature quite clear. For example, if a specific cancer is invariably fatal, and its diagnosis is clear, we may have confidence in historical controls from the literature if the new treatment results in, for example, a 25% survival.

What happens when poorly controlled trials are carried out? Physicians, especially uncritical physicians, may begin to believe the results of sloppy trials, especially when repeatedly poorly controlled trials arrive at the same conclusion: that the innovative therapy is a winner. As Hugo Muench has taught us, nothing improves the performance of an innovation more than lack of controls.[1]

Performing a poor trial has serious long-run drawbacks. First, the results of a weak trial may foreclose—for a long period—the possibility of a good evaluation by a strong trial. Second, a weak trial may leave a well-established yet ineffective therapy in place for years to come. The losses associated with applying ineffective or less effective therapies to large populations soon outweigh 1000-fold the costs of careful trials.

History of Trials

Most of the early investigations affecting choice of treatment took advantage of accidental or incidental deviations from standard treatments rather than being planned experiments. The sixteenth century military surgeon Ambrose Paré became famous for his report of an unplanned comparison of treatments of battlefield wounds. The standard French practice at that time was to pour boiling oil over the injury. In 1537 at the Battle of Villaine, Paré and his assistants found their oil supply exhausted. They used an alternative treatment consisting of a mixture of eggs, oil of roses, and turpentine. On early morning rounds the next day, Paré found those treated with the alternative mixture "feeling but little pain, their wounds neither swollen nor inflamed . . . having slept through the night. The others to whom I had applied the boiling oil were feverish with much pain and swelling about their wounds." Today, we would call this investigation a quasi-experiment, or perhaps, a natural experiment.

Preplanned clinical trials were rare until well into the twentieth century. In the nineteenth century many advances in surgery resulted from the rise of the modern hospital, influenced in so many ways by the work of Florence Nightingale, as well as the discovery and widespread use of general anesthetics, and the introduction of antiseptic and, later, aseptic surgery. In some instances, as in anesthesia, the effectiveness of the innovation was dramatic enough to be convincing without resort to careful evaluation. Yet, the work of Lister and his successors on sepsis, although of equal or perhaps greater importance, was less dramatically convincing to surgeons. For example, here are some of Lister's early data:

	Ordinary dressings	Lister's method	Totals
No blood poisoning	9	7	16
Blood poisoning	5	3	8
Totals	14	10	24

In Lister's time, people did not know how to analyze such a simple 2 × 2 table, and the discussion in British journals and newspapers was lively. The lack of a careful comparative trial of competing surgical techniques using modern statistical methods led to a period of 15 to 25 years of bitter controversy on the prevention of surgical infection.

We owe many of our current ideas about the proper way to conduct a practical field trial, and particularly the concept of randomization, to R. A. Fisher and his associates at the British Agricultural Experiment Station at Rothamsted. Fisher's data consisted of the yields of crops grown in small plots treated differently—for example, with different fertilizers or different doses of a given fertilizer. Analyzing such data was difficult because even if plots were treated in the same way, crop yields in the various plots varied because of differences in soil quality, drainage, or exposure to sun. Some of these differences were quite large, and there was a need for an unbiased method of allocating fields to treatments.

In 1923 Fisher and MacKenzie first proposed the idea of randomization and, in 1935 in his textbook, *The Design of Experiments*, Fisher suggested that his method might be applied to experiments in humans.

In 1931 Amberson et al. performed a randomized clinical trial to evaluate treatments for tuberculosis, and in 1948 the British Medical Research Council published a randomized clinical trial demonstrating the effectiveness of streptomycin in the treatment of tuberculosis.

The leadership of John Goligher taught surgeons that randomized trials are valuable instruments. Goligher and his colleagues randomized patients to surgical treatments for peptic ulcer disease. His studies clarified the role of vagotomy and drainage procedures and choice of postgastrectomy reconstructions. Perhaps Goligher's most important contribution was the credibility he gave to the concept of randomized trials as an element of surgical practice.[2]

Random Does Not Mean Haphazard

By a randomized controlled trial, we mean a planned experiment to assess the effectiveness of treatments by comparing the outcomes in subjects drawn from the same population and allocated to two or more treatment groups by a random method. Randomization of a large enough group of patients provides the theoretical basis for assuming that the treatment groups were initially comparable in terms of both known and unknown confounding factors. In using the term "random" we do not mean haphazard or unplanned, but a deliberate choice based on probabilities. In the simplest problem, we want each possible sample to have the same probability of being drawn. Setting the probabilities lends strength to analyses based on statistical methods and protects the investigators from various biases.

Errors

Statisticians often speak of type I and type II errors, usually in the context of testing whether a new treatment differs from a standard or, more generally, whether differences might reasonably be thought to be negligible. In confirmatory statistical analysis, exemplified by significance tests, we may well ask at what rate per experiment we will falsely claim that a difference exists even when the two therapies are equal in effect. Such a false claim is called a type I error. This rate is associated with the significance level of the test, often chosen to be .05. When the observed difference falls beyond the .05 level, we say the result is significant, while admitting that we are risking a 5% frequency of a type I error.

Failing to recognize a difference when one is present is called a type II error. Given the method of testing for the difference and the significance level chosen, say .05, then what is the probability that we will fail to recognize a true difference, that is, make a type II error? This probability depends, of course, on the size of the true difference—larger differences are not as likely to be missed in our sample as smaller ones.

For a given significance level, we can control the rate of type II errors for a given difference in performance of the tests by adjusting the sample sizes. Thus the rates of type I and type II errors we will accept are important considerations in designing investigations.

Ideally, we would have no error of either kind. To assure this requires infinite sample sizes.

To put a small touch of reality back into the discussion, no one believes that two different therapies have *exactly* the same performance rates, but we might feel they were so close that we couldn't afford to measure their difference, or that very small differences were negligible from a clinical point of view. Thus, a declaration of no significant difference does not promise zero differences.

Trials that Convince

Over the past generation in medicine and surgery, we have come to agree that, when well-executed, a randomized controlled trial provides the strongest evidence available for evaluating the relative effectiveness of the interventions tested.

We know how to conduct clinical trials that provide strong information about the relative effectiveness of two or more therapies. Most controversies with clinical trials arise from investigators' desire to modify or avoid some requirement of the classical randomized controlled trial design. They worry that it will be difficult to get enough patients, that some will think randomization is unfair, or may wish to substitute historical experience for a control group or to avoid some other requirement or strengthening feature. In some situations, requirements can be relaxed with little or no harm to the trial, but often what seems acceptable to some investigators will not satisfy later readers of the trials' reports.

The randomized controlled trial and its analysis have been developed to protect investigators from untoward influences including their own biases that might invalidate the data and the conclusions to be drawn. If we could be sure that a particular biasing influence does not threaten the study at hand, we might not need to take advantage of the aspect of the trial that protects against that influence. For example, if you knew that all experimental units were the same and there was no variation from one unit to another, you would not have to randomize.

What if the investigators' assumptions about the trial are not shared by readers? The trial loses its ability to convince; readers will criticize the design and conduct of the trial. The trial will fail, even if it gives an answer that is ultimately accepted as being right, because its failure to convince other clinicians means it will fail to affect clinical practice.

Strengthening Features

Some of the strengthening features of randomized controlled trials are as follows.

Use of a prespecified explicit question.
Clearly defined conditions for admission to the trial.
Defined therapies.
Entrance of patients into the trial prior to allocation to treatment groups.
Blindness to treatment (by patient, experimenter, and evaluator if feasible).
Systematic evaluation and follow-up of both treatment and control groups.
Adequate sample size (for power to discriminate when treatments differ in their performance).
Appropriate statistical analyses of outcomes and side effects.
Careful, complete reporting.

TABLE 14.1. The key elements of a study protocol for a prospective controlled randomized trial.

1. Background and description of the clinical problem
2. Clearly defined question(s) or hypotheses
3. Reasons for the need to perform the designed study
4. Description of the type of the study
5. Definition of the study population
   Inclusion criteria
   Exclusion criteria (escape and dropout)
6. Definition and description of intervention and control group
7. Type and execution of the randomization
8. Reasons for and execution of blinding
9. Sample size estimates
10. Data of the study
    Definition of basic data of patients
    Definition of endpoints of the study
    Data collection, quality assurance, and quality-control
    Data analysis (tests of hypotheses, descriptive statistics)
    Data protection
11. Ethical considerations (informed consent)
12. Description and schedule for a single patient (logistics)
13. Organizational structure of the study
14. References
15. Forms and data handling for a single patient

Reprinted with permission from Neugebauer E, Rothmund M, Lorenz W. Kunstruct Strukture und Praxis Perspectives Klinische Studies. Chirurg 60:203–13 1989, Springer-Verlag Heidelberg, FRG.

To provide the strengthening features of the randomized controlled design, careful planning is necessary before starting a trial. The study protocol must fulfill scientific, ethical, and organizational requirements, so that the trial can be conducted efficiently. The protocol should be developed before the beginning of subject enrollment and should remain essentially unchanged throughout the study. The key elements of a study protocol are outlined in Table 14.1.

Innovation

Goligher points out that innovations in treatment start out as good ideas, sometimes one's own, or ideas suggested by others, but not well worked out or ever evaluated. Goligher's next step is possibly the hardest: the generation of energy and enthusiasm to test the idea, to demonstrate whether it works by using laboratory studies or animal experimentation, and then "... by a cautious pilot clinical study on selected volunteer patients, who have had clearly explained to them the respective potential advantages and disadvantages of the innovation."[3]

New ideas, even new ideas with good theoretical or laboratory support, most frequently turn out to be useless. Often very small clinical experience will convincingly demonstrate that this is so. Much less commonly, the idea will be quickly and convincingly recognized as a revolutionary success, and will rapidly go into clinical practice. A much more likely possibility is that the idea will look somewhat promising, suggesting the need for a more careful evaluation of its efficacy. Ordinarily it is at this point that consideration of a means of careful evaluation arises, and the thought occurs that the innovative measure should be compared to the best standard treatment by a clinical trial.

Trials are difficult and time-consuming, and they require a genuine commitment on the part of the investigators and their associates—a commitment of enthusiasm, energy, and discipline, as well as resources in terms of time and money. Most trials ought to require a relatively large number of cases, and the investigators must assure an adequate number of patients in a relatively short period of time. *Trials that take many years to complete run the risk of being overtaken by new developments in diagnosis or therapy, which make them difficult to finish or irrelevant.* Most research teams find the discipline of a trial irksome, and the required enthusiasm and energy difficult to maintain over long periods.

Sometimes the collaboration of a number of institutions across the world is required. Some problems, particularly those involving truly rare conditions, simply cannot be studied by clinical trials, even large multicentered ones. Many other problems will be judged of insufficient importance to warrant the effort.

Deciding to Start a Trial

Because of a trial's requirements and the commitments its planners must make, one must consider the proper role for randomized clinical trials. In an ideal world with unlimited resources of patients, personnel, and money, all innovations might be assessed by trials. Since none of us live in that world, we must prioritize our efforts, and make the best use of our resources.

The first requirement for a trial is that the physicians and surgeons who participate be honestly ignorant of the comparative merits of the treatments they propose to compare, if they are to recruit patients for a trial. At the same time, they must have a proper skepticism about the state of their real knowledge, not confusing mere prejudice with knowledge. Even careful and thoughtful people frequently have been found to be much too confident of what they think they know.[4]

The potential investigators must believe that the treatments may differ in outcome, and that these differences may be clinically important. There are too many important problems in medicine and surgery to expend resources on issues we do not expect to matter. It is often hard to be sure about what will matter in clinical practice, or how much it might matter. Finally a trial's planners must believe that a trial is feasible with the resources of patients, enthusiasm, personnel, and money that can be made available.

Structure of a Prospective Controlled Randomized Trial: The Study Protocol

When the decision to run a trial has emerged, trial planners meet to develop a study protocol. The study protocol provides detailed specification of the trial procedure.

What Is the Clinical Problem?

A description of the background and the clinical problem explains why the trial is needed and how it builds on the experience gained from previous research.[5]

What Is the Question?

Although a trial may have several purposes, we explicitly define a principal question in advance. This question serves to guide planning of the whole study. The principal question should be the one the investigators are most interested in answering and is the question on which the sample size of the study is based. We frame the principal question in the form of a testable hypothesis.[6]

Consider problems of multiplicity. If a number of questions are investigated, a statistical problem arises. If we look at a large enough number of questions in a single investigation, inevitably some of them will display an unusual outcome. If we compare a number of treatments, even if they are truly equivalent, sampling variation alone would make some of them look better than others. Similarly, when individual institutions are compared in a cooperative multi-institutional therapeutic trial, even if they are equivalent in excellence, sampling variation will make some look much better than others.

One way of asking many relevant questions and causing problems of multiplicity is to use multiple endpoints. For example, in a controlled trial of coronary bypass surgery, are we preventing death, first myocardial infarctions, second myocardial infarctions, or angina? All these may be legitimate endpoints, but usually one is fundamental and the others are side interests. If that is true, explicitly naming the primary endpoint in advance strengthens statistical appraisal and clarifies suitable experimental design. Analysis becomes more complicated when there are two endpoints or more because larger samples are required to maintain power.

We may well want to look at additional questions and analyses that suggest themselves in various ways after the data analysis has begun. This is information we are not anxious to throw away, but it may be quite difficult to know how much value we should place on the answers we get. With a statistical test chosen on the basis of a peek at the data, it is hard to say what the properties of the test are because every set of data has unusual features. Thus, it may be difficult to say whether a rare event has occurred if a test of significance is chosen from a large number of possibly related tests. These problems are not unique to randomized controlled trials; they can occur with equal or greater impact in any statistical study.

Why a Further Study?

After the primary question has been framed, we review and analyze the published literature on the issue. Several approaches to systematically reviewing previous work are outlined in Chapter 9. As a result of the literature analysis, we formulate a convincing statement of the need for the suggested trial on the primary question.

Type of Trial?

The type of trial is determined by the kind of principal question posed. Schwartz and Lellouch[7] distinguish two different kinds of questions that trials frequently ask.[8] The first kind asks for scientific demonstration of efficacy or superiority: Will operation A produce better results than operation B? This is sometimes called an *explanatory* trial, or an *efficacy* trial; it seeks to compare the effects of treatments with close control under ideal or restricted circumstances.

The explanatory or efficacy trial seeks to determine whether the treatment can work under the best circumstances. Such a trial might restrict its admission of patients to those most likely to respond well, and it may call for elaborate monitoring, regulation of treatment, or more frequent follow-up.

The second kind of question deals with *pragmatic* management or clinical effectiveness under wider conditions more nearly like ordinary clinical practice. The *pragmatic* or *effectiveness* trial, sometimes called a management trial, asks the question: Can this procedure or treatment be generalized easily to practice?

A pragmatic or effectiveness trial is likely to accept a wider spectrum of patients, perhaps treated by a varied group of surgeons or practitioners. Its treatments usually strive to replicate clinical practice to obtain a better estimate of the overall usefulness of a therapeutic maneuver in widespread use.

Who Are the Patients?

A trial's protocol should specify the conditions for admission to the trial, that is, which patients or subjects are eligible for admission. The inclusion/exclusion criteria must be clearly defined.

Later readers of published reports will almost always want to assess whether the findings of a trial can be generalized to another patient group, or applied to individual patients seen in their own practices. Such extrapolation requires specific information about who the subjects of a trial were and how they were selected. Published reports that lack this information make generalizing a trial's findings to groups other than the subjects themselves very difficult.

What Are the Treatments?

Each therapy must be clearly defined. We ought to know what will be done, how it will be done, and by whom.

Allocation to Treatment Groups

Patients must be entered into the trial before the choice of therapy is made. Determination of admission to a study after treatment assignment is known may bias subject selection. Those in the know may push forward or hold back potential subjects, as a result of conscious or unconscious prejudice about treatment assignment. Assignments based on birthdays, odd or even chart numbers, or alternate arrival often tip the assignment in advance and allow bias to creep in.

Assignment of treatments using published random number tables reduces bias in clinical trials. Frequently, known prognostic factors are used to stratify patients prior to randomization. This can help to achieve balance among treatment groups—at least with respect to known factors. The exact procedure used should be specified so that readers can be assured that the randomization was reliable. The time of randomization and the chosen procedure must be explained and described in detail.

Blindness?

Studies should be blinded to the extent possible. Ideally, the patient, the physician giving the treatment, and the person doing the evaluation should not know what treatment is given. Some degrees of blindness may not be feasible, especially in surgical trials (consider a trial of amputation vs. medical treatment), but blindness is an important strengthening feature and should be used wherever possible. For example, histological slides, x-rays, or laboratory tests can be read by a physician blinded to the patients' treatment allocation.

The protocol should state which parts of the study are blinded and should tell how to assure that the blinding conditions are met.

Power and Sample Size

The probability of detecting an event of given size in a comparative study is called the "power." The larger the sample size and the larger the size of the treatment effect, the greater is the power. Power also depends on study design, on the statistical techniques of analysis, and on the significance level, chosen by the investigators. Smaller significance levels give smaller power.

It is important to concentrate on sample size because it is, at least, partially under the control of the investigator. One way to think about power is that it quantifies the probability of detecting a substantial improvement and also the probability of missing one—the probability of a type II error.

A fundamental question that must be faced by investigators planning a clinical trial is: How many patients are needed? Beginning investigators will want to seek the advice of a statistician experienced in clinical trial design. There are various published formulas and tables for determining the number of patients necessary to meet the trial's principal objectives, but seemingly minor changes in trial design may make a given formula or table inapplicable. For example, sample size and power calculations can differ depending on the question being asked and on whether the outcome measure is dichotomous (e.g., success or failure) or a quantitative measurement. Standard textbooks[5,9] ordinarily devote one or more large chapters to sample size and power determinations.

How large is the usual treatment group in a clinical trial? Zelen drew a systematic sample of clinical trials reported in the journal *Cancer* and concluded that the usual size is about 50.[10] Mosteller and associates[11] examined 285 samples from randomized clinical trials in three areas of cancer. The median sample size was 9 for studies of multiple myeloma and chronic myelocytic leukemia, 7 for studies of gastrointestinal cancer, and 25 per treatment group for randomized trials of breast cancer. In all these distributions, sample sizes larger than 200 were rare. Only 7% of the samples exceeded 200. Small trials have very low power. Why is power important? Weak trials, trials with very low power, can fail to detect even big improvements in performance.

Freiman et al[12] document the risk of missing substantial improvements when a trial's power is low. They investigated 71 clinical trials that reported no statistically significant difference between the therapies. They looked at the 90% confidence intervals to see whether substantial improvement might have been missed because of the breadth of the intervals. These intervals contained potential 25% improvements in 57 comparisons and potential 50% improvement in 34 comparisons. The designs were so weak that they left open the possibility that such sizable improvements would be missed.

Emerson et al. found that only 5% of published reports of surgical trials disclose the trial's power to detect treatment differences.[13] This suggests that investigators, as well as editors, referees, and readers, fail to appreciate the importance discussions of power should hold for readers.

Data of the Study

Baseline Assessment

To describe study subjects accurately, baseline data should reflect the condition of the subjects before the start of the intervention. The protocol defines the appropriate baseline measures and their assessment. In general, they consist of socioeconomic and demographic characteristics, and medical data with attention to known risk or prognosis factors. Published baseline data allow readers to evaluate whether the study groups were really comparable before intervention started (randomization, except in truly large trials with many hundreds of patients in each group, does not guarantee balance between comparison groups). Imbalance in important characteristics can yield misleading results.

Beside comparability, baseline assessment offers opportunities for stratification and subgrouping. Stratification can be done at the time of allocation to treatment or during analysis.[14] The definition of subgroups normally relies on baseline data, not data measured after intervention. Subgroup analysis in most cases serves only to generate new hypotheses for subsequent testing.

Inclusion/Exclusion Criteria and Study Endpoints

A key element in study documentation is the assessment of the inclusion/exclusion criteria and study endpoints. Study endpoints are response variables measured during the course of the trial that answer the questions of the study (see Chapter 17). The methods for measurement must be described in detail. If a number of methods are available, the protocol should state the reasons for the choice of a particular method (e.g., practicability, reliability, validity).

Data Collection, Quality Assurance, and Control

To have data collected completely as possible, develop a data handling form for each patient. All data should be clearly defined in terms of how, when, and by whom they are to be collected. To minimize observer variation and to increase the quality of the data, a training course for standardization of the assessment of response variables may be necessary.

Analysis of the Data

Variation among individual patients, physicians, institutions, and other sources of variability outside the investigator's control usually require statistical inference to evaluate the outcome of a clinical trial. In terms of statistical tests of significance, we gain control much more readily by prespecified analyses of the significance level of the investigation than by postspecified analyses. If we know what questions we want to ask, we can specify the statistics to be used, choose the significance level we feel would be appropriate and convincing to others, and discuss other properties of the statistical test—all in advance.

The protocol should specify the statistical methods to be used and how they are to be applied (See Chapter 15).

Data Protection

The increasing use of electronic data processing raises problems of data security. Investigators must devise methods (e.g., passwords, separate data files for baseline data, response variables, and hard copies in secure places) to ensure data protection.

Ethics

The study must be ethically performed. Conflicts may arise between a physician's perception of what is good for a patient and the needs of the trial. In such instances, the needs of the subject must predominate. Informed consent is essential (see Chapter 12).

Schedule for a Single Patient (Logistics)

Before creating data handling forms for a single patient, trace the path of an individual patient coming through the study. Consider special arrangements and personal relationships as well as specific organizational structures within the institution.

Organization for the Trial

The organization should be as straightforward as possible and should avoid overlapping tasks. A simple team consists of the leader of the study, who is closely connected with the study secretary. The study secretary is responsible for collecting the data from physicians and nurses at each patient's bedside. Depending on the type of the study, a data monitoring committee may be necessary. Commonly, an advisory group gives professional expertise or experience of scientists on special parts of the protocol. All members of the team must keep abreast of the study's progress and work well together.

References

A study protocol may contain a list of the relevant references.

Data Handling Forms for a Single Patient

After completing the protocol, the investigator must develop data forms for each patient.

Collaborative Trials

Most clinical trials, like most biomedical research, have their genesis as individual, investigator-initiated ideas that come from individual scholars or small groups of interested collaborators. Many clinical trials are rather small for what they seek to do; that is, they have relatively few patients in each treatment arm of the trial. Small trials usually have low power, and a low-powered trial will reliably identify only large differences between treatment arms.

One solution is to organize a multi-institutional collaborative trial. Joining groups of investigators together to work on a trial can increase power by enlarging treatment groups and accelerating the rate of recruitment, but it also brings its own problems.

Multicentered collaborative trials require special care in their planning and execution. There are problems in assuring that the patients and treatment in Toronto are the same as in Boston or Berlin, and special efforts must be made to maintain investigator enthusiasm, accurate recording of events, and all the myriad issues that cause problems, even in trials in single institutions. We have now had a good bit of experience at such large enterprises. A number of groups are set up to function as coordinating centers and advisers for such trials, but multicentered trials are usually very expensive to organize and conduct.

Over the past few decades, groups of investigators have joined together to coordinate long-term programs of treatment evaluations by randomized clinical trials. Some of these groups take responsibility for broad areas of medicine and surgery, such as the regional oncology groups sponsored by the U.S. National Cancer Institute (e.g., the Eastern Cooperative Oncology Group, Southwestern Oncology Group, etc.). Others may be organ specific, such as the U.S. National Surgical Adjuvant Breast Cancer Program, or the North American Lung Cancer Study Group.

These government-funded, collaborative research groups represent one of the most important scientific resources of North American medicine and surgery. These groups have developed long-term mechanisms for data collection, review, and analysis by a relatively constant group of collaborators. They incorporate statistical and design consultation at the outset of each project from statisticians who have a well developed sense of the history and problems of the group and its particular strengths and aptitudes. Through surveillance of the basic science literature, the members are able to recognize new treatments appropriate for evaluation using their cooperative group. Much of their success comes from the fact that their organization takes advantage of continuing experience. They mount clinical trials that build on the results of the trials just completed. Their organization permits a targeted, systematic approach to the evaluation of treatment in their areas of interest. Continued development and growth of this system is likely to prove advantageous for surgery in the future.

When the original hypothesis for which the cooperative group was formed has been tested, there is a temptation for funding agencies to dismantle the group used in the trial. Dismantling a well functioning collaborative group is a very expensive step when the start-up cost of reconstituting a group for the next testable treatment question is taken into consideration. Strategies should be developed to protect well functioning cooperative groups from decommissioning and to incorporate, insofar as it is possible, the routines of data gathering and analysis into the ordinary practice of surgical care in the collaborating institutions. The Cleveland system, reported by Neuhauser[15] and discussed in more detail below, represents a more stable form of investigative instrument, so constructed that the start-up costs of a trial are minimized because the data management, patient allocation, and other technical components become part of the standard practice of the hospital. We must develop similar techniques for preserving multi-institutional collaborative trial groups and make these less expensive to maintain when not in active use.

Future Directions: Making Trials Easier

Even small trials are difficult to organize and they consume resources in terms of investigators' energy, enthusiasm, time, and money. Is there any way to make randomized clinical trials less difficult, more practical? Certainly, we should not want to do this by sacrificing precision or any of the strengthening features of design or conduct that lend credibility to a trial's conclusions or increase the generalizability of its findings to other patients in other places.

There is some parallel with our experience in the large-sample surveys that were so extraordinarily difficult to organize two generations ago. Great blunders occurred with some frequency, and surveys were not contemplated except for major issues, where the need clearly warranted the cost involved. Then, social scientists established institutions devoted in large measure to conducting sample surveys. Efficient methods were developed and surveys became easier to perform, because sample survey specialists had appropriate methods and personnel who were familiar with the necessary techniques and ready to perform both large and small surveys on commission.[16] Since surveys became more practical, they have become common and increasingly relied on by governments, universities, scientific and medical institutions, large corporations, economists, physicians, social scientists, and the public at large. For most purposes, sample surveys have replaced the census.

Duncan Neuhauser has described a somewhat analogous development for randomized clinical trials. He points out that many large hospitals are divided into subunits consisting of groups of physicians and nurses who care for groups of patients, and that new patients are frequently assigned to such teams by some sort of systematic allocation, frequently by rotation, to equalize the workload of the groups. The 700 bed Cleveland Metropolitan General Hospital has four such teams on the general medical service. Beginning in 1981, all new patients have been allocated among these teams at random. As Neuhauser points out:

> In every hospital, hundreds of changes in the organization and delivery of medical care are made in the belief that such changes provide better care and/or more efficient care. Only a small fraction of these changes are carefully evaluated to show whether this belief is correct.[15]

Neuhauser and his associates have used the hospital's teams to systematically evaluate a series of treatment changes. They institute changes on two of the four teams, selected at random, while the other two remain unchanged, as controls. To increase the comparability of teams, the hospital allocates new physicians to each team at random, and they remain with their team for their three years of training. A variety of medical care innovations, tested by this system, seem to have been very well received in the hospital. Treatment evaluations are much more easily and efficiently organized and conducted, largely because the system is in place and ready to go with only a little extra effort when the introduction and assessment of an innovation is contemplated.

Many of the Cleveland innovations might not have been judged important enough for careful evaluation, let alone a randomized clinical trial; but with an effective evaluation system already in place, a clinical trial seemed practical. Some extra work is required to organize each trial: approval must be sought from the appropriate ethics committee, a protocol must be drafted (to specify the new treatment, endpoints, follow-up, analysis, etc.), agreement must be obtained from the various collaborators, and consent must be sought from patients. Nevertheless, with the Cleveland system in place and ready to go, many trials seem more feasible.

Many of the Cleveland trials have posed such questions as: "Does feedback to physicians of the costs of the laboratory tests they employ reduce their use of tests?" and "Does the deployment of specialized intravenous therapy teams reduce the incidence of phlebitis?" It seems likely that this system, or variants, could also be used to evaluate other treatment innovations by asking questions like "Which measures are more effective in reducing pain after operation?" or "Which of two operations is more effective?" Perhaps people would be less anxious about participating as subjects in a trial of a new operation if they knew it were the standard treatment on the service to which they had been randomly assigned upon admission to the hospital.

Informed Consent

Patients in the Cleveland system are not explicitly told that their allocation to a team was determined by a random method, but informed consent is obtained for those innovations determined by the hospital ethics committee to be intrusive (e.g., consent is obtained for the obtaining of a venous blood sample, required in a study of diagnostic screening for diabetes).

This approach is similar to the idea for randomization expressed by Zelen.[17] Zelen suggested that to compare the best standard treatment A with experimental treatment B, the investigator follow the protocol for deciding patient eligibility. He randomizes all eligible patients to two groups: "seek informed consent" and "do not seek informed consent." Members of the second group are given the best standard therapy and are followed for outcome. Members of the "seek informed consent" group are advised that they have the opportunity to receive the experimental therapy if they wish to participate in the clinical trial. As usual, the patient receives a full explanation of benefits and risks. Some patients give consent and receive treatment B; others decline and presumably receive treatment A. The final comparison is between the outcome of the two consent groups, rather than outcomes from A versus B in the "seek consent" group. Thus, if few patients are willing to accept B, then the power of the experiment would be very weak—yet so would the classical clinical trial, if few patients were willing to consent to one of the treatments.

The Cleveland system appears to offer an innovative, practical idea for making clinical trials easier to organize, and it deserves careful exploration by surgeons and physicians from other specialties.

The idea has already spread beyond the Cleveland Metropolitan General Hospital. For example, at University Hospitals of Cleveland, ambulatory patients are randomly assigned to one of two teams of physicians, and a trial has been performed to see if it is more effective to have nurse practitioners rather than resident physicians screen for colon cancer.

Other hospitals are beginning to join in some collaborative efforts, although there has been little or no real coordination.

Since other institutions are exploring this system, the formation of consortia of hospitals or of clinical or surgical services at a number of institutions might result. With appropriate collaborative mechanisms in place, we might organize groups that are able to undertake the design and execution of clinical trials of surgical therapies in a way that would take advantage of previous experience and build on economies of scale. Many specific problems would remain to be worked out, but the concept offers a particularly fruitful area for development and research that might have substantial payoff for both surgical investigators and patients.

Current Status; Evaluation in Surgery

Although surgeons are often criticized, frequently unjustly, for the quality of their evaluations of both standard and innovative surgical treatments, the record shows that clinical trials in surgery are being done frequently and, on the whole, well.[18] Surgical leaders around the world are concerned with good clinical evaluation and research, are actively pursuing both, are gaining increasing support from practicing surgeons, and merit our support and applause for their efforts.

A significant advance in public appreciation of randomized trials in surgery was gained through the publicity associated with the trials of limited surgery for breast cancer. Further public education, and systematic education of surgeons in the value and proper conduct of randomized trials, will facilitate their application.

Acknowledgments. This chapter is adapted from McPeek B, Mosteller F, McKneally MF, Randomized clinical trials in surgery [Int J Technol Assess Health Care, 1989;5:317–32]. We have also drawn, in part, on some of our earlier work appearing in references 4, 11, 13, 16, and 19–22.

References

1. Bearman JE, Loewenson RB, Gullen WH. Muench's Postulates, Laws, and Corollaries, or Biometricians' Views on Clinical Studies, Biometrics Note 4. Bethesda, MD: Office of Biometry and Epidemiology, National Eye Institute, National Institutes of Health, 1974.
2. Goligher, JC, Pulvertaft CN, Watkinson G. Controlled trial of vagotomy and gastro-enterostomy, vagotomy and antrectomy, and subtotal gastrectomy in elective treatment of duodenal ulcer: interim report. Br Med J 1964;1:455–60.
3. Goligher J. The skeptical surgeon. Ann R Coll Surg (Engl) 1984;66:207–10.
4. Gilbert JP, McPeek B, Mosteller F. Statistics and ethics in surgery and anesthesia. Science 1977;198: 684–89.
5. Pocock S. Clinical Trials–A Practical Approach. New York: Wiley, 1983.
6. Friedman LM, Furberg CD, De Metz DL. Fundamentals of Clinical Trials, 2nd ed. Littleton, MA: Publishing Co., 1985:1–307.
7. Schwartz D, Lellouch J. Explanatory and pragmatic attitudes in clinical trials. J Chronic Dis 1967;20: 637–48.
8. MacRae KD. Pragmatic versus explanatory trials. Int J Technol Assess Health Care 1989;5:333–39.
9. Meinert CL. Clinical Trials–Design, Conduct, and Analysis. New York: Oxford University Press, 1986.
10. Zelen M, Gehan E, Glibwell O. Biostatistics in cancer research. In: Importance of Cooperative Groups, Hoogstralen B, ed. New York: Mason, 1980:291–312.
11. Mosteller F, Gilbert JP, McPeek B. Reporting standards and research strategies for controlled trials. Controlled Clin Trials 1980;1:37–58.
12. Freiman JA, Chalmers TC, Smith H. The importance of beta, the type II error, and sample size in the design and interpretation of the randomized controlled trial. N Engl J Med 1978;290: 690–94.
13. Emerson JD, McPeek B, Mosteller F. Reporting clinical trials in general surgical journals. Surgery 1984; 85:572–79.
14. Shapiro S, Louis A, eds. Clinical Trials: Issues and Approaches. New York: Dekker, 1982.
15. Neuhauser D. The Metro firm trials and ongoing patient randomization. In: Statistics, a Guide to the Unknown, 3rd ed., Tanur JM, et al., eds. Pacific Grove, CA: Wadsworth and Brooks/Cole, 1989.
16. Hoaglin DC, Light RJ, McPeek B, Mosteller F et al. Data for Decisions. Cambridge, MA: Abt Press, 1982;997–99.
17. Zelen M. A new design for randomized clinical trials. N Engl J Med 1979;300:1242–45.
18. Schwartz D, Flamant R, Lellouch J. Clinical Trials. New York: Academic Press, 1980.
19. Gilbert JP, McPeek B, Mosteller F. Progress in surgery and anesthesia: benefits and risks of innovative therapy. In: Costs, Risks, and Benefits of Surgery, Bunker JP, Barnes BA, Mosteller F, eds. New York: Oxford University Press, 1977;124–169.
20. O'Young J, McPeek B. Quality of life variables in surgical trials. J Chronic Dis 1987;40:513–22.
21. Miller JN, Colditz GA, Mosteller F. How study design affects outcomes in comparisons of therapy. II. Surgical. Stat Med, 1989;8:455–66.
22. Louis TA, Mosteller F, McPeek B. Timely topics in statistical methods for clinical trials. Annu Rev Biophys Bioeng 1982;11:81–104.

Additional Reading

A variety of textbooks and journal articles are now available to guide those undertaking or evaluating a trial. An especially readable book, *Clinical Trials: Issues and Approaches*, edited by Stanley Shapiro and Thomas A. Louis,[14] deals with the controversies, design, analysis, and methodology of clinical trials. This will be appreciated by both novices and experts.

While there is general agreement about the conduct of a randomized clinical trial and about what constitutes a good trial, the field is by no means static. Many thoughtful, innovative ideas appear each year. The official journal of the Society for Clinical Trials, *Controlled Clinical Trials*, began publication in 1980 and deals with all aspects of clinical trials.

Emerson JD, McPeek B, Mosteller F. Reporting clinical trials in general surgical journals. Surgery 1984;85: 572–79.

Freiman JA, Chalmers TC, Smith H. The importance of beta, the type II error, and sample size in the design and interpretation of the randomized controlled trial. N Engl J Med 1978;290:690–94.

Gilbert JP, McPeek B, Mosteller F. Statistics and ethics in surgery and anesthesia. Science 1977;198:684–89.

Meinert CL. Clinical Trials—Design, Conduct, and Analysis. New York: Oxford University Press, 1986.

Mosteller F, Gilbert JP, McPeek B. Reporting standards and research strategies for controlled trials. Controlled Clin Trials 1980;1:37–58.

Pocock S. Clinical Trials—A Practical Approach. Chichester, New York: Wiley, 1983.

Schwartz D, Flamant R, Lellouch J. Clinical Trials. New York: Academic Press, 1980.

Shapiro S, Louis TA, eds. Clinical Trials: Issues and Approaches, New York: Dekker, 1982.

15

Clinical Biostatistics: An Overview

M.S. Kramer

Most clinical investigators approach statistics in one of three ways: (1) total avoidance, (2) mindless "number crunching" often facilitated by ready access to microcomputers with statistical software packages, or (3) blind faith in the advice of statistical consultants. Unfortunately, none of these approaches is particularly conducive to research of high quality and utility.

The main objective for this chapter is to provide the surgical researcher with sufficient background to become an informed consumer of biostatistics. The discussion is not intended to replace either professional statistical advice or standard texts. The emphasis is on conceptual understanding, rather than technical facility; the use of algebraic notation and mathematical formulas will be kept to the strict minimum required for clarity. A number of clinical examples are included to illustrate the concepts discussed, including several from general surgery and the surgical subspecialties. Careful reading of the chapter should help demystify a subject for which unfamiliarity all too often leads to one of the unfortunate consequences cited above.

Introduction

Variables

The attributes or events measured in a research study are called *variables*, since they vary (take on different values at different times in different subjects). Variables are measured according to two broad types of measurement scales: continuous and categorical.

Continuous variables (also called dimensional, quantitative, or interval variables) are those consisting of continuous integers, fractions, or decimals, in which equal distances exist between successive intervals. Age, systolic blood pressure, and serum sodium concentration are all examples of continuous variables.

Categorical variables (also called discrete variables) are those in which the measured attribute or event is placed into one of two or more discrete categories. Categorical variables may be either *dichotomous* (two categories) or *polychotomous* (three or more categories). Examples of dichotomous variables include vital status (dead vs. alive), treatment (surgical vs. medical) in a two-arm clinical trial, yes versus no responses to a question, and sex. Polychotomous variables can be either nominal or ordinal. *Nominal variables* consist of named categories that bear no ordered relation to one another (e.g., hair color, identity of operating surgeon, country of origin). With *ordinal variables*, the categories are ordered or ranked. Unlike continuous variables, the intervals between categories need not be equal. For example, postoperative pain might be measured using the following four ranked categories of severity: none, mild, moderate, and severe.

The different types of variable are summarized in Table 15.1.

Most clinical research studies involve measurement of variables in *groups* of study subjects. The groups are defined by such characteristics of interest to the study as the presence or absence of a certain disease or the use of one kind of treatment versus another. The primary statistical analysis often consists of a comparison of a given variable of interest (e.g., survival, blood pressure, postoperative infection) between the study groups. When the study variable is continuous, the overall value for the group is usually taken as the average (or *mean*) value for the individuals in the group. When the variable is categorical, the comparison between groups is based on the *rate* (proportion) of group members having the attribute.

Populations and Samples

Neither an investigator nor the public he or she intends to benefit is exclusively interested in results that apply *only* to the subjects participating in a given study. Unless the study subjects are representative of some *target population* of interest, the results will have little meaning. Since, for reasons of feasibility, the entire target population can rarely be studied, some sampling procedure, whether explicit or implicit, must usually be employed. Inferences about the target population will be valid only to the extent that the sample is *representative* of that population.

The best way of ensuring representativeness is by *random sampling*, in which a random number table or some other procedure based on pure chance (e.g., rolling a die or flipping a coin) is used to create the study sample. When random numbers are used, a 50% sample can be obtained by selecting all subjects corresponding to even (or odd) numbers. (For a 10% sample, those whose numbers are divisible by 10 are chosen, etc.) *Systematic* (e.g., alternate, every tenth) *sampling* may result in a representative sample, but if there is any inherent ordering in the population, the sample may be distorted (nonrepresentative). The most common method of sampling is called *convenience sampling*, in which a group of study subjects who either happen to show up or are readily accessible to the investigator are chosen for study. For feasibility reasons, convenience sampling is often unavoidable, but it then becomes difficult to identify the target population that such a sample represents.

Another important aspect of sampling is *sampling variation*, which refers to the chance variation in a sample statistic such as the mean (for continuous variables) or rate (for categorical variables). A small sample might, just by chance, have a mean or rate that differs considerably from that of the entire population, even if the sample is truly random. Repeated small samples from the same population are likely to exhibit considerable sampling variation. In contrast, repeated samples that are large enough to include almost all members of the population would yield sample means or rates very close to the population value and to each other. In other words, sampling variation is inversely related to the sample size.

Description Versus Statistical Inference

Descriptive statistics are intended to summarize a set of individual measurements for a study sample. No contrasts or statistical inferences are made; the data are presented for their own sake. Continuous variables are described by summary measures of central location and spread. Mean urine output and median survival time are examples of central location statistics. Standard deviation and percentile ranges are the kinds of statistics used to describe spread. Rates (e.g., survival rate or treatment success rate) are the descriptive statistics most commonly used for categorical variables.

TABLE 15.1. Types of variable (with examples).

I. Continuous (systolic blood pressure)
II. Categorical
  A. Dichotomous (vital status: dead vs. alive)
  B. Polychotomous
    1. Nominal (country of origin)
    2. Ordinal (severity of postoperative pain: none, mild, moderate, severe)

Statistical inference is a process by which data from samples are used to make inferences about populations. It comprises two principal activities: parametric estimation and significance testing. In *parametric estimation*, inferences are drawn about *parameters** (mathematical descriptors such as the rate, mean, relative risk, slope, correlation coefficient, or standard deviation) in a population based on *parametric estimators* obtained in a sample. This activity includes the estimation of *confidence intervals* around sample statistics. In *significance testing*, *P* values (probabilities) are calculated based on hypotheses about the effect (and direction of effect) of one variable on another.

It must be emphasized that statistical inference is not the same thing as *analytic inference*. Statistical inference *assumes* that the sample is obtained randomly from (and is therefore representative of) the target population. It is based purely on sampling variation and concerns the role of chance in extrapolating the sample results to the population. In analytic inference, we also draw conclusions about a target population based on evidence adduced in a sample, but the basis for inference is the absence of bias in the design and execution of the study.

*Many people use the term "parameter" as a synonym for "variable." Although this is common in everyday parlance, we will avoid it in this chapter and restrict the use of "parameter" to its accepted statistical meaning.

TABLE 15.2. Age distribution of 250 postcholecystectomy patients.

Age (years)	Number (%) of patients
16-20	2 (0.5)
21-25	2 (0.5)
26-30	5 (2.0)
31-35	9 (3.6)
36-40	17 (6.8)
41-45	31 (12.4)
46-50	83 (33.2)
51-55	46 (18.4)
56-60	35 (14.0)
61-65	20 (8.0)
Total	250 (100)

Descriptive Statistics and Data Display

Continuous Variables

Perhaps the most informative method for summarizing and displaying a set of measurements for a continuous variable is constructing a *frequency distribution*. This is accomplished by categorizing the continuous data (i.e., breaking down the range of observed values into a series of successive categories) and counting the number of study subjects whose measurements fall within each category. The frequency distribution can be displayed in either tabular or graphic form. The usual graphic form is the *histogram*, a bar graph in which the rate for each category is proportional to the *area* of the corresponding bar. If the investigator wants the *heights* of the bars to reflect the rates for each category, he or she needs to ensure that the *width* of each bar (i.e., the upper minus the lower limit for each category) is the same.

Suppose you want to describe the age distribution of 250 patients undergoing cholecystectomy in your surgical department within a given time period. If you choose ten 5-year age categories, the results might look like those shown in Table 15.2. The corresponding histogram appears in Figure 15.1. Because there is a total of only 9 patients in the three youngest age categories, it might be advisable to "collapse" them into a single category, 16–30 years. In that case, the height of the corresponding histogram bar should be 3, rather than 9, so that the total area of the bar remains proportional to the overall rate for the enlarged category:

$$(3)(15) = 45 = (2)(5) + (2)(5) + (5)(5)$$

In addition to these tabular and graphic methods, continuous variables can often be summarized using simple statistics that describe the distribution of individual values in the sample. Three major characteristics of the distribution are usually described: central tendency, shape, and spread.

Three measures are in common use for describing central tendency: the mean, the median, and the mode. The *mean* (or average) is the sum of all values divided by the number of values. The *median* is the value of the middle member of the group. The median is preferred to the mean as a measure of central tendency when the distribution is asymmetrical. Length of hospital stay is a good example; it has a fixed lower bound but no upper bound. The *mode*, that is, the peak of the frequency distribution, is the value that appears most often. It is the least used of the three measures of central

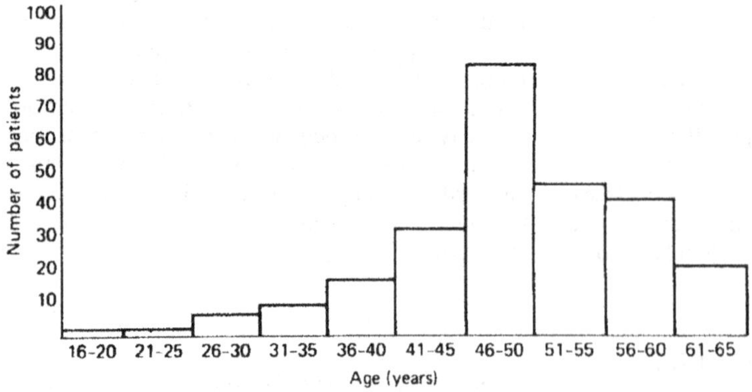

FIGURE 15.1. Age histogram for 250 postcholecystectomy patients.

tendency because it is not readily manipulated mathematically.

The calculation of each of these three measures is illustrated below for the serum creatinine measurements (in mg/dl, arranged in ascending order) in a sample of 15 patients:

0.3, 0.6, 0.6, 0.7, 0.8, 0.8, 0.8, 0.9, 1.0, 1.0, 1.1, 1.3, 1.4, 1.6, 2.1

mean = 15.0/15 = 1.0 mg/dl
median = 8th value = 0.9 mg/dl
mode = 0.8 mg/dl

The main characteristics of the shape of a frequency distribution are the number of peaks (modes) and the degree of asymmetry. A distribution with two modes is referred to as *bimodal*, one with three modes as *trimodal*, etc. The asymmetry characteristic is called *skewness*. A distribution is said to be skewed to the right when the mean exceeds the median and skewed to the left when the median exceeds the mean.

Four types of statistics are commonly used to describe the spread of a distribution: range, percentile ranges, variance, and standard deviation. The *range* is the interval between the lowest and highest value in the distribution. A *percentile range* is an interval between two percentile points. Thus, the inner 90 percentile range includes all values between the 5th and 95th percentiles; the inter quartile range includes those between the 25th and 75th percentiles. The *variance* is defined as follows:

$$\text{variance} = \frac{\Sigma(x_i - \bar{x})^2}{n - 1}$$

where x_i = the individual values
$\bar{x}$ = the mean (average) value of the study group
n = the sample size (the number of subjects in the study group)
Σ = the Greek symbol used to denote summing all the $(x_i - \bar{x})^2$ for each x_i in the group

The *standard deviation* (SD) is the square root of the variance:

$$\text{SD} = \sqrt{\frac{\Sigma(x_i - \bar{x})^2}{n - 1}}.$$

The quantity $n - 1$ is called the *degrees of freedom*. The rationale for its use is based on the fact that, for a given mean $\bar{x}$, $n - 1$ x_i's are considered free or independent, since the nth value of x is determined by $\bar{x}$ and all the other x_i's. The standard deviation can also be expressed as a proportion, or percentage, of the mean value. This entity SD/$\bar{x}$ is called the *coefficient of variation*.

The range and percentile ranges can be used for any distribution, regardless of its shape. The standard deviation is best reserved for sample data that are distributed fairly symmetrically around the sample mean, because it is affected by extreme (very high or very low) values. It is most appropriate when the distribution is what statisticians call *normal*.

The *normal*, or *Gaussian, distribution* is the most important distribution in statistics. This is the well-known bell-shaped curve that not only describes the distribution of many traits (e.g., height, blood pressure, intelligence) in the general population, but also serves as the basis for the inferential statistics of means to be discussed below.

The standard deviation is a particularly useful descriptor of spread for data that are normally distributed, because the proportions of values that lie within intervals defined by multiples of the SD are known:

68.3% lie within $\pm$ 1 SD from the mean
95.4% lie within $\pm$ 2 SD from the mean
99.7% lie within $\pm$ 3 SD from the mean

Despite these attractive properties, it must be emphasized that the term "normal," when used to describe this distribution, has absolutely nothing to do with the usual clinical connotation of the word indicating absence of disease.

Another statistic is often encountered in the medical literature as a descriptor of spread: the *standard error of the mean* (SEM). It is defined as

$$\text{SEM} = \left(\frac{\text{SD}}{\sqrt{n}}\right)$$

where n is the sample size (number of subjects in the study group).

Because the SEM decreases with increasing sample size, it is *not* a good descriptor of the spread of a distribution, despite its popularity. A large sample with a high standard deviation may have a small standard error. Since the standard error is always smaller than the standard deviation, it tends to give the impression that the spread of the data is less than it really is. Consequently, it may be favored by authors who wish to minimize, rather than illustrate, the variability of their data.

The SEM is actually the SD of a distribution of *means* obtained in repeated sampling from a population. As we shall see later, it is important in making inferences based on sample means. As a descriptor, however, its use should be avoided.

TABLE 15.3. Four steps in research.

1. Statement of research hypothesis
2. Study design
3. Data collection
4. Statistical analysis

Categorical Variables

A categorical variable is best described by the rate, or proportion, of study subjects falling within each category of the variable. Suppose you are interested in describing the outcome in the sample of 250 cholecystectomy patients mentioned earlier. If the outcome of interest is the (dichotomous) presence or absence of right upper quadrant pain 6 months postoperatively, the result can be expressed as a proportion or percentage. Thus, if 140 patients are pain-free at 6 months, the overall rate for the sample is 140/250, or 56%. Although such a result could be represented visually in a table or graph, a single rate or percentage is usually sufficient to convey the information. The proportion of patients still experiencing pain is, of course, $1 - 140/250 = 110/250$, or $100 - 56\% = 44\%$.

When rates for a polychotomous variable are described, tables and graphs are often helpful. Suppose your 6-month follow-up variable comprises the following four ordinal categories: more pain, no change (from preoperative pain status), less pain, and no pain. (Assume that this scale has specific criteria that produce reproducible, valid measurements.) The hypothetical results in the 250 study patients can then be described as follows: 15/250 (6%) with more pain, 25/250 (10%) with no change, 70/250 (28%) with less pain, and 140/250 (56%) (as above) with no pain. The sum of the proportions must equal 1, and that of the percentages, 100%. When many categories are involved, the use of a table, histogram, or pie chart can often aid the reader to appreciate the relative proportions in each category. A pie chart achieves the same effect as a histogram by dividing a circle into slices that correspond in size to the respective proportions.

Statistical Inference

Formulating and Testing a Research Hypothesis

There are four steps in the execution of a research project (see Table 15.3). The first is the statement of a *research hypothesis*. The research hypothesis is what the researcher thinks might happen. It can usually be posed in the form of a statement or question. Consider a clinical trial of medical versus surgical (coronary artery bypass grafting) therapy in patients with left main stem coronary obstruction. The research hypothesis might be expressed as a statement: "Surgery leads to longer survival than medical therapy" or as a question: "Does surgery lead to longer survival than medical therapy?"

The second step in carrying out a research project is the *design* of a study that will test the research hypothesis adequately and without bias. After the design has been carefully laid out, the study is begun and the *data* are *collected*—the third step. The fourth step is the *statistical analysis* of the data.

Besides the description and display of the data, the analysis usually involves statistical inferences, particularly about the effect of such variables as treatment or disease on some health outcome in the target population of which the study sample is representative. The two basic approaches to statistical inference are hypothesis-testing (calculation of P values) and estimation of confidence intervals around the observed (sample) measure of effect. The remainder of this section and the two sections that follow focus on hypothesis testing.

In the traditional approach, the researcher tests for statistical significance by examining the data obtained in the study with respect to a *null hypothesis*. The null hypothesis is a theoretical construct, postulating that there is no effect of a given variable on the study outcome. When two groups are being compared, the null hypothesis states that the two groups are random samples from target populations with the same mean or proportion.

Note that the null hypothesis is usually quite different from the research hypothesis. The investigator plans the research because he or she thinks a difference exists between the two groups or is suspicious enough that it might exist to make such a study worthwhile. The null hypothesis is a "straw man" that provides a reference for examining the significance of the data obtained. For our coronary bypass example, the null hypothesis is that there is no difference in survival among patients with left main stem coronary obstruction who receive surgery and those who receive medical therapy.

The null hypothesis can be the same as the research hypothesis if the researcher believes, or wants to demonstrate, that there really is no difference between the two groups. In general, however, the research and null hypotheses are entirely different. Once this distinction is clear, the testing of the null hypothesis becomes the basis for assessing the statistical significance of an observed difference.

Testing the Null Hypothesis

Let us restrict our discussion to the consideration of data obtained from two study groups (samples). We wish to determine whether the difference obtained between the two groups is statistically significant—that is, whether their underlying target populations have different means or proportions. We begin testing the null hypothesis by assuming it to be true (i.e., that the two groups are both random samples from target populations with the same mean or proportion). We then calculate the probability of obtaining a difference at least as large as the observed difference between the two study groups under that assumption. In other words, we calculate the probability of obtaining the observed difference *by chance* if the two groups are random samples from populations with the same mean or proportion. This probability is called the *P value*.

If P is less than a certain amount (by convention, .05), we consider the null hypothesis to be sufficiently unlikely to reject it. Conversely, we are unwilling to reject the null hypothesis if P is $> .05$ because we do not consider it sufficiently unlikely. Rejecting the null hypothesis means that we conclude that the two study groups are not random samples from populations with the same mean or proportion (i.e., that they arise from populations with different means or proportions). The P value "cut off point," or threshold, for rejection of the null hypothesis, should be established a priori. This threshold is called the *α-level* and is conventionally set at .05.

Although .05 has come to be the accepted α-level for most studies in the medical and scientific literature, there is nothing "magic" about it. The difference between a P value of .04 and .06 is very small. The sensible scientist will keep such distinctions in their proper place and will not discard results if the P value is above .05, nor automatically accept them as proven merely because the P value is below .05. It is a fact of life, however, that the difference between P values of .04 and .06 can result in a paper being accepted or rejected for publication.

We may be wrong in rejecting the null hypothesis even if $P < .05$, but we would consider the probability of being wrong acceptably low. A P value of .05 simply indicates that the results obtained could have occurred by chance 5% of the time when the null hypothesis is true. Once out of every 20 times, on average, rejecting the null hypothesis when the P value is .05 will result in an error; that is, we will be rejecting the null hypothesis when it is true. This type of error is called a *Type I error*, and we run the risk of making it whenever we reject the null hypothesis. The lower the P value, the lower the risk. With a P value of .001, there is only one chance in a thousand of making a Type I error.

Because clinical investigation is usually expensive and time-consuming, studies are often used to answer several questions at once (i.e., to test several hypotheses). Interventions may be compared for multiple outcomes, or a variety of clinical, sociodemographic, or treatment factors may be examined for their effects on one or more outcomes. When many tests of significance are performed, some significant differences are likely to arise by chance. In fact, for every 20 independent tests of the null hypothesis, one, on average, will result in statistical significance just by chance. If 100 tests are carried out and 10 are associated with P values less than .05, it is impossible to know which of the 10 are mere chance findings and which represent "truly" significant differences.

To protect against a plethora of Type I errors, some statisticians advocate dividing the α-level required to reject the null hypothesis by the number of tests performed. Because many of the outcomes are associated with one another, the probability of their joint occurrence is usually greater than the product of their individual probabilities; that is, they are not statistically independent. Consequently, such a procedure may be overly conservative and may tend to attribute true differences to chance. At the very least, the investigator should indicate the number of tests performed in addition to the number achieving statistical significance and should moderate his inferences accordingly.

Multiple hypothesis testing becomes an even greater problem when the research hypotheses arise post hoc (i.e., after the data have been collected) rather than a priori. When descriptive statistics are used to *generate* hypotheses for statistical testing, the calculated P values do not accurately reflect the true probability of a difference occurring by chance. After all, it is virtually certain that *some* differences will occur by chance. Betting on a horse after a race is not usually rewarded at the ticket window. Similarly, performing a statistical test of significance on data because they "look" different will result in significant P values that bear no relation to the chance occurrence of a difference hypothesized a priori.

Regardless of whether we are correct in rejecting the null hypothesis, an observed difference that is *statistically significant* may or may not be *clinically important*. Suppose a study comparing serum sodium concentration in two groups of patients yields means in the two groups of 140.2 and 139.9 meq/l. The difference of 0.3 meq/l is clinically trivial, even though with large sample sizes such a difference might be statistically significant. The clinical importance of the observed difference is a *clinical*, not a *statistical*, decision. Never let a colleague, statistician, or editor convince you that a low (i.e., significant) P value can compensate for a difference that is too small to be useful to you or your patients. As we shall see, clinically important differences can fall short of achieving statistical significance, just as clinically trivial differences can occasionally be statistically significant.

We have already discussed the important distinction between the research hypothesis and the null hypothesis. We have also indicated that the research hypothesis can be put in the form of a statement or a question. Let us now consider the *directionality* or *nondirectionality* of the research hypothesis and what it implies in terms of testing for statistical significance (testing the null hypothesis).

In *directional* hypothesis testing, the research hypothesis not only implies that the two groups under investigation will be different but also indicates the direction of the difference. For example, in our study of surgical versus medical therapy for patients with left main stem coronary disease, the research hypothesis is that surgery is *better* (leads to longer survival) than medicine. In *nondirectional* hypothesis testing, the investigator still examines two groups of subjects for a difference but may have no a priori knowledge of which group will fare better. Asked in nondirectional terms, our example would read as follows: *Which* treatment leads to longer survival, surgical or medical? It cannot be overemphasized that if the research hypothesis implies a certain direction (i.e., if the investigator has a strong suspicion that one treatment is better than the other or that the outcome will be better in one group), this must be stated *before* the research is actually carried out, in other words, *before* any data are collected.

The P values listed in most statistical tables are associated with *nondirectional* testing of the null hypothesis; that is, the probability of obtaining the observed difference whether Treatment A is better than Treatment B or vice versa. This is called a *two-sided* test of the null hypothesis. (It is also called a *two-tailed* test, because the distributions of test statistics used to test the null hypothesis often contain two tails, and the P value is equal to the area under the curve of these two tails.)

When the research hypothesis is *directional*, a *one-sided (one-tailed)* test of the null hypothesis can be used. It is essential that the observed difference be in the expected direction (i.e., the direction hypothesized in the directional research hypothesis). If the investigator suspects that Treatment A is better than Treatment B, but the data show the reverse, the derived P value will be highly misleading. The investigator would then do better to refrain from reporting any P value, explaining instead that the direction of the difference was opposite to the one hypothesized. To obtain a one-sided P value, we simply divide the P value listed in a two-sided statistical table by 2.

When in doubt, it is better to use a two-sided test, since this is the more conservative approach. If the research hypothesis is nondirectional, a two-sided test *must* be used. When the research hypothesis is directional and the results are concordant with the direction predicted, a one-sided test can be justified. This distinction can be important, because dividing a P value by 2 (e.g., $P = .08$ to $P = .04$) can create a "statistically significant" ($P < .05$) result, which can often determine the fate of a scientific paper.

Type II Error and Statistical Power

So far, we have talked about what happens when P is less than .05 and about rejecting the null hypothesis. When P is greater than .05 (or some other chosen α-level), we do not reject the null hypothesis. The fact that the chance probability of obtaining the observed difference is greater than .05 does not, however, prove that the null hypothesis is correct. It merely says that the probability is not low enough to reject it. Failing to reject the null hypothesis does not validate it.

If P equals .10, for example, the probability of obtaining the observed difference, under the assumption that the null hypothesis is true, remains unlikely (this is equivalent to a horse with 9-to-1 odds winning a race); but by convention, we do not consider it unlikely *enough* to reject the null hypothesis. Whenever we accept the null hypothesis (i.e., whenever the P value is not low enough to reject it), we risk making another sort of error. This is called a *Type II error*, and it can occur only when the null hypothesis is not rejected. This is important to remember. When we reject the null hypothesis, we run the risk of making a Type I error and the probability of our doing so is equal to the P value. When we do not reject the null hypothesis, we run the risk of a Type II error—that is, the null hypothesis might still be untrue and the study groups are not samples from target populations with the same mean or proportion. These relationships are illustrated in Table 15.4.

The magnitude of the observed difference may be clinically important even if it does not achieve statistical significance. This is especially likely to occur when the sample size is small. Suppose our coronary artery bypass trial included only 3 patients in each group. Because sampling variation is very large with such small sample sizes (see earlier discussion), even if all 3 patients die in one group and all 3 survive in the other, the difference would not be statistically significant. Thus, any investigator who wants to argue that two groups are *not* different merely needs to restrict the number of study subjects to guarantee that no statistically significant difference will be found. The argument remains unconvincing, however, because the risk of a Type II error is high.

The probability, β, of a Type II error can be calculated by constructing an *alternative hypothesis* in which the observed difference is compared to some difference determined a priori to be of potential clinical importance. $1-\beta$ is called *statistical power* and is the probability of detecting some specified, potentially important difference. If a researcher wants to "prove" the null hypothesis (i.e., if the research hypothesis is that no difference exists between the study groups), he or she needs to show that the probability of the alternative hypothesis being correct is very low. The higher the statistical power, the lower the risk of missing (failing to detect) a difference that is potentially clinically important. In other words, to *validate* rather than just fail to reject the null hypothesis. Type II error must be minimized. The probability of committing a Type II error is determined by the magnitude of the hypothesized difference under the alternative hypothesis, the magnitude of the observed difference, the sample size, and (for continuous variables) the variability of the data. Since sample size is the only one of these determinants that is directly controllable by the investigator, sample size is the most important consideration in the planning of a research project for an investigator who wishes to minimize the possibility of a Type II error and maximize statistical power.

An Alternative Approach: Estimation of Confidence Intervals

Recent clinical literature tends to de-emphasize hypothesis testing and P values in favor of estimating confidence intervals around such sample measures of effect as difference in means or proportions, relative risk, slope, and correlation coefficient. Estimating a confidence interval does not require postulation of a null hypothesis. Consequently, the resulting inference allows greater flexibility than the all-or-none decision about whether to reject the null hypothesis.

The confidence interval represents the range in which the effect measure in the target population is likely to fall, based on the data obtained in the study sample. The term "likely" refers to the probability that repeated random samples from the target population would result in an effect measure

TABLE 15.4. The two errors of hypothesis testing (H_0 = null hypothesis).

		Truth	
		H_0 False	H_0 True
Inference	Reject H_0	Correct	Type I error
	Do not reject H_0	Type II error	Correct

falling within the estimated interval. For a 95% confidence interval, the probability is .95, for a 99% confidence interval the probability is .99, and so on. For a difference in means or proportions, a confidence interval is usually expressed as the sample estimate of the difference plus or minus a given value.

Inferential Statistics of Means

Repetitive Sampling and the Central Limit Theorem

Suppose we chose a random sample from some infinitely large source population with known mean μ and standard deviation σ, determined the sample mean $\bar{x}$, replaced the sample, then chose another random sample of the same size, and so on.* What distribution would the *means* of those repeated samples have? It turns out that if n, the size of each sample, is large enough, then the $\bar{x}$'s form a normal distribution, regardless of the distribution of the source population. The mean of this *sampling distribution* of $\bar{x}$'s is the same as the population mean μ; its standard deviation (called the standard error of the mean, or SEM) is $\sigma/\sqrt{n}$.

These interesting and useful facts derive from the *central limit theorem*, one of the pillars of statistical theory. What requirements must be met for the central limit theorem to apply? The main requirement is that n be large enough. How large is "large enough" depends on the distribution of the source population. If it is very close to normal, n can be as small as 2 or 3; if it is quite non-normal (particularly if highly skewed in one direction), n may have to be 50 or even 100.

*Although avoiding excessive use of algebraic symbols is desirable, a certain minimum is required for clarity and economy of expression. The usual convention is to use lowercase Roman letters to indicate sample statistics and lowercase Greek letters for the corresponding population parameters. The sample and population means are usually represented by x and μ, and the standard deviations by s and σ, respectively.

These properties of the central limit theorem would be of theoretical interest only if their application depended on actual repetitive sampling. In the real world of clinical investigation, the investigator has no chance to observe or make use of the distribution of means of repeated samples from a target population. The central limit theorem, however, tells us the mean and standard deviation of the normal distribution that *would* result from repetitive sampling.

By comparing the actual mean obtained in a study sample with the mean and standard deviation of the theoretical sampling distribution of means, the investigator can determine the likelihood (i.e., the probability) of obtaining such a sample, assuming that it originated from the source population of the theoretical sampling distribution. Thus, he or she can calculate a *P* value representing the probability that the sample mean observed would occur in random sampling from a source population with a given mean and standard deviation.

Unfortunately, the use of the normal distribution to test the statistical significance of a difference between a single sample mean and a known population mean depends on knowing the population standard deviation, σ. To test the significance of a sample mean when σ is unknown, a different sampling distribution, the so-called *t-distribution*, is required. The *t*-distribution was discovered by William S. Gossett, a statistician working at the Guinness Brewery in the early years of this century. To avoid a possible adverse reaction by his employer, Gossett published his observations under the name of Student. Most of Gossett's experiments involved small samples from unknown source populations, and he found that the normal distribution was unsatisfactory for making inferences about the means of his samples.

The *t* sampling distribution differs from the normal sampling distribution in that, although its mean is the same (namely, the population mean μ), its standard error, $s/\sqrt{n}$, uses the *sample* standard deviation s, rather than the population standard deviation σ. Like the normal distribution, the *t*-distribution is bell-shaped. Its two "tails," however, are higher than the tails of the normal distribution. Thus, the calculated *P* values, which correspond to the area under the curve of the tails, are higher (i.e., less significant) for a given difference between the sample and population means.

Unlike the normal distribution, there is a different *t*-distribution according to the number of degrees of freedom ($n - 1$). For small samples, the difference from the normal distribution is quite marked. For large samples ($n \geq 30$), the *t*-distribution is quite close to the normal distribution, and the latter can be used for making inferences.

Statistical Inferences Using the *t*-Distribution

As mentioned in the preceding section, the *t*-distribution (or, for large samples, the normal distribution) can be used to test for a statistically significant difference between a sample mean and a known population mean. It can also be used to construct a confidence interval around a sample mean. Such a confidence interval consists of the sample mean plus or minus a multiple of the sample standard error and represents the range in which the investigator can be "confident" that the true population mean lies. A 95% confidence interval represents the range in which the population mean can be expected to lie 95% of the time, based on the sample mean and standard error. An investigator who wants to be more confident (e.g., 99%) needs to extend the interval. Formulas for calculating such intervals are provided in several standard biostatistics texts.[1-5]

The most common use of the *t*-distribution is in testing the significance of a difference in two sample means, or in estimating a confidence interval around the observed difference. If one were to randomly choose two samples at a time from a given (hypothetical) source population, replace the two samples, choose two new samples of the same size, and so on, the *differences* between the two sample means would be normally distributed, provided the source population and sample size do not grossly violate the assumptions of the central limit theorem. In the real world, when investigators wish to test for a statistically significant difference between the means of two study groups, or estimate a confidence interval around the difference, they use the observed difference in means and the standard error of the difference. Under the null hypothesis that the two study groups represent random samples from source populations with the same mean, they can then test the observed difference using the *t*-distribution.

This is the so-called *Student's t-test* (after Gossett) for unpaired (or independent) samples. In effect, the *t*-test compares the magnitude of the observed difference to the variability of the difference as represented by the standard error. If the size of the difference is large with respect to its standard error, the calculated *P* value will be small ($< .05$), the null hypothesis is rejected, and the difference is declared statistically significant. The formula for the *t*-test, as well as instructions for using the t-tables for determining P values and estimating confidence intervals, are provided in the previously cited texts.[1-5]

When two study groups represent matched pairs, the *paired t-test* is a statistically more efficient technique. A matched pair analysis of means is appropriate whenever (1) each subject from one study group is matched to a subject from the other group or (2) the same subject receives each of two study maneuvers. An example of the first type might be a comparison of blood pressure reduction with arterioplasty versus medical therapy in patients with hypertension caused by renal artery obstruction, in which the patients were pair-matched for age, sex, pretreatment blood pressure, and the presence or absence of pretreatment cardiac decompensation. The second type is represented by the crossover trial. In a clinical trial comparing two oral antihypertensive agents, for example, each patient might be tried sequentially on the two agents. Differential treatment of paired organs represents another example of this type, as illustrated by the use of one topical antiglaucoma agent in one eye and a second antiglaucoma drug in the other eye of patients with bilateral disease.

In the paired t-test, statistical significance (or estimation of a confidence interval) is based on the differences observed between the two values for each pair. The pairing results in greater statistical efficiency (i.e., a smaller sample size is required to demonstrate statistical significance and confidence intervals are narrower) because the variability between members of a pair is typically less than that of two unrelated subjects. By eliminating or greatly reducing all sources of intrapair variability *other* than that caused by the study maneuver, any given mean difference will have a greater chance of achieving statistical significance. Formulas for the paired t-test and for estimation of confidence intervals can be found in previously cited texts.[1-5] Crossover trials require several additional statistical considerations, and the interested reader is referred to an excellent review.[6]

Calculating Sample Sizes

In the planning (design) stage of clinical investigation, one of the most important questions the researcher needs to ask is "How many patients (or rats, tissue culture samples, etc.) do I need to study?" To be protected against a Type II error and, in particular, against obtaining a difference that may be clinically important but not quite statistically significant, the investigator must specify, in advance, the difference in means considered clinically worth detecting and the statistical power ($1-\beta$, where β is the probability of a Type II error) desired to detect this difference. The investigator must also estimate (perhaps by consulting the results of previous studies) the standard deviation expected in the sample. Formulas are provided in standard texts.[1,2,4,5]

A far greater (often two- to four-fold) sample size is usually required to protect against Type II error than to demonstrate statistical significance. Consequently, the temptation to ignore Type II error is strong, especially when patients are involved, because the calculated sample sizes are smaller and therefore easier to achieve at a single center over a reasonable period of time. Despite its attractions, such a practice is perilous because the investigator may well find it impossible to make *any* inference at all.

Let us take another look at our study of arterioplasty versus medical therapy for renovascular hypertension. Suppose the surgeon–investigator specifies a difference of 10 mm Hg in diastolic blood pressure as a clinically important difference worth detecting. He estimates his sample standard deviation and, ignoring Type II error, calculates his required sample size. But suppose the study is then carried out with the calculated sample size and the results show a 9 mm Hg difference favoring surgery. Because the sample size calculation was based on a 10 mm difference, the 9 mm difference is not statistically significant. The surgeon may not consider the 9 mm difference to be clinically important, but how sure can he be that the true difference (under the alternative hypothesis) is not 10 mm or even larger? Not very sure, unfortunately, and he can say neither that there is a clinically important difference nor that there is not. The dangers of this Scylla and Charybdis can be avoided only by considering Type II error (statistical power) in the sample size calculation.

Many investigators, faced with the results above, would be tempted to enroll additional patients in the study in an effort to achieve statistical significance for the 9 mm Hg difference. There are two problems with such an approach. First, repeated significance testing increases the risk of detecting a significant difference by chance alone (i.e., of committing a Type I error). If results are repeatedly analyzed, the P values calculated from the t-tests will underestimate the true risk of a Type I error (see the discussion of multiple significance tests). Second, if the null hypothesis is in fact true, subsequent results may show a difference smaller than 9 mm Hg, and the difference may fail to achieve statistical significance despite the larger sample size.

Nonparametric Tests

The t-test (paired or unpaired) is the significance test of choice in comparing two means, provided the requirements of the central limit theorem are met. Unless sample sizes are quite small, however, the underlying source populations may exhibit considerable departure from normality without disturbing, to an important degree, the sampling distribution of means or difference in means. In statistical parlance, we say that the t-test is *robust*. Many investigators who have had some exposure to statistics have the quite mistaken notion that the t-test can be used only when source populations are normally distributed. Such is not the case.

When the requirements of the central limit theorem are grossly violated, alternative analytic strategies are required. This is particularly likely to occur with small samples from highly skewed source populations. Variables with zero as the obligatory lower boundary often exhibit skewed distributions, with many low values and fewer and fewer high values extending out into a long tail. Examples include length of hospitalization and the dose of drug required to produce a given clinical effect.

Faced with a highly skewed distribution, the investigator has two main choices. He or she can either *transform* the native data in a way that normalizes the distribution (e.g., by taking their logarithms), or use a *nonparametric* test. Nonparametric tests differ from the t-test and other *parametric tests* because they do not depend on using sampling distributions of parametric estimators (such as the mean) obtained in samples to make inferences about the corresponding population parameters. In other words, they require no assumptions about underlying distributions.

To use a nonparametric test of two continuous variables, the actual magnitudes are ignored and only the *ranks* (i.e., relative magnitudes) are used to calculate statistical significance. In the unpaired test (the *Mann–Whitney U test*),[1,5,7,8] each member of one study group is compared to every member of the other group, and a "winner" is declared for each comparison. The total number of wins in each group (called the U statistic) is calculated and then compared to the totals that would be expected if the wins were distributed by chance. In the *Wilcoxon signed rank test* (a paired test),[1-3,5,7] the magnitudes of the differences (ignoring the sign) between each matched pair are ranked (assigning the rank 1 to the smallest difference) and the sums of the ranks are compared in those pairs with positive differences and those with negative differences. Under the null hypothesis, these sums should be equal and the actual result can be referred to the chance-expected distribution of sums around a median of 0.

Although nonparametric tests of means have the advantage of requiring no assumptions, the use of relative magnitudes or ranks rather than actual values may result in a loss of statistical efficiency and, therefore, in more conservative statistical inferences. To maximize statistical efficiency, it is sometimes preferable to use the t-test, even if prior logarithmic or other transformation of highly skewed data is required.

Comparing Three or More Means

So far, we have restricted our discussion to testing the statistical significance of a difference in two means. To compare the means of three or more groups, the investigator uses a procedure called a *one-way analysis of variance* (ANOVA). The assumptions are similar to those required for the t-test, and the null hypothesis is that the groups are equivalent (i.e., they represent random samples from the source populations with the same mean). In essence, the procedure divides the total variance (the square of the standard deviation) of all study subjects into two portions: (1) that part accounted for by differences among the groups (the intergroup variance), and (2) that part accounted for by differences between subjects within the same group (the intragroup variance). The larger the former relative to the latter, the less likely it is that the differences among group means are due to chance.

The primary result of a one-way ANOVA is a P value representing a test of the null hypothesis. If P is less than .05, we conclude that the group means are not equivalent. If the investigator is interested in finding out which groups are responsible for the overall difference, pairs of groups can be compared two at a time, but P values must be adjusted to account for multiple testing. Different procedures are available for carrying out such secondary analyses, and the interested reader may wish to consult an appropriate reference.[1]

Sometimes, an investigator may wish to study the effects of two or more treatments or other study factors simultaneously. In the example of arterioplasty versus medical therapy in renovascular hypertension, the investigator may be interested in studying the effect of gender, as well as treatment, on the outcome (diastolic blood pressure). Although a separate t-test could be performed for males and females, a *two-way analysis of variance* provides greater statistical efficiency and an opportunity to test for gender effects independent of treatment. Provided the sample size is sufficient to yield adequate numbers in each subgroup, ANOVA methods can be extended (three-way, four-way, etc.) for larger numbers of study effects.

Control for Confounding Factors

In many clinical investigations, a simple comparison of two or more group means may be biased by confounding differences between groups. Consider once again our example of arterioplasty versus medical therapy for renovascular hypertension, in which the major outcome is diastolic blood pressure 6 months after initiating treatment. If the surgical group has lower pretreatment blood pressure, on average, than the medical group, a lower posttreatment diastolic pressure in the surgical group might be due to the pretreatment difference rather than the surgery. Such a confounding effect could even occur in a randomized trial, in which patients were randomly assigned to medical versus surgical therapy, if the random treatment assignment yielded a maldistribution of pretreatment blood pressures, unlikely as that would be.

We have already mentioned one way of controlling for such a confounding factor, namely pairwise matching. For example, each surgical patient could be matched by pretreatment diastolic pressure (e.g., $\pm$ 5 mm Hg) with a medical patient, and a paired t-test could be used to test for a significant difference. A second strategy would be to stratify all study patients according to the confounder (e.g., 90–99 mm Hg, 100–109 mm Hg, $\geq$ 110 mm Hg) and then compare the stratum-specific group means.

The most convenient strategy, in this day of prepackaged software, may be to *adjust* the group means according to the outcome each subject would have if he had the mean value of the confounder. (This adjustment assumes that the relationship between the confounder and the outcome is known, e.g., pretreatment and posttreatment diastolic pressures, respectively, in our example. Most frequently, a linear correlation is assumed. Linear correlation will be considered in greater detail below.) This procedure is called *analysis of covariance* (ANCOVA) or covariate adjustment and can be used for any number of continuous and dichotomous categorical variables.[1,9] It can be combined with the study of multiple study effects by using multiple-way ANCOVA.

Inferential Statistics of Rates and Proportions

Comparing Two Proportions

When the outcome variable under analysis is categorical rather than continuous, the main statistical procedure is a comparison of rates (proportions) rather than means. When there are two study groups and the outcome variable is dichotomous, the comparison is between two proportions. As an example, consider a comparison of postoperative wound infection rates in patients treated preoperatively with broad spectrum antibiotics and those treated with placebo. Suppose we randomized treatment assignment in 500 consecutive laparotomy patients, with 240 receiving the antibiotic and 260 receiving the placebo, and that the subsequent infection rates were 7/240 (2.9%) and 15/260 (5.8%), respectively. The data can be displayed in a 2 × 2 (fourfold) table, as shown in Table 15.5. The row totals are the total numbers of patients receiving antibiotic and placebo; the column totals are the total numbers of patient with and without wound infections. In 2 × 2 tables, the greater the difference between two proportions (e.g., the proportions of antibiotic and placebo recipients with postoperative wound infections), the greater the association of the columns with the rows. In our example, we are interested in testing whether there is a statistically significant association between postoperative wound infection (columns) and preoperative treatment (rows), in other words, a statistically significant effect of preoperative treatment on postoperative wound infection.

Table 15.5. Postlaparotomy wound infection after preoperative antibiotic versus placebo.

	Infection	No infection	
Antibiotic	7	233	240
Placebo	15	245	260
	22	478	500

To test for such an association, we establish a null hypothesis of no association and then assess the probability that the observed association arose solely by chance. (This is equivalent to saying that the two treatment groups arose by random sampling from source populations with the same infection rate.) Because the null hypothesis of no effect indicates that the columns should be independent of the rows, we thus calculate the frequency we would *expect* in each of the four cells of the 2 × 2 table under the null hypothesis of statistical independence. If the observed frequencies differ sufficiently from the frequencies expected under the null hypothesis, we reject the null hypothesis and conclude that the columns and rows are not independent (i.e., that they are associated).

How do we calculate the expected cell frequencies? The probability that two independent events will both occur is the product of their individual probabilities. [For example, the probability of simultaneously obtaining a heads on a coin flip and a 6 on a die role is $(1/2)(1/6) = 1/12$.] The probability of being in a given row is the same as the proportion of the total sample N lying in that row (i.e., r_i/N), the row total divided by the total sample size. Similarly, the probability of being in a given column is c_j/N. Thus the probability of being in a given cell (i.e., the two independent events of being in a given row *and* a given column) is $(r_i/N)(c_j/N)$, or r_ic_j/N^2. The expected cell frequency (E_{ij}) is then simply the probability of being in a given cell times the total sample size: $E_{ij} = (r_ic_j/N^2)(N) = r_ic_j/N$. For the example shown in Table 15.5, the expected frequency for the upper left cell (antibiotic recipients with postoperative wound infections) is calculated as follows:

$$E = \frac{(240)\,(22)}{500} = 10.6$$

In each cell of the table, we now have both an observed (O) and an expected (E) frequency. The only thing we lack is a statistical method for comparing the Os with the Es to see whether we should reject the null hypothesis.

χ^2 (chi-square) is a statistic with a known frequency distribution that allows us to calculate P values from observed (O_{ij}) and expected (E_{ij}) cell frequencies. It is defined as follows:

$$\chi^2 = \Sigma \frac{(O_{ij} - E_{ij})^2}{E_{ij}}$$

It can be calculated by computing the expected frequency (E_{ij}) for each cell, subtracting it from the observed frequency (O_{ij}) in the table, squaring the resulting difference, dividing by the expected frequency, and then summing this ratio over all four cells in the table. (Various algebraically equivalent, but computationally more convenient, formulas for calculating χ^2 are found in most statistics texts.[1-3,5,10]) The larger the value for χ^2, the more the observed frequencies differ from those expected under the null hypothesis and the smaller (i.e., the more significant) the P value.

As with the t-distribution, a different χ^2 distribution exists for each different number of degrees of freedom. For χ^2, however, the number of degrees of freedom is based not on the total sample size, but on the number of rows and columns:

$$\text{degrees of freedom} = (r - 1)\,(c - 1)$$

where r is the number of rows and c is the number of columns.

For a 2×2 table, degrees of freedom $= (2 - 1)(2 - 1) = 1$. This makes intuitive sense, because the marginal (row and column) totals are considered to be fixed in calculating the expected cell frequencies. With fixed marginals in a 2×2 table, the value in any one cell automatically determines the other three.

The theoretical χ^2 frequency distribution is a smooth, continuous curve. Because observed frequencies are discrete, so are the calculated values of χ^2. When N is very large, many more values are possible for O_{ij} and thus for χ^2, and the distribution of calculated values begins to approach the theoretical distribution. A wound infection rate of 7 out of 240 might represent any number from 6½ to 7½; that is, a similar group of 2400 patients would have observed frequencies anywhere from 65 to 75. Some statisticians feel that when N is small a *continuity correction* is required to compensate for the failure of the discrete possible values to closely approximate the continuous distribution. In 1934 Yates decided to subtract 1/2 from the absolute value of each $O_{ij} - E_{ij}$ to provide a better approximation. The resulting χ^2 with continuity correction (χ^2_c) is defined as follows:

$$\chi^2_c = \Sigma \frac{(|O_{ij} - E_{ij}| - \frac{1}{2})^2}{E_{ij}}$$

where $|\ \ |$ indicates absolute value (i.e., a minus sign becomes positive). χ^2_c is then interpreted in the same way as the uncorrected χ^2 at 1 degree of freedom (χ^2_c is used only for comparing two proportions).

The continuity correction results in smaller values for χ^2 and, consequently, in statistical inferences that are more conservative. In other words, the null hypothesis is less likely to be rejected. The lower risk of Type I error must be balanced against a greater risk of Type II error. For large samples, the continuity correction is probably unnecessary, but for small samples the P values obtained using χ^2_c will be closer to the exact probability calculated using a purely stochastic (chance-based) model.

When expected cell frequencies are very small (<5), the χ^2 test, even with the continuity correction, should be avoided. The statistical test of choice in such a situation is the *Fisher exact probability test*.[1-3,5,10] The P values calculated with the Fisher exact test are derived from a pure stochastic model based on permutation theory. The test requires laborious computations if performed by hand but is expeditiously executed by programs that are readily available in most statistical software packages. The test first examines all the 2 × 2 tables possible by chance, given the fixed marginal (row and column) totals, then determines the number of such tables with results at least as extreme (i.e., with the rows and columns associated to at least as great a degree) as those observed. Since each table is equally likely to occur by chance under the pure stochastic model, the *P* value is simply the number of tables with equal or greater association divided by the total possible number of tables.

Like the comparison of two means, the estimation of confidence intervals represents an alternative approach to statistical comparison of two proportions. Instead of testing how consistent an observed difference in proportions is with a "true" state of no difference, the confidence interval indicates how big the "true" difference is likely to be. The estimation procedure is based on the normal approximation of the binomial distribution (see next section), and is described in several standard texts.[1-3,10]

A comparison of two proportions can also be based on their *ratio*, rather than their difference. In clinical trials or cohort studies, such a comparison usually consists of the ratio of the proportion of subjects in the two study groups p_1 and p_2 who develop a given outcome: p_1/p_2. This ratio is called the *relative risk* (*RR*). Thus the results of the postlaparotomy wound infection trial, tabulated in Table 15.5, can be summarized in terms of the relative risk of infection in antibiotic- versus placebo-treated patients as 7/240/15/260 = 0.51. In case-control studies, the corresponding measure is the *odds ratio* (*OR*), which is the ratio of the odds (*p*/1-*p*) of exposure to the suspected causal agent or maneuver in subjects with the outcome (cases), to the odds in those without the outcome (controls).

If *RR* (or *OR*) is greater than 1, exposure is associated with an increased risk of the outcome. If *RR* (or *OR*) is less than 1, exposure is associated with a significantly decreased risk of (i.e., protection against) developing the outcome. Accordingly, the *RR* = .51 for postoperative wound infection in antibiotic-treated (relative to placebo-treated) patients indicates the degree of protection (i.e., reduction by approximately one-half) afforded by the antibiotic. The statistical significance of an *RR* or *OR* can be tested using the χ^2 test or the Fisher exact test or by estimating a confidence interval around the observed value using one of several procedures.[10,14]

Calculating Sample Sizes

To ensure adequate statistical power to detect a given difference in proportions and exclude such a difference if no significant difference is found, statisticians usually rely on a formula based on the normal distribution. The normal distribution can be used as a basis for this calculation because the pure stochastic model produces a frequency distribution, called the *binomial distribution*, that closely approximates the normal distribution, provided the expected cell frequencies are all 5 or more.

Assuming an α-level of .05, the investigator must specify two additional components to permit the sample size calculation: p_1 and p_2 the proportions he or she estimates in the two groups, such that $p_1 - p_2$ represents the minimum threshold for a clinically important difference; and $1 - \beta$, the statistical power desired to ensure that a difference as large as $p_1 - p_2$ in the hypothetical source population will be detected. Once these components have been specified, the investigator may use a standard formula[1,2,5,10] or consult the derived tables provided by Fleiss.[10]

Comparing Three or More Proportions

The χ^2 test is easily extended to comparison of three or more proportions, although this is not the case with χ^2_c or the Fisher exact text. χ^2 is still defined as $\Sigma(O_{ij} - E_{ij})^2/E_{ij}$ and is interpreted at $(r - 1)(c - 1)$ degrees of freedom. When the outcome variable is ordinal, however, the χ^2 test does not take account of the inherent order among the categories used to measure the variable. It merely tests the significance of the observed versus expected differences across all the $r \times c$ cells of the table.

Consider a 6-month follow-up comparison of ankle swelling (none, mild, or severe) in patients with ligamentous injuries treated with surgery versus those treated conservatively (cast only). With a χ^2 test, none, mild, and severe are treated as simple nominal, nonordered categories of swelling. Such a test of mere association between columns and rows may be statistically inefficient, because it fails to account for the *direction* of the association. The χ^2 test makes no distinction between results showing more instances of severe swelling with casts and more instances of mild and no swelling with surgery (surgery clearly better than casts) versus those showing more instances of mild swelling with surgery and *both* more instances of severe *and* more instances of nonswelling with casts (surgery more likely to produce intermediate results).

One alternative to the χ^2 test that does take order into account is the Mann-Whitney test. This test is the same nonparametric test described previously and is based on comparing the ranks, or relative magnitudes, of all subjects in both groups. With only three categories in our example,

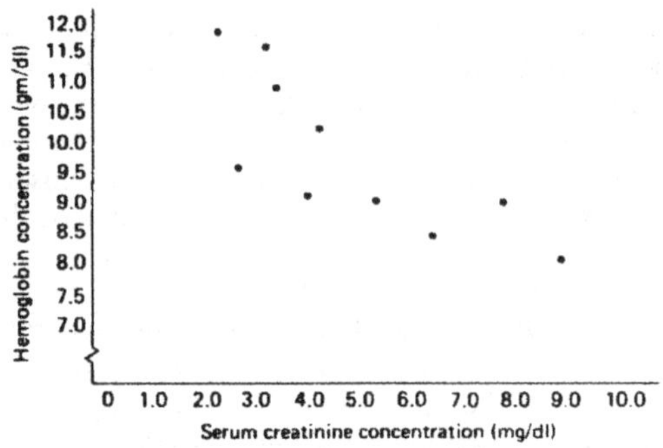

FIGURE 15.2. Hemoglobin and serum creatinine concentrations in 10 patients with chronic renal failure.

there will be many ties, but the procedure may nevertheless provide an improvement in efficiency over the χ^2 test.

Control for Confounding Factors

Comparisons of proportions, like comparisons of means, can be biased by confounding differences between the study groups. In our study of surgical repair versus casts in patients with ligamentous ankle injuries, a result showing less swelling in the surgically treated group at 6-month follow-up would be biased if the patients in that group were younger, on average, than those in the group treated with casts. Surgeons might be understandably reluctant to operate on older patients with such injuries, but the younger patients might be expected to do better regardless of treatment. A fair test of the treatment effect should control for the confounding effect of age.

Because our discussion can be greatly simplified by focusing on dichotomous outcomes, we shall "dichotomize" ankle swelling as absent or mild (clinically unimportant) versus severe (clinically important). One way of controlling for the confounding effect of age would be to pair-match surgically and nonsurgically treated patients by age (e.g., $\pm$ 5 years). A matched-pair χ^2 test, called the *McNemar test*, can then be performed and the result can be interpreted in the same way as the usual χ^2 test.[1-4,10,11] A second strategy would be to stratify the study group by age category (e.g., ≤ 40 years vs. > 40 years) and then calculate the stratum-specific χ^2's or an overall χ^2 weighted by the size of the individual strata, the *Mantel–Haenszel χ^2 test*.[1,5,10,11]

In the case of multiple confounders, two multivariate adjustment techniques are most commonly used: *discriminant function analysis* and *multiple logistic regression*. The latter is generally preferable, because the validity of the former depends, to some extent, on the assumption of normally distributed source populations. Both techniques are beyond the scope of this chapter, but the interested reader will find excellent discussions in two of the references cited at the end of this chapter.[12,13]

Linear Correlation and Regression

Linear Correlation

A comparison of proportions is really a test of association between two categorical variables: study group (e.g., antibiotic vs. placebo) and outcome (presence or absence of postoperative wound infection). Even a comparison of means can be thought of as a test of association between a categorical variable (study group, e.g., surgery vs. medical therapy for renovascular hypertension) and a continuous variable (the study outcome, e.g., posttreatment diastolic pressure). But how do we measure the association between two continuous variables? The usual strategy is to examine the extent to which the relation between the two can be described by a straight line, that is, the extent of their *linear correlation*.

Linear correlation measures the degree to which an increase in one continuous variable is associated with an exactly proportional increase or decrease in a second continuous variable. Consider a scatter diagram (Fig. 15.2) depicting the hemoglobin and serum creatinine concentrations in 10 patients with chronic renal failure. If every point fell exactly on a straight line, the two variables would be perfectly correlated.

The *Pearson correlation coefficient*, abbreviated by the letter r, is a descriptive statistic indicating the extent of linear correlation. It ranges in value from -1 to $+1$, with 0 representing no correlation, -1 a perfect inverse correlation (negatively sloping line), and $+1$ a perfect positive correlation (positively sloping line) between the two variables. For our hemoglobin–creatinine example, $r = -.78$, indicating a strong inverse correlation. It should be stressed that r indicates the extent of *linear* correlation only. Two continuous variables may have a very close relation but poor linear correlation (e.g., a U-shaped or quadratic relation).

Dependent and Nondependent Relationships

In examining the linear relation between two continuous variables, we can often deduce, on biological grounds, whether one variable is *dependent* on the other or whether the two are *nondependent*. In our chronic renal failure example, hemoglobin is being tested for its dependence on renal function (as represented by serum creatinine). We certainly do not believe that the creatinine depends on the hemoglobin; this type of dependency makes no biologic sense. Hemoglobin concentration is called the *dependent variable* and serum creatinine the *independent variable*. (It is as if the creatinine were allowed to vary independently, and the hemoglobin then depended on the observed value of creatinine.) By convention, the independent variable is usually represented by the x-axis and the dependent variable by the y-axis.

In contrast to the dependent relation between hemoglobin and creatinine, consider the relation between blood urea nitrogen (BUN) and creatinine. The two are usually highly positively correlated because both are tests of renal function, even though other factors (e.g., state of hydration for BUN and muscle mass for creatinine) prevent the correlation from being perfect. Although both variables depend on renal function, neither depends on the other and the relation between the two is nondependent. In a graphical display of the relationship, either could be represented by the y-axis. The decision that a relationship is dependent or nondependent arises from *clinical*, not *statistical*, reasoning.

Since the correlation between two variables is rarely perfect (i.e., r rarely equals $+1$ or -1), we are often interested in measuring the extent to which the relation between the two is explained by a straight line. To do this, we make use of a concept known as *explained variance*.

We can interpret r in these terms by measuring the proportion of total variance in one variable that is due to its linear relation with the other. In our example of hemoglobin and creatinine, we can divide the variance in hemoglobin into (1) a component due to the linear relation between hemoglobin and creatinine and (2) a component due to undetermined causes, including random variation. It can be shown that r^2 equals the proportion of variance in either variable that is due to its linear correlation with the other. In our example, $r = -.78$, and $r^2 = .61$. Our interpretation of this value of r^2 is that the relation between hemoglobin and serum creatinine "accounts for" 61% of the variance in hemoglobin.

Linear Regression

Linear regression is the process of fitting a straight line to bivariate continuous data. Given two continuous variables, x and y, we wish to determine the parameters a and b in the equation: $\hat{y} = a + bx$, where $\hat{y}$ indicates the estimated value of y, based on x. In this general equation for a straight line, a is the intercept (the value of y when $x = 0$) and b is the slope (the amount of change in y per unit change in x). Another name for b is the *regression coefficient*.

In our example of hemoglobin (y) and creatinine (x),

$$\hat{y} = 12.04 - 0.49x$$

This means that, on average, for every increase in serum creatinine concentration of 1 mg/dl, the decrease in hemoglobin concentration is 0.49 g/dl, at least over the range of measurements shown in Figure 15.2. (It is hazardous to extrapolate the linear relation between x and y beyond the observed ranges of x and y.)

Because the relation between hemoglobin and creatinine is a biologically dependent one (since renal function, as represented by the serum creatinine, affects the hemoglobin concentration, rather than the converse), we have *regressed* hemoglobin on creatinine. This is the usual practice we regress one variable on another—that is, we regress y (the dependent variable) on x (the independent variable).

Interpretation of r and b

We now have two different descriptive statistics, or coefficients, to describe the extent of linear relation between two continuous variables x and y. The correlation coefficient r is useful for describing the degree of linear closeness (linear correlation) between x and y, irrespective of which is dependent or independent. A major advantage of r is that it remains the same regardless of units. In our example, $r = -.78$ whether creatinine is measured in milligrams per deciliter or millimoles per liter. The one disadvantage of r is that it is not useful for *predicting* y from x.

To predict y from x, regression is required. Unlike r, the value of the regression coefficient b will change with changes in the units in which x and y are measured. The value of b in our example would be entirely different from -0.49 if creatinine were measured in millimoles per liter instead of milligrams per deciliter.

The extent to which a relationship between variables can be described by a straight line is denoted by r, whereas b is the rate of change in y for every unit rise in x. Interpretation of the two coefficients is contrasted by the three regression lines shown in Figure 15.3. Each of the three regressions is represented by a perfectly straight line (i.e., $r = 1$

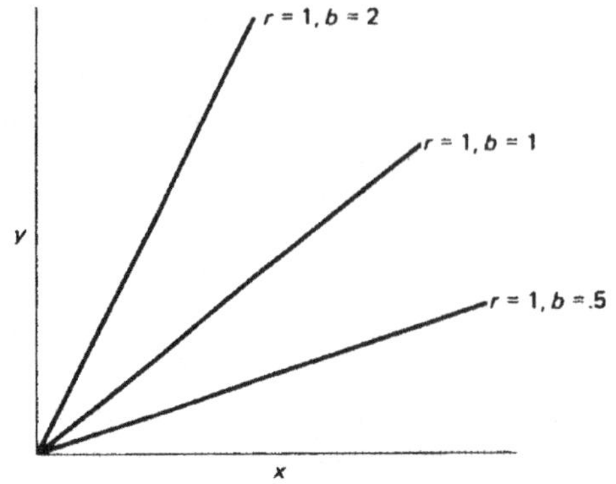

FIGURE 15.3. The distinction between r and b.

for all three). The slope b differs considerably, however.

Thus r and b are descriptive statistics that denote different aspects of the linear relation between two continuous variables x and y. When $r = 0$ or $b = 0$, there is no linear relation between x and y. When values different from 0 are obtained in a study sample, we need to ask ourselves whether the difference might have arisen by chance.

Since r and b are calculated from samples, we must turn to statistical inference to provide inferences about the linear relation between x and y in the underlying target population. We can test for the statistical significance of r or b by postulating the null hypothesis that ρ (the population correlation coefficient) or β (the population regression coefficient) is equal to 0. Standard statistical texts[1,2,5,9] provide a formula for carrying out a t-test on either r or b (the result is the same with either coefficient). It should be emphasized, however, that the statistical significance of r or b is heavily dependent on the sample size. With very large samples, even small degrees of correlation may yield P values below .05. A procedure for estimating a confidence interval around r is given in reference 5.

Control for Confounding Variables

A third (or more) variable can confound the linear relation between two continuous variables. Although matching or stratification can be used to control for such confounding factors, a powerful multivariate statistical technique exists for simultaneous control of any number of confounders: *multiple linear regression*. Multiple regression also allows the investigator to assess the separate unconfounded effects of several independent variables on a single dependent variable.

The multiple linear regression technique models the dependent variable y as a linear function of all the independent variables (x_i's):

$$\hat{y} = a + b_1x_1 + b_2x_2 + b_3x_3 + \cdots + b_nx_n$$

The x_i's may be any continuous or dichotomous variables, and the b_i's are the corresponding regression coefficients. Each b_i is adjusted simultaneously for the linear relation between its corresponding x_i and every other x_i, as well as the linear relation between the other x_i's and y. An overall r^2 can be calculated for the model; it represents the proportion of the total variance in y accounted for by its linear relation with all the x_i's. Further details are available in standard texts.[1,8,12]

Correlation Between Two Ordinal Variables

The two-group comparison for an ordinal variable using the Mann–Whitney U test was mentioned earlier. When two ordinal variables are measured in each study subject, the investigator may be interested in measuring the correlation between the two. In this situation, using the *Spearman rank correlation coefficient*, r_s, may be preferable to a χ^2 test. The Spearman technique compares the ranks for each of the two variables for each subject. The smaller the sum of the squared differences in ranks, the greater the correlation between the ranks, and the higher the value of r_s. The magnitude of r_s can vary between -1 and $+1$ and is interpreted in the same way as the usual Pearson correlation coefficient, r. The formula for computing r_s, as well as tables for testing its statistical significance, are available in standard references.[2,5,9]

Concluding Remarks

Familiarity with statistical principles and techniques is invaluable for the researcher, from the earliest planning stages to the final proofreading of a manuscript already accepted for publication. Although many surgical investigators will choose to consult or collaborate with one or more statistical colleagues, some background is essential if such consultation or collaboration is to be both useful and efficient. Few statisticians are trained in the nuances of clinical medicine and the subtle processes that influence physicians' decisions. Statistically bereft clinicians who put themselves entirely at the mercy of a biostatistician do so at their own peril. The results may be mathematically sound but clinically irrelevant or, if relevant, incomprehensible and therefore of no practical value to a clinical audience.

The surgical researcher should know at least enough to be an informed consumer, if not a producer, of statistics. As a general principle, investigators should avoid using any statistical technique whose purpose *and* interpretation they do not understand. Although they usually need not be familiar with statistical theories and mathematical derivations, when these are required (e.g., in examining the validity of assumptions underlying certain tests), professional statistical help is essential.

References

1. Armitage P, Berry G. Statistical Methods in Medical Research, 2nd ed. Oxford: Blackwell Scientific Publications, 1987.
2. Colton T. Statistics in Medicine. Boston: Little, Brown, 1974.
3. Swinscow TDV. Statistics at Square One. London: British Medical Association, 1976.
4. Ingelfinger JA, Mosteller F, Thibodeau LA, Ware JH. Biostatistics in Clinical Medicine. New York: Macmillan, 1983.
5. Kramer MS. Clinical Epidemiology and Biostatistics. Heidelberg: Springer-Verlag, 1988.
6. Louis TA, Lavori PW, Bailar JC, Polansky M. Crossover and self-controlled designs in clinical research. N Engl J Med 1984;310:24–31.
7. Smart JV. Elements of Medical Statistics. Springfield, IL: Charles C Thomas, 1963.
8. Moses LE, Emerson JD, Hosseini H. Analyzing data from ordered categories. N Engl J Med 1984;311: 442–48.
9. Snedecor GW, Cochran WG. Statistical Methods, 7th ed. Ames: Iowa State University Press, 1980.
10. Fleiss JL. Statistical Methods for Rates and Proportions, 2nd ed. New York: Wiley, 1981.
11. Kleinbaum DG, Kupper LL, Morgenstern H. Epidemiologic Research: Principles and Quantitative Methods. Belmont, CA: Lifetime Publications, 1982.
12. Kleinbaum DG, Kupper LL. Applied Regression Analysis and Other Multivariable Methods. North Scituate, MA: Duxbury Press, 1978.
13. Anderson S, Auquier A, Hauck WW, Oakes D, Vandaele W, Weisberg HI. Statistical Methods for Comparative Studies: Techniques for Bias Reduction. New York: Wiley, 1980.
14. Miettinen OS. Simple interval-estimation of risk ratio. Am J Epidemiol 1974;100:515–516.

16

Case Studies for Learning Basic Biostatistical Concepts

R.C.-J. Chiu and D.S. Mulder

Clinical investigators are finding it increasingly necessary to employ biostatistical concepts and methodologies in their experimental designs, data analyses, and reports. Grant applications and manuscripts submitted for publication are now routinely reviewed for their statistical validity, often by professional statisticians. Even clinicians not engaged in research must understand some basic biostatistical concepts to be able to evaluate the scientific advances published in their own professional journals.

Although the importance of being able to understand biostatistical concepts is recognized by virtually all of us, many—possibly most—surgeons and new surgical investigators find biostatistics difficult, threatening, or boring. "Statistics made easy" treatises are full of mathematical formulas many clinicians left behind decades ago during their undergraduate years. Such terms as *regression* or *significance* have different connotations in clinical and statistical usage:

Surgeon: "There has been a *significant regression* in tumor size following the adjuvant therapy" (translation: the tumor became considerably smaller).

Statistician: "Linear *regression* analysis showed *significant* correlation between posttreatment tumor size and total dosage of adjuvant therapy" (translation: $Y = 2x + 3.2$, $P < 0.02$, $r = 0.86$).

This chapter illustrates a few basic biostatistical concepts with a minimal use of mathematical language. While the discussions are neither rigorous nor profound, they may make learning these concepts relatively painless for those with limited prior expertise in this area. To give the discussions a sense of relevance, we will use surgical case studies as examples. Real examples from the literature would be ideal but, since most would be selected to demonstrate fallacies and errors, using such examples might provoke considerable distress among the authors of the original articles. Saying it is not our intent "to impugn the motives or integrity of the investigator or to deride the quality of what appears in the medical literature"[1] might not provide much solace to the criticized authors. Accordingly, and for the sake of brevity and clarity, we have opted to used fictionalized cases: names, numbers, and disease conditions have been altered; but most examples are based on published articles or manuscripts submitted to journals for publication. We cannot say "Any similarity you may find is purely coincidental."

Why Do We Need Biostatistics?

Biostatistical concepts and methodologies help us to avoid fallacies in numerical reasoning and give us some assurance that the conclusions we have drawn from our data are correct.

Example 1

An acupuncturist claims his treatment for arthritis is more effective than physiotherapy. As proof, he produces 10 patients who testified that acupuncture was indeed superior.

The acupuncturist chose 10 patients whose results were favorable to his conclusion. What about the dozens of others who did not testify? Bias may be obvious or subtle. Carrying out a study in a way that avoids bias is the *first objective* of a study design that will permit accurate conclusions to be drawn. The ultimate approach to avoiding bias is to design a prospective, randomized double-blind study so that neither the investigators nor the subjects know to which experimental group subjects are assigned; neither can become biased, even subconsciously. In real life, it is not possible to perform every study this way, but every effort should be made to do so, if at all possible. If ethical considerations preclude such a study, you must clearly recognize the limitations on what you can infer, scientifically, from a less rigorous study.

Example 2

We tried our new orthopedic procedure in 10 cases, with successful outcome in 8. Of 10 matched patients with similar conditions, the old operation was successful in only 5. The new operation is clearly an improvement over the traditional therapy.

This conclusion may be true, but the number of patients (10 in each group) and the difference in the number of successes (3 cases) are small. The apparent improvement in results with the new operation may be due to chance (i.e., luck); the next few cases treated by the old procedure might be more successful. In statistical jargon, one cannot reject the null hypothesis that the results of the two operations are the same. By proper calculation (e.g. chi-square test; $x^2 = 1.978$, df = 1), one can show that the probability (*P* value; $P > .15$) of the authors' conclusion being wrong (type I or alpha error) is quite high (in this case > 15%). This illustrates why the *second objective* in biostatistical analysis is to assure that the conclusion is not based on chance, alone. In other words, the probability that the authors' conclusion cannot be reproduced, repeatedly, must be sufficiently low; by convention this must be < 5% of the time (or $P < .05$). Conversely, the conclusion should be right more than 95 times out of 100.

Example 3

Results of this new test given to 100 representative subjects from our community of 50,000 showed the titers to be normally distributed. The 95% confidence limits, calculated from mean plus or minus standard deviation, were then used as the normal values of this test in our community.

The *third objective* of biostatistical inference is to be able to extrapolate and generalize the results obtained from a relatively small number of sample subjects, to the whole population these subjects represent.

Many pitfalls must be recognized and avoided if the three objectives are to be achieved.

Sample Versus Population

Example 4

Admission records accumulated over a 10-year period, in a large general hospital computer were reviewed. Gastrointestinal hemorrhage was the diagnosis in 1.2 per 1000 admissions in Caucasian patients, while it was 6.1 per 1000 in nonwhite patients. It is concluded that GI hemorrhage is more common in nonwhites.

The difficulty, here, is the assumption that the ratio of admissions of whites to nonwhites in this hospital is the same as it is in the general population. Suppose nonwhites are admitted only half as often as whites for such things as cosmetic surgery; this would reduce the denominator, with a consequent increase in prevalence. Before you can extrapolate and generalize the finding to the whole population, you must ensure that the sample appropriately represents the particular population. Studies such as this one can be of interest to hospital administrators, but they are often not valid in estimating disease prevalence.

Is It "Normal?"

Example 5

Among 200 patients undergoing cardiac surgery, half of the patients were randomly selected to receive protease inhibitors to reduce postoperative blood loss. In the control group, average blood loss in the first 24 hours postop was 980 ± 186 ml; two patients were reexplored for major hemorrhage. Comparison was carried out using Student's *t*-test . . .

The statistical expression "mean ± standard deviation" (mean ± SD) indicates a confidence level. Two standard deviations above and below the mean values represents approximately 95% of a population. A "normal" or "bell shaped" frequency distribution (i.e., a Gaussian distribution) is implicit in this expression. By definition, the mean (sum of data, divided by number of items in sample) is the same as the median (the middle datum when the data are ranked in order of magnitude); data greater than mean and less than mean are distributed symmetrically and taper off at both ends. When the data obtained are "normally" distributed, confidence limits and such statistical tests as the *t*-test and analysis of variance are valid. If the frequency distribution of the data is not normal, "nonparametric" statistical methods are required (e.g., Mann–Whitney *U* test; Wilcoxon signed-rank test).

In Example 5, a few patients with massive hemorrhage required reexploration. They caused the mean value for blood loss to increase considerably, because the median values for both groups were only in the 600 ml range. The distribution curve is skewed to the right (i.e., the figure is larger), the curve is not symmetrical, and the mean (in the 800–900s) is not equal to the median (in the 600s). Consequently, both the expression of mean $\pm$ SD and the use of t-tests are inappropriate; nonparametric tests should have been employed.

It is prudent to plot the data to make sure that their distribution approximates the normal before you use parametric tests. Parametric tests can only be used if the distribution is normal; nonparametric methods are more generally applicable, regardless of whether the distribution of data is normal.

Incomplete Follow-ups

Example 6

To date, we have implanted 1890 mechanical and 1422 bioprosthetic cardiac valves in the mitral position. The follow-up period ranged from 12 years to 6 months. Among mechanical valve patients, 22% developed valve-related complications at the mean of 5 $\pm$ 1.2 years postop. In comparison, only 18% of bioprosthetic valve cases had valve-related complications occurring at 6.7 $\pm$ 2.2 years. Our results with mitral bioprosthesis is therefore encouraging.

This statement embodies a number of problems. The length of follow-up is different for each patient and is simply too short, in many cases, to determine whether and when the patient will develop valve-related complications. The true failure rate and time to failure could be known only when all the patients had been followed until death or valve failure.

Life table (or actuarial) analysis is the appropriate biostatistical representation to use for this sort of follow-up study. This method allows you to take account of dropouts (death, lost for follow-up) and shorter follow-up periods, if there are not too many. You can also calculate confidence limits based on the sample size, and compare the statistical significance of the differences at each follow-up interval. Many journal editors now require life table analysis for mortality or morbidity data; 5-year survivals or mean survival times are not acceptable.

Another method is to use the number of person-months or person-years. You could say there is one valve-related complication per certain person-month of follow-up, but you must be careful not to use these units (i.e., person-months or person-years) as the numbers for calculating the tests of significance. One person-year can also be 12 person-months. This is a good example of using an inappropriate sample unit for statistical calculations. Another example is doing 10 measurements each for five patients, and using the 50 data obtained to calculate the tests of significance. When uncertainty about appropriateness arises, obtain statistical consultation.

Good Versus Better

Example 7

A new modified Cooper's ligament repair for inguinal hernia, previously described, was carried out in 867 patients. With a minimal follow-up of at least 2 years, the recurrence rate was only 1.4%. Consequently, we believe that this technique is the procedure of choice for inguinal hernia.

The results are good, but you cannot tell whether the new technique is any better than others because there is no comparison group. The results may be better than most of those described in the literature, but it is not clear that the patients are comparable; the authors' series may have more young patients and fewer recurrent hernias. The conclusion that the new technique is the procedure of choice is more a statement of faith than of fact.

Comparing an Apple with an Orange

Even in the pioneering days of clinical cardiac transplantation, the benefit of this procedure was thought to be evident.

Example 8

In one series, in the early 1970s, 57 patients with end-stage heart disease entered a transplant program; 15 eventually underwent 16 cardiac transplantations, as donor organs became available after an average waiting period of 22 days. The mean survival after transplant was 111 days; without transplant, patients lived for an average of only 74 days. Even when the waiting period was subtracted from the transplant survival time, the prolongation of life, although limited, was clearly demonstrated.

Since the transplanted and nontransplanted patient groups came from the same pool of terminal heart disease cases, and assignment to each group was dependent on organ match and not on severity of disease, the comparison seems to be fair, at first glance. Some patients were so sick, however, that they died shortly after entering the transplant program and did not live long enough to receive a donor organ. Since they did not undergo transplantation, they automatically belonged to the nontransplant group. Consequently, the study design had a built-in bias against the nontransplant group. Comparison is valid only when you are comparing like with like.

Young Versus Old

Example 9

It is well known that the incidence of breast cancer is higher in the daughters of breast cancer patients. Our data establish that such daughters develop their breast cancers at a younger age than their mothers did. To date, we have found a total of 182 pairs of mothers and daughters with breast cancers by examining our cancer registry data. The mean age at diagnosis for the mothers is 59.7 years, for the daughters, 47.5 years. The 12.2-year difference is highly significant.

This study design also introduces a hidden bias (i.e., age). By selecting mother-daughter pairs, the authors embarked on a comparison of two cohorts of patients with different ages. In so doing, they effectively excluded many daughters who will develop breast cancer at an older age. Appropriate data can be obtained only by studying pairs who have all grown older and died from breast cancer, or other causes (see also discussion under "Incomplete Follow-up").

To Pair or Not to Pair

Example 10

In two groups of 10 patients each with Crohn's disease, the effect of two different diets in reducing the frequency of bowel movements was studied. The group receiving the elemental diet had fewer bowel movements than the group on the control diet, but the difference did not achieve statistical significance ($P > .3$) because of the relatively small sample size and the considerable variations in individual patients.

When two groups are compared, it is easier to establish a statistically significant difference if (a) the mean values are wide apart, (b) the spread of data in each group (variance or standard deviation) is small, and (c) the sample size is large (i.e., many patients studied). When you get a result whose type I (alpha) error does not achieve the significant level (i.e., $P < .05$), you cannot readily draw the conclusion that the two groups do not differ, because of the type II (beta) error problem discussed later.

The investigator would have had a higher likelihood of confirming his hypothesis about elemental diet reducing the frequency of bowel movement if he had used a paired design for the study—that is, if he had fed each patient one diet, and then the other. The results obtained in each patient under the two diets can be compared, statistically, and then pooled for all patients (paired tests). This reduces the problem of dealing with individual differences within each group.

A crossover design, in which the first group receives diet A, then B, while the second group receives diet B and then A, would be a further refinement, since it avoids possible bias due to temporal changes. Such designs are particularly helpful when it is difficult to recruit a large number of subjects.

Paired design cannot be used in all types of study; it would be difficult, or impossible, to use it to compare operative versus nonoperative therapies for any single disease.

Association Fallacy

Example 11

Review of autopsy records showed that 8% of patients who died of trauma had clinically unrecognized pulmonary embolism. This rate is much lower than the 31.2% seen in all other autopsy cases during the same period in our hospital ($P < .05$; χ^2 test).

Critical examination of this report revealed that the autopsy rate for patients who died of trauma with medicolegal implications was nearly 100%, while the rate for patients dying in the hospital, as a whole, was only 22%. By selecting autopsy records as the basis for study, a differential entry rate for study was built in and led to a fallacious conclusion, known in statistics as Berkson's fallacy.[2] Be wary of this problem when it appears likely that differential admission to a study about the presence of association could occur. The differential admission rate must be known, and taken into account, to permit correct calculation of association. The χ^2 test result shown above is misleading.

Association Versus Cause and Effect

Example 12

To study the mechanism of gastric erosions caused by nonsteroid anti-inflammatory drugs, we measured gastric motility and pressure changes in the rat, with a balloon, and correlated their magnitudes with the size and number of erosions developed. The data showed that the development of erosions is due to high pressure zones developed in the gastric mucosa following the administration of these drugs.

Statistical evidence of association does not establish a cause and effect relationship, and you should be careful about implying such a relationship in your conclusions. To prove cause and effect can often be difficult and frustrating. Medical scientists are familiar with Koch's postulates about what is required to prove that a particular microorganism is the cause of particular disease, but there is no generalized and infallible principle that readily proves cause and effect. See Chapters 13 and 14.

Generating a dose–response relationship will not prove, but will definitely strengthen, an argument that cause and effect may underlie an observed association. Ultimately, establishing causality may require an understanding of the biological, chemical or physical nature of the relation. Nevertheless, strong evidence of association may, in itself, be highly valuable clinically (e.g., smoking and lung cancer).

Sample Size: No Difference or Not Enough Cases?

Example 13

To compare the patency rates of in situ versus reversed vein grafts for below the knee femoropopliteal artery bypass, we restudied 25 patients in each group with arteriography 2 years after their operations. The difference between the failure rates of 28% and 36%, respectively, were not statistically significant ($P > .5$). We conclude that in situ vein grafts offer no advantage in such bypasses.

Example 13 illustrates a very common problem and error encountered in studies showing differences between comparison groups that fail to reach statistical significance (i.e., $P > .05$). Failure to show statistically significant difference is often considered to be proof that there is no difference.

In fact, failure to show difference indicates (a) that the two groups are indeed not different (the null hypothesis is correct); or (b) that the two groups are different but not enough patients were studied to demonstrate it. A bit of bad luck—probability or chance—masked the underlying difference. The study in Example 13 is inconclusive; it neither showed a difference nor proved its absence. Such studies are not very helpful, but they demonstrate why a statistician always looks at the sample size when evaluating a study design.

If you study numerous cases and find no difference between groups, you can be sure there is no true difference. Logistically, however, there is a limit to how many you can study, so how many is enough? That depends on how much risk you wish to take when you declare there is no difference, (i.e., how big a type II or beta error).

A type II error of 20% means that when you conclude "two groups studied are not different," your statement is at least 80% accurate (i.e., 100% − 20% = 80%). This figure, 80%, is called the "power" of the study. It is important that you calculate the sample size required, before you undertake an investigation, to achieve the desired beta error and power for your study. Otherwise, if the alpha error (P value) does not reach significance, you may end up with an inconclusive study. Whenever you read an article reporting a negative result, you should ask whether the sample size was big enough to permit the investigators to draw such a conclusion. See Chapter 14.

For the same power of statistics, sample size can be smaller if (a) the difference you are looking for between the groups is large (e.g., to show a 50% reduction in mortality, from 50% to 25%, you may need a sample size of < 100 cases; from 2% to 1% might require thousands of cases), and (b) the spread of data within each group (standard deviation) is small.

How can you know the magnitude of the difference and the degree of spread in your data *before* you begin your study? You cannot know! Then how do you calculate the sample size ahead of time? You must make an "educated guess" by basing your estimates on studies reported by others, or on your own preliminary studies. Clearly stating how your assumptions were made is an important part of successful grantsmanship. The difference you are looking for between the groups depends, in great measure, on what magnitude of difference you would consider "clinically significant." The sample size calculation is seldom absolute and usually depends, to a considerable extent, on the clinical judgment of the investigator(s).

Ways Out of Small Sample Size

Reduce the Noise

Example 14

In a large multicenter randomized prospective controlled study comparing medical therapy with coronary artery bypass in patients with coronary artery disease, no difference in longevity was detected. Significant improvement in survival time was established, however, in one surgically treated subgroup of patients with left mainstem coronary artery occlusion.

The degree and number of coronary artery occlusions, cardiac functional reserve, age, etc. vary widely among patients with coronary artery disease and affect their prognoses and responses to therapy. These variations, or "noises," can obscure the difference you are looking for in your study. Selecting a subgroup of more uniform and high-risk patients will reduce the noise and allow you to establish significant difference between comparison groups with a smaller sample size (discussed under Example 13). If you cannot study large numbers of subjects, you will be more likely to get significant results if you study a subgroup with the stipulated characteristics. The price you pay for using this strategy is that your conclusion cannot be generalized to a wider population (see discussion under "Sample Versus Population").

Tune Up the Sensitivity

Example 15

Fifty patients were randomly assigned to receive, or not receive, intravenous hyperalimentation of 10 days' duration prior to undergoing surgery for esophageal cancer. There was no difference in postoperative mortality or morbidity, but the total exchangeable potassium to sodium ratio, representing the lean body mass, increased by 8.6% ($P < .05$) in the hyperalimentation group.

Negative studies (no difference between comparison groups) may be very important, but investigators frequently say it is easier to get studies with positive results published. If you establish a significant difference, sample size becomes a less important issue. One way to achieve significant difference is to fine tune the endpoint and use more sensitive indicators to look at the difference.

In Example 15, the exchangeable K/Na data were more sensitive than mortality and morbidity figures, but the price paid for adopting this strategy was a possible reduction in clinical relevance. How important is it for patients to have 8.6% more lean body mass if it does not improve mortality and morbidity? In pathophysiological studies, such sensitive parameters are valuable endpoints, but their meaning for the clinical management of patients should be considered in the appropriate perspective.

The difference between "statistical" and "clinical" significance is an important issue for clinicians. Statistical significance simply means that it is highly unlikely that the described results are due to chance alone; it does not indicate that the observed differences are, or are not, clinically meaningful. That is a matter of clinical judgment.

Computer-Generated Significance

Example 16

Three hundred items of data, generated on each patient during his or her stay in our intensive care unit, were stored in our computer. Each item on a given patient was statistically compared with that patient's survival or death, within 30 days of admission, to determine which item(s) could predict the outcome. We were surprised to find that a number of unexpected items achieved statistical significance as predictors.

Nowadays, it is easy to have a computer store large amounts of data and spew out the results of numerous tests for significance. The danger in this approach is that spurious "significance" will likely be found by chance. Even if all 300 items in Example 16 are unrelated to patients' survival or death, we are accepting a 5% alpha error each time we do a significance test. Consequently, we could get up to $300 \times 0.05 = 15$ significant items by chance alone. Be on guard against such a "fishing expedition," with no clear hypothesis to prove, when you are tempted to misuse the availability and power of computer technology.

Problems Unique to Surgical Investigators

Example 17

Patient entry into a multicenter study, comparing surgical versus medical therapy for incomplete small bowel obstruction, was based on agreed clinical criteria and was followed by random assignment to either of the two treatment groups. The clinical status of 29% of the patients originally assigned to the medical therapy group did not show sufficient improvement or became worse, and they were subsequently operated upon. These patients were still considered to have been medically treated, in our analysis of the results, according to the "intent of therapy" principle.

Although this sort of argument is common in high-powered clinical trial circles and appears to be accepted by most biostatisticians, it perplexes surgeons. How can a patient initially treated medically, but requiring surgery for clinical improvement, still be credited as a medical success? Nonsurgical studies can follow a crossover design in which one group receives treatment A followed by B and a second group receives treatment B followed by A; surgical studies cannot use this strategy. A patient who has been treated medically can be transferred to surgical therapy, but once the patient has had surgery, the operation cannot be undone and the patient reassigned to medical therapy alone. Methodologists are still debating this issue; many surgeons remain skeptical.

Example 18

Controversy continues over which surgical procedure gives best results for patients with reflux esophagitis. Advocates of each procedure report good results, without adequate controls. A clinical trial comparing Allison and Nissen repairs is planned in our hospital; patient selection and follow-up protocols have been agreed upon. How can our study design and analysis take account of the differing levels of expertise in the performance of the different operative procedures by the participating surgeons?

There is no easy solution to this problem. Operative trials are unlike drug trials; the skill of the surgeon, an important variable, is difficult to quantify. We suggest a design in which patients are randomized, not as a whole group, but for each surgeon. Each surgeon, with his own particular operative skill, operates on two groups of patients so randomized, and the success and failure rates are calculated for each surgeon. The data from all the participating surgeons are then combined to obtain greater statistical power (e.g., Mantel–Haenszel χ^2 test). Such statistical methods are available and are often used to combine data from a multicenter trial. Each surgeon is considered to be a trial center. Unique problems require unique solutions!

Conclusions

Personal computers and a variety of statistical programs are making statistical calculations easy and accessible, but they tell us neither which test to use nor what the numbers mean. An understanding of biostatistical concepts helps you to comprehend and evaluate the surgical literature, design and analyze a clinical study or laboratory experiment, foster more rigorous scientific thinking, and develop a mind that is critical but not skeptical. We believe that biostatistical training should be a regular part of the education of all of tomorrow's clinicians. Whether you are using biostatistics or a scalpel, it is important that you know when to call in an expert consultant to avoid costly mistakes.

References

1. Colton T. Statistics in Medicine. Boston: Little, Brown, 1974.
2. Berkson J. Limitations of the application of fourfold table analysis to hospital data. Biometrics 1946;2:47.

Additional Reading

Bailar JC, Mosteller F. eds. Medical Uses of Statistics. Waltham, MA: NEJM Books, 1991.

Kirklin JW, Barratt-Boyes BG. Surgical concepts, research methods, and data analysis and use. In: Cardiac Surgery. New York: Wiley, 1986:177–204.

The authors recommend this chapter for the serious student wishing to learn more about data analysis, particularly as applied to cardiac surgery. This chapter deals at length with such topics as incremental risk factors, multivariate analysis, analysis of time-related events, and actuarial methods. It provides programs for programmable hand-held calculators and details of the mathematical rationale for such statistical analyses as confidence limits for proportions, the Kaplan–Meier actuarial methodology, and proportional hazards linear models.

17

Endpoints for Clinical Studies: Conventional and Innovative Variables

S. Wood-Dauphinée and H. Troidl

Two well-dressed gentlemen were on their way home from a party where they had obviously dined and wined too well. One was on his knees systematically examining the sidewalk beneath a streetlight. His friend volunteered, helpfully: "I'm sure I heard your keys drop back here where it's dark!" The searcher replied: "I know, but what's the use of looking back there where I can't see when it's so much easier here in the light?"

This chapter discusses flashlights for finding keys in the dark. Surgical treatment is not always dramatically lifesaving. Its aim is to improve quality of life and halt the ravages of disease that quietly and relentlessly erode comfort and dispel happiness. Patients come to surgeons for relief from discomfort and pain of gallbladder disease or heartburn that accompanies reflux esophagitis, not to have their abnormal laboratory findings corrected.

As clinicians, we inquire about decrease in discomfort following surgery, note improvement in appetite or ability to sleep throughout the night, and record any such changes on our patients' charts. When data are collected for research purposes, however, this important information is left in the dark. Instead, we collect mortality figures, survival times, postoperative complications, laboratory test results, and other similar data. Perhaps we do so because such data are easily found under the street light.

Because pain, functional limitation, and overall well-being are perceived as being difficult to measure, we turn to variables we can measure even if they have little bearing on the symptoms that brought the patient to see us in the first place. The fact that an outcome variable is easy to measure reliably does not enhance its usefulness if it assesses the wrong thing. Resorting to such approaches is unnecessary because it really is possible to measure the effects of treatment in terms of variables like discomfort, disability, and dissatisfaction, to document the true value of surgery, and to assess the effectiveness of innovative treatment.

Variables in General

Variables are measurable attributes of patients or of the process of care that differ from one individual to another. Identifying the differences or changes in particular variables in groups of patients subjected to different treatments and discovering what causes them is the essence of clinical research.

Patient variables include sociodemographic characteristics like age, sex, and marital status; clinical information like the type and stage of disease, signs, and symptoms; and laboratory measurements like hematocrit, body weight, and x-ray findings. Patient variables also include physical, emotional, and social functioning; personal aspects of daily living; and attitudes toward life, illness, and the health care process.[1] Table 17.1 lists patient variables of potential use in surgical studies.

Treatment variables are interventions by health professionals intended to effect a cure, prolong life, alleviate suffering, improve function, or otherwise ameliorate the quality of life. They include pharmaceutical, surgical, rehabilitative, and other approaches to care, and the way such approaches are organized and delivered to patients. They are usually documented in terms of operative procedure, therapeutic regimen, length of hospital stay, or the skill and experience of those providing treatment. Examples of some treatment variables related to surgical studies are listed in Table 17.2.

The selection of appropriate patient and treatment variables depends on the question under investigation, the nature of the clinical disorder, and the cultural setting of the study. Care must

TABLE 17.1. Examples of patient variables in surgical studies.

Socio-demographic	Clinical	Sociopersonal
Age	Diagnosis	Physical performance
Sex	Disease stage	Emotional performance
Marital status	Disease localization	Cognitive performance
Socioeconomic status	Signs	Social performance
Educational level	Symptoms	Body image
Occupation	Comorbidity	Beliefs
Religion	Complications	Attitudes
Place of residence	Laboratory data	Functional status
Nationality	Radiographic data	Health status
Ethnic origin	Angiogram information	Quality of life
Employment status	Endoscopic information	Suffering

TABLE 17.2. Examples of treatment variables in surgical studies.

Related to surgery	Related to adjunct treatments
Type of surgery	Anesthetic technique
Extent of surgery	Postsurgical nursing care
Timing of surgery	Drug therapy
Skill of the surgical team	Chemotherapy
Use of mechanical devices	Radiotherapy
	Physical therapy
	Nutritional therapy

be taken at the outset to identify and record all pertinent variables. Patient variables may be described by direct observation or examination, by test results, by behavior that appears to reflect an underlying trait, or by a self-report from the patient. It is particularly important to record clinical variables related to prognosis; for example, if tumor stage and location are known to affect outcome, they must be included. Aspects of the care process suspected of influencing the results of treatment must also be systematically documented.

The interaction between patient and treatment variables is the focus of primary interest. Treatment variables are said to be independent because they can be manipulated by the investigator and are presumed to alter certain patient variables. Patient variables that change and reflect the effect of a therapeutic intervention are called dependent or outcome variables.

All variables used in a study, whether independent or dependent, must be defined in operational terms. An operational definition puts the variable in terms that are concrete, observable, and measurable, and dictates how it will be employed in the study. For example, if you are including "overweight" patients in a trial, this variable could be defined as a set percentage above the standardized weight for age, sex, height, and body build, a specified skin fold thickness, or a positive response to the question "Do you feel that you are overweight?" This approach to defining yields a measurable score, assures consistency, and permits replication of the study.

Outcome Variables in Clinical Studies in Surgery

In 1967 White[2] listed five outcome variables that describe much of the spectrum of health states: death, disease, discomfort, disability, and dissatisfaction. Death has been used as an endpoint in many studies because preventing premature death is an eminent therapeutic goal, and death is easily recognized and reported. When death occurs in relation to a surgical intervention, the major issues are the specific cause of death and whether it could have been prevented. The duration of survival following an operative procedure for a condition known to lead eventually to death, and operative or late mortality are obviously useful outcome variables, but if they are the only endpoints measured, other important consequences for those who survive may be missed.

Disease manifests itself as a combination of physical signs, subjective symptoms, and abnormal test results. Such deviations from normal may be the result of the disease process, its complications, or therapy. When the impact of care is being assessed, the aspects of morbidity that are of interest will vary with the nature of the disease. In cancer, local recurrence and distant metastasis are significant; in peripheral vascular disease, information on distal pulses, flow rates, and pain during ambulation is required; in urological conditions, data on urinary output, glomerular filtration rates, or frequency are required. Whether a surgeon is attempting to cure or to palliate, one or more manifestation(s) of the particular disease may be selected as endpoints for a surgical study.

Discomfort is such a salient feature of disease that it merits its own category. Discomfort includes symptoms like pain, nausea, dyspnea, depression, anorexia, anxiety, and fatigue, and is important to both patient and physician. The presence, absence, or severity of discomfort is a meaningful outcome for investigators trying to determine the effects of a surgical procedure. Although measures of discomfort were seldom used as outcome variables in

TABLE 17.3. Ranking the importance of outcome variables in surgical situations.

Clinical situation	Surgical examples	Ranked importance of outcome variables[a]
Impaired quality of life but not life threatening	Hernia Gallstones Lacerated meniscus Peripheral arterial occlusion	Discomfort > Disability > Disease > Dissatisfaction > Death
Impaired quality of life and life threatening; surgery prolongs life but increases morbidity	Stoma for colitis Amputation for vascular disease Transplantation	Discomfort > Disability > Disease > Dissatisfaction Death
Different therapeutic approaches; similar operative mortality, complications, and survival	Arterial occlusion: bypass vs. profundaplasty Stomach cancer: different reconstructions	Discomfort > Disability > Dissatisfaction Disease > Death
Trade off between better quality of life and increased therapeutic risk	Colitis: stoma vs. pelvic pouch Coxarthrosis: conservative vs. endoprosthesis	Discomfort > Death > Disability > Dissatisfaction > Disease >
Palliation	Esophageal carcinoma Pancreatic carcinoma	Discomfort > Disability > Dissatisfaction > Disease > Death

[a]Read > as "more important than."

older studies, relief of discomfort is now appearing in the literature and is being advocated as a criterion of successful treatment.[3,4] This outcome will become increasingly important in the assessment of the efficacy of surgical results by hospitals, insurers, and government agencies.

Disability[5] refers to a decrease in the normal competence of individuals to perform activities like caring for themselves, moving about their environment, and going about their daily lives at home, at work, or during recreational or social pursuits. Outcome variables reflecting the physical dimensions of disability have been reported in the surgical literature[6-8] for many years, but endpoints relating to social and emotional components have been much less common. This discrepancy reflects not only the difficulty of assessing the social and emotional components of disability, but also the absence of their consideration in traditional medical education programs, which viewed disease in terms of a biomedical model; treatment was directed at modifying biologic mechanisms, and outcome measures were chosen accordingly.[9] Because the multidimensional characteristics of disease and response patterns are now better understood, the newer health models include physical, emotional, and social components. Studies using all of them as endpoints are now appearing in the surgical literature.[10-14]

Dissatisfaction with the process of care, or its results, has been widely discussed in the literature, and its measurement is currently regarded as a necessary component in any evaluation of quality of care.[15] Several scales have been designed for the purpose,[16-18] but patients' perceptions of surgical care and its results are just starting to be addressed in reports of surgical studies.[19-20] These perceptions are increasing in importance to consumers, payers and readers of the literature.

Table 17.3 presents an attempt by one author (HT) to rank the importance of these outcome variables in a spectrum of surgical situations.

Selecting Outcome Variables

Although our understanding of the causes and mechanisms of disease is growing constantly, and positive accomplishments of therapeutic interventions are numerous, Feinstein[21] has pointed out that much of the information used to substantiate these achievements has been gathered from clinical information that provides only anatomical, physiological, or biochemical data about disease. Fletcher and Fletcher[22] determined that 90% of published articles documenting outcomes of disease used biologic data obtained by diagnostic tests. Although clinical phenomena form much of the basis of daily practice, relatively little attention has been paid to them.

Measurement of clinical parameters is appropriate for several reasons. Patients generally seek help because of the presence of symptoms. Clinicians listen to the complaint while taking a history, perform a physical examination to elicit signs of the disease, and order related tests. While the test results are obviously important, clinicians frequently rely on signs and symptoms as indications for surgery. Hot and swollen knees, specific bowel sounds or their absence, pain, and disability guide surgeons in their decisions to operate.

Surgery also involves an agreement by patients to accept the risk and pain associated with surgery in the hope that it will alleviate their symptoms and improve their quality of life. Patients threatened by cancer submit to radical operations to evade or delay premature death even though the radical surgery may be followed by a significant decrease in the quality of their lives. Because it is difficult to convey to patients what their lives will be like following an operation, variables designed to record the course of recovery after operation must be included as endpoints in studies of treatment. For instance, almost every operation is followed by a recovery phase during which the patient feels worse and quality of life variables recorded during this period would make the operation seem less effective. This problem can be overcome by making measures of patients' status at specific points during the course of recovery. Armed with such concrete information, surgeons can give patients a more accurate picture of what to expect following an operation.

In surgery, there are often tradeoffs when deciding which specific operation to carry out. For instance, surgeons could perform a Brook's ileostomy or a pelvic pouch for patients with colitis. The first procedure means a permanent opening in the abdominal wall, but it also means less risk, fewer complications and the possibility of less disability in the long term. Conversely, the pouch is aesthetically more appealing but surgically more difficult. In this situation, surgeons must understand the specific manifestations of the tradeoff so that the patient can be presented with an accurate picture. Only by systematically assessing appropriate outcomes in a series of patients who have undergone a specific operative technique can surgeons communicate accurate information about the consequences of their treatments.

Physiologic or anatomic variables, such as arterial blood gas determinations, hemoglobin or electrolyte levels, and tumor size, are important parameters in tracking the course of a disease or searching for more efficacious treatment. They hold little meaning for patients unless they are related to significant clinical events in their lives.[9,23] Accordingly, the evaluator of a treatment should choose outcome variables that reflect patient-important values as well as the usual laboratory findings. Patients are primarily interested in having symptoms alleviated and functional ability restored so that they can continue the routines of daily living.

Advocating clinical data as outcome measures raises the issue of "hard" versus "soft" data. Traditionally, hard data were chosen because they were "objectively" acquired and "quantifiable" in terms of an established scale, and could be "accurately" reproduced or stored for analysis.[24] Standard hard data include death or survival and information obtained through radiography, CT scanning, endoscopy, cardiac catheterization, biochemical analysis, etc. Patients' reports of symptoms or their attitudes toward illness and the health care system, and measures of functional capabilities are considered to be imprecise, variable, and nonreproducible (i.e., suspect or soft). In truth, extensive evidence suggests that much of the hard information in the literature is softer than we like to think.[25] Most studies assessing the reproducibility of cardiovascular, gastrointestinal, or respiratory signs, the interpretation of diagnostic procedures, or the diagnosis or need for a specific treatment have demonstrated considerable disagreement.[26] In contrast, many of the outcomes regarded as being soft are really as solid as, or more reliable than, those long accepted as hard.

Several methods exist to acquire harder data in soft areas.[21,26-30] One way uses procedures developed through social science research for the design of standardized questionnaires and indices to assess symptoms, functional performance, and overall well-being. This approach requires special skills and knowledge. Data on such clinical signs as heart murmurs, joint swelling, organ enlargements, and blood pressure are made more consistent or reliable by repeated assessments by the same person or by two or more individuals in accordance with specified criteria or standards. A similar routine can be used for diagnostic tests. The system for staging dysplastic changes in biopsy specimens from patients with ulcerative colitis illustrates the use of this approach to develop standards or criteria.[31]

Reproducibility of results is enhanced by recording the precise findings of the physical examination and the clinical impression or the diagnosis inferred from the findings. Reporting hematuria, flank pain, and abdominal mass is more conducive to agreement than simply stating a diagnosis of renal carcinoma, and it provides data for comparisons of initial findings in groups of patients subjected to different interventions. Diagnoses should be based on information from several sources, the history, and physical and test results.

Assessments made with simple aids like tape measures, pupil gauges, eye charts, or goniometers are more reproducible than casual estimations. These more precise findings can be verified by checking them against existing records of other clinical examinations or the results of diagnostic tests. Patient evaluations or test interpreters should be blind to the treatment regimen of the patient and to the specific purpose of the study, if possible. Ways of making clinical data more reliable are summarized in Table 17.4.

Some types of hard data are based on endpoints that occur infrequently and, as a consequence, large sample sizes are required to obtain statistical significance. If, for example, death is chosen as the principal outcome in the study of a surgical procedure and it occurs only rarely, a large number of patients will be required.[25] You should choose other more frequent outcomes, provided they are related to the primary objective of the study. A study comparing survival following different surgical approaches to ruptured appendix might use in-hospital mortality as a principal endpoint. If relief of symptoms is the aim of a surgical intervention in patients with chronic pancreatitis, endpoints reflecting a change in pain and general health status are appropriate. Cancer surgery performed for palliative purposes has more to do with the quality of survival than with its quantity. Hence, relief of symptoms and quality of life are the appropriate outcomes to measure and report.

Investigators may be strongly tempted to generate a list of all the relevant outcome variables for a study and measure each of them. This is not only time-consuming and expensive, but potentially fatiguing for patients. It also has methodological and statistical implications. If multiple endpoints are used, the probability of your finding one that demonstrates a difference increases. With 20 measures and a planned level of statistical significance of .05 or less, at least one measure should demonstrate such a difference by chance alone.[32] Statistical procedures are available to correct the problem just described, but they dramatically increase the sample size requirements and complexity of the study.[32]

Related to the use of multiple endpoints is the issue of employing a battery of specific measures chosen to reflect different dimensions of one outcome. For instance, if one wishes to assess the impact of a surgical procedure on health, suffering, or quality of life, there may not be an appropriate instrument able to do this. Consequently, the investigator will have to identify the specific dimensions within the global endpoint and select a valid and reliable tool to measure each of them.[33] Using quality of life as an example, one might choose physical capacity, emotional performance, the capability of performing social roles, and such important symptoms as pain, fatigue, and depression.

Table 17.4. Suggestions for making clinical data more reliable.

Repeat evaluation and assess agreement.
Evaluate according to specified criteria.
Record precise physical findings.
Use appropriate assessment aids.
Use blind evaluators.
Verify findings against other data sources.

Source: Ref. 30, p. 39.

While comprehensive, this approach has the practical, methodological, and statistical problems mentioned earlier. Moreover, interpretation of the data may be problematic if the measures do not present a consistent picture of results.[33] In this case, the researcher is faced with weighing the evidence to determine whether the intervention has really had a positive or negative impact; controversy may follow. Currently, investigators working with Alzheimer's, stroke, cancer and cerebral palsy patients are in the process of validating batteries of tests that will provide a summary score—thereby alleviating some of the difficulties of multiple endpoints. Studies of this nature for surgical problems have yet to be implemented.

Few guidelines are available, but we favor Abramson's advice to "choose as many as necessary and as few as possible."[34] Sometimes it is necessary to use a battery of tests to measure the more complicated outcomes, such as quality of life or general well being, but the most widely accepted procedure is to select one variable from the group of possible dependent variables and make it the primary focal point for assessing the treatment effect.[27,35] A few other outcome variables may be added to reflect the different impact areas of the intervention. If you are comparing dialysis and kidney transplantation for end-stage renal disease, you could choose quality of life as the principal endpoint and document specific symptom relief and length of survival as subsidiary outcomes. Establish a hierarchy of outcomes, choose the most relevant, and add a few others according to their importance.

The outcome variables chosen by other investigators are in the literature, but your own clinical expertise and knowledge of the intervention and your study's objectives are your best guide to what is pertinent and important. Remember to consider how common the outcome is in terms of future

TABLE 17.5. Guidelines for selecting endpoints.

Make sure your endpoints are related to the primary objective of your study. (Measure pain following surgery for chronic pancreatitis rather than hypoglycemia)
Choose endpoints that have a high probability of being influenced by the intervention. (Assess relief of discomfort following gallbladder surgery.)
Be certain your endpoints will occur frequently among the patients under study. (For minor investigative surgery, select outcomes such as postoperative pain, nausea, and fatigue, NOT mortality.)
Incorporate sociopersonal and clinical as well as laboratory outcomes. (Functional status, anxiety, anal sphincter pressure measurements.)
Choose as few endpoints as possible to assess the study objectives. Prioritize when possible.
Be sure your endpoints are important for future clinical management.
Be certain your endpoints can be accurately measured. (Run checks on accuracy and reproducibility.)
Make sure the endpoints chosen can be reproduced by the other investigators. (Choose published standardized scales and indices.)

clinical management, how likely it is that the outcome will be influenced by the intervention being assessed,[36] and how measurable the outcome currently is. Table 17.5 lists the guidelines for selecting study endpoints.

Methodologic Criteria of Measuring Instruments

Although the term "measuring instrument" is commonly associated with mechanical devices, it is also used to describe laboratory and physical tests, questionnaires, and scales and indices of various types. Carefully developed measuring instruments should include information about the methodologic criteria that must be met to ensure satisfactory measurement. Reliability, validity, and responsiveness are some of the measurement criteria.[37-39] Researchers also need to be concerned with how practical the instruments are and on which populations they have been used.

Reliability

Reliability is the extent to which a measure obtains similar results when the presence or magnitude of a stable characteristic is repeatedly determined. As a consequence, it reflects the random error inherent in the measurement process. Some degree of variation, or error, attributable to the measuring instrument or the individual making the observation is unavoidable; there is always some disagreement among clinicians about physical findings or the interpretation of laboratory data.[26,40] Measurement errors can lead to serious consequences like missed diagnoses, mislabeling of patients, increased sample size, and incorrect study conclusions.[41,42] A measure is said to be reliable when its variation or random fluctuation due to errors is small.

Test–retest reliability refers to the stability of a result when the measure is repeatedly determined under similar conditions. For instance, laboratory values from the analysis of the same sample should be similar if the test is redone. When human judgment is required to assess the presence of a physical finding, interpret x-rays, or complete a questionnaire, both interrater reliability (the ability of more than one rater to obtain similar results) and intrarater reliability (the ability of one rater to obtain similar results when a test is repeated under identical conditions) become important. When a measuring instrument includes several items summed to a total score, we must ask how the items are related to each other and to the whole instrument. An example of such an instrument would be one that contained a number of items reflecting the severity of pain. Internal consistency is the degree to which the various items within the instrument, designed to measure the same characteristic, are scored similarly by respondents.

Although each type of reliability testing is not appropriate for every type of instrument or intended use (Table 17.6), a standardized instrument or procedure should provide information on the aspects of reliability that are applicable. Reliability is usually expressed as a decimal value (< 1). It indicates the proportion of information a score contains rather than the amount of random error within it. Although no universally acceptable values are set, reliability is considered high if the coefficient is .80 or above, moderate if it is between .60 and .79, and questionable if it is below .60.[43]

Validity

Validity is the extent to which an instrument actually measures what it claims to measure, that is, the relation between what is observed and reported, and the real situation.

TABLE 17.6. Assessment of instrument reliability.

Method	For estimation of	Information
Test–retest	Stability of results	Laboratory data Presence, absence, or severity gradings of physical signs Questionnaires, scales, or indices assessing symptoms, function, well-being, or satisfaction if the characteristic is stable
Interrater reliability	Reproducibility of results by different raters	Diagnostic test interpretations; presence, absence, or severity of physical signs
Intrarater reliability	Reproducibility of results by a single rater over repeated observations	Questionnaires, scales, or indices assessing symptoms, function, or well-being
Internal consistency	Relation of individual components of an instrument to each other and to the overall content of the instrument	Multiple-item questionnaires, scales, or indices assessing symptoms, functional capacity, well-being, or satisfaction

TABLE 17.7. Approaches to assessing the validity of paper instruments.

Type of validation	Purpose	Procedure
Content	To estimate whether the instrument represents the spectrum of content of the characteristic being measured	Inspection of instrument
Criterion related	To compare the results of a new instrument with a criterion or "gold standard"	Comparison or correlation of scores from the two measures
Construct	To assess the meaning of an instrument in terms of its hypothesized or theoretical basis	Comparison with external variables related to the construct

For laboratory measures, ensuring validity is less difficult than it is for measures assessing abilities, attitudes, or behaviors. In the laboratory, quality control techniques are used to establish and maintain accuracy. For example, each instrument is calibrated by comparing its accuracy with a known standard. In some laboratories, 50% of all the tests performed are for calibration purposes.[23] In some countries, analytical variance is monitored through interlaboratory surveys, and certification is dependent on satisfactory performance.[44]

The validity of clinical observations can be similarly established by comparing the observed measure to some accepted standard. The pulse rate, obtained by palpation and a watch, can be compared to the heart rate recorded simultaneously by an ECG monitor; the existence of a peptic ulcer, suspected on the basis of a clinical history, can be confirmed by direct viewing through a fiberoptic endoscope.

For many clinical measures, such as pain, functional ability, and quality of life, there are no physical criteria by which to judge validity. They are, nevertheless, appropriate outcome variables for clinical studies and instruments like questionnaires, and scales must be employed. Establishing the validity of such instruments is achievable by using methods already established by social scientists (Table 17.7)

When they are selecting a scale or index as an outcome tool, investigators should be concerned with content validity—that is, how well the tool measures or represents the various components of the characteristic being assessed. A close examination of the individual components and the overall content will disclose what is being measured, and what the responses will mean.[39] A judgment can then be made as to whether changes caused by an intervention will be reflected in the scores. Trying to measure something that an intervention cannot alter is a waste of time, money, and effort.

Researchers should also check how a measure performs in relation to other measures assessing similar or related characteristics: when this comparison is made against a "gold standard" (i.e., a formally validated and/or a highly accepted measure), the measure is said to have criterion-related validity. For example, if a new measure of dyspnea correlated highly with pulmonary function tests, criterion-related validity would be deemed to exist. For many clinical outcomes, there is no criterion or "gold standard," and investigators developing measures for them have had to evaluate their construct validity. This involves assessing the essence of the measure in terms of its theoretical basis. An instrument designed to measure "independence" should demonstrate strong correlations with other measures assessing self-care styles, indoor and community mobility, and employment or financial status. A "trauma impact index" should yield similar scores for accident victims sustaining comparable injuries. All minor accidents should get a low score, and major multiple-organ injuries associated with shock and loss of consciousness should yield high scores.

Responsiveness

The importance of responsiveness—the ability of an instrument to detect changes, especially clinically important changes, over time in individuals or in groups of subjects—has been recently recognized in the health measurement literature.[45-47] A responsive instrument for assessing pain would, for example, display appropriate changes in score when a patient reports decreased discomfort. In theory, a valid and reliable measure should be sensitive enough to detect clinical changes, but responsiveness is also related to scaling precision and how much movement within scale categories is required before the score changes.

In controlled studies, the required degree of responsiveness is related to the clinical changes that may occur following an experimental intervention. If the group receiving the intervention is expected to do much better than the control group, a high degree of responsiveness is not necessary; if the anticipated difference is small, greater sensitivity is required. The aim is to choose an instrument capable of detecting real and clinically important differences.

Published reports have only begun to discuss the responsiveness of a measure, and it must most often be appraised on its content and scaling system.

Applicability

The applicability of a measuring instrument is the appropriateness of its use with a proposed study population. For example, the Quality of Life Index,[48] initially developed for cancer patients, was subsequently validated on patients with other chronic diseases of varying severity, using three languages in several geographic areas. This kind of information allows you to assess whether the instrument is appropriate for your intended use. Surgeons should assess applicability carefully, because many scales and indices have been created for use in patients with chronic disease and have not been tested on surgical populations.

The prevalence of the outcome variable has a bearing on the applicability of an instrument to your proposed study sample. One group of investigators found, in the course of constructing a battery of functional status measures for use in a general population, that fewer than 1% of participants reported any limitations in such basic physical activities as personal care or indoor mobility.[49] This outcome variable obviously should not be chosen for a study in such a population, nor operative mortality as the primary endpoint in a study comparing different types of hip arthroplasty.

Practicality

The final criterion, practicality, becomes important only when you have decided that the instrument is acceptable in terms of its other properties. You should assess it from your patients' point of view and from your own.

Can good compliance be anticipated, or is the burden imposed on patients by the process of making the measurement unreasonable? Does the measure involve a painful procedure? Will obtaining the information take so long that patients will become fatigued? Are there so many questions that patients will never answer them all if the instrument is self-administered? Is the instrument anxiety provoking because it invades privacy or raises sensitive issues? The answers to these and other similar questions are particularly important if it is necessary to evaluate patients on several occasions. Serious consideration of these aspects of the instrument should reduce losses due to patient withdrawal or refusal to be evaluated.

The burden for you and your colleagues should be similarly assessed. What type of data collection procedure does the instrument demand? Does it need patient evaluation or direct observation? Are interviews required, or can patients do a self-assessment? If it is to be administered by a staff member, what skill or knowledge must this person possess? Is this individual already available, or would intensive training beyond that necessary to achieve rater reliability be required? Will a chart audit or other form of information retrieval be necessary? For laboratory measures, is the instrument available, or would it have to be purchased specifically for the investigation? How expensive is it? Are paper instruments available and standardized in the language of the patients? Is the instrument easily understood and storable, or does it require complicated mathematical manipulations or coding reversals for computation? Can the data be stored and interpreted easily? Each additional procedure increases the difficulty, the time requirement, and the possibilities for human error. In sum, mode of data collation, its cost, and the burden it imposes must be taken into account.

Do not consider creating a new instrument unless you have the necessary time, resources, and expertise; this is a difficult procedure and a scientific

TABLE 17.8. Considerations for determining the usefulness of an instrument for your research project.

Has the instrument been shown to be reliable enough over time or between observations for the intended use?
If the instrument has multiple items, has the relationship among the items been evaluated?
Does the content of the instrument reflect what you hypothesize the intervention will alter and therefore what you wish to measure?
If a gold standard or criterion is available, how does the instrument relate to it?
Has validity been demonstrated through wide acceptance and use, or by formal construct validation testing procedures?
Do the instrument and its scoring system seem to be responsive enough to detect anticipated clinical changes?
Has the instrument been developed or used in a patient population similar to yours?
Is the instrument practical in terms of patient compliance and professional burden?

investigation in its own right. Table 17.8 lists guidelines for determining the usefulness of an instrument for your research.

Approaches to Assessing Outcomes

Measures of Symptoms

In practice, clinicians evaluate signs and symptoms separately and then aggregate the results to arrive at a diagnosis. In research, individual signs and symptoms are evaluated to determine whether and how they are influenced by the care process.

Because pain is one of the most distressing symptoms and the one for which relief is most often sought, medical practitioners frequently wish to assess it. Surgeons are particularly interested in monitoring pain in the postoperative period, and over time, and in using it to evaluate treatment effectiveness. While several approaches to measuring pain are available, rating scales and questionnaires have been most commonly employed. Both verbal rating scales and visual analogue scales have been used in surgical studies. The visual analogue scale (Fig. 17.1) is a simple bar, usually 10 cm long, representing the range of pain from none to the worst possible. The verbal rating scale (also Fig. 17.1) comprises five to seven categories reflecting different intensities of pain; the patient is asked to choose the most appropriate word description for his or her pain. The psychometric properties of these scales have recently been reviewed.[50] Both have demonstrated acceptable reliability, validity, and responsiveness in a variety of studies, including some on postoperative patients.[51-52] The scores they obtain correlate highly, but patient preference varies between the two formats.

The main problems with rating scales is that they fail to portray the complexity of pain.[50] In 1975 Melzack[53] reported the McGill Pain Questionnaire (MPQ) for measuring the sensory, affective, and evaluative qualities of pain. Patients are asked to choose from specific groups the descriptive adjectives that most closely describe their pain. Since intensity is the most prominent feature of pain, a separate scale is used to record this variable when the question is posed. The Present Pain Intensity (PPI) Index is recorded on an equal-interval scale of 1 to 5 with each number representing a descriptive word in the range of mild to excruciating. Completion of the MPQ provides three scores: the Pain Rating Index (PRI), based on the rank values of the words and their assigned points; the total number of words chosen; and the PPI. In 1987 Melzack[54] also published the Short-Form McGill Pain Questionnaire (SF-MPQ), which includes the PPI and a visual analogue scale.

The MPQ has been widely used in clinical studies of several pain syndromes including those experienced by postsurgical patients.[55-58] It takes an interviewer 15 to 20 minutes to administer it on the first occasion, but up to 50% less time for repeat evaluations. Patients find it acceptable and comply readily. A recent review[50] of the psychometric properties of the MPQ found strong evidence to support its reliability and validity. The SF-MPQ takes 2 to 5 minutes to complete, correlates highly with the MPQ, is sensitive to clinical change and is easily understood by patients.[54] The PPI Index can be administered in less than a minute and has been suggested as an acceptable alternative to the entire questionnaire.[59]

Table 17.9 was compiled mainly from information contained in *Measuring Health: A Guide to Rating Scales and Questionnaires*.[60] It presents selected instruments and approaches for assessing pain.

Increasing attention is being given to nausea as a side effect of chemotherapy for cancer. Although many assessment procedures have been reported, none of the new scales and indices being developed can currently be regarded as well-standardized.[67] Melzack and coworkers[68] have proposed a nausea questionnaire that looks useful. Words chosen from categories of ranked descriptors are used to measure the subjective qualities and intensity of the nausea experienced. An Overall Nausea Inten-

Visual Analogue Scale

At the present time, I would rate the pain I am experiencing as:

No Pain [ ] The worst possible pain

Place an X within the bar at the spot you feel describes your pain at the present time.

Verbal Rating Scale

At the present time I would rate the pain I am experiencing as :

☐	☐	☐	☐	☐
No pain	Mild pain	Moderate pain	Severe pain	Intolerable pain

Place an X in the box that best describes your pain at the present time.

FIGURE 17.1. Formats of pain rating scales.

sity Scale similar to the PPI Index and a visual "no nausea" to "extreme nausea" analogue scale are included to provide three measures of the subjective features and intensity of nausea. The three assessments correlate closely with one another and with the responses to specific chemotherapy drugs, as judged by physicians and nurses. The Nausea Rating Scale demonstrates satisfactory internal consistency and discriminates between the effects of drugs known to provoke severe nausea and those that stimulate a much milder response. In a recent study,[57] the Nausea Scale was able to document the intensity of postoperative nausea associated with anesthesia.

Increased levels of anxiety are often linked to being ill or being faced with surgery—a situation entailing pain or, possibly, death. As a consequence, researchers have been interested in assessing the anxiety associated with an operation and determining whether a surgical intervention will alleviate anxiety in patients who submit to surgery for a chronic problem. The Spielberger State-Trait Inventory[69] has frequently been employed with surgical patients.[70-73] According to the theory underlying the Inventory, trait anxiety refers to relatively stable individual differences in being disposed to anxiety (i.e., how generally anxious we are on a day-to-day basis). On the other hand, state anxiety is the response to a specific stressful situation that normally decreases when the situation is resolved. The instrument consists of two separate 20-item self-report questionnaires in which each

TABLE 17.9. Selected measures for assessing pain.[a]

Authors	Measure	Dimensions included	Rater	Time	Reliability	Validity	Comments
Huskisson: 1974 (61)	Visual analogue scale	Intensity	Patient	30 seconds	XXX	XX	Widely used clinically and in research
Melzack: 1975 (53)	Verbal (5 point) rating scale	Intensity	Patient	< 1 minute	X	X	May be as useful as entire MPQ (59)
Melzack: 1975 (53)	McGill Pain Questionnaire	Sensory; affective; evaluative	Patient	15–20 minute	XX	XX	Useful for chronic and acute pain
Melzack: 1987 (54)	Short-Form McGill Pain Questionnaire	Sensory; affective; evaluative	Patient	5–10 minute	XX	XX	Useful when MPQ takes too long
Pilowsky et al: 1983 (62)	Illness Behavior Questionnaire	Emotional/behavioral responses to pain	Patient	15–20 minute	XX	XX	Used with coronary bypass patients (63)
Black and Chapman; 1976 (64)	SAD Index	Somatic, anxiety & depressive responses to pain	Physician				Used only as a clinical tool
Tursky et al: 1982 (65)	Pain perception profile	Intensity; unpleasantness; type	Behavior therapist				Used mainly in research
Zung: 1983 (66)	Pain and distress scale	Emotional and behavioral responses to pain	Patient	5–10 minute	XX		Used only with acute pain

[a]Symbols: X weak, XX adequate, XXX excellent, reliability/validity.
Source: Compiled mainly from information contained in McDowell I, Newell C. Measuring Health. A Guide to Rating Scales and Questionnaires. New York: Oxford University Press, 1987:229–68.

item is scored on a scale of 1 to 4, reflecting intensity. The measure has acceptable internal consistency and test–retest reliability,[69,74] and it correlates highly with other measures of anxiety.[69]

Visick[8] proposed another approach to the assessment of symptoms as outcomes following gastrectomy for peptic ulcer. In 1968 Goligher and colleagues[75] published the results of a study in which they used a modification of the Visick instrument that attempted to clarify the criteria for each symptom category without altering the overall concept of Visick's classification scheme. Since then, other minor modifications have been made[76] and the instrument has been applied to patients with gastric cancer.[77] Hall and colleagues[78] have assessed its intraobserver reliability and found high agreement on the absence or presence and severity of symptoms, but quite low agreement on the overall Visick gradings before extensive discussion with the raters. After discussion, interrater agreement was acceptably high, but the raters' gradings were quite different from those made by the patients on themselves. Hall and colleagues concluded that the most reliable method of assessing the status of the ulcer patient, after surgery, is simply to record the presence or absence of specific symptoms.

Measures of Physical Function

Although the appraisal of functional performance is common in patients who are elderly or undergoing rehabilitation, many other patients have a disease, disorder, or injury that leads to temporary or permanent structural or functional impairment. The addition of a functional descriptor to other clinical outcome measures provides greater insight into the overall results of any surgical intervention.

Many measures of functional performance focus on the activities and skills of daily living (ADL). The Katz Index of ADL[79,80] was developed through studies of large numbers of patients with various diagnoses. Six ADL dimensions—bathing, dressing, toileting, transferring, continence, and feeding—are used, and scoring is on an ordinal scale that bifurcates according to whether the patient can perform a task independently. The Index takes account of the number of activities the patient can perform and the order in which self-care capabilities are lost or regained. The theoretical basis of the instrument is the authors' contention that the pattern of recovery from a disabled state parallels the normal sequence of development in a child. Functional abilities are categorized by an overall score that ranges from A (independent) to G (dependent). A high coefficient of reproducibility has been reported,[81] and concurrent validity has been demonstrated,[82] by comparing the instrument to two widely accepted ADL scales, the Barthel Index[83] and the Kenny Self-Care Evaluation.[84] Although the Katz Index is the least sensitive of the three to change,[82] it has been widely used to describe and classify the functional performance of patients in clinical studies.

Various scales have been devised to assess specific joints and their function pre- and postoperatively.[85-87]

Kettlekamp and Thompson[88] have developed a knee scale that combines clinical expertise, biomechanical principles, and statistical analysis. Two scales were developed and tested on post-osteotomy and postarthroplasty knees, then compared with each other and with a previously determined clinical classification. The one chosen sums to 103 points. It contains items on pain, function, range of motion, instability, and deformity; it is short and easy to complete; and it contains only clinical variables obtained routinely during a knee examination. Although relatively little information is available about the validity or reliability of this instrument, it has been used in clinical studies and has demonstrated change between the pre- and postoperative states.[89-91]

In 1949, Karnofsky[7] developed what has become one of the most widely used clinical scales for measuring the overall ability of patients to perform physical activities. The scale comprises 11 categories that cover the functional spectrum from dead to normal, with scores that range from 0 to 100. The categories are major groupings that classify patients' current performance in relation to self-care, general activities, and work. The scoring can be completed by the patient or a health care professional in a few minutes. Professional interrater reliability has been shown to range from moderate[92] to low,[93] especially when the scores are corrected for chance agreement, and there is considerable disagreement between the patients' self-ratings and the physicians' ratings.[93] Hutchinson and colleagues[93] feel that the defects in the scale could be easily corrected by providing specific criteria and having only one performance activity in each category.

Measures of Well-Being

Instruments designed to assess well-being are based on the World Health Organization concept of health,[94] which includes physical, social, and psychological dimensions. Their objective is to produce a single summary score for an attribute that is multidimensional.[95] To capture the full spectrum of daily functioning, several investigators have developed measures of health status.[38,96-100]

One such measure, the Sickness Impact Profile (SIP),[97] is based on the concept that sickness-related dysfunction is manifested by behavioral changes that are quantifiable. The physical and psychosocial dimensions of the SIP encompass 136 items grouped into 12 categories.[101] Each item is a first-person statement of a specific dysfunction currently being experienced as a consequence of illness, and each has been weighted on the basis of an estimate of the relative severity of the stated dysfunction.[102] The SIP, which can be completed by an interviewer or the patient, is reported to be acceptable to patients even though it takes 20 to 30 minutes to complete. It has also been validated in Spanish[103] and used with a Spanish-speaking population.[104] It has been used in studies of low back pain, cancer, arthritis and hip replacement,[11,101,104-106] and has demonstrated consistently acceptable levels of interrater and test–retest reliability, as well as internal consistency in test trials and field applications.[107,108] The SIP distinguishes groups of patients with small degrees of clinical distinctiveness and is a useful measure of the behavioral impact of illness.

Assessing quality of life as an outcome of a disease process or a therapeutic intervention is currently popular in the literature, but its use as an endpoint in comparative studies has mainly been in chronic conditions when insignificant differences in survival are anticipated, or when a treatment is known to increase survival while incurring substantial morbidity.[109]

Health-related quality of life generally entails physical, social, and psychological components. The physical component includes self-care, mobility, common daily activities, sexuality, and freedom from discomfort. Social functioning involves relationships with family and friends, leisure, recreational and work activities, and the fulfillment of social and cultural roles. Psychological

TABLE 17.10. Selected health-related quality of life measures.[a]

Authors	Dimensions	Response format/raters	Applications	Validity	Reliability	Comments
Spitzer et al; 1981	Daily activities; self-care, health; support; outlook	5 items: 0–3 scale/patient, clinician significant others	Cancer, cardiac, transplantation, terminally ill, and ICU patients	XX	XX	Most useful to document net effects of disease and management over time
Padilla et al; 1983	Physical condition; daily activities; personal attitudes	14 items: visual analogue scales/patients	Cancer patients	X	X	Unable to locate usage by other authors
Padilla et al; 1985	Physical, social psychological well-being; treatment response (surgical)	24 items: visual analogue scales/patient	Colostomy patients	X	X	Unable to locate usage by other authors
Schipper et al; 1984	Daily functioning; symptoms; satisfaction	22 items: 1–7 scale/patient	Cancer patients	XX	XX	Presented on tear sheets to be returned by patients
Priestman & Baum, 1976	Physical functioning, physical and psychological symptoms; personal relationships	Variable number of items; visual analogue scales/patient	Cancer patients	X	X	Extensively used by other investigators

[a]Symbols: X = present; XX = strong feature.
Source: Table compiled from information contained in Williams JI, Wood-Dauphinée S. Assessing quality of life: measures and utility. In: Quality of Life and Technology and Assessment, Mosteller F, Falotico-Taylor J, eds. Washington, DC: National Academy Press, 1989:65–115.

functioning has cognitive, perceptual, and emotional constituents that include how a patient copes with a perceived problem to diminish the associated stress.

A recent review of the assessment of quality of life in surgical studies[110] has revealed that most attempts to assess it rely on narrative documentation,[111-113] proxy measures such as the total time spent in hospital during the final months of life,[114] the ability to work,[13,115] or a battery of measures, each of which assesses a different dimension felt to influence life's quality.[11,14,116,117] Perhaps the best example of this approach is found in a study by Sugarbaker et al.[11] In a controlled clinical trial designed to compare the quality of life of limb sarcoma patients treated by amputation or by limb-sparing surgery plus radiation and chemotherapy, quality of life was determined by measures of the activities of daily living, health status, psychosocial adjustment to being sick, pain, mobility, social relationships, and financial implications. More precise measurement of this construct has received considerable attention. Well-standardized instruments are available,[10,118-122] but have seldom been used in surgical studies.

The Quality of Life (QL) Index devised by Spitzer and coworkers[48] is an exception. This index has a questionnaire format that addresses five equally weighted factors related to the patient's mood, perception of his or her own health, self-care ability, work capability, and social interaction with family and friends. The main part of the QL Index sums to 10 points, but there is also a one-dimensional visual analogue scale (Uniscale) that portrays the overall estimate. The QL Index can be completed by the patient, or be administered by an interviewer or a health professional who knows the patient well, in less than 5 minutes. It was initially developed for cancer patients but has been validated for patients with other diseases and has been found to be acceptable to patients and health care providers. The QL Index's content, criterion and construct validity, responsiveness to change over time, and interobserver reliability in English and French have been demonstrated.[123] It has been used successfully in surgical studies of gastric cancer,[124] end-stage renal disease,[125] and diabetes.[126] Another surgical study,[127-128] however, encountered difficulty with the ability of the index to discriminate between two groups of patients subjected to differ-

TABLE 17.11. Psychometric properties of established measuring instruments for clinical endpoints.[a]

Instrument	Reliability	Validity	Responsiveness	Practicality
McGill Pain Questionnaire	XX	XX	X	X
Nausea Questionnaire	X	X	X	XX
State-Trait Anxiety Inventory	XX	XX	X	X
Visick Scale	X			XX
Katz Index of ADL	XX	XX	X	XX
Knee Scoring Scale		X	X	X
Karnofsky Index	X	XX		XX
Sickness Impact Profile	XX	XX	XX	X
Quality of Life (QL) Index	XX	XX	X	XX

[a] Symbols: X = present; XX = strong feature.

ent reconstructive techniques following total gastrectomy and systematic lymphadenectomy in patients with gastric cancer. Differences were found in survival and in a disease-specific quality of life measure designed for the study.

During the past few years, a group of researchers at McMaster University, in Canada, have concentrated on developing disease-specific quality of life measures for use in clinical trials,[129] and have published instruments for use in patients with inflammatory bowel disease,[130] chronic lung disease,[131] and breast cancer.[132] Each measure has been carefully developed in terms of disease-specific content and has been assessed for reliability, validity, and responsiveness to clinical change. While further testing has been advocated, each has performed at an acceptable level in a clinical study.

Any discussion of quality of life measures would be incomplete without reference to the work of the European Organization for Research and Treatment of Cancer (EORTC). This international group has been both promoting the incorporation of quality of life measures into cancer clinical trials and developing quality of life measures applicable across cancer types and treatment settings.[133] EORTC proposes a modular approach, in which each questionnaire would contain a core set of items assessing functional status, psychological distress, social interaction, common symptoms of cancer and its treatment, perceived health status, and general quality of life. The core would be supplemented by additional items focusing on symptoms and treatment side effects specific to different cancer types. The EORTC Core Quality of Life Questionnaire and Lung Cancer-Specific Module has been published; information on measures assessing quality of life in patients with melanoma or breast, prostatic, and gastrointestinal cancers is expected in the near future.

Table 17.10, compiled from information contained in Quality of Life and Technology Assessment,[134] presents a selection of health-related quality of life measures of interest to surgeons.

Table 17.11 provides an overview of the known psychometric properties of the established measuring instruments described in this chapter.

Final Comment

The instruments described in this chapter were compared to flashlights for illuminating dark areas where "keys" will be found. We are convinced that much is now known in this area; the development and regular use endpoint measuring instruments will help patients and investigators.

Our conviction about the importance of broadening the choice of endpoints in surgical studies does not imply that mortality, and technologically acquired data, should be ignored or abandoned; they make significant contributions to advancing our understanding of disease. We do suggest that the validity and reliability of these so-called hard measures be questioned, because the difference between them and measures labeled "soft" are not nearly as great as we are inclined to believe. Valid, reliable, and practical measures of functional capacity, overall well-being, and quality of life will increase our comprehension of the impact of disease and the results of treatment.

References

1. Spitzer WO, Feinstein AR, Sackett DL. What is a health care trial? J Am Med Assoc 1975;233: 161–63.
2. White KL. Improved medical care statistics and health services system. Pub Health Rep 1967;82: 847–54.
3. Graham C, Bond S, Gerkovich M, Cook M. Use of McGill Pain Questionnaire in assessment of cancer pain replicability and consistency. Pain 1980;8: 377–87.

4. Melzack R, O'Fiesh JG, Mount BM. The Bromptom mixture: effects on pain in cancer patients. Can Med Assoc J 1976;115:125–29.
5. World Health Organization. International Classification of Impairments, Disabilities, and Handicaps. Geneva: WHO, 1980.
6. Criteria Committee of the New York Heart Association. Diseases of the Heart and Blood Vessels. Nomenclature and Criteria for Diagnosis. Boston: Little, Brown 1964:112–13.
7. Karnofsky DA, Burchenal JH. Clinical evaluation of chemotherapeutic agents in cancer. In: Evaluation of Chemotherapeutic Agents, Macleod CM, ed. New York: Columbia University Press, 1949; 191–205.
8. Visick AH. A study of the failures after gastrectomy. Edinburgh: Ann R Coll Surg, 1948;3:266–84.
9. Fries JF. Toward an understanding of patient outcome measurement. Arthritis Rheum 1983;26: 697–704.
10. Gough R, Furnival CM, Schilder L, Grove W. Assessment of the quality of life of patients with advanced cancer. Eur J Cancer Clin Oncol 1983; 19:1161–65.
11. Sugarbaker PH, Barofsky I, Rosenberg SA, Gianola FJ. Quality of life assessment of patients in extremity sarcoma clinical trials. Surgery 1982; 91:17–23.
12. Troidl H, Kusche J. Lebensqualität nach Gastrektomie: Ergebnisse einer randomisierten Studie zum vergleich Oesophago-jujunostomie nach Schlatter mit dem Hunt–Laurence–Rodino Pouch. In: Das Magenkarzinom. Methodik klinischer Studien and therapeutischer Ansatze, Rohde H, Troidl H, eds. Stuttgart: Thieme, 1984.
13. LaMendola WF, Pellegrini RV. Quality of life and coronary artery bypass surgery patients. Soc Sci Med 1979;13A:457–61.
14. Williams NS, Johnston D. The quality of life after rectal excision for low rectal cancer. Br J Surg 1983;70:460–62.
15. Lebow JL. Consumer assessment of the quality of medical care. Med Care 1974;12:328–37.
16. Hulka BS, Zyzanski SJ, Cassel JC, Thompson SJ. Scale for the measurement of attitudes toward physicians and primary medical care. Med Care 1970; 5:429–35.
17. Mangelsdorff AD. Patient satisfaction questionnaire. Med Care 1979;17:86–90.
18. Taylor PW, Nelson-Wernick E, Currey HS, Woodbury ME, Conley LE. Development and use of a method of assessing patient perception of care. Hosp Health Serv Admin 1981;26:89–103.
19. Light HK, Solheim JS, Hunter GW. Satisfaction with medical care during pregnancy and delivery. Am J Obstet Gynecol 1976;122:827–31.
20. Pineault R, Contandriopoulos A-P, Valois M, Bastian M-L, Lance J-M. Randomized clinical trial of one-day surgery: patient satisfaction, clinical outcomes, and costs. Med Care 1985;23:171–82.
21. Feinstein AR. An additional basic science for clinical medicine: IV. The development of clinimetrics. Ann Intern Med 1983;99:843–48.
22. Fletcher RH, Fletcher SW. Clinical research in general medical journals. A 30-year perspective. N Engl J Med 1979;301:180–83.
23. Fletcher RH, Fletcher SW, Wagner EH. Clinical epidemiology—the essentials. Baltimore: Williams & Wilkins, 1982.
24. Feinstein AR. An additional basic science for clinical medicine: II. The limitations of randomized trials. Ann Intern Med 1983;99:544–50.
25. Feinstein AR. Clinical biostatistics: XLI. Hard science, soft data, and the challenges of choosing clinical variables in research. Clin Pharmacol Ther 1977;22:485–98.
26. Koran LM. The reliability of clinical methods, data and judgments. N Engl J Med 1975;293:642–46, 695–701.
27. Feinstein AR. Clinical biostatistics: XLV. The purposes and functions of criteria. Clin Pharmacol Ther 1978;24:479–92.
28. Feinstein AR. Clinical biostatistics: XLVI. What are the criteria for criteria? Clin Pharmacol Ther 1979;25:108–16.
29. Department of Clinical Epidemiology and Biostatistics, McMaster University. Clinical disagreement: II. How to avoid it and how to learn from one's mistakes. Can Med Assoc J 1980;123: 613–17.
30. Sackett DL, Haynes RE, Tugwell P. Clinical Epidemiology. A Basic Science for Clinical Medicine. Toronto: Little, Brown, 1985.
31. Riddell RH, Goldman H, Ransohoff DF, Appelman HD, Fenoglio CM, Haggett R, Ahren C, Correa P, Hamilton SR, Morson BC, Sammers SC, Yardky JH. Dysplasia in inflammatory bowel disease: standardized classification with provisional clinical applications. Human Pathol 1983;14:931–68.
32. Smythe H, Helewa A, Goldsmith CH. Selection and combination of outcome measures. J Rheumatol 1982;9:770–74.
33. Guyatt GH, Veldhuyzen Van Zanten SJO, Feeny DH, Patrick DL. Measuring quality of life in clinical trials. Can Med Assoc J 1989;140:1441–47.
34. Abramson JH. Survey methods in community medicine. Edinburgh: Churchill-Livingston, 1979.
35. Pocock SJ. Current issues in the design and interpretation of clinical trials. Br Med J 1985;290: 39–42.
36. Bombardier C, Tugwell P. A methodological framework to develop and select indices for clinical trials: statistical and judgmental approaches. J Rheumatol 1982;9:753–57.
37. Jette AM. Concepts of health and methodological issues in functional assessment. In: Functional assessment in rehabilitation medicine, Granger CV, Gresham GA, ed. Baltimore: Williams & Wilkins, 1984:46–64.
38. Sackett DL, Chambers LW, MacPherson AS, Goldsmith CH, Maculey RG. The development and

application of indices of health: general methods and a summary of results. Am J Public Health 1977;67:423–28.
39. Ware JE, Brook RH, Davies AR, Lohr KN. Choosing measures of health status for individuals in general populations. Am J Public Health 1981;71: 620–25.
40. Department of Clinical Epidemiology and Biostatistics, McMaster University. Clinical disagreement: I. How often it occurs and why. Can Med Assoc J 1980;123:499–504.
41. Haynes RB, Sackett DL, Tugwell P. Problems in the handling of clinical and research evidence by medical practitioners. Arch Intern Med 1983;143: 971–75.
42. Fleiss JL. The design and analysis of clinical experiments. New York. Wiley, 1986.
43. Makrides L, Richman J, Prince B. Research methodology and applied statistics: 3. Measurement procedures in research. Physiother Can 1980;32: 253–57.
44. Whitehead TP. Quality control techniques in laboratory services. Br Med Bull 1974;30:237–42.
45. Deyo RA, Inui TS. Toward clinical applications of health status measures: sensitivity of scales to clinically important changes. Health Serv Res 1984; 19:275–89.
46. Guyatt G, Walter S, Norman G. Measuring change over time: assessing the usefulness of evaluative instruments. J Chronic Dis 1987;40:171–78.
47. Deyo RA, Centor RM. Assessing the responsiveness of functional scales to clinical change: an analogy to diagnostic test performance. J Chronic Dis 1986;39:899–906.
48. Spitzer WO, Dobson AJ, Hall J, Chesterman E, Levi J, Shepherd R, Battista RN, Catchlove BR. Measuring the quality of life of cancer patients. A concise QL-Index for use by physicians. J Chronic Dis 1981;34:585–97.
49. Stewart AL, Ware JE, Brook RH. Construction and Scoring of Aggregate Functional Status Measures: Vol. I, Rand Health Insurance Experiment Series, R-225 1-1-HHS. Santa Monica, CA: Rand, 1982.
50. Reading AE. Testing pain mechanisms in persons in pain. In: Textbook of Pain, Wall PD, Melzack R, ed. New York: Churchill-Livingstone, 1989:269–80.
51. Sriwatanakul K, Kelvie W, Lasagna L, Calimlim JF, Weis OF, Mehta G. Studies with different types of visual analogue scales for measurement of pain. Clin Pharmacol Ther 1983;34:234–39.
52. Melzack R, Torgerson WS. On the language of pain. Anesthesiology 1971;24:50–59.
53. Melzack R. The McGill Pain Questionnaire: major properties and scoring methods. Pain 1975;1:277–99.
54. Melzack R. The Short-Form McGill Pain Questionnaire. Pain 1987;30:191–97.
55. Reading AE, Hand DJ, Sledmere CM. A comparison of response profiles obtained on the McGill Pain Questionnaire and an adjective checklist. Pain 1982;6:375–83.
56. Van Buren J, Kleinknecht RA. An evaluation of the McGill Pain Questionnaire for use in dental pain assessment. Pain 1979;6:23–33.
57. Cohen MM, Tate RB. Using the McGill Pain Questionnaire to study common postoperative complications. Pain 1989;39:275–79.
58. Taenzer P. Postoperative pain: relationships among measures of pain, mood and narcotic requirements. In: Pain Measurement and Assessment, Melzack R, ed. New York: Raven Press, 1983:111–18.
59. Finch L, Melzack R. Objective pain measurement: a case for increased clinical usage. Physiother Can 1982;34:343–46.
60. McDowell I, Newell C. Measuring Health. A Guide to Rating Scales and Questionnaires. New York: Oxford University Press, 1987.
61. Huskisson EC. Measurement of pain. Lancet 1974; 2:1127–31.
62. Pilowsky I, Spence ND. Manual for the Illness Behavior Questionnaire (IBQ), 2nd ed. Adelaide, Australia: University of Adelaide, 1983.
63. Pilowsky I, Spence ND, Waddy JL. Illness behavior and coronary artery bypass surgery. J Psychosom Res 1979;23:39–44.
64. Black RG, Chapman CR. SAD Index for clinical assessment of pain. In: Advances in Pain Research and Therapy, Vol. I, Bonica JJ, Albe-Fessard D, eds. New York: Raven Press, 1976:301–5.
65. Tursky B, Jammer LD, Friedman R. The Pain Perception Profile: a psychological approach to the assessment of pain report. Behav Ther 1982;13: 376–94.
66. Zung WWK. A self-rating pain and distress scale. Psychosomatics 1983;24:887–94.
67. Morrow GR. The assessment of nausea and vomiting. Past problems, current issues and suggestions for future research. Cancer 1984;53(Suppl):2267–80.
68. Melzack R, Rosberger Z, Hillingsworth ML, Thirlwell M. New approaches to measuring nausea. Can Med Assoc J 1985;133:755–59.
69. Spielberger CD, Gorsuch RL, Lushene RE, Manual for the State-Trait Anxiety Inventory (Self-Evaluation Questionnaire). Palo Alto, CA: Consulting Psychologists Press, 1970.
70. Johnston M. Anxiety in surgical patients. Psychol Med 1980;10:145–52.
71. Auerbach SM. Trait-state anxiety and adjustment to surgery. J Consult Clin Psychol 1973;40:264–71.
72. Martinez-Urrutia A. Anxiety and pain in surgical patients. J Consult Clin Psychol 1975;4:437–42.
73. Johnston M, Carpenter L. Relationship between preoperative anxiety and postoperative state. Psychol Med 1980;10:361–67.
74. Rule WR, Traver MD. Test-retest reliabilities of State-Trait Anxiety Inventory in a stressful social analogue situation. J Pers Assess 1983;47:276–77.
75. Goligher JC, Pulvertaft CN, de Dombal FT, Conyers JH, Duthie HL, Feather DB, Latchmore

AJC, Shoesmith JH, Smiddy FG, Willson-Pepper J. Five-to-eight-year results of Leeds/York controlled trial of elective surgery for duodenal ulcer. Br Med J 1968;2:781–87.
76. Emas S, Fernstrom M. Prospective, randomized trial of selective vagotomy with pyloroplasty and selective proximal vagotomy with and without pyloroplasty in the treatment of duodenal, pyloric and prepyloric ulcers. Am J Surg 1985;149:236–43.
77. Troidl H, Menge K-H, Lorenz W, Vestweber K-H, Barth H, Hamelmann H. Quality of life and stomach replacement. In: Gastric Cancer, Herfarth CH, Schlag P, eds. Berlin: Springer Verlag, 1979: 312–17.
78. Hall R, Horrocks JC, Clamp SE, de Dombal FT. Observer variation in results of surgery for peptic ulceration. Br Med J 1976;1:814–16.
79. Katz S, Ford AB, Moskowitz RW, Jackson BA, Jaffe MW, Cleveland MA. Studies of illness in the aged. The Index of ADL: a standardized measure of biological and psychosocial function. JAMA 1963; 185:914–19.
80. Katz S, Downs TD, Cash HR, Grotz RC. Progress in the development of the Index of ADL. Gerontologist 1970;10:20–30.
81. Sherwood SJ, Morris J, Mor V, Gutkin C. Compendium of measures for describing and assessing long-term care populations. Boston: Hebrew Rehabilitation Center for the Aged. In: Assessing the Elderly. A Practical Guide to Measurement, Kane RA, Kane RL, eds.. Lexington, MA: Lexington Books, D.C. Heath, 1981:45.
82. Donaldson SW, Wagner CC, Gresham CE. A unified ADL evaluation form. Arch Phys Med Rehabil, 1973;54:175–80.
83. Mahoney FI, Barthel DW. Functional evaluation: the Barthel Index. MD State Med J 1965;14:61–65.
84. Schoening HA, Iversen IA. Numerical scoring of self-care status: a study of the Kenny Self Care Evaluation. Arch Phys Med Rehabil 1968;49: 221–29.
85. Harris WH. Traumatic arthritis of the hip after dislocation and acetabular fractures: treatment by mold arthroplasty. J Bone Joint Surg 1969;51-A: 737–55.
86. Larson CB. Rating scale for hip disabilities. Clin Orthop Relat Res 1963;31:85–92.
87. Neer CS, Watson KC, Stanton FJ. Recent experience in total shoulder replacement. J Bone and Joint Surg 1982;64-A:319–37.
88. Kettlekamp DB, Thompson C. Development of a knee scoring scale. Clin Orthop Related 1975;107: 93–99.
89. Hejgaard N, Sandberg H, Hide A, Jacobsen K. Prospective stress radiography in 38 old injuries of the ligaments of the knee joint. Acta Orthop Scand 1983;54:119–25.
90. Murray DG, Webster DA. The variable axis knee prosthesis. J Bone Joint Surg 1981;63-A:687–94.
91. Short WH, Hootnick DR, Murray DG. Ipsilateral supracondylar femur fractures following knee arthroplasty. Clin Orthop Relat Res 1981;158: 111–16.
92. Yates JW, Chalmer B, McKegney FP. Evaluation of patients with advanced cancer using the Karnofsky Performance Status. Cancer 1980;45:2220–24.
93. Hutchinson TA, Boyd NF, Feinstein AR. Scientific problems in clinical scales as demonstrated in the Karnofsky Index of Performance Status. J Chronic Dis 1979;32:661–66.
94. World Health Organization: Constitution of the World Health Organization. Basic Documents. Geneva: WHO, 1948:2.
95. Boyle MH, Torrance GW. Developing multiattribute health indexes. Med Care 1984;22:1045–57.
96. Brook RH, Ware JE, Davies-Avery A, Stewart AL, Donald CA, Rogers WH, Williams KN, Johnston SA. Overview of adult health status measures fielded in Rand's Health Insurance Study. Med Care 1979;17(Suppl 7):1–131.
97. Gilson BS, Gilson JS, Bergner M, Bobbitt RA, Kressel S, Pollard WE, Vesselago M. The Sickness Impact Profile. Development of an outcome measure of health care. Am J Public Health 1975;65: 1304–10.
98. Grogono AW, Woodgate DJ. Index for measuring health. Lancet 1971;2:1024–26.
99. Kaplan RM, Atkins CJ, Timms R. Validity of a quality of well-being scale as an outcome measure in chronic obstructive pulmonary disease. J Chronic Dis 1984;37:85–95.
100. Patrick DL, Bush JW, Chen MM. Toward an operational definition of health. J Health Soc Behav 1973;14:6–23.
101. Bergner M, Bobbitt RA, Carter WB, Gilson, BS. The Sickness Impact Profile: development and final revision of a health status measure. Med Care 1981;19:787–805.
102. Carter WB, Bobbitt RA, Bergner M, Gilson BS. Validation of an interval scaling: the Sickness Impact Profile. Health Serv Res 1976;11:516–28.
103. Gilson BS, Erickson D, Chavez CT, Bobbitt RA, Bergner M, Carter WB. A Chicano version of the Sickness Impact Profile (SIP). Cult Med Psychiatr 1980;4:137–50.
104. Deyo RA, Diehl AK. Measuring physical and psychosocial function in patients with low-back pain. Spine 1983;8:635–42.
105. Deyo RA, Inui TS, Leininger J, Overman S. Physical and psychosocial function in rheumatoid arthritis. Arch Intern Med 1982;142:879–82.
106. Deyo RA, Inui TS, Leininger JD, Overman SS. Measuring functional outcomes in chronic disease: a comparison of traditional scales and a self-administered health status questionnaire in patients with rheumatoid arthritis. Med Care 1983;21:180–92.
107. Bergner M, Bobbitt RA, Pollard WE, Martin DP, Gilson BS. The Sickness Impact Profile: validation of a health status measure. Med Care 1976;14: 57–67.
108. Pollard WE, Bobbitt RA, Bergner M, Martin DP, Gilson BS. The Sickness Impact Profile: reliability

of a health status measure. Med Care 1976;14:146–55.
109. Schipper H. Why measure quality of life? Can Med Assoc J 1983;128:1367–70.
110. Wood-Dauphinée S, Troidl H. Assessing quality of life in surgical studies. Theor Surg 1989;4:35–44.
111. McLeod RS, Fazio VW. Quality of life with continent ileostomy. World J Surg 1984;8:90–95.
112. Bennett RC. Long-term follow-up of surgical adrenalectomy for breast cancer. Aust NZ J Surg, 1983;53:415–519.
113. Meyers S. Assessing quality of life. Mt Sinai J Med 1983;50:190–92.
114. Scharschmidt BF. Human liver transplantation: analyses of data on 540 patients from four centers. Hepathology 1984;4(Suppl I):958–1019.
115. Westaby S, Sapsford RN, Bentall HH. Return to work and quality of life after surgery for coronary artery disease. Br Med J 1979;2:1028–31.
116. Drettner B, Ahlbom A. Quality of life and state of health for patients with cancer of the head and neck. Acta Otolaryngol 1983;96:307–14.
117. Trudel L, Fabia J, Bouchard J-P. Quality of life of 50 carotid endarterectomy survivors: a long-term follow-up study. Arch Phys Med Rehabil 1984; 65:310–12.
118. Schipper H, Levitt M. Measuring quality of life: risks and benefits. Cancer Treatment Rep 1985; 69:1115–25.
119. Priestman TJ, Baum M. Evaluation of quality of life in patients receiving treatment for advanced breast cancer. Lancet 1976;2:899–901.
120. Coates A, Dillenbeck CF, McNeil DR, Kaye SB, Sims K, Fox RM, Woods RL, Milton GW, Solomon J, Tattersall MH. On the receiving end: II. Linear Analogue Self Assessment (LASA) in the evaluation of aspects of the quality of life of cancer patients receiving therapy. Eur J Cancer Clin Oncol 1983;19:1633–37.
121. Selby PJ, Chapman J-A-W, Etazadi-Amoli J, Dalley D, Boyd NF. The development of a method for assessing the quality of life of cancer patients. Br J Cancer 1984;50:13–22.
122. Schipper H, Clinch J, McMurray A, Levitt M. Measuring the quality of life of cancer patients: the Functional Living Index—Cancer: development and validation. J Clin Oncol 1984;2:472–83.
123. Wood-Dauphinée S, Williams JI. The Spitzer Quality of Life Index: its performance as a measure. In: The Effect of Cancer on Quality of Life, Osaba D, ed. Boca Raton, FL: CRC Press, submitted.
124. Köster R, Gebbensleben H, Stützen B, Salzberger B, Ahrens P, Rhode H. Quality of life in gastric cancer. Karnofsky's scale and Spitzer's index in comparison at the time of surgery in a cohort of 1081 patients. Scand J Gastroenterol 1987; 22 (Suppl 133):102–6.
125. Parfrey PS, Vavasour H, Bullock M, Henry S, Harnett JD, Gault HM. Symptoms in end stage renal diseases: dialysis vs transplantation. Transplant Proc 1987;19:3407–09.
126. Nakache R, Tydén G, Groth CG. Quality of life in diabetic patients after combined pancreas-kidney or kidney transplantation. Diabetes 1989;38:40–42.
127. Troidl H, Kusche J, Vestweber K-H, Eypasch E, Maul V. Pouch versus esophagojejunostomy after total gastrectomy. World J Surg 1987;11:699–712.
128. Kusche J, Vestweber K-H, Troidl H. Quality of life after total gastrectomy for stomach cancer. Results of three types of evaluative methods. Scand J Gastroenterol 1987;22(Suppl 133):96–102.
129. Guyatt GH, Bombardier C, Tugwell P. Measuring disease-specific quality of life in clinical trials. Can Med Assoc J 1986;134:889–95.
130. Guyatt GH, Mitchell A, Irvine EJ, Singer J, Williams N, Goodacre R, Tompkins C. A new measure of health status for clinical trials in inflammatory bowel disease. Gastroenterology 1989;96:804–10.
131. Guyatt GH, Berman L, Townsend M, Pugsley SO, Chambers LW. A measure of quality of life for clinical trials in chronic lung disease. Thorax 1987; 43:773–78.
132. Levine MN, Guyatt GH, Gent M, DePauw S, Goodyear MD, Hryniuk WM, Arnold A, Findlay B, Skillings JR, Bramwell VH, Levin L, Bush H, Abu-Zahra H, Kotalik J. Quality of life in stage II breast cancer: an instrument for clinical trials. J Clin Oncol 1988;6:1798–1810.
133. Aaronson NK, Bullinger M, Ahmedzia S. A modular approach to quality-of-life assessment in cancer clinical trials. Recent Results Can Res 1988;111:231–49.
134. Williams JI, Wood-Dauphinée S. Assessing quality of life: measures and utility. In: Quality of Life and Technology Assessment, Mosteller F, Falotico-Taylor J, eds. Washington, DC: National Academy Press, 1989:65–115.

18

Risk and Prognosis

S.A. Marion and M.T. Schechter

Risk and Prognosis: The Concepts

An understanding of the natural history of treated and untreated disease is essential to the physician, is an area of utmost concern to patients, and is the basis of most decisions about management. The clinician faces numerous questions about the risk of certain events and the natural history of various disease states. Given a patient of a certain age and sex, what is the probability that symptomatic coronary heart disease will develop in the next 5 years? Given such a patient, together with the results of certain diagnostic maneuvers, what is the probability that significant coronary heart disease is already present? Given a set of characteristics of a coronary bypass surgery candidate, what is the probability that he or she will survive at least 5 years after surgery?

Much scientific research is a quest to better characterize or estimate the probabilities that particular events will occur.[1] Rational clinical decision making requires sound estimates of the probability of various possible events occurring along each available therapeutic path.

The questions posed in the opening paragraph illustrate certain points about the concept of probability. The first is that, to be useful in clinical practice, the probability should refer to very specific circumstances—the more specific the better. Planners estimating the demand for coronary care beds might find it interesting to consider the probability that a person selected at random from their country's adult population will develop clinically significant coronary heart disease in the next 5 years, but this probability would be of little value to a clinician. The patient seeking consultation has certain known characteristics, such as age, sex, and a medical history that will affect the probability, sometimes profoundly. In clinical practice, what is desired is a probability estimate that is specific to a given set of circumstances.

The second aspect of probability is specificity of outcome. To define a probability, one must clearly state exactly which events are to be counted. The easiest outcome to measure is death; its correct definition may be disputable, but the fact seldom is. But even here, specificity is required regarding the time period involved. Every one dies eventually; to provide useful information, an estimate of the probability of death must refer to a specified time interval, such as the next 5 years. For other outcomes, there is the additional problem of arriving at a precise and useful definition of the event itself. The probability of developing coronary heart disease will be different depending on how its presence or absence is defined. Minimal evidence, as defined by small abnormalities on coronary angiogram versus a 50% occlusion, will result in a higher probability. The definition chosen needs to be precise and clinically relevant.

The same examples also illustrate three different clinical purposes for which estimates of probability are useful: risk evaluation, diagnosis, and prognosis. Given individual circumstances of age, sex, life style, occupation, etc., *risk evaluation* considers the probability that an apparently healthy person will develop certain disease states within specified intervals of future time. Given individual circumstances, together with the results of diagnostic maneuvers and tests, *diagnosis* considers the probability that an individual currently has a specified disease. Given the same set of circumstances (age, sex, etc.) and a specified disease state, *prognosis* addresses the question of the probability of important clinical events in the future. Diagnosis is discussed in Chapter 19; evaluation of risk and prognosis is the focus of this chapter.

The characteristics, called "factors," that appear to affect risk and prognosis fall into three groups: modifiable determinants, nonmodifiable determinants, and markers. Determinants of risk and prognosis are the factors that are causally related to the outcome or event of interest. Serum cholesterol is believed to be causally related to risk of subsequent coronary artery disease and is therefore called a determinant. Serum cholesterol, smoking, and blood pressure are modifiable determinants of coronary heart disease risk, whereas age and family history are nonmodifiable determinants. Markers are associated with increased or decreased risk, or better or worse prognosis, but are not causally related. The association seen in North America between alcohol consumption and increased risk of lung cancer is believed to be due, not to alcohol being a cause of lung cancer, but to the strong association between alcohol consumption and cigarette smoking. Individuals who consume more alcohol tend, on average, to smoke more cigarettes; modifying their alcohol consumption without changing their smoking behavior would not change their risk of lung cancer. Accordingly, alcohol is a marker of risk, not a determinant.

Why Study Risk and Prognosis?

We study risk and prognosis to obtain estimates of the probability of occurrence of important health related events. A patient with coronary artery disease may need to choose medical management or coronary bypass surgery; the probability of survival for various time periods, for each option, is a factor that should enter into the decision. If the probabilities are uniformly better with one strategy, and other factors such as pain are similar, the rational choice is the alternative with the higher probability of survival.

Life is rarely so simple; the survival may be better with medical management over the short term (weeks to months) but better with surgical management over the longer term; the side effects may be quite different and difficult to compare. Decision analysis is a formal method for weighing all the options and choosing the one of greatest benefit, but the details of the calculations are beyond the scope of this chapter. The crucial point is that the probabilities of such important events as death or recurrence of disease are fundamental to making informed decisions in the context of formal decision analysis and in routine clinical practice. The example that we have chosen relates to prognosis, but the principle is equally valid in risk evaluation.

Measures of Risk and Prognosis

Suppose we are following a homogeneous population—that is, a population in which the major determinants of the outcome of interest are approximately the same for all its members—for a particular outcome, over time. The outcome of interest, generally called the "critical event," might be recurrence of breast cancer, myocardial infarction, postoperative pulmonary embolism, or death. Probabilities are estimated by taking the observed *proportion* that experiences the critical event.

For example, consider a sample of 2000 patients for whom the critical event is deep vein thrombosis (DVT) in the postoperative period after total hip replacement. Half were treated with prophylactic heparin; half were not. Table 18.1 presents the hypothetical results from such a study. The columns labeled "Events" show the number of critical events on each successive day in the untreated and treated groups respectively. Because 16 patients in the untreated group developed DVT *on day 5*, our estimate of the single day probability is 16/1000 (i.e., 0.016 or 1.6%). These daily probabilities have been plotted as a histogram in Figure 18.1. Because 40 patients in the untreated group developed DVT *by day 5*, our estimate of the cumulative probability at day 5 is 40/1000 (i.e., 0.040 or 4.0%). These cumulative probabilities have been plotted in Figure 18.2.

Even with the large hypothetical sample of 2000 individuals, the estimated daily probabilities exhibit considerable fluctuation (Fig. 18.1). The cumulative probabilities are more stable, and it is often preferable to present the data in this form. The complement of the cumulative probability (1 − the cumulative probability) plotted over time, called the *survival curve*, is a commonly presented summary of the data. It represents the probability of reaching a given point in time without experiencing the critical event.

An important distinction should be made concerning the probability of events. The probability, faced at the outset by all persons in the untreated group, of suffering a critical event precisely on day 12 (10/1000, or 1.0%), is not quite the same as that faced on day 12 by those who begin day 12 without having developed a DVT. To calculate the latter probability, we remove from the denominator individuals who developed a DVT on days 1 through 11 and obtain a probability of 10/866 or 1.2%. In epidemiology this is called a *rate*—a special kind of proportion calculated by including in the denominator only people who are truly at risk at the beginning of the interval in question. Since the rate also depends on the length of the time

TABLE 18.1. Hypothetical data regarding occurrences of deep vein thrombosis in the first 21 days following hip surgery in 1000 patients treated with heparin and 1000 patients not treated.

	Untreated				Treated				
Day	Events	Prob. (%)	*N*	Rate (%)	Events	Prob. (%)	*N*	Rate (%)	Relative rate (rate ratio)
1	1	0.1	1000	0.10	1	0.1	1000	0.10	1.00
2	7	0.7	999	0.70	1	0.1	999	0.10	0.14
3	9	0.9	992	0.91	3	0.3	998	0.30	0.33
4	7	0.7	983	0.71	6	0.6	995	0.60	0.85
5	16	1.6	976	1.64	2	0.2	989	0.20	0.12
6	19	1.9	960	1.98	7	0.7	987	0.71	0.36
7	22	2.2	941	2.34	3	0.3	980	0.31	0.13
8	16	1.6	919	1.74	5	0.5	977	0.51	0.29
9	13	1.3	903	1.44	2	0.2	972	0.21	0.14
10	11	1.1	890	1.24	3	0.3	970	0.31	0.25
11	13	1.3	879	1.48	3	0.3	967	0.31	0.21
12	10	1.0	866	1.15	4	0.4	964	0.41	0.36
13	3	0.3	856	0.35	1	0.1	960	0.10	0.30
14	6	0.6	853	0.70	0	0.0	959	0.00	0.00
15	7	0.7	847	0.83	2	0.2	959	0.21	0.25
16	3	0.3	840	0.36	2	0.2	957	0.21	0.59
17	2	0.2	837	0.24	0	0.0	955	0.00	0.00
18	4	0.4	835	0.48	2	0.2	955	0.21	0.44
19	1	0.1	831	0.12	0	0.0	953	0.00	0.00
20	1	0.1	830	0.12	0	0.0	953	0.00	0.00
21	1	0.1	829	0.12	0	0.0	953	0.00	0.00

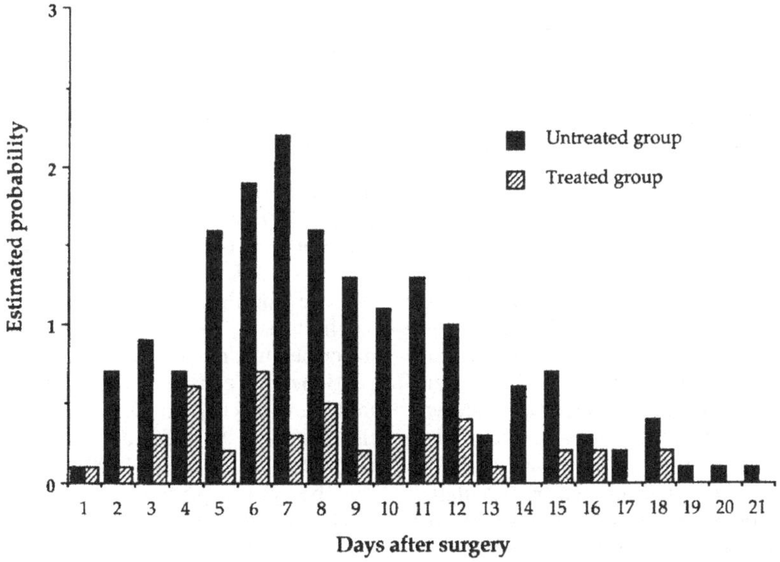

FIGURE 18.1. The daily probability of developing deep vein thrombosis in the postoperative period in treated versus untreated groups.

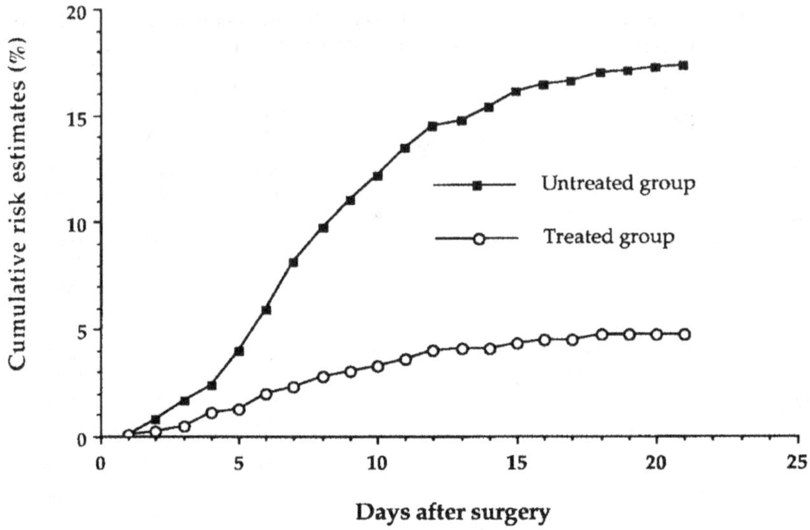

FIGURE 18.2. The cumulative risk estimate of developing deep vein thrombosis in the postoperative period in treated versus untreated groups.

interval, it is customary to recognize this explicitly by expressing the rate in units:

(number of critical events) per (number of persons at risk) per (unit of time)

or

(number of events) per (person-unit of time at risk) In our example, the denominator would be person-days at risk.

The rate is a more accurate measure of risk than the proportion, considered previously. However, there is an unfortunate confusion in terminology. To some, "risk" corresponds to the cumulative probability plotted in Figure 18.2. When there is a possibility of confusion, the unambiguous term "*hazard*" is used. It is the probability of an individual experiencing an event in a short time interval, given that the event has not already occurred to that individual before the start of the interval. The hazard for an interval is estimated by calculating the observed rate for that interval. In keeping with common usage, we will use "risk" both for the cumulative probability and for the hazard.

The next step is to compare risk or prognosis in the treated and untreated groups, but *remember that the data are hypothetical* and are presented solely to illustrate the concepts under discussion. From inspection of the data, it seems clear that the risk of DVT is reduced with heparin prophylaxis. This is most apparent in the cumulative risk estimates, which illustrates their usefulness in this type of comparison. How do we quantify the difference in prognosis in the two populations? How do we rule out the possibility that the observed difference is simply due to chance?

The simplest approach is to look at the final results of the whole 3-week period of follow-up (i.e., the risk of DVT with heparin is 47/1000 or 4.7%; without it, 172/1000 or 17.2%). We then calculate the ratio of the two risk estimates—4.7/17.2, or 0.27—called the *relative risk*. This means the risk with heparin is only 0.27 of the risk without it; or inversely, the risk without heparin is 1/0.27 or 3.7 times higher than with it. To rule out the possibility that the observed difference might have arisen by chance, we use the methods described in Chapter 15. To compare the two proportions, we construct the corresponding 2 × 2 table, and calculate a χ^2 statistic and a p value. In this instance, $\chi^2 = 82$, and $p < .001$. (i.e., there is less than 1 chance in 1000 that a relative risk of the observed magnitude would occur by chance).

The relative risk has become the most commonly used measure for comparing two risks, but others are available. One is *excess risk*—the arithmetic difference between the two risks. In our example, the excess risk in those not given heparin, compared to those receiving it, is 17.2% − 4.7% = 12.5%. This may be interpreted as the net risk of DVT attributable to failure to treat with heparin. The excess risk is sometimes called the *attributable risk*, but this term is used for several different

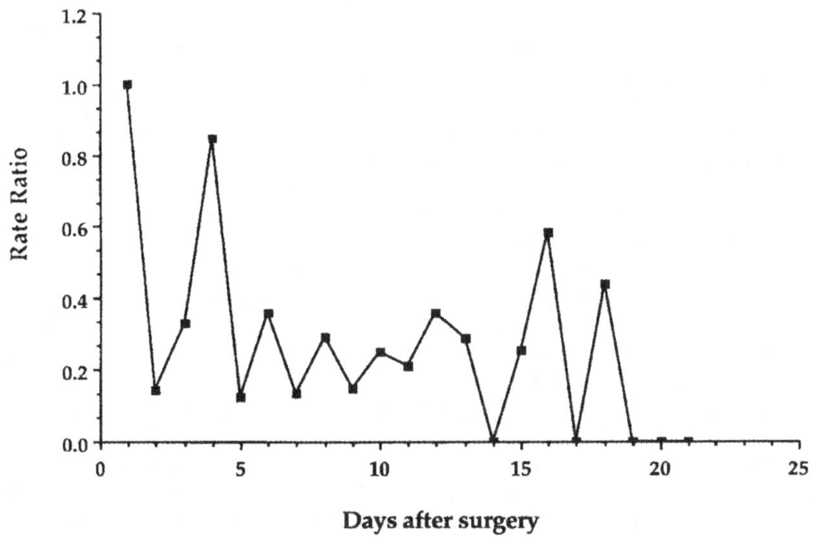

FIGURE 18.3. The rate ratio of developing deep vein thrombosis in the postoperative period in treated versus untreated groups.

measures and is best avoided. Another measure is the *attributable proportion exposed*—the excess risk divided by the risk in the higher risk group. It is interpreted as the proportion or fraction of the risk that is avoidable by treatment, or attributable to nontreatment. In our example, it is 12.5%/17.2% = 72.7%; that is, about 73% of the risk could be avoided by treatment with heparin. The attributable proportion exposed is sometimes also called the attributable risk.

Using the relative risk for the whole follow-up period as the summary measure to compare prognosis in the two groups is problematic in that the calculation is based only on the final cumulative counts of events and ignores everything that happened in between. It focuses on the cumulative probability, but rates are better measures of risk. Another approach is to calculate the *relative rate* or *rate ratio*, the ratio of the rates for the two groups for each successive time interval (one day in our example). These rate ratios are plotted in Figure 18.3. Because the number of events entering into the calculations for each time interval is quite small, rate ratios exhibit considerable instability, as shown in the figure. This can be circumvented by assuming that, aside from random fluctuation, there is really a constant underlying value known as the *relative rate*. This premise about a constant underlying relative rate is a viable assumption under many circumstances, and is called the *proportional hazards* assumption. It allows one to summarize the relative rates over time with a single number, the summary relative rate.

Calculation of the summary relative rate from the individual time interval data will not be detailed here. One approach to it, the Mantel–Haenszel technique, produces a summary relative rate and a χ^2 test of whether it is significantly different, statistically, from 1. For our data on DVT, the summary relative hazard is 0.25, and the corresponding χ^2 is 80 (again $p < .001$). A summary relative hazard of 0.25 suggests that, on average, the heparin group experienced a risk of DVT about 25% of that of the nonheparin group. In this instance, the summary relative rate of 0.25 and the relative risk of 0.27 (i.e., the ratio of the cumulative risks) are almost identical. This will generally be true if the cumulative risk over the whole follow-up period is fairly small; in our example, it is 17.2% in the higher risk group. If the cumulative risk over the follow-up period is large, say 50%, the two methods will usually produce quite different estimates, with the cumulative probability method producing estimates that are biased toward 1.

Incomplete follow-up is an important issue in studies that involve monitoring participants over time. Participants may withdraw, become inaccessible by moving away, or cease to be at risk for the critical event because of death or some other intercurrent event. In many studies, recruitment is staggered over time, and participants may be at various uncompleted stages of follow-up when the study terminates. Any individual who does not undergo the critical event and is not followed for the maximal period is said to be *censored*. Censoring, for one or another of the reasons above, often affects a considerable fraction of the study participants. Because simply dropping them from the analysis would waste a great deal of useful data, the method of Kaplan and Meier and actuarial life table methods have been developed for estimating survival curves from incomplete data.

The essential approach in such methods is the inclusion of all individuals followed for any length of time up to the point of being censored; after that, they are no longer considered to be at risk and this fact is reflected in the rate calculation. In the DVT example, suppose that on the 10th day, 10 subjects in the untreated group developed DVT, another 3 died of cardiac arrest, and 2 others were transferred to another facility and lost to follow-up. All 15 would be considered to be no longer at risk for DVT after day 10 and would be removed from the rate calculations beyond that point.

In using these techniques of survival analysis, we must make the assumption that loss to follow-up occurs at random or, at least, is not confounded with the relationship of primary interest (e.g., the relationship between deep vein thrombosis and heparin therapy in our example discussed). For further discussion, consult monographs on survival analysis.[2]

Method of Analysis

Under measures of risk and prognosis, we discussed methods of analysis in the somewhat idealized circumstances of comparing two homogeneous groups followed over time, where the proportional hazards assumption is valid. We now turn to more realistic situations, in which the sample being followed is heterogeneous with respect to such important prognostic variables as age and sex—the situation of greatest interest to clinicians, who naturally wish to tailor their risk and prognosis statements to the circumstances of an individual patient.

One method is to divide the sample into homogeneous subgroups and carry out a separate analysis for each. The problem with this approach is that, unless the original sample is very large, the subsamples become so small that meaningful conclusions cannot be drawn and random fluctuation will completely obscure the effects of interest. Nevertheless, when the sample is large enough, separate analysis of each subgroup is a viable approach and has the advantage of not relying on any assumptions about the relationship among the subgroups. An illustration of this approach is provided in Chapter 29, Figure 29.2 where the survival of various treatment and age subgroups following therapy for breast cancer is shown.

When the total sample is not large enough to support separate subgroup analyses, a regression model can be used. This type of analysis, in contrast to independent analysis of each subgroup, depends on making an assumption that the way in which risk or prognosis varies across subgroups can be described by fairly simple mathematical equations. Suppose the subgroups of interest are defined by age. We might assume that the logarithm of the risk is directly proportional to the age, at least over the range of ages that are of practical importance in a particular context. Such an assumption allows the experience of individuals with different ages to be combined in one analysis.

Now suppose that, in our hypothetical DVT study, the treated and untreated groups were not similar with respect to age and that age is a determinant of risk of DVT. A straightforward comparison of the risk of DVT between the groups would not be fair if it did not take account of age differences. Two regression models are presented, one corresponds to the cumulative risk approach and the other to the rate approach.

If the focus is on cumulative risk, logistic regression is the appropriate model. It takes the form:

$$\log\left(\frac{p}{1-p}\right) = b_0 + b_1 \times (\text{age} - \text{age}_0) + b_2 \times (rx)$$

where p is the cumulative risk (or probability) of DVT over the whole follow-up period; "age" is the age in years; age_0 is a constant reference age, such as the mean age of all subjects; and rx is 1 for those on heparin and 0 for those not on heparin. The coefficients b_0, b_1 and b_2 are unknown quantities (parameters), which are estimated from the actual follow-up data. The detailed method of estimating the parameters from the data will not be addressed here except to say that the method most commonly used is called the "maximum likelihood" method and is available in a variety of statistical software packages. The primary interest in this model is the estimated value of b_2. It turns out that $\exp(b_2)$, the exponential of b_2, is an estimate of the relative risk of DVT in those treated with heparin compared to those not treated. By including the term "$b_1 \times (\text{age} - \text{age}_0)$" in the model, we have managed to compensate for the age differences in the sample. The estimate of the relative risk obtained is, in a sense, an average over all age groups and is said to be adjusted for age. It should be noted that the equation above explicitly assumes a linear relationship between age and the quantity $\log\left(\frac{p}{1-p}\right)$, called the "logit" of the risk. Although this is unlikely to be exactly true, it may be approximately true in the range of ages in the sample. Using this equation to calculate the risk for a new individual is acceptable, if his or her age falls in the same range. The equation should not be used to extrapolate to ages outside the range represented in the sample data.

If the focus is on rates, the appropriate regression model is called Cox regression. The model takes the form:

$$\log(\theta) = b_1 \times (\text{age} - \text{age}_0) + b_2 \times (rx)$$

where "θ" is the summary relative rate (hazard) for an individual, compared to someone of reference age not on heparin treatment. The similarity to the logistic equation is evident. There is no b_0 term but, otherwise, the coefficients have a similar interpretation. Again $\exp(b_2)$ is the summary relative rate adjusted for the differences in age. There is an explicit assumption that the logarithm of the relative rate varies linearly with age and, as above, this is often a reasonable assumption for the range of ages in the sample. There is also an assumption that the relative rate is constant over time—the same "proportional hazards" assumption mentioned when the summary relative rate was defined, earlier. Cox regression is also able to cope with censored data.

There are many sophisticated elaborations of the logistic regression and Cox regression models, including incorporation of additional terms to allow adjustment for individual characteristics, such as sex or socioeconomic status, possible interactions among factors, and (in the Cox model) variation of the relative hazard over time.

Methodological Issues

Knowing what will likely happen to our patients with given conditions, or after certain operative procedures, is fundamental to sound clinical decision making, but we must depend on observations from past studies to guide us now, and we must hope that the estimates of what will happen are valid *and* applicable to our own patients.

Earlier, we discussed some fundamental concepts associated with the natural history of disease and presented methods of calculating various measures of risk. We now turn to methodological issues associated with studies of prognosis, basing our discussion on the framework used in Chapter 10, "Critical Appraisal of Published Research": WHY, WHO and WHEN, WHAT, HOW and HOW MANY.

WHY: Clarifying the Purpose

Whenever you are assessing a natural history study, begin with an evaluation of the investigator's stated purpose. Studies that state hypotheses in advance are more reliable than studies that pursue hypotheses after the fact; and studies investigating a single prespecified endpoint are more credible than studies investigating many outcomes, as dictated by the data. In a natural history study, if you follow a group of people and assess them for a multitude of outcomes, there is a strong probability that one or more of the outcomes will be statistically high (or low) by chance. This is analogous to the conduct of multiple comparisons between the treatment and control groups in clinical trials. In the context of natural history studies, it might be termed the "multiple-outcomes problem."

Studies that test hypotheses after the fact are more likely to use retrospective methods. Be extra vigilant when a prognosis study is conducted retrospectively, that is, when historical data are used to assess outcomes in a population. Such studies can be carried out retrospectively in a valid fashion, but they are made much more difficult by the many pitfalls confronted when groups of patients are assembled retrospectively for follow-up studies.

WHO and WHEN: Assembling the Cohort

Ideally, the way to study prognosis is to assemble a group of individuals who share common features and observe what happens to them over time; such a group is usually called a "cohort" (Chapter 13). Assembling an appropriate cohort is undoubtedly the most critical step in this type of research. Failure to negotiate this step successfully can doom the study to producing hopelessly biased results that will be useless or, even worse, seriously misleading.

WHO and WHEN remind you of the need to consider the precise nature of the cohort being studied. Who, exactly, is being investigated? When, in the natural history of their condition, have they been sampled? The general principle is that you should assemble a cohort consisting of a *representative* spectrum of people with the condition in question who are at a *homogeneous* and *early* point in its natural history.

The representativeness of the cohort will ultimately determine how generalizable the results will be. The important factors affecting representativeness include the type of patients in the catchment area of the study, the nature of the settings in which the patients are sampled (e.g., primary, secondary, or tertiary), and the mechanisms of presentation or referral that bring the patients into the sampling frame. If, in a study of outcomes in ulcerative colitis, a cohort is assembled by reviewing charts and collecting all people admitted to a given hospital with a diagnosis of ulcerative colitis during a specified period, several sampling biases could be at work to make the cohort nonrepresentative. First, only cases severe enough to require hospital admission are being sampled; individuals with milder disease, managed within their communities, are not adequately represented in the cohort. This biases the results toward worse outcomes. Second, the hospital's referral pattern could play a role: a tertiary care center may admit only the most difficult or intractable cases—another bias toward poor outcomes (unless the study's intent is to examine the natural history of ulcerative colitis in hospitalized tertiary care patients).

The simple way to avoid any bias is to set the sampling frame to target the patient population the study intends to investigate. If the aim is to study the entire spectrum of patients with a given condition, it might sample newly diagnosed patients with the condition at all primary care settings, emergency rooms, and hospitals in a given catchment area. If the intention is to study only hospitalized patients, the sample can be restricted to all hospitals in the catchment area.

How the sample is constructed may seem esoteric to some, who may also consider it an unlikely source of appreciable empirical differences. The importance of the sampling frame has been vividly demonstrated, however, in studies investigating whether children with febrile seizures have an increased risk of recurrent nonfebrile seizures in later life. Ellenberg and Nelson[3] (1980) showed that studies in which children were sampled from hospital clinics and tertiary referral units provided estimates of recurrence ranging as high as 76.9%, whereas all studies that sampled children through primary care settings and in the general population found recurrence rates under 5%.

All persons in a cohort under study *must* be homogeneous with respect to where they are in the natural history of their illness. The need for uniformity can best be appreciated by considering what would arise in its absence. What meaning could be derived from the 5-year mortality rate observed in a group of patients who have had bowel cancer for as little as 1 or 2 years, or as long as 15 or 20 years? To whom could such a mortality rate be validly generalized? On the other hand, the 5-year mortality rate observed in a group of people, whose diagnoses of bowel cancer had all been made within the prior year, could be reasonably applied to anyone at the same stage of the illness. To repeat, homogeneity gives the measurement of time internal consistency within the cohort and makes the cohort's experience generalizable to others at the same point in the natural history of a disease. Without such uniformity, the observed incidence rates are not reliable and are simply a function of the relative proportions of the various stages of illness that happen to fall within the cohort in question.

It is equally important that all persons in the cohort be observed onward from an early point in the natural history of the illness. The are two reasons for this. First, early observation allows for a characterization of the entire natural history of the illness. Second, and more importantly, it avoids potential biases associated with assembling cohorts at later points in time.

Consider a study of the subsequent rate of stroke in patients with hypertension. Suppose all patients currently under treatment for hypertension at a few primary care clinics, and who have not had stroke, are identified and followed forward in time. This sample includes patients who have been treated for hypertension for many years and are still under treatment. This is known as a prevalent cohort, because it includes prevalent cases (i.e., all existing cases at a particular point in time). To appreciate the potential biases, fully, consider those not captured in this sample. First, it will tend to miss the patients who were at highest risk and had a stroke soon after developing hypertension. As a consequence, the sample will overrepresent "survivors" who may be more "stroke-resistant"—the study would then underestimate the true risk of stroke. It will also tend to exclude those with very mild hypertension that responded to diet, weight loss and/or exercise (i.e., essentially was cured by the time of the sampling). Thus, the sample will overrepresent persons with more severe hypertension who require long-term treatment and will lead to an overestimation of the risk of stroke. Both examples illustrate what might be termed "migration bias".

Migration bias occurs when cohorts are assembled later in the natural history of a disease, because doing so raises the possibility that some members have migrated from the cohort as a result of early ill effects or early cure. Although we might argue that these effects work in opposite directions and might cancel each other, it would depend on the relative weights of the two forms of migration. Using an incident cohort of individuals assembled at an early and uniform point in the natural history of an illness is much preferable to relying on chance.

There are usually several points in the natural history of a disease from which to choose an inception point for a cohort. For studying the natural history of an illness, two obvious inception points are the time of onset of symptoms and the time of first diagnosis; each has advantages and disadvantages. Time of onset of symptoms is more closely related to the true biologic onset of the illness, but it may not be reliably documented and cannot be truly validated. Establishing the inception point for a person with ulcerative colitis may be impossible: How can we tell whether an episode of abdominal pain and diarrhea 5 years prior to diagnosis was truly the first episode of the illness or simply a transient infectious gastroenteritis? In contrast, time of first diagnosis is usually well documented on medical charts and accompanied by confirmatory diagnostic evidence, but diagnosis may be separated from the biologic and clinical onset of the illness by varying amounts of time attributable to delays in seeking medical help, or to differences in access to diagnostic facilities.

To study prognosis following a particular surgical procedure, the time of operation is an obvious choice for the inception point of a cohort. The sampling required to obtain such a cohort *must* be carried out in a way that ensures that all persons undergoing the procedure are represented; any form of sampling at a later postoperative point would be subject to bias because those with perioperative or early postoperative events could be missed. It may surprise you to learn that the time of surgery is not necessarily the best inception point for a prognosis study of a surgical intervention. Consider a study of prognosis in cardiac transplantation patients. If we were to assemble a cohort of patients at the time of surgery, only those who survived long enough for a donor to be found would be captured; those with very severe disease who died waiting for a donor would be missed. If we wish to study the policy of attempting to perform a transplant rather than the surgery itself, outcomes during the preoperative waiting period ought to be included and attributed to the policy of attempting to perform a transplant. A preferable inception point might, therefore, be the point at which the patient is deemed eligible for transplant and is entered on the waiting list. Although not perfect, this inception point is much more uniform than the date of surgery, which is influenced by the availability of donors and applicable only to those who survive to undergo the procedure. Use of this inception point converts the study into an investigation of the natural history of what might be termed "transplant-eligible end-stage cardiac disease."

Sometimes, it is possible to choose an inception point that is too early in the natural history of the disease. Consider a study of prognosis in women with breast cancer. For convenience, it is tempting to assemble a cohort of all women detected as having breast cancer at an initial visit to a mammography screening program. Although the results of such a study will be generalizable to all women with similarly detected cancers, they will not be applicable to the vast majority of women whose cancers are detected clinically in the community.

The fundamental goal of screening is to enhance the benefit of therapy by implementing it at an earlier stage in the natural history. Even if screening had no beneficial effect on outcome, however, the experience of the screen-detected cohort will not be generalizable to community-detected populations. First, earlier detection will automatically lengthen survival following detection, but this longer survival accrues to the length of time patients carry the diagnosis, not to their life spans—an effect known as "lead time bias." Second, a more subtle effect stems from the fact that the cancers that are most amenable to detection at an initial screening visit have the longest detectable phase prior to clinical detection and tend to be the slowest growing. Accordingly, the prognosis for women detected as having breast cancer at an initial screening visit will appear to be more favorable than for women diagnosed in the community because slower growing, less fulminant cancers will have been overrepresented in our cohort sample. This effect is known as "length bias." An inception point that is too early—as would occur with screen detection—may yield results that are not generalizable to the illness as it is customarily diagnosed.

WHAT: Defining the Endpoints

This criterion reminds the reader to consider precisely what endpoint is being studied. Outcomes *must* be so clearly defined that the reader of a report will know exactly what was being measured and what must be measured to reproduce the study. This principle applies no less to a study of prognosis than to any other type of biomedical investigation. Even when the outcome is as unambiguous as death, there may be problems if the analysis depends on distinguishing differences in its etiology (e.g., cardiovascular vs. cerebrovascular); death certificates are notoriously unreliable for such purposes. The need for clear criteria is even more marked when the endpoint is less incontrovertible than death. A study of prognosis following femoral–popliteal bypass grafting that uses loss of graft patency as its endpoint will need a precise definition of this outcome.

HOW: Monitoring for the Endpoints

Once a clear definition of the endpoint has been identified, you should consider how occurrences of the endpoint were monitored. In general, surveillance for the endpoint of interest, in a natural history study, should be carried out in a uniform fashion and should be performed, when possible, by individuals who are blind to the prior history or relevant risk factors in the study.

When surveillance is not carried out in a uniform fashion, surveillance bias (so-called) is possible. Consider a prognosis study following a particular operative procedure in which a cohort of patients is assembled and monitored. In the perioperative period, patients are classified as being high and low in risk on the basis of a profile of associated risk factors; high-risk patients are subsequently followed at a specialized clinic. Clinically, it is an excellent idea to provide specialized follow-up for the high-risk patients, but it will likely bias the results in terms of prognosis; the high-risk individuals will likely receive closer scrutiny, more frequent evaluation, and earlier and more frequent diagnostic tests.

The net effect of this differential intensity in follow-up is that events may be uncovered more frequently or, at the least, endpoints may be detected earlier in the closely followed group. In either case, the incidence of later endpoint events may be artifactually elevated as a result of this surveillance bias. Even in the absence of a specialized clinic, if those who are conducting the follow-up are aware of the risk status, it may influence them to scrutinize the high-risk persons more carefully for the outcome (i.e, a diagnostic suspicion bias). Similarly, when ambiguous events occur or uncertain diagnostic test results are present, knowledge of the prior status may influence interpretation of the diagnostic test or categorization of the event (i.e., an expectation bias). All these effects can be minimized if (a) the follow-up is conducted in a uniform fashion that simulates routine clinical follow-up in intensity, and (b) interpretations are made by individuals who are blind to the particular risk status of patients.

HOW MANY: Completeness of Follow-up and Methods of Analysis

The final criterion, HOW MANY, alerts you to some of the quantitative issues surrounding natural history studies. How many of the subjects were followed completely and how many were lost to follow-up are crucial questions. We have already discussed the methods of analysis that are applicable when there is incomplete follow-up; they usually "censor" the data on any individuals who are lost to follow-up at the time of their last known status; that is, they are not considered to be at risk beyond that point. Although this assumption helps to provide more precise estimates of the incidence of outcome events and maximizes use of the information gained in the study, the estimates will be unbiased only if similar subsequent courses are experienced by those who were lost to follow-up and those who were followed completely. Our knowledge of prognosis in persons who volunteer for studies and in those who comply with study protocols suggests that this is unlikely to be true.

There are several strategies for dealing with this problem. If the proportion of persons lost to follow-up is small, a bias that will seriously distort the estimates is unlikely; if it is not, you can try to gauge how different the persons lost to follow-up are from those who were not lost. If you have baseline demographic information and data on prognostic factors, and you can show that they are similar for those followed and those lost, you have some circumstantial evidence that the bias may not be very severe.

Another strategy is to explore the boundaries of the potential bias by assuming the best and worst possible outcomes in those who were lost—sometimes referred to as best- and worst-case scenarios, respectively. Suppose that, in a 10-year follow-up study of mortality in persons subjected to a particular surgical procedure, approximately 20% of the cohort was lost prior to completion of the study; whether they lived or died beyond the last point of contact with them is not known. Conventional methods of survival analysis, which censor such persons at the last point of contact, provide unbiased estimates *if* these persons have a subsequent mortality experience similar to that of those who were followed completely. Now consider the two possible extremes. The worst-case assumption is that every person who was lost to follow-up died just after the point of last contact; survival analysis using this assumption will provide a maximum estimate of mortality for the cohort in the worst-case scenario. The other extreme is to assume that every person lost to follow-up survived the entire study period; survival analysis using this assumption will provide a minimum estimate of mortality in the best case scenario. The truth will likely be somewhere in between.

If the extremes lie in a particular direction, they may help to strengthen your conclusion. If the observed mortality in the 10-year mortality study following the surgery remains low, even in the worst case scenario, you can remain relatively confident it is low despite the incomplete follow-up. Conversely, if the observed mortality remains high, even in the best-case scenario, you can remain confident that in the conclusion that mortality is high.

In studies of prognosis in which analytic comparisons are being made, you should ensure that issues of statistical significance are addressed satisfactorily. Suppose a study reports the 5-year survival probabilities of a certain class of heart disease patients are 50% and 60% with medical management and surgical management, respectively. Because these are estimates from a finite data set, they are subject to random error. Could such an observed difference in prognosis easily arise by chance alone, or is there a real difference? The statistical methods provide a p value, which may be interpreted as the chance that a difference of the observed magnitude could have arisen by chance alone (i.e., the "null" hypothesis of no true difference). Confidence intervals around probabilities should be provided, to permit an appreciation of the range of values compatible with the data.

When a prognosis study reports a statistically significant difference in outcomes between two cohorts, the canny reader will immediately question whether it is clinically significant. Clinically trivial differences in the probabilities of critical events can be statistically significant when large cohorts are involved. Conversely, when a study finds no statistically significant difference in the probability of certain outcomes between cohorts, the reader should immediately ask whether the cohorts were large enough to provide adequate power for important differences to have been detected. When a difference in prognosis is found, it may have arisen because of other differences between the two groups. Inequalities in socioeconomic status or in severity of disease are almost certain to be present if random allocation to the two groups was not used. Statistical methods are available to allow the prognosis associated with the method of management to be separated from, or adjusted for, other differences between two groups, if the other factors influencing risk or prognosis are known and have been accurately measured. Nevertheless, the possibility remains that an unrecognized factor is present, or a recognized factor is being poorly measured ("misclassified"). The only convincing way to deal with this possibility is to perform a randomized controlled trial, in which the random allocation is expected to apportion unrecognized factors about equally between the two groups.

Summary

Evaluation of risk and prognosis involve estimating the probability of future events, given present circumstances. Risk evaluation refers specifically to the probability of future disease or injury in apparently healthy individuals; prognosis refers to the probability of future health-related events in individuals who already have a disease or injury. The term "risk" is also generally used in both contexts. To estimate risk in simple situations, proportions and rates are used. To compare risk between two groups, relative risk and the summary relative rate are available. A useful graphic technique is to present a survival curve for the study sample, or a set of survival curves for different subgroups. Statistical hypothesis testing can be carried out using the ordinary χ^2 test for a 2×2 table, or the more sophisticated Mantel–Haenszel summary χ^2 statistic.

For more complex situations, in which the populations being compared are not homogeneous, logistic regression and Cox regression are used. Censoring (loss to follow-up) is a commonly encountered complication. The survival curve can be estimated in this situation by the Kaplan–Meier method, and the summary relative rate, adjusted for confounding factors, by Cox regression.

A methodological framework has been provided for assessing the quality of an article reporting a study of prognosis (or for planning such a study). WHY reminds the reader to begin, *always*, with an evaluation of the investigator's stated purpose. In general, studies that state hypotheses in advance are more reliable than studies that pursue hypotheses after the fact, and studies that investigate a single prespecified endpoint are more credible than studies that investigate many outcomes, as dictated by the data. WHO and WHEN remind the reader that, in a natural history study, it is crucial to consider the precise nature of the cohort being studied. Who, exactly, is being investigated, and when in the natural history have these subjects been sampled? The general principle is that a cohort ought to assemble a *representative* spectrum of people with a particular condition who are at a *homogeneous* and *early* point in its natural history. Failure to construct such an inception or incident cohort can bias a study beyond repair.

WHAT reminds the reader to consider precisely what endpoint is being studied. The primary outcomes must be clearly defined so that the reader will know exactly what is being measured. The HOW criterion pertains to how occurrences of the endpoint were monitored. Surveillance for the endpoint of interest in a natural history study should be carried out in a uniform fashion and should be performed, whenever possible, by individuals who are blind to the prior history or relevant risk factors in the study. Failure to perform uniform and blinded surveillance should alert the reader to the possibilities of surveillance bias, diagnostic suspicion bias and expectation bias.

The final criterion, HOW MANY, is meant to alert the reader to some of the quantitative issues surrounding natural history studies. How many subjects were lost to follow-up and how they were handled in the analysis are crucial questions. Techniques of survival analysis can utilize censored observations, but losses to follow-up are assumed to have similar subsequent experiences. Best-and worst-case scenarios can be used to explore the boundaries of any possible bias. Like studies of therapeutic interventions, prognosis studies should explore the statistical significance of important differences, should assess whether statistically significant differences are clinically meaningful, and in the case of negative hypothesis tests, should document adequate power to have detected important differences if they were present.

References

1. Knaus WA. The science of prediction and its implications for clinicians today. Theo Surg 1988;3:93–101.
2. Lee ET. Statistical Methods for Survival Data Analysis. Belmont, CA: Wadsworth, Lifetime Learning Publications, 1980.
3. Ellenberg JH, Nelson KB. Sample selection and the natural history of disease: studies of febrile seizures. JAMA 1980;243:1337–40.

Additional Reading

Beslow NE, Day NE. Statistical Methods in Cancer Research: Vol. II, The Design and Analysis of Cohort Studies. Lyons, France: International Agency for Research on Cancer, 1982.

Buck N, Devlin HB, Lunn JN. Report of a confidential inquiry into perioperative deaths. The Nuffield Provincial Hospitals Trust/Kings Fund, 1988.

Cooper JB, Newbower RS, Long CD, McPeek B: Preventable anesthesia mishaps: a study of human factors. Anesthesiology 1978;49:399.

Ellenberg JH, Nelson KB. Sample selection and the natural history of disease: studies of febrile seizures. JAMA 1980;243:1337–40.

Kleinbaum DG, Kupper LL, Morgenstern H. Epidemiologic Research: Principles and Quantitative Methods. Belmont, CA: Lifetime Publications, 1982.

Knaus WA. The science of prediction and its implications for clinicians today. Theo Surg 1988;3:93–101.

Kramer MS. Clinical Epidemiology and Biostatistics. Berlin: Springer-Verlag, 1988.

Lee ET. Statistical Methods for Survival Data Analysis. Belmont, CA: Lifetime Learning Publications; Wadsworth, 1980.

Lunn JN, Devlin HB: Lessons from the confidential enquiry into perioperative deaths in three NHS regions. Lancet 1987;2(8572), 1384–1386.

McPeek B, Gasko M, Mosteller F. Measuring outcome from anesthesia and operation. Theor Surg 1986;1: 2–9.

Rothman KJ. Modern Epidemiology. Boston: Little, Brown, 1986.

Sackett DL, Haynes RB, Tugwell P. Clinical Epidemiology: A Basic Science for Clinical Medicine. Boston: Little, Brown, 1985.

19

Evaluation of the Diagnostic Process

M.T. Schechter

Yerushalmy's pioneering work[1] on observer variability in the interpretation of chest roentgenograms initiated a still-expanding interest in the evaluation of the diagnostic process. He introduced the terms *sensitivity* and *specificity* as measures of the validity of diagnostic tests, and an entire methodology, including the concept of *predictive value*, has developed in response to the geometric growth in and reliance on diagnostic testing in clinical practice.

Diagnostic Test Validity

Clinicians use diagnostic tests to ascertain whether a disease is present. For example, you can use a gallium scan to test for the presence or absence of an intraabdominal abscess, or mammography to help you determine whether a palpable lump is malignant.

The disease state that a diagnostic test is meant to detect is sometimes referred to as the *target disease*. The *validity* of a diagnostic test refers simply to its ability to register an abnormal result for patients in whom the target disease is present, and a normal result for patients in whom the target disease is absent. An ideal diagnostic test would exhibit both these behaviors; that is, it would register abnormal results only for patients who have the target disease, and normal results only for patients who are free of the target disease. Such a diagnostic test would be perfect in the sense that its results would be perfectly predictive of absence or presence of the target disease. Unfortunately, most diagnostic tests do not perform this well, and a number of concepts and techniques have been developed to gauge just how satisfactorily a given diagnostic test performs.

To judge how well a test performs in detecting a target disease in certain patients, we need some way of determining the truth about the disease's presence or absence in the same patients. To judge the capabilities of the gallium scan in diagnosing intraabdominal abscess, we need to know whether such abscesses are present in a group of patients so that we can compare this information with the results obtained by means of the gallium scan. We could use the findings of laparotomy, and subsequent pathological confirmation of an abscess, as the determinant of the true target disease state. Similarly, we could use the results of laparotomy, as the determinant for the presence of intraperitoneal injury, to assess the performance of peritoneal lavage as a diagnostic maneuver. To assess mammography as a means of detecting malignant breast tumors, we could use pathological examination of the tumor as our determinant. The method used to confirm the presence or absence of the target disease in such determinations is known as the *gold standard*; it should be the best clinical standard currently available.

When surgical exploration and pathological confirmation are part of the usual clinical management, they are obvious choices as gold standards; when they are not, other standards must be used. To determine the validity of fibrinogen leg scanning as a diagnostic test for deep vein thrombosis (DVT), the best clinical standard currently available is venography. Consequently, the results of this radiological procedure are usually used as the gold standard for the presence or absence of DVT. Similarly, to check the validity of such tests as radionuclide angiography in the detection of coronary artery stenoses, where surgical confirmation is available only in the relatively small number of patients who come to bypass surgery, coronary angiography is often used as the gold standard.

Figure 19.1 sets out the structure of a diagnostic test assessment in general terms. In essence, we merely compare the diagnostic test result (abnor-

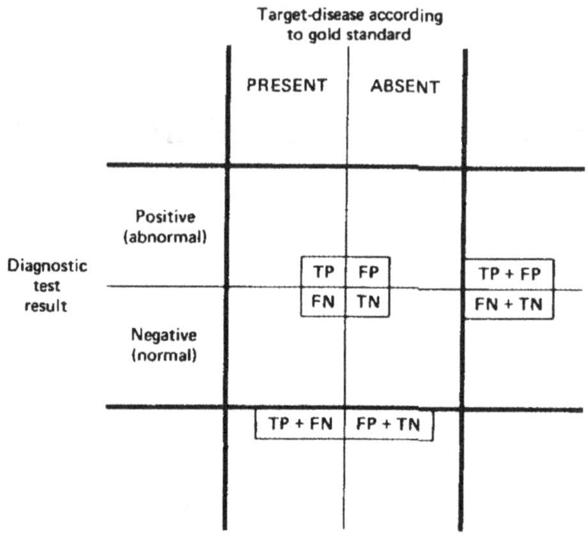

FIGURE 19.1.

mal vs. normal) with the gold standard result for the target disease (present vs absent). By convention, the test result is set out in the rows of a 2 × 2 table, while the gold standard result is displayed in the columns. Adoption of this arbitrary convention will help you to recall some of the definitions we will come to later.

The upper left hand cell displays the number of patients who have the disease, according to the gold standard, and also have positive test results; that is, the test correctly identifies them as having the target disease. Such patients are called *true positives* (TP). The lower right-hand cell displays the number of patients who do not have the disease and have negative test results, the *true negatives* (TN). Taken together, the true positives and true negatives constitute all the patients in whom the diagnostic test is correct. The greater the proportion of patients found in these two groups, the more accurate the diagnostic test.

The patients who fall into the two remaining cells give rise to whatever uncertainty there is. The number in the upper right-hand cell represents the patients who do not have the disease but who have erroneously positive test results. These patients are called *false positives* (FP). The costs of this type of error are the unnecessary further investigations and treatments that might be undertaken and the effects of falsely labeling the patient. The number in the lower left-hand cell represents the patients who have the disease, but erroneously negative test results, *false negatives* (FN). The costs of this type of error are the morbidity and mortality associated with lack of immediate treatment. We have completed the table by adding the rows and columns: TP + FN, FP + TN, TP + FP, FN + TN.

Sensitivity is defined as the proportion of those with the disease who have a positive test result. This is sometimes shortened to "positivity in disease." Sensitivity is a measure of how well the test performs at detecting the disease when it is present. It can be calculated from the first column of the table by the formula:

$$\text{sensitivity} = \frac{TP}{TP + FN}$$

Specificity is defined as the proportion of those who do not have the disease who have negative test results—sometimes referred to as "negativity in health." Specificity is a measure of how well the test performs at registering negative results when the target disease is absent. It can be computed from the second column of the table by the formula:

$$\text{specificity} = \frac{TN}{FP + TN}$$

If you prefer the terminology of conditional probabilities, *sensitivity* is the conditional probability of a positive test given the presence of disease, and *specificity* is the conditional probability of a negative test given the absence of disease. These latter definitions are included only because you may encounter them in the literature.

Let us consider a diagnostic test assessment, adapted from Foti et al.,[2] of a radioimmunoassay serum test for prostatic acid phosphatase (PAP) meant to detect prostatic carcinoma. Foti and his colleagues used 113 patients with prostatic carci-

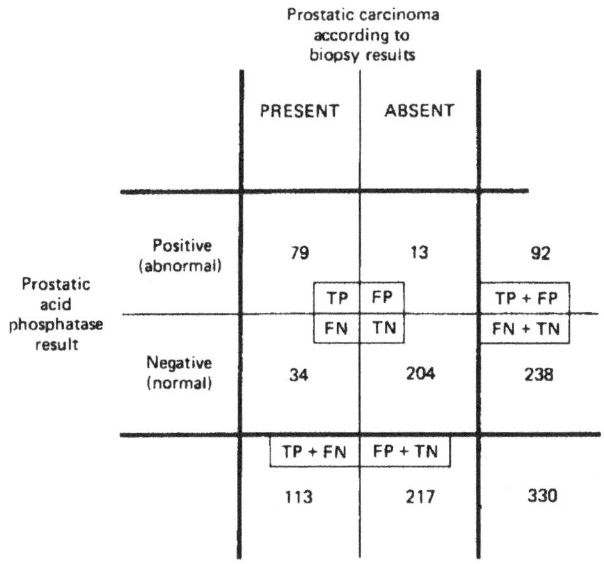

FIGURE 19.2.

noma, confirmed by the gold standard of surgical biopsy, and 217 individuals free of prostatic cancer. The latter group consisted of normal individuals and patients with benign prostatic hyperplasia, previous prostatectomy, gastrointestinal disorders, or nonprostatic cancer. Sera from the 330 individuals were assessed by the assay for the presence of PAP and each specimen was characterized as positive (abnormal) or negative (normal). The results were compared with the true prostatic cancer status of the 330 individuals to produce Figure 19.2.

In the 113 patients with prostatic carcinoma, the PAP test was positive in 79, for *a sensitivity* of 79/113 or 0.70. A *sensitivity* of 0.70 or 70% prompts the inference that, given 100 patients with prostatic carcinoma, the test will detect approximately 70 of them, and miss about 30. The latter figure, derived by subtracting the *sensitivity*, in percent, from 100, is known as the *false negative rate*.

In the 217 patients who did not have prostatic carcinoma, the test was negative in 204, i.e., a *specificity* of 204/217 or 0.94. A *specificity* of 0.94 or 94% suggests that, given 100 patients without prostatic carcinoma, the test will be negative in about 94 of them and falsely positive in the remaining 6. The last figure, obtained by subtracting the specificity, in percent, from 100, is known as the *false positive rate*.

Sensitivity and *specificity* are measures of a diagnostic test's validity; the higher these values are, the better the test is at detecting the presence and absence of disease, respectively. The higher the sensitivity is, the lower the false negative rate is; that is, the lower the chances are of missing the target disease when it is present. The higher the specificity is, the lower the false-positive result when the target disease is absent. The PAP test, with a sensitivity of 70% and a specificity of 94%, exemplifies high specificity with only moderate sensitivity.

Diagnostic Test Utility (Usefulness)

To calculate sensitivity and specificity, you *must* know the true presence or absence of the target disease. This was illustrated earlier by the 113 patients in whom biopsy had already established the actual presence of prostatic carcinoma. In many clinical situations, we do not know whether the target disease is present or absent. If the results of a gold standard were available, there would be no need for another diagnostic test.

In clinical practice, we are often confronted by additional problems when the presence of the target disease is uncertain. First, given that a patient has a positive test result, we need to know what the probability is that the target disease is present—that is, the *positive predictive value* (PPV) of the test. The PPV reflects how certain we may be about the presence of the target disease in patients with a positive test result. Similarly, for patients with negative test results, we need to know the probability that the target disease is absent, the *negative*

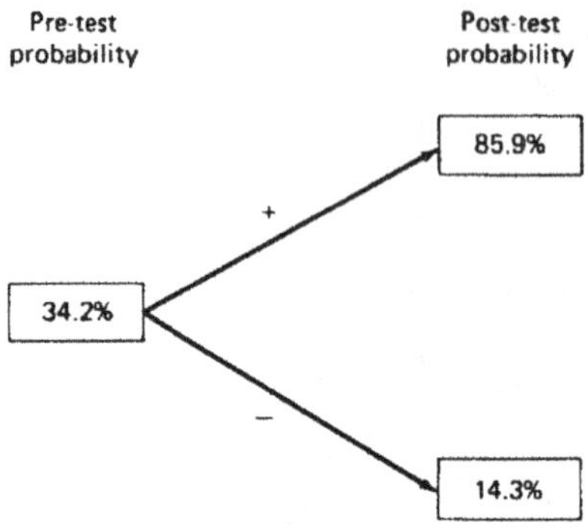

FIGURE 19.3.

predictive value (NPV). The higher the PPV, the better the test is at "ruling in" the disease when the test result is positive; the higher the NPV, the better the test is at "ruling out" the disease when the test result is negative. Whereas sensitivity and specificity measure the test's intrinsic abilities to detect the presence and absence of the target disease, respectively, the predictive values measure the test's utility in clinical practice.

Consider a typical patient drawn at random from the entire group of 330 individuals in the study by Foti and his colleagues (Fig. 19.2). Suppose we do not know whether the individual has prostatic carcinoma, as would be true in clinical practice, and we are going to rely on the PAP assay for the answers. Since 113 of the 330 individuals in the study have prostatic carcinoma, we know there is a probability of 113/330 or 34.2% that our randomly chosen individual has the disease. This measure of the proportion of diseased patients within the total population is known as the *prevalence* and is calculated using the formula:

$$\text{prevalence} = \frac{\text{TP} + \text{FN}}{\text{TP} + \text{FN} + \text{FP} + \text{TN}}$$

The numerator (TP + TN) is the total number of individuals with the disease (i.e., the sum of the cells in the left-hand column of Fig. 19.2); the denominator is the total number of participants (i.e., the sum of all four cells in Fig. 19.2). Since there is a 34.2% chance that our typical patient, drawn at random from the sample, has prostatic cancer prior to undergoing the PAP test, the prevalence is also referred to as the *pretest probability* or *pretest likelihood* of the disease.

Let us now see how well the PAP test performs at predicting the presence or absence of disease in our typical patient by supposing that his test result is positive. Since there are 92 patients with positive test results, of whom 79 actually have prostatic cancer, there is a 79/92 or 85.9% chance that our patient has prostatic carcinoma given a positive test. This is the PPV for this population (Fig. 19.2), that is,

$$\text{PPV} = \frac{\text{TP}}{\text{TP} + \text{FP}}$$

Since the PPV represents the probability of a patient having a given disease when the test result is positive, it is also referred to as the *posttest probability of a positive test* (PTL+). In this case, the PPV (or PTL+) is substantially higher (85.9%) than the pretest probability of 34.2% and the test has performed very well at "ruling in" prostatic carcinoma by markedly increasing the probability of its presence when the test is positive.

Now, suppose the PAP result in our randomly chosen individual is negative. Since there are 238 patients with negative test results, of whom 204 do not have the disease, there is a 204/238 or 85.7% chance that our subject is free of prostatic carcinoma given a negative test. This is the negative predictive value (NPV) for this population (Fig. 19.2), that is,

$$\text{NPV} = \frac{\text{TN}}{\text{FN} + \text{TN}}$$

This NPV of 85.7% represents the probability of not having the disease when the PAP result is negative. If there is an 85.7% chance of not having the disease, there is a 14.3% chance of having it; subtracting the NPV from 100 gives the probability of having the disease even when the test is negative—the *posttest probability of a negative result*. As you might anticipate, the probability of having the disease after a negative test (14.3%) is lower than the pretest probability of disease (34.2%). Consequently, the negative test result has contributed to "ruling out" prostatic carcinoma by decreasing the probability of the presence of the disease from 34.2% to 14.3%.

You may have noticed an asymmetry. The *positive predictive value* (PPV) and the *posttest probability of a positive test* (PTL+) are synonymous, but the *negative predictive value* (NPV) and the *posttest probability of a negative test* (PTL−) are not. The NPV refers to the probability of the disease being absent in those with a negative result, while the PTL− refers to the probability of the disease being present in those with a negative result. Although the two quantities are not the same, they are strictly related, since they sum to 100% and one can be easily derived from the other.

The results of the PAP test in this particular population can be depicted by a diagnostic tree diagram (Fig. 19.3). Such representations are very useful in clinical decision analysis, the science of structuring clinical decisions. The patient enters the test at the left of the diagram with a pretest probability of prostatic carcinoma of 34.2%. If the test is positive, this probability rises to the posttest probability of a positive test (85.9%); if the test is negative, this probability falls to the posttest probability of a negative test (14.3%). The test appears, therefore, to provide some potentially useful information in this population. For patients with positive results, the probability of disease is sufficiently high (85.9%) to warrant biopsy and possible surgical exploration; but if the results are negative, the probability of disease is sufficiently low (14.3%) that such patients may be followed, or given another noninvasive test, if one is available.

On the basis of the sensitivity and specificity results of Foti and his colleagues, many concluded that the PAP radioimmunoassay could serve as an effective screening test for the early detection of prostatic cancer. In an editorial accompanying the report of Foti et al., Gittes stated: "The grim finding has been that, overall, 90% of cases are first detected when they have already metastasized. The clear implication of the accompanying report is that mass screening on the basis of a blood test alone can reverse this gloomy experience."[3] The popular press reported that a new blood test promised to do for prostatic cancer what the Papanicolaou smear had accomplished for cancer of the cervix.

The *utility* of a test refers to its usefulness and its ability to affect patient care positively in a specific clinical situation. It can be judged only in relation to a *particular* clinical situation; a relatively good sensitivity and specificity do *not* suffice to establish the clinical utility of a given test in *any* situation. Although sensitivity and specificity measure intrinsic qualities of a test's validity, and may be assumed to remain relatively stable in different clinical situations, the predictive values and posttest probabilities can change drastically. Since the predictive values and posttest probabilities depend very heavily on the pretest probability (prevalence), changes in prevalence can lead to marked changes in the predictive values and the clinical utility of a test. In other words, to adequately assess a diagnostic test for a specific clinical purpose, you must analyze it in relation to that particular purpose.

The original analysis of the PAP assay was carried out in a population of patients in whom the prevalence of prostatic cancer was 34.2%—hardly representative of the usual screening situation. Three years after the report of Foti et al., Watson and Tang presented their analysis of the PAP test as a screening test for prostatic cancer.[4] On the basis of national data for the United States for 1964, these authors assumed that the prevalence of prostatic carcinoma among white American men was 35 cases per 100,000. They then used the PAP test's established sensitivity and specificity of 70% and 94%, respectively, to calculate its predictive values in the screening situation.

To make these calculations, you begin by putting the hypothetical population of 100,000 as the total at the lower right-hand corner of the 2 × 2 table (TP + FP + FN + TN) (Fig. 19.4A). Since there are an estimated 35 cases among this hypothetical group, the sum at the bottom of the left hand column (TP + FN) should read 35. It follows that the sum of the right hand column (FP + TN) should be 100,000 − 35 = 99,965 (Fig. 19.4A). Of the 35 men who have prostatic cancer, the test will be positive in about 70% (sensitivity), that is, approximately 25, and this quantity can be entered in the TP cell (Fig. 19.4B). The remainder, 35 − 25 = 10, can be entered in the FN cell. Similarly, of the 99,965 men without prostatic carcinoma, the test will be negative in about 94% (specificity), that is, approximately 93,967, and this quantity can be entered in the TN cell (Fig. 19.4C). The remainder, 99,965 − 93,967 = 5998, is entered in the FP cell (Fig. 19.4C). The table can be completed by simply adding the row totals (Fig. 19.5).

We can now calculate the predictive values and posttest probabilities for the screening situation. The positive predictive value (PPV) (or PTL+) is TP/(TP + FP) or 25/6023, that is, 0.42%. The negative predictive value (NPV) is TN/(TN + FN) or 93,967/93,977, that is, 99.99%. Consequently, the posttest probability of a negative test, obtained by subtracting the NPV from 100%, is 0.01%. The probability of prostatic carcinoma prior to the test (the pretest likelihood or prevalence) was set at 35/100,000 or 0.035%.

Figure 19.6 is a diagnostic tree diagram summarizing these results for the screening situation. The average asymptomatic man, who would be screened by such a test, approaches the test at the left of the diagram with a pretest probability of prostatic cancer of 0.035% (35 chances in 100,000). If his test is positive, the probability rises to only 0.42% (1 chance in 240). Even with a positive test result, the chance of having prostatic cancer is still extremely slim, and it would be hard to justify further invasive testing. Obviously, the test is of little clinical help when it is positive in a screening situation.

Moreover, since approximately 6% (6023/100,000) of all white American men would have positive PAP screening tests, any policy of investigating positives further would involve the needless testing of significant numbers of healthy men. If the test is negative,

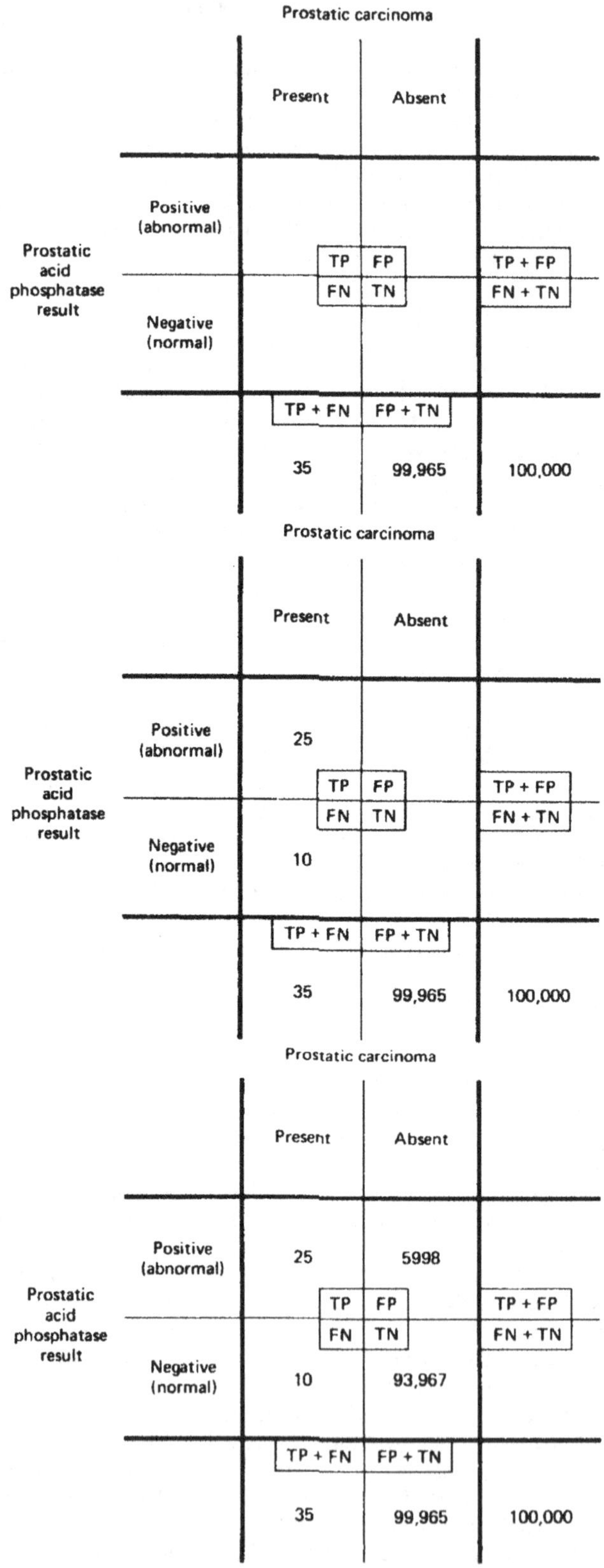
Prostatic carcinoma
Present
Absent
Positive (abnormal)
Prostatic acid phosphatase result
Negative (normal)
TP FP
FN TN
TP + FP
FN + TN
TP + FN
FP + TN
35
99,965
100,000
Prostatic carcinoma
Present
Absent
Positive (abnormal)
25
Prostatic acid phosphatase result
Negative (normal)
10
TP FP
FN TN
TP + FP
FN + TN
TP + FN
FP + TN
35
99,965
100,000
Prostatic carcinoma
Present
Absent
Positive (abnormal)
25
5998
Prostatic acid phosphatase result
Negative (normal)
10
93,967
TP FP
FN TN
TP + FP
FN + TN
TP + FN
FP + TN
35
99,965
100,000

FIGURE 19.4.

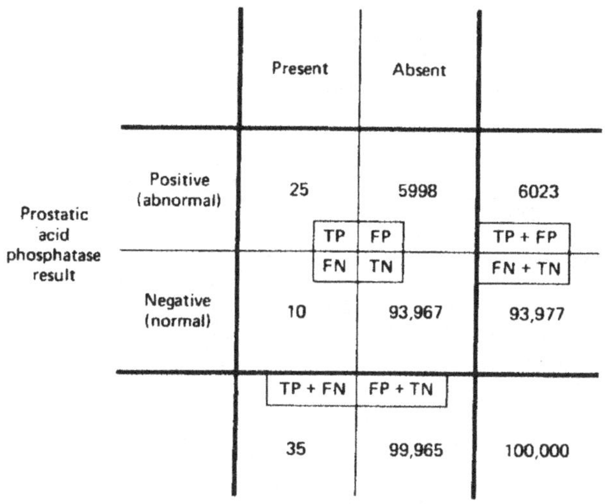

PPV = TP/(TP + FP) = 25/6023 = .0042 or 0.42%
NPV = TN/(TN + FN) = 93,967/93,977 = 0.9999 or 99.99%

FIGURE 19.5.

the probability of disease falls to 0.01% (10/100,000). Although one could argue that the test is useful in the screening situation, since it virtually rules out prostatic carcinoma when it is negative, this decrease in probability is of little benefit because the disease is exceptionally rare in the given population (35/100,000).

Our example illustrates the relation between posttest likelihoods and pretest likelihoods. In the diagnostic analysis carried out by Foti et al., the posttest likelihoods of a positive and negative test were relatively high (85.9% and 14.3%, respectively) because the pretest likelihood was high (34.2%) prior to the test. In the screening analysis carried out by Watson and Tang, the posttest likelihoods of a positive and negative test were extremely low (0.42% and 0.01%, respectively) because the pretest likelihood was very low (0.035%) prior to the test. The pre- and posttest likelihoods can be linked by a mathematical expression known as Bayes' theorem. The following are two of many equivalent expressions for Bayes' theorem:

$$\text{PPV} = \frac{\text{P}\cdot\text{SENS}}{(\text{P}\cdot\text{SENS}) + (1 - \text{P})\cdot(1 - \text{SPEC})}$$

$$\text{NPV} = \frac{(1 - \text{P})\cdot\text{SPEC}}{(1 - \text{P})\cdot\text{SPEC} + \text{P}\cdot(1 - \text{SENS})}$$

where P, SENS, and SPEC represent the pretest probability, sensitivity, and specificity, respectively, in decimal (e.g., 0.80) rather than percent (e.g., 80%) format. The different expressions used for Bayes' theorem have the common feature of portraying the posttest probabilities or predictive values in terms of the pretest probability. They all demonstrate how dependent the former values are on the latter value, and they provide a method for calculating posttest probabilities and predictive values for a given diagnostic test and a given pretest probability. You are encouraged to calculate the predictive values for the PAP test in the screening situation by setting P at 0.00035, SENS at 0.70, and SPEC at 0.94, in the formulas above. You should derive the predictive values that were obtained before, except for possible slight differences due to rounding error. These formulas pro-

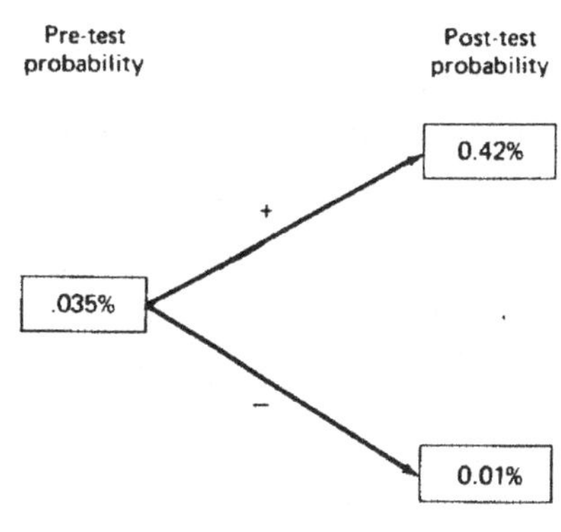

FIGURE 19.6.

vide an attractive alternative to the series of calculations and tables we went through, earlier, to derive the predictive values and posttest probabilities (Figs. 19.4A–C, 19.5). Bayes' theorem, in whatever form, is a relatively straightforward method of deriving the predictive values and the posttest likelihoods that are central to the consideration of clinical utility. This type of analysis is sometimes referred to as "Bayesian analysis."

The PAP radioimmunoassay illustrates several fundamental things about diagnostic tests:

1. Sensitivity and specificity measure the validity (accuracy) of a diagnostic test. They have no direct bearing on its clinical utility.
2. The clinical utility of a test is best assessed by considering its predictive values and posttest probabilities in a specific clinical situation.
3. Predictive values and posttest probabilities depend very heavily on the pretest probability (prevalence) of disease and, as a consequence, on both the clinical situation and the patient population in which a test is applied. This differs greatly from the popular misconception that test results are definitive (i.e., positive tests imply that patients are diseased and negative tests that they are not) and that the conclusions to be drawn from test results are independent of the patient who is tested.

The Assessment of Diagnostic Tests

New diagnostic tests and technologies are being developed at a constantly increasing rate; we have, for example, the prostatic acid phosphatase (PAP) test, positron emission tomography (PET), and magnetic resonance imaging (MRI). These new tests and techniques must be evaluated before they enter into widespread clinical use, and the medical literature contains more and more articles about their "assessment."

Guidelines for the Assessment of New Tests or Techniques

The Purpose of the Diagnostic Test

Any proper assessment of a diagnostic test begins with a clear statement of its proposed clinical purpose. The prostatic acid phosphatase radioimmunoassay test illustrates how a clinical test may perform well in one situation (diagnosis) and fail in another (screening). The proposed clinical function dictates how the assessment should be carried out.

Clinical tests serve five different clinical functions: diagnosis, screening, staging, monitoring, and triage. *Diagnosis* is the "ruling in" or "ruling out" of a disease in a patient in whom the disease is clinically suspected (e.g., coronary angiography for detecting coronary artery disease in a patient with angina). *Screening* refers to the presumptive detection of a given disease in a group of individuals who are asymptomatic for, and not suspected of having, it (e.g., mammography for the presumptive detection of breast cancer in middle-aged women). *Staging* is the use of a clinical test to gauge how far a disease has advanced as a guide to treatment (e.g., mediastinoscopy to determine the resectability of a lung cancer). *Monitoring* uses a test to assess and adjust ongoing therapy (e.g., prothrombin times to monitor the effect of anticoagulant therapy). *Triage* refers to the use of a test to determine which patients should receive further invasive testing (e.g., Doppler studies to determine which patients should have cerebral angiography).

Accordingly, you must state the type of patient, the intended clinical setting, and the purpose of a test before you embark on any assessment of it. The importance of these requirements will become more apparent as we continue.

The Spectrum and Number of Patients

When you are choosing the patients who will participate in a diagnostic test assessment, observe the rule: *the type of patient used in the assessment of a test should replicate the type of patient for whom the test is intended in clinical practice.* Unfortunately, this rule is not always followed. To carry out an assessment, you require a population with the target disease to estimate sensitivity, and a population free of the target disease to estimate specificity. You may be tempted to use an already identified group with established, florid disease as the diseased group, and a group of normally healthy controls as the nondiseased group. A moment's thought should convince you that such disparate groups would not challenge the clinical test with the wide spectrum of patients you and others will face in normal clinical practice. A test proposed for *diagnosis* should be assessed in a wide range of patients suspected of having the target disease or other diseases often confused with the target disease. A *screening* test should be challenged with asymptomatic individuals like those it will be applied to in clinical practice.

The use of obviously diseased and healthy individuals as cases and controls will spuriously inflate both sensitivity and specificity values, since these

these individuals will likely have positive and negative tests, respectively. If you start with a statement of the test's proposed function, the proposed type of patient in whom it is to be used, and the proposed setting for its use, you merely need to assemble, consecutively, all the patients matching the specified profile who are seen in the appropriate setting(s) over a sufficient interval of time. The use of consecutive patients minimizes the possibility of introducing bias into the selection of patients and replicates the spectrum of patients the test will be applied to in its eventual clinical use.

If you wish to assess a new diagnostic test for DVT for use when patients first present themselves at the primary care level, consider using every consecutive patient who consults his or her family practitioner, or arrives at a local emergency room, with a swollen calf and suspected DVT over a specified interval of time. Such a group will include patients who actually have DVT, in varying degrees of severity, and some who have confusing disorders, such as ruptured Baker's cysts or superficial thrombophlebitis. The performance of the test in such a group of patients will accurately reflect its performance in similar groups in similar primary care settings. If you propose to assess a *screening* test for the early detection of prostatic carcinoma, you should state that the test is proposed for use in elderly men who are both asymptomatic and clinically normal, and then assess it in a large population of such individuals.

Too often, inadequate numbers of patients are used. An investigator may assess a test in 25 diseased individuals, find that 20 of them have positive results, and conclude that the sensitivity is 80%. Although this is technically the best estimate for sensitivity based on the data, the 95% confidence limits around it are very wide (64% to 96%): see Chapter 15). The investigator should take the conservative approach and use the lower limit (64%) as the estimate of sensitivity but, more often than not, the sensitivity is simply stated as being 80%. The result is an overestimation of test validity. The only acceptable exception to the use of sufficient numbers of patients to ensure precise estimates occurs when a test for a rare target disease is being assessed and the number of available patients is inescapably small.

The Gold Standard

The *gold standard* is the set of criteria used by investigators to determine which patients are truly diseased and which are not. These criteria have a crucial impact on the 2 × 2 table and on the determination of the sensitivity and specificity of a test. Gold standards may be definitive (e.g., histopathological results from biopsy, surgery, or autopsy) or may simply be the results of other diagnostic tests currently accepted as standards for the diagnosis of the target disease in question. In certain situations, the gold standard may be a complex of symptoms, signs, and test results (e.g., the classification systems for the diagnosis of rheumatoid arthritis, systemic lupus erythematosus, and rheumatic fever). In diagnostic test assessments, it is critically important that the gold standard be well-defined, repeatable, and accepted as a current clinical standard for the diagnosis of the target disease. Anyone who reads a report on a diagnostic test assessment will want to know how the test will perform at detecting the presence or absence of the target disease in relation to the gold standard. If the gold standard is not well-defined or does not represent the current standard for diagnosis of the target disease, the assessment will be of little use because it will not be directly applicable to clinical practice. For example, since autopsy results or surgical findings are not usually available for patients with coronary artery disease (CAD), the results of coronary angiography are widely accepted as the clinical standard for diagnosis. Consequently, if you wish to assess the performance of a new test in the diagnosis of CAD, you might well utilize coronary angiography as your external gold standard for verifying the presence or absence of CAD in each patient; the angiographic criteria you use to establish the presence of CAD should be explicitly stated in your assessment report. Such explicit statements should include such clear, repeatable criteria as "a stenosis of greater than 75% seen on independent review by two cardiologists" and avoid such vagueness as "any abnormality seen on angiography." Describe the exact methods used to carry out the gold standard so that readers can determine whether the gold standard, as used in your study, corresponds with the one in use in their clinical settings.

The Diagnostic Test

An exact detailed description, as prescribed for your gold standard, is equally necessary for the diagnostic test you are assessing; that is, you must describe explicitly your test methodology, the conditions under which the test was performed, and how the patients were prepared. Supply enough detail to enable your readers to perform the diagnostic test exactly as you did in your assessment.

When the test produces a quantitative result (e.g., the concentration of a serum constituent), you should assess its precision. The variability produced by the test technology can be assessed by comparing the results for several samples taken from the same patient at the same time; the intrapatient variability can be assessed by comparing the results for samples taken from the same patient at different times. The sensitivity, specificity, and predictive values should be calculated at several threshold values (e.g., the value that separates normal from abnormal results). When you choose a single threshold value, your choice should be justified.

If the test produces a qualitative result that requires interpretation (e.g., CT scans must be interpreted by a radiologist), state clear and repeatable interpretation criteria. In addition, assess both the inter- and intraobserver variability in the interpretative component of the test by presenting the same consecutive panel of test results to two or more observers for independent review, and to a single observer for independent review on two or more separate occasions.

Independence

When each patient in your sample has undergone the diagnostic and gold standard tests, the results are compared in a 2 × 2 table (Fig. 19.2) to determine the test's validity and utility.

The diagnostic test and the gold standard test *must* be independent. Each patient *must* undergo both tests, that is, the diagnostic test result must not influence the selection of who is to have the gold standard test. The process should be triple-blinded if possible: that is, those who perform the tests, those who interpret them, and those who undergo them (the patients) should be kept "blinded" until both tests have been performed and interpreted. The various individuals who perform, interpret, or undergo the diagnostic test should be unaware of the gold standard results, if possible. Conversely, the various individuals who perform, interpret, or undergo the gold standard test should be unaware of the diagnostic test results, if possible. If this independence is not maintained, expectation bias can occur and can result in a spurious increase in the derived sensitivity, specificity, and predictive values. This is especially true when there is a significant subjective patient component or a significant interpretive component to the diagnostic test.

Assessment of Validity and Utility

When you have produced a 2 × 2 table, derived sensitivity, specificity, and predictive values, and concluded the test is useful, if the values are reasonably high, you may think your job is finished. A proper assessment, however, goes on to consider the predictive values, the posttest probabilities, and their significance in the clinical situation proposed for the test. Since these values depend very heavily on the prevalence of the target disease in your patient sample, as determined by the gold standard, you must assess whether this prevalence is reasonably close to the true prevalence of the same disease in the proposed target population. This will almost certainly be so if you obeyed the principle of using all consecutive patients who are like those for whom the test is intended and who arrived at one or more settings similar to those in which use of the test is envisaged.

If the prevalence in your patient sample is not a realistic estimate for the target population, recalculate the predictive values and posttest probabilities on the basis of a more realistic prevalence. You can do this easily by using Bayes' theorem with the new prevalence value (P), and the derived sensitivity (SENS) and specificity (SPEC). Your assessment of clinical utility should center on whether the test provides enough information, on the basis of predictive values and posttest likelihoods, to cause a change in management. The radioimmunoassay test for PAP failed in the screening situation because the posttest likelihoods of a positive and negative test were not sufficiently different from the pretest likelihood (prevalence) to affect any management decisions. A proper assessment, based on a realistic prevalence, could have demonstrated this in the initial analysis before the use of PAP as a screening test had been suggested.

When you assess clinical utility and the impact of the predictive values and posttest likelihood on clinical decisions, you must consider the consequences for false positives and false negatives. If the target disease is frequently fatal and a treatment exists that markedly alters the outcome (e.g., intraabdominal bleeding, subdural hematoma, bacterial meningitis), false negatives are extremely undesirable and a high sensitivity is required. A high sensitivity value has the effect of markedly reducing the posttest likelihood of a negative test (i.e., the negative predictive value is raised) and provides reasonable certainty that the target disease is absent when the test is negative. If you are screening for a disease that is not immediately fatal if missed, for which no effective treatment is available, and/or for which the costs of labeling and further investigation of positives are high (e.g., cystic fibrosis in newborns), you will want to keep the number of false positives to a minimum, and a high specificity will be required. A high specificity has the effect of markedly increasing the posttest likelihood of a positive test (i.e., the positive predictive value is raised) and provides reasonable certainty that the target disease is present when the test is positive.

In general, the impact of posttest likelihoods and predictive values on clinical decisions cannot be assessed without reference to the subsequent management of and consequences for positives and negatives.

References

1. Yerushalmy J. Statistical problems in assessing methods of medical diagnosis with special reference to x-ray techniques. Public Health Rep 1947;62:1432–49.
2. Foti AG, Cooper JF, Hershman H, Malvaez RR. Detection of prostatic cancer by solid-shape radioimmunoassay of serum prostatic acid phosphatase. N Engl J Med 1977;297:1357–61.
3. Gittes R. Acid phosphatase reappraised. N Engl J Med 1977;297:1398–99.
4. Watson RA, Tang DB. The predictive value of prostatic acid phosphatase as a screening test for prostatic cancer. N Engl J Med 1980;303:497–99.
5. Bayes T. An essay toward solving a problem in the doctrine of chance. Philos Trans R Soc London 1763;53:370–418.

Additional Reading

1. Department of Clinical Epidemiology and Biostatistics, McMaster University. How to read a clinical journal: II. To learn about a diagnostic test. Can Med Assoc J 1981;124:703–10.
2. Department of Clinical Epidemiology and Biostatistics, McMaster University. Interpretation of diagnostic data (six parts). Can Med Assoc J 1983;129: 429–32, 559–64, 587, 705–10, 832–35, 947–54, 1093–9.
3. Diagnostic tests. In: Clinical Epidemiology and Biostatistics. Kramer MS, ed. Berlin:Springer-Verlag, 1988:201–19.
4. Feinstein AR. On the Sensitivity, Specificity and Discrimination of Diagnostic Tests, in Clinical Biostatistics. St. Louis: CV Mosby, 1977;214–26.
5. Galen RS, Gambino SR. Beyond Normality: The Predictive Value and Efficiency of Medical Diagnoses. New York: Wiley, 1975.
6. Griner PF, Mayewski RJ, Mushlin AL, et al. Selection and interpretation of tests and procedures: principles and application. Ann Intern Med 1982;94: 557–600.
7. McNeil BJ, Keeler E, Adelstein SJ. Primer on certain elements of medical decision making. N Engl J Med 1975;293:211–15.
8. Schechter MT, Sheps SB. Diagnostic testing revisited: pathways through uncertainty. Can Med Assoc J 1985;132:755–60.
9. Sheps SB, Schechter MT. The assessment of diagnostic tests. A survey of current medical research. JAMA 1984;252:2418–22.
10. Sox HC Jr. Probability theory in the use of diagnostic tests. Ann Intern Med 1986;104:60–66.
11. Vecchio TJ. Predictive value of a single diagnostic test in unselected populations. N Engl J Med 1966; 274:1171–73.
12. Weinstein MC, Fineberg HV. Clinical Decision Analysis. Philadelphia: Saunders, 1980.

20

Scaling, Scoring, and Staging

M.E. Charlson, N.A. Johanson, and P.G. Williams

The world of scales often appears to be murky, filled with inscrutable jargon and even more incomprehensible analytic techniques. Clinicians planning clinical research must take a common-sense approach to the use of scales or indices. A scale like a thermometer is an instrument to measure clinical phenomena; a score is a value on the scale in a given patient. Clinical scales provide a standardized, repeatable measure of a patient's condition or functional status, just as thermometers provide a standardized repeatable measure of temperature.

Scale Anatomy

From the simplest to the most complex, scales have similar structures. Scales consist of one or more elements or questions and their answers. The answers may be either dichotomous, yes/no, or rank-ordered. The simplest scales consist of only one element. Complex scales many contain many elements, organized into domains of interest. For example, physical function might be one domain, and psychosocial function another. In assessing a scale, first inspect its constituent parts.

Ranks for an Individual Scale Element or Question

The simplest scale addresses only one question. For example, a scale for rating peripheral edema ranges from 1+ to 4+. To use this scale in clinical research, we must clearly define the individual ranks. For example, 1+ edema might be defined as noticeable only after digital pressure applied for more than 10 seconds. We define each of the other ranks, 2+ through 4+ in a way that is both clear and mutually exclusive. In clinical practice, the difference between grades 2+ and 3+ may not appear to be critical. However, if you study the response of patients to two different diuretic regimens after a shunt procedure and want to assess peripheral edema as one outcome, you would need to clearly define ranks with no confusion between them. If one observer rates a patient as having 1+ edema and another rates the same patient as having 3+ edema, you will not have meaningful results. If 2+ and 3+ peripheral edema are truly indistinguishable, the scale should not force an artificial division.

Other problems arise if the ranks are not *mutually exclusive*. For example, one disability status scale[1] has ranks for no, minimal, moderate, and severe disability but uses a separate rank for patients who require a cane or crutches to walk. Clinically, however, the extent of disability and the requirement for assisting devices are separate phenomena. How would one classify a patient who has minimal disability but requires a cane?

The ranking must yield a *clinically sensible, hierarchical order*. The scale should progress in an orderly way from least to most, or best to worst. Generally, we take hierarchical progression for granted. For example, the TNM staging systems[2] rank local disease as stage I, locally advanced disease as II, regional extension as III, and metastatic disease as IV. It would create confusion if regional extension was I; local disease, II; and metastases, III. In the disability scale cited above, the lack of mutual exclusivity precludes ranking in a defined hierarchical manner. In summary, a scale element or question must assess a single type of qualitative phenomena, have ranking that is clearly defined and mutually exclusive, and be arranged hierarchically.[3]

Scale ranks must encompass a range of responses relevant to the patients being studied; that is, *the scale must have an adequate range* for the patient population. Consider weighing patients. The usual adult scale is not useful for a baby, nor will it be useful for a patient who weighs 350 pounds. The same phenomenon occurs with indices – the index must encompass a range that is relevant to the patients studied. For example, there are a number of scales that measure strenuous physical activity.[4] However, if you used one of these scales to compare patients before and after total hip replacement, you might find that there was no change, since few patients are likely to play basketball or to jog either before or after this operation. Since the activities measured are more than most patients are likely to do, such a scale could not reasonably be expected to change in response to total hip replacement. On the other hand, if you used the Activities of Daily Living (ADL) scale,[5] which measures patients' ability to dress, wash, and generally care for themselves, there also may be little postoperative change, because most patients undergoing hip replacement were at the highest level of that scale before operation. In short, a scale's range in relation to the patients under study must be adequate to permit detection of both improvement and deterioration. If patients are clustered at the top or bottom of the scale before treatment, it may be impossible to detect improvement for those at the top, or deterioration in those at the bottom.[6]

Scale Questions or Elements

While the simplest scales contain only one question or element and are designed to measure only one phenomenon, more complicated scales consist of a number of separate elements or questions that cover different issues. For example, the New York Heart Association classification has four ranks of physical function in relation to angina – ranging from no angina on strenuous exertion to angina at rest. In contrast, the Goldman cardiac risk scale for noncardiac surgery patients is a complicated scale that incorporates nine different elements, including age, presence of congestive failure, severity of congestive failure, and others.[8] The responses to each of the elements are assigned weighted scores, which are then summed to arrive at a total score for each patient. For example, age greater than 70 years has a weight of 5, and a recent myocardial infarction has a weight of 10.[7] A patient with both would have a total score of 15 and would be assigned to the class 3 risk group. This scale is simpler than some others because it predicts one outcome – cardiac morbidity and mortality in the perioperative period.

Other scales include not only multiple questions or elements, but different domains, such as psychosocial, physical, or emotional function. However, your basic approach to a scale should remain the same, regardless of how complicated it is. You should review the questions and see if they are relevant to what *you* want to measure. You must assess the possible responses to the questions to ensure they are clear and mutually exclusive, and decide whether the range is sufficient to assess your patient population. Finally, you must review how the elements are aggregated to see if the combinations are sensible.

What Do You Want the Scale to Do?

A scale may serve three basic functions: prediction, evaluation, or description.[9] Predictive scales divide patients into groups that have prognostic importance over time; many predictive scales are called staging systems. Evaluative scales evaluate change or stability in a population over time, and particularly, the effect of a therapeutic intervention. Descriptive scales describe and contrast populations at a single point in time; they discriminate between those with and without condition X. The type of scale you need differs substantially depending on how you want to use it.

Predictive Scales

Let us suppose you are conducting a clinical trial to study the effect of two different topical antibiotics on the survival of burn patients. Patients randomized to the two different treatments must, before treatment, have an equal likelihood of survival. If their risk were not equal (e.g., if one group contained a larger proportion of patients with greater than 50% second and third degree burns),[9] it would be difficult to tell at the end of the trial whether any differences in survival between the groups were due to the prognostic imbalance or to differences in the efficacy of the therapy. Therefore, you would want to stratify patients prior to randomization according to their likelihood of survival; to help do this, you could use a scale (i.e., the percentage and depth of injury of involved skin) that predicts survival with reasonable accuracy. The importance of predictive scales or staging systems has long been recognized in studies of cancer patients. For example, a breast cancer trial that randomized patients with local disease and those with distant metastases, without stratifying them and balancing them according to stage, would not be clinically sensible because the prognoses of the patients are so different. In fact, randomizing them together might obscure rather than clarify the effects of treatment, because treatment effect could be completely opposite for the two groups. Experience with trials in cancer patients has shown that an effective treatment for patients of one stage may be ineffective for those of another. This underscores the importance of using predictive scales or prognostic staging systems in studies of treatment effectiveness. Apart from oncologic staging systems, predictive indices for survival have been developed for burn patients,[1] for trauma patients,[2,10-12] and for postoperative ICU patients.[13,14] The scoring system for burns,[1] the abbreviated injury score,[2-5] and scale for ICU patients,[7,14] have been demonstrated to predict patients' survival. A method of classifying comorbid conditions has also been developed for use in longitudinal studies.[6]

However, scales designed for prediction may not serve well to evaluate the effects of therapy. For example, the percent involvement might not be useful in evaluating the response to two different approaches to skin grafts. The Child's classification for cirrhosis,[15] which has clear prognostic importance, might not be helpful in evaluating the response to shunts.

Evaluative Scales

Let us assume that you wish to compare porous ingrowth hip prostheses versus cemented metal implants with respect to long term patient outcomes, in particular, the patient's physical function. To measure the impact of therapy, you need to assess the patient on at least two occasions—preoperative and postoperatively. You would want to choose a scale that could measure changes in physical function related to operation. First, the scale should measure phenomena in some way related to physical function and the hip. Second, the scale should show improvement when the patient gets better, and deterioration if the patient worsens. To evaluate the effect of therapy, the patient's preoperative scale rank would be compared with his postoperative score. The outcome of interest is a change in an individual patient; the aggregate mean preoperative scores compared to postoperative scores would be of little value, because fundamentally you want to know how many patients improved, or worsened, or stayed the same. Relatively few evaluative scales have been developed specifically for surgical patients. However, some scales that have been developed for other uses may be useful for surgical patients. The Arthritis Impact Measurement Scale (AIMS) is one such example.[16,17]

Descriptive Scales

Both predictive and evaluative scales imply that the status of patients will be observed at two points in time; predictive scales must accurately forecast how the patient will do, and evaluative scales must be able to distinguish patients who have changed clinically from those who have not. Descriptive scales are designed to characterize patients at a single point in time. We use such indices to compare one group of patients with another. The Karnovsky classification of performance status in oncologic studies is an example of a scale that was developed for a descriptive purpose.[18] The American Society of Anesthesiologists' classification of physical status and the New York Heart Association classification of angina[19] are examples of scales developed primarily for descriptive purposes.[20] Another example of a descriptive scale is the Organ Injury Scaling System for the spleen, liver, and kidney.[21]

Scale Physiology: Reproducibility, Validity and Responsiveness

Not only are the purposes of the three types of scales distinct, but the design requirements of predictive, evaluative, and descriptive studies and scales differ. The distinctions are crucial, because indices designed for one purpose will not necessarily work for another purpose.

All scales must first be reproducible—that is, they must have minimal intraobserver and interobserver variability. (Translation: The scale gives scores within reasonable range of variation on repeated administrations to the same patient by the same and by different observers.) If reproducibility is poor, the scale will be useless for any purpose. Second, a scale must be a valid measure of what it is supposed to be measuring. The requirements for validity differ according to the scale's purpose. Predictive scales must be useful in predicting outcomes—their prognostic validity. Descriptive scales must distinguish between different populations. Evaluative scales must correlate with the results of other methods of assessing outcome; if patients score better, there should be ways of confirming that they are indeed better. Third, evaluative scales have an additional requirement— responsiveness. If the patient's condition changes, they should change; if the patient does not change, they should not change. We usually do not emphasize responsiveness sufficiently. Let's look at these issues in scale physiology one at a time.

Reproducibility

Reproducibility issues associated with scales are similar to those we encounter every day with the reproducibility of clinical data. Most biologic variables we want to measure are not static, but fluctuate and change. For example, pulse, blood pressure, urine output, and serum sodium constantly change throughout a day. The fluctuations are partly random and partly reflect efforts to maintain homeostasis. The usual range of values through which these variables fluctuate differs for different people. A runner may have a pulse that ranges from 40 to 60 during usual activity, while someone else may have a usual pulse that ranges from 70 to 90. Apart from moment to moment variability, there are often patterns of changes or trends on a daily, monthly, or seasonal basis. These variations also occur in responses to scales. Patients evaluated at the end of a tiring day may be ranked worse than would have been the case if they had been evaluated that morning.

Scales must have unambiguous questions with enough detail to ensure that the same question will be more likely to receive the same answer. For example, a question about whether a patient has pain on walking will have better reproducibility if specific conditions are considered, such as pain after climbing one flight of stairs.

The circumstances of measurement must be the same. Consider blood pressure. First, the conditions under which we take the measurement are important in minimizing inter- and intraobserver variability. The measurements should be made in the same position, with the same cuff size, applied at the same arm position, using the same deflation rate, and viewing the meniscus in the same way.[22] Second, the sequence of measurement is important. On the second or third measurement, the patient's blood pressure is usually lower than on the first measurement.[23] The results may be different if we scale or score at the end of an exhaustive evaluation, or at the beginning. If the index involves asking the patient to respond to questions, we must use the same wording—varying, or "ad libbing" the questions may adversely effect reproducibility. Furthermore, responses may differ if they are given by the patient, a spouse, or the surgeon. If the scale calls for patient responses, the investigator must not supply the answers. If it is designed to be read to the patient or filled in by the patient, those procedures should be followed. In short, the way we give indices must be operationally defined with sufficient precision to permit the repitition of subsequent measurements in identical circumstances.

Finally, we must ensure that the patient has *not* changed clinically when the reproducibility of the measurements is being assessed. If you were trying to establish reproducibility of an index designed to measure hip function, it would be foolish to test it before and after hip replacement, because you would expect the patient to change between the assessments. We must establish reproducibility in stable, nonchanging patients.

Even if the circumstances of measurements are standardized and the patient is stable, there may still be differences among different observers or among the reports of one observer on several occasions. One must recognize problems with reproducibility and plan strategies to reduce variability. Contrary to popular belief, observer variability is as much a problem with "hard" data from radiologic and pathologic tests as it is with "soft" data in scales.[24,25] One key question associated with scales is who does the measurement. With clinical scales, particularly for the evaluation of outcomes, the surgeon often is the observer. There may be a natural tendency for surgeons to rate postoperative assessments as improved. Therefore, perhaps one should have someone not involved with the treatment assess the patient. Many studies use, "blinded" assessors, who are unaware of the patient's treatment.

There are several ways to assess the reproducibility of scales. Without going into detail, most rank-ordered scales should be assessed using a statistic called kappa, not percent agreement. Percent agreement does not take into account agreement that occurs by chance alone. If you flip a coin, you will be right 50% of the time whether you call heads or tails. Similarly, when scales are used, some ratings agree simply by chance. The kappa statistic takes this into account and reports the agreement beyond chance.[26]

In summary, assessing reproducibility addresses the following question: Is the scale measurement the same on repeated administrations when the patient has not changed?

Validity

Validity asks whether the scale measures the phenomena it is supposed to measure. The assessment of validity differs according to the purpose of the scale.

This issue is usually fairly straightforward with predictive scales. They are valid if they predict the outcome they are supposed to predict. If patients are classified according to Goldman's cardiac risk class, patients in class I should have lower cardiac morbidity and mortality than those in class IV.

Note, however, that none of the predictive scales separate patients perfectly according to outcome. For example, the cardiac risk index score cannot reliably identify two groups of patients: the ones who will die and the ones who will live. Prediction is never perfect.

Does the scale identify a range from those most likely to live to those most likely to die? If you had proposed a new scale to predict the likelihood of postoperative wound dehiscence, you might first evaluate all patients undergoing abdominal surgery to assess their status on your scale. Validation of the scale would require that you show that a larger proportion of patients in the highest risk group in your scale had wound dehiscence than those in the lower risk groups.

With descriptive scales, the question of validity is somewhat circular. Descriptive scales are constructed because there is no standard method of assessing the phenomena you want to measure. Yet, scale measurements at a single point in time should have a reasonable relationship to other related assessments. For example, a patient in New York Heart Association class IV (i.e., angina at rest) should not be able to walk one mile without stopping and should not achieve a maximal treadmill exercise test. The validity of descriptive indices is generally established by their relation to other measures directed at the same qualitative phenomena at the same point in time.

With evaluative scales, the issue of validity is more complex. First, does the scale, on its face value, appear to be qualitatively correct? It is tempting to choose measures that are very precise, but if they do not measure the phenomena you are actually interested in, that precision is useless. For example, if you used pulse rates to measure preoperative anxiety, you would get very precise numbers; however, the pulse rates may or may not relate to anxiety. Second, the scale should measure the phenomena that you believe to be clinically important. For example, a hip score designed to assess patients undergoing total hip replacement that measured only range of motion and did not assess of walking ability or pain, would not be very useful because it does not capture the most clinically relevant outcomes. Physicians and patients may place different weights on outcomes. We must consider whether a scale takes into account the issues most important to the patient. For example, most scales include pain, because the extent of pain is extremely important to most patients—despite its "subjectivity."

Responsiveness

A responsive scale shows change when the patient changes, and no change when the patient is stable. The requirement for responsiveness is distinct from those for reproducibility and validity. A scale may be reproducible and valid, but unresponsive to change. For example, the New York Heart Association classification may be reproducible and valid. However, let us say that we want to use it to measure outcome after coronary artery bypass surgery. You assess patient classes preoperatively and postoperatively and find that most patients did not change. Perhaps the gradations in the scale are too gross to measure change.[27] Consider weighing patients on a vehicle scale that measures only in hundreds of pounds. If you used that device to assess weight loss with dieting, you would be unable to demonstrate that weight loss had occurred. Even if every patient had lost weight, you would be unable to show it because your measurement device is unresponsive to change. To be useful for evaluation of response to treatment, a scale needs responsiveness. Many predictive and descriptive scales have yielded disappointing results because their basic anatomical design is not suited for evaluation.

Many indices have been modeled after scales developed by psychologists to measure personality characteristics and intelligence. Designed to characterize the differences between populations in cross-sectional studies, such scales contained many questions and required 30 minutes or more to administer. Scales that had been shown to be reproducible and valid were then used to evaluate the effect of therapeutic interventions. Often these single-state scales showed no difference before and after treatment, even when everyone agreed that the patient had indeed changed. This occurred because the scales were designed to discriminate between large populations by including many items, many of which would not be expected to change when the patient changed.[28] This structure impairs their ability to discern change and to evaluate response to therapy.[29] For example, when surgical patients were evaluated preoperatively and postoperatively with the Sickness Impact Profile, a widely used descriptive scale,[30] the instrument was able to detect only patients who were worse. It was unable to detect improvement.[31] Recently, this scale has been modified to improve its responsiveness for head injury patients.[32]

Single-State Versus Transition Scales

Most evaluative scales are single-state scales, designed to be administered twice: we use the same scale once before treatment and once after treatment. We attribute any differences in score between the two administrations to treatment effect. Another type of scale is a transition scale.

With a transition scale, patients are asked at the second evaluation whether they are better, the same, or worse than they were at the time of the first evaluation. This type of scale mimics the way we, as clinicians, actually assess patients. An example is a scale developed to measure dyspnea.[33] At the baseline administration, we ask the patient to respond to three different elements (level of functional impairment secondary to shortness of breath, magnitude of task resulting in shortness of breath, and magnitude of effort resulting in shortness of breath) and each element receives a rating from 0 (= most severe) to 4 (= unimpaired). The ratings for each element are added to form a baseline score. On the second administration, the patient is asked how much deterioration or improvement has occurred compared to the baseline state for each element, ranging from −3 to +3 level change. We sum the transition ratings on the different elements to arrive at a transition score.

Patient-Specific Indices

To take into account the wide variation in activities of different patients (i.e., questions about grocery shopping or mowing the lawn or playing golf will not be relevant to all patients), patient-specific indices of change have been developed. For example, a patient-specific index of physical function[33] has patients identify one or more physical activities they do frequently and consider to be the most demanding in terms of physical effort. Each patient's response forms the basis for subsequent assessments of change. For example, if a patient says "walking up subway stairs" at the initial evaluation, at the subsequent assessment we ask the patient about whether there has been a change in his ability to walk up subway stairs (i.e., better, the same, or worse; if better, how much better). You can see that this follows the transition scale model. Patient-specific indices have been developed to measure changes in dyspnea, fatigue, emotional function, and mastery as outcome measures in trials involving patients with congestive heart failure and chronic pulmonary disease.[34] Additionally, the model has been used to develop disease-specific measures of quality of life or function for a number of other conditions, for example, inflammatory bowel disease.[35]

Scale Use

The Clinically Important Difference

What is a clinically important difference in score? All too often, articles report that one group of patients had a mean score that was 2.6 points higher than the other group, but no data are provided to permit the reader to understand what this difference in score actually means. The investigator needs to provide a context so that readers can interpret scores and changes in scores. For example, one study of adult health described a 10 point difference on the physical subscale as being equivalent to the effect of mild, chronic osteoarthritis.[36] We must define the minimal clinically important difference for each single state scale. Standards for defining clinically important differences have been developed for transition scales.[37]

Quality of Life

The Example of Coronary Artery Bypass Grafts

The issues become more complex when measuring the overall quality of life. Consider the issue of quality of life using the example of coronary artery bypass graft surgery. When many studies of prognosis after coronary artery bypass graft (CABG) were begun, the work in the area of defining and measuring health status or quality of life was in its infancy. There were only a few scales available for investigators to use, for example, the Karnovsky scale[38] and Katz's ADL scale.[39] Neither scale appeared to be optimal to investigators accustomed to quantitating luminal obstruction or ejection fraction. Furthermore, most patients were too well to have quality of life or function measured by an ADL instrument designed for assessing outcomes in elderly patients and nursing home residents. In the mid-1970s, a series of instruments was developed based on the World Health Organization definition; health status or quality of life was defined operationally by physical, mental, and social function.[40] Most scales developed to assess quality of life included specific measures of physical and psychosocial function, but not mental function.

Why is quality of life important in studies of CABG patients? The Coronary Artery Surgery Study (CASS)[41] and the European cooperative study[42] suggest that patients with left main and triple vessel disease survive longer with surgical rather than medical treatment. Among patients with less extensive disease, survival in the medical and surgical groups was similar. Given the similarity in survival of patients with less extensive disease, the effect of therapy on quality of life (i.e., on physical, mental and psychosocial function) became the critical question.[43]

The CASS study operationally defined quality of life according to disease-related items (i.e., chest pain, congestive failure, hospitalization, or drug treatment) and activity-related items (i.e., limitations in daily activities, recreational activities, and employment).[41] Surgically treated patients had less chest pain, better exercise tolerance, and fewer limitations in daily activities.[44] In general, after CABG chest pain decreased significantly, yet the New York Heart Association and Canadian cardiovascular classifications did not change. (These scales were insensitive to postoperative improvement).[45] Other studies focused on return to work to assess quality of life after CABG. They found that employment status is not usually altered by CABG[40]; the most optimistic studies report a net gain in employment of only about 10% after CABG.[46-48] For example, patients who were not working before CABG generally did not return to work. Younger patients and those with more education were more likely to return to work postoperatively. In an important but small study that helps to explain these findings, post-CABG patients were asked whether they *wanted* to work[49]; ironically, patients ranked returning to work as least important to their quality of life after CABG. Family relationships, relief of symptoms, and increased physical activity were more important to patients.[50] The emphasis on return to work as a major method of assessing quality of life after CABG is understandable given the pressure to prove that CABG is more effective than medical therapy and that this benefit is worth the additional cost.[51] Demonstrating that patients resumed work would have provided a powerful argument for cost-effectiveness. Other important aspects of quality of life have received less attention than return to work.[52,53] This paradoxical situation arose because of the perceived difficulties in defining and measuring quality of life.

Function and Health Status: Generic Measures

The problems of such indices have been reviewed extensively in other publications.[54-56] There are currently a wide variety of indices available. The Quality of Well-Being scale[57] and the Quality of Index[58] require the least time to administer. While some data on responsiveness and the minimal clinically important difference of these scales are available, we need more studies of this important issue. For cardiopulmonary disease[31] and arthritis patients,[16] disease-specific instruments are available. We can now measure quality of life or health status with available instruments that are designed for different patient groups, including both physical and psychosocial function, and have been shown to be reproducible, valid, and responsive to change.

Choosing a Scale, Designing and Testing Your Own

When evaluating a scale for its appropriateness for use in your own research, decide whether it focuses on the elements relevant to the outcomes you are interested in. You may find that there is no scale that directly addresses the issues that concern you. In this case, you may feel that a few additional elements combined with an existing scale would fit your needs or that a minor transformation of an existing scale would be appropriate. Alternatively, you may feel that you have to start from scratch, that there is nothing available which is relevant to your research questions.

You can develop your own scale, based on your own clinical knowledge and experience. For those undertaking such a task, more detailed understanding of the issues is key.[59] Common sense will enable you to choose questions and responses that cover the various outcomes of interest, and are valid at face value. You then need to pilot test your scale to see whether patients understand your questions and to assure that the response ranges are appropriate. You may find that there are redundant elements which can be dropped to yield a briefer instrument. The scale then needs to undergo testing to ensure its reproducibility and validity. If you want to use it to evaluate the effect of therapy, you must make certain that it is responsive. (See also Chapters 17, 18, and 19.)

References

1. Hauser SL, Dawson DM, Lehrick JR et al. Intensive immunosuppression in progressive multiple sclerosis. N Engl J Med 1983;308:173–80.
2. International Union Against Cancer (UICC). TNM Classification of Malignant Tumours. Geneva: International Union Against Cancer 1974:51–55.
3. MacKenzie CR, ME Charlson. Standards for the use of ordinal scales in clinical trials. Br Med J 1986; 292:40–43.
4. Taylor HL, Jacobs DR, Schucker B, et al. A questionnaire for the assessment of leisure time physical activities. J Chronic Dis 1978;31:741–55.
5. Katz S, Ford AB, Moskowitz RW, et al. Studies of illness in the aged: the index of ADL, a standardized measure of biological and psychosocial function. JAMA 1963;185:914–19.
6. Charlson ME, Pompei P, Ales KL, et al. A new method of classifying prognostic comorbidity in longitudinal studies: development and validation. J Chronic Dis 1987;40:373–83.
7. Goldman L, Caldera DL, Nussbaum SR, et al. Multifactorial index of cardiac risk in noncardiac surgical procedures. N Engl J Med 1977;297:845–50.

8. Kirshner B and G Guyatt. A methodologic framework for assessing health indices. J Chronic Dis 1985;38:27-36.
9. Committee on Medical Aspects of Automobile Safety. Rating the severity of tissue damage. JAMA 1971:215:277-80.
10. Kirkpatrick JR, and Youmans, RL. Trauma Index: an aide in the evaluation of injury victims. J Trauma 1971:11:711-14.
11. Committee on the Medical Aspects of Automotive Safety. Rating the severity of tissue damage: the comprehensive scale. JAMA 1972;220:717-20.
12. Baker SP, O'Neill B, Haddon W, et al. The injury severity score: a method for describing patients with multiple injuries and evaluating emergency care. J Trauma 1974;14:187-96.
13. Knaus WA, Wagner DP, Draper EA. Relationship between acute physiologic derangement and risk of death. J Chronic Dis 1985;38:295-300.
14. Knaus WA, Draper EA, Wagner DP, et al. An evaluation of outcome from intensive care in major medical centers. Ann Intern Med 1986;104:410-18.
15. Conn H, Lindenmuth W, Mayu C, et al. Prophylactic portocaval anastomosis. Medicine 1972;51:27-40.
16. Meenan RF, Anderson JJ, Kasiz LE, et al. Outcome assessment in clinical trials: evidence for the sensitivity of a health status measure. Arthritis Rheum 1984;27:1344-52.
17. Liang M, Larson MG, Cullen KE, et al. Comparative measurement efficiency and sensitivity of five health status instruments for arthritis research. Arthritis Rheum 1985;28:542-47.
18. Karnofsky DA, Burchenal JH. The clinical evaluation of chemotherapeutic agents in cancer In: Evaluation of Chemotherapeutic Agents, MacLeod DM, ed. New York: Columbia University Press 1949; 191-205.
19. Criteria Committee of the New York Heart Association. Diseases of the Heart and Blood Vessels: Nomenclature and Criteria for Diagnosis, 6th ed. Boston: Little, Brown, 1964:112-13.
20. Dripps RD, Lamont A, Ecknehoff JE. The role of anesthesia in surgical mortality. JAMA 1961;178: 261-66.
21. Moore EE, Shackford SR, Pachter HL, et al. Organ Injury Scaling System: Spleen, Liver and Kidney. J Trauma 1989;29:1664-66.
22. Kirkendall WM, Feinleib M, Freis ED, et al. American Heart Association recommendations for human blood pressure determinations by sphygmomanometer. Hypertension 1981;2:509-19A.
23. Armitage P, Fox W, Rose GA, et al. The variability of measurements of casual blood pressure: II. Survey experience. Clin Sci 1966;30:337-44.
24. Boyd NF, Wolfson C, Moskowitz M, et al. Observer variation in the interpretation of xeromammograms. J Natl Cancer Inst 1982;68:357-63.
25. Feinstein AR, Gelfman NA, Yesner R, et al. Observer variability in the histopathologic diagnosis of lung cancer. Am Rev Respir Dis 1970;101:671-84.
26. Spitzer RL, Cohen J , Fleiss JL, et al. Quantification of agreement in psychiatric diagnosis: a new approach. Arch Gen Psychiatr 1967;17:83-87.
27. Goldman L, Cook EF, Mitchell N, et al. Pitfalls in the serial assessment of cardiac functional status. J Chronic Dis 1982;35:763-71.
28. Guyatt G, Walter S, and Norman G. Measuring change over time: assessing the usefulness of evaluative instruments J Chronic Dis 1987;40:171-78.
29. Kirshner B, Guyatt G. A methodologic framework for assessing health indices. J Chronic Dis 1985; 38:27-36. A classic article providing a framework for thinking about the use of scales.
30. Bergner M, Bobbitt RS, Carter WB, et al. The Sickness Impact Profile: development and final revision of a health status measure. Med Care 1981;19: 787-805.
31. MacKenzie CR, Charlson ME, DiGioia D, et al. Can the Sickness Impact Profile measure change? An example of scale assessment. J Chronic Dis 1986; 39:429-38.
32. Temkin N, McLean A, Dikmen S, et al. Development and evaluation of modifications to the Sickness Impact Profile for head injury. J Clin Epidemiol 1988;41:47-57.
33. Mahler DA, Weinberg DH, Wells CK, et al. The measurement of dyspnea: contents, interobserver agreement and physiologic correlates of two new clinical indexes. Chest 1984;85:751-58.
34. Guyatt GH, Berman LB, Townsend M, et al. Should study subjects see their previous responses? J. Chronic Dis 1985;38:1003-7.
35. Guyatt G, Deyo RA, Charlson ME, et al. Responsiveness and validity in health status measurement. J Clin Epidemiol 1989;42:403-8.
36. Brook RH, Ware JE, Rogers WH, et al. Does free care improve adult health? Results from a randomized controlled trial. N Engl J Med 1983;309: 1426-33.
37. Jaeschke R, Singer J, Guyatt G. Health status measurement: ascertaining the minimal clinically important difference. Clin Res 1989;37:315A.
38. Karnovsky DA, Abelmann WH, Craver LF, et al. The use of nitrogen mustard in the palliative treatment of carcinoma. Cancer 1948;1:634-56.
39. Katz S, Ford AD, Moskowitz RW, et al. Studies of illness in the aged. JAMA 1963;185:914-19.
40. World Health Organization. The constitution of the World Health Organization. WHO Chron 1947; 1:29.
41. CASS Principal Investigators and Their Associates. Myocardial infarction and mortality in the coronary artery surgery study (CASS) randomized trial. N Engl J Med 1984;310:750-58.
42. European Coronary Surgery Study Group. Long term results of prospective randomized study of coronary artery bypass surgery in stable angina pectoris Lancet 1982;ii:1173-80.
43. Hampton JR. Coronary artery bypass grafting for the reduction of mortality: an analysis of the trials Br Med J 1984;289:1166-70.

44. CASS Principal Investigators and Their Associates. Coronary Artery Surgery Study (CASS): a randomized trial of coronary artery bypass surgery quality of life in patients randomly assigned to treatment groups. Circulation 1983;68:951–60.
45. National Institutes of Health Consensus Development Conference Statement. Coronary artery bypass surgery: scientific and clinical aspects N Engl J Med 1981;304:680–84.
46. Niles NW, Vander Salm TJ, Cutler BS. Return to work after coronary artery bypass operation. J Thorac Cardiovasc Surg 1980;79:916–21.
47. Symmes JC, Lenkei SC, Berman ND. Influence of aortocoronary bypass surgery on employment. Can Med J 1978;118:268–70.
48. Gutman M, Knapp D, Pollock M, et al. Coronary artery bypass patients and work status Circulation 1982;66(Suppl III):33–41.
49. LaMendola WF, Pellegrini RV. Quality of life and coronary artery bypass surgery patients. Soc Sci Med 1979;13A:457–61.
50. Flynn MK, Frantz R. Coronary artery bypass surgery: quality of life during early convalescence. Heart Lung 1987;16:159–67.
51. Doubilet R, Weinstein MC, McNeil BJ. Use and misuse of the term "cost effective" in medicine. N Engl J Med 1986;314:253–56.
52. Fletcher AE, Hunt BM, Bulpitt CJ. Evaluation of quality of life in clinical trials of cardiovascular disease. J Chronic Dis 1987;40:557–66.
53. Stanton BA, Jenkins CD, Savageau JA, et al. Functional benefits following coronary artery bypass graft surgery. Ann Thorac Surg 1984;37:286–90.
54. Feinstein AR, Josephy BR, Wells CK. Scientific and clinical problems in indexes of functional disability. Ann Intern Med 1986;105:413–20.
55. O'Young J, McPeek B. Quality of life variables in surgical trials. J. Chronic Dis 1987;40:513–22. A review of the experience with surgical trials.
56. McDowell I, Newell C. Measuring Health. A Guide to Rating Scales and Questionnaires. New York: Oxford Univ Press, 1987. A detailed description and critique of many different health status measures.
57. Kaplan RM, Bush JE, Berry CC. Health status: types of validity and the index of well being. Health Serv Res 1976;11:478–507.
58. Spitzer WO, Dobson AJ, Hall J, et al. Measuring the quality of life of cancer patients. J Chronic Dis 1981;34:585–97.
59. Feinstein AR. Clinimetrics. New Haven, CT: Yale University Press, 1987.

Additional Reading

Knaus WA. The science of prediction and its implications for the clinician today. Theor Surg 1988;3: 93–101.

21

Using Computers in Research

S.W. Dziuban, Jr., G.G. Bernstein, and R.G. Margolese

Today, computers can help scholars in more ways than ever before, but those who have never used them often have questions about how computers can help, and how to get started using them. The goal of this chapter is to provide awareness, direction, and perspective in the face of rapidly changing computer options and products.

While the general advice we provide should be helpful, there is no substitute for your own experience. If it appears that computers might help in your work, jump in and use them. We hope this chapter will help you decide where and how to jump.

Uses for Computers in Research

Are computers always helpful? Would your research improve if you used one? What specifically can a computer do to help you?

"Using computers," like "doing surgery," is not an end in itself, but a means to an end. A computer is a tool to help you accomplish a specific task; its value can be measured by how much easier, quicker, more efficient, or more effective it makes your work. (See also Section III, Chapter 38.)

The justification for a computer can be that it reduces the time or effort required to achieve given results, or that it can help you produce better results than other methods, although it may cost more in time or effort. Computer methods are certainly of no help if they take more time and effort than paper methods without any added benefit.

The use of a computer is most successful when it is driven by a specific need. A motivating need helps a new computer user climb the learning curve.

Reviewing the Literature and Organizing References

Access to electronic literature data bases permits review of scientific and medical literature. The primary advantage is the speed of searching an enormous reference base with a focus that is as specific as you wish to make it. As your references accumulate, you can organize them in a computer program known as a reference manager.

Electronic Literature Searches

One commonly used data base is the U.S. National Library of Medicine MEDLINE, which contains more than 5 million references. Each reference citation contains such key items as title, author(s), journal, and abstract, but not usually the complete text of the article. (See Chapter 7, above.)

The MEDLINE database is searched using terms that get matched to the stored content of the references. Usually the first search is too broad or too narrow and must be modified to obtain exactly what you want. It can be refined by using such logical (Boolean) combination terms as "*and*," "*or*," and "*not*" with several search words, or by using the results of a previous search with new words. Figure 21.1 is an example of refining and focusing taken from a real search.

Although a search can be based on a "free text" match using any words, it is often helpful to take advantage of the fact that MEDLINE references have all been classified by the National Library of Medicine, using the Medical Subject Headings (MeSH). The MeSH is a list of categories using standardized terminology, which can be more reliable since different authors use highly variable wording. By searching for the appropriate MeSH

You travel home one evening thinking about the unusual patient problem you saw, a bilateral congenital diaphragmatic hernia. At home, you decide to a quick search; your personal computer dials the number and connects you to MEDLINE using your private password. Using the MEDLINE database from 1966 to the present, you first search for any articles containing the words "diaphragmatic hernia."

Search #1: Diaphragmatic hernia
Result #1: 1436 documents found

There are too many articles; you need to refine the search. Probably some references about acquired hernias are included, which you don't want. You next search for those articles from result #1 that contain the word "congenital."

Search #2: 1 and congenital
Result #2: 506 documents found

Better, but still too many articles. You wonder how many of these articles in result #2 contain the word "bilateral."

Search #3: 2 and bilateral
Result #3: 20 documents found

Fine! You can easily scan the titles and abstracts of 20 articles. You print a copy of the citations and abstracts. Tomorrow you will have the interesting ones copied from the bound journals. The entire process required less than ten minutes, although you might easily spend more time if you get absorbed in different searches.

FIGURE 21.1. Example of an electronic literature search.

categories, you can quickly retrieve most relevant references. This is often a good way to start a search, or to pursue a search that seems difficult to pin down. Lists of the MeSH are available in most medical libraries or from the U.S. National Technical Information Service.

Personal computers can access MEDLINE and other data bases through telephone lines using a modem. This service is typically sold as a subscription service [e.g., through the Bibliographic Retrieval Service (BRS Colleague)]. There is a membership fee and a usage charge based on connect time and the number of articles retrieved. BRS offers other on-line medical data bases, such as indexes (e.g., *Current Contents*), special topic collections (e.g. cancer literature), complete text of selected medical journals and textbooks, and other general reference sources (e.g., *Books in Print*, and the Index to U.S. Government Publications).

More recently, the MEDLINE data base has become available on CD-ROM (compact disk–Read-Only Memory)—a laserdisk similar to the audio compact disks. This CD-ROM requires a special disk reader, attached as an accessory to a personal computer. The disk is updated monthly and is usually maintained in a local central facility, such as the library. Once this investment has been made, users can take turns accessing the data base without incurring repeated charges from the commercial information services.

Reference Manager Programs

Reference manager programs build your own local data base of the articles you have selected as important. The reference data (title, journal, authors, abstract, comments) can be entered, filed, and searched by criteria similar to those given above. Although the data can be entered by the computer keyboard, it is possible and easier to transfer the data directly from a disk file using some reference managers. (See Chapter 8, above.)

Reference managers can also print lists of stored citations in different formats to suit different journal styles (e.g., "A.B. Author" vs. "Author, AB"). These citation lists can be appended to a manuscript; the need to type them over again in a new format for each different journal submission is eliminated.

Computerized Measurement and Control

Computers can be used to measure or control other signals or processes during research experiments by means of specialized software and hardware adapter boards designed to be compatible with a given type of computer—usually microcomputers or minicomputers.

Computer Data Acquisition

Data acquisition is a general process in which the computer "reads" an external signal and converts it to internal digital numbers. The external signal might be digital (i.e., binary on–off state) or any continuously varying analog waveform, such as a tracing of left ventricular pressure from a transducer. Analog signals are measured using an analog-to-digital (A/D—pronounced "A-to-D") converter that "samples" the level of a continuously varying analog signal at discrete time points. The values of the discrete points form a digitized signal that is really a series of numerical values (see Figure 21.2).

The primary advantage of A/D conversion is that the series of numerical values can be further processed within the computer, for example, to perform analyses that would be more difficult or impossible using the original analog waveform. For some types of data analysis, particularly on complex physiologic signals, A/D conversion is the only practical way to accomplish the desired analyses.

Analog-to-digital conversion is a relatively technical research use of computers. Be forewarned that it is advisable to consult an engineer or electrophysiologist to ensure that the system is doing what is desired of it; there are pitfalls involving transducers, amplifiers, grounding, filtering, A/D converter resolution, and sampling rates. For example, the sampled points must be close enough to reproduce the shape of the waveform faithfully; the required "sampling rate" depends on how rapidly the measured signal is changing—specifically, its high-frequency components. When the sampled points are close enough, the approximation is excellent; when they are not, "aliasing" results and the data can be very misleading.

Another aspect of A/D conversion is that digitized data are not necessarily easier to handle. A large number of data points are generated when a rapidly changing signal is sampled. For example, hemodynamic waveforms might be sampled at 200 points per second; digitizing four channels for 30 seconds would produce 24,000 data values. This mass of digitized raw data rarely provides the final answer to the question of interest. The effort required to review the data, process them to yield the appropriate results, and control for processing errors is large and involves more work than the actual process of acquisition. It can be worthwhile, however, if the results justify the investment.

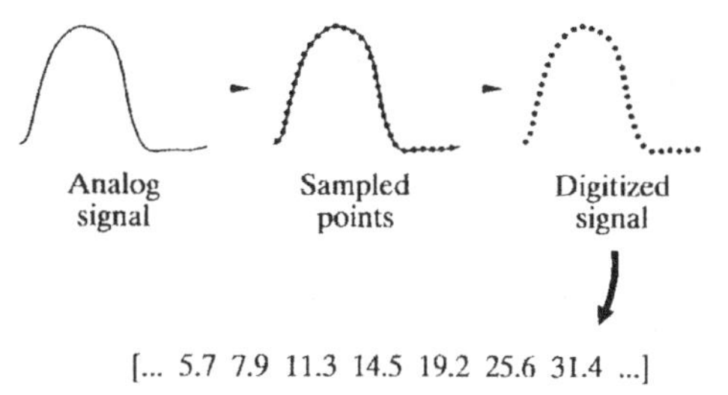

FIGURE 21.2. Analog signals are measured using an analog-to-digital converter that "samples" the level of a continuously varying analog signal at discrete time points. The values of the discrete points form a digitalized signal that is reallly a series of numerical values.

A simpler form of data acquisition is done with digitizing tablets that allow the researcher to quantify a graphic curve or surface area by tracing it with a special pen and tablet—for example, you can integrate the surface area of a tissue sample, or the area under a pressure tracing curve. These tools are similar to those described below under computer mice.

Computer Control in Experiments

Computers can send control information to instruments or other devices, as digital or analog signals (D/A conversion). These signals are used alone, or with signals sent back to the computer, to control and monitor instruments or experimental study processes.

Although computerized control is used less commonly than acquisition in research, it has definite applications in neurosciences and psychology (e.g., stimulus–response studies) and with experimental instruments and mechanisms. Menu-driven programs have made it easier to implement computer acquisition and control without deep expertise in computer programming, but they are still highly technical.

Some standard protocols permit communication between computers and instruments; for example, the General Purpose Instrument Bus (GPIB) allows a new patient ventilator with a built-in computer to connect to other computers using the GPIB standard. Data measured within the ventilator, such as the respiratory rate, volume, and pressure, can be transferred through the GPIB interface to another computer for study of patient ventilatory mechanics. Many different patient monitoring devices now use internal computers, but they do not usually adhere to any standard interface for

In the first non-normalized (incorrect) design, the data are spread out in four columns. The column headings contain implicit information about the data, namely the time the measurement was taken:

Patient no.	Pulse #1	Pulse #2	Pulse #3
101	80	72	90
102	75	88	100

To record other measurements at different times, the design must be changed (i.e., new columns must be added). If some patients don't have measurements at a given time, there are missing data values. It is more difficult to separate and sort the data.

In the normalized (correct) design, the data are stored in fewer columns, having generic names, and all information is stored in the data for each row. This creates a larger number of entries but offers more flexibility:

Patient no.	Visit no.	Date	Pulse
101	1	01-Mar-90	80
101	2	01-Apr-90	72
101	3	03-May-90	90
102	1	04-Feb-90	75
102	2	15-Mar-90	88
102	3	15-Apr-90	100

FIGURE 21.3. The concept of normalized data base structure.

their data transfer to other instruments or computers. Such standards have been proposed and will no doubt be accepted across the industry.

Analysis of Experimental Data or Studies

Microcomputers have put powerful tools for analysis of numerical or categorical data into researchers's hands (e.g., data bases, spreadsheets, statistical packages).

Data Bases

Storing and retrieving information in a data base is a traditional research use for computers. Data base applications with more friendly software design requiring less programming have proliferated in the microcomputer world. Many individuals or small departments now maintain records of patients and their diagnoses, treatments, operations, and outcomes on data base packages.

The most important factor in getting what you want from a data base is the design of the data structure or relationships. Because data base methods are so flexible, they can store or express data in many different ways with individual advantages and limitations. Simpler data bases use a "flat file" structure that can be represented as tabular entries on a sheet of paper with lines and columns. Other structures include the "hierarchical" and the "relational"; they are more complex and powerful.

Before you enter any data, define the structure and planned content of the data base to achieve the end result you want. The flexibility offered by data base programs allows the use of different designs; one might have a significant advantage over the others. One important consideration is "normal form," or normalized structure, which usually offers advantages of flexibility in manipulating and analysing the data; this concept is illustrated in Figure 21.3.

It is often difficult to make a data base work properly, or to predict exactly how it will be used before you have an opportunity to try it. To start, test the data base with a small amount of data, work out the wrinkles, and proceed with expansion when you know it is working properly. If you wish to revise a data base later in response to new questions, it may be difficult to modify data already entered.

Data collection and entry account for most of the cost of maintaining a data base and most of the errors. Because invalid or corrupt data are much more difficult to catch after entry, it is cost efficient to expend effort in providing quality control or "entry checks"; for example, in data fields involving text words (e.g., diagnoses), require all entries to be restricted to a valid set of words. Store a list of valid entries in a table and have the data base program automatically reject any that are not

An operating room keeps the surgical log on a data base to get "better case retrievals." But the operative procedure name has no entry controls or checks. The log is voluminous and contains the following scattered entries:

January 3	Left lower lobectomy
January 11	Resection right lower lobe
January 22	Right upper and middle lobectomies
January 31	Left upper lobecty

Searching for the number of "lobectomy" cases in January will produce the following erroneous result:

One case: January 3 Left lower lobectomy

The other three cases were not found because they did not literally match the term being searched.

FIGURE 21.4. Example in inaccurate data retrieval with "bad" entries.

included in the table. This prevents typographical errors or word sequence changes from becoming bad entries (Fig. 21.4) that could be missed in searches because they don't match a correctly formatted entry.

Spreadsheets

Electronic spreadsheets, developed primarily in the world of micro-computers, are relatively recent arrivals on the computer scene. Spreadsheets are electronic versions of ruled paper worksheets, which evolved as flexible tools for analysis of budgets, production figures, or other business data. For many people, this microcomputer application ranks second only to word processing.

A spreadsheet appears as a two-dimensional layout of rows and columns; each row–column intersection is one "cell"; each cell contains a number or text value. Formulas can be used to process the contents of certain "input" cells to create values for new "result" cells. Different input cell data or assumptions can be evaluated immediately, to allow comparison of different data results or scenarios.

Most spreadsheets offer automatic graphing of their data in such different formats as bar, line, or pie graphs. In early spreadsheet products, the graphic capabilities were more suited to business uses (e.g., high–low charts for stock market results), and most graphs fell short of the quality required for publication. Newer versions have added multiple x–y plots, statistical formulas, regression curve calculations and higher quality graphics output.

Because of their broad familiarity and ease of use, spreadsheets have become common and convenient tools for storing, reviewing, and analyzing numerical results. Users often find that their convenience offsets other limitations in their capabilities, especially for preliminary review of data and for making informal graphs for a quick look at data plots.

Statistical Packages

True statistical packages can perform sophisticated analyses on large or complex data sets; they are generally more complex and relatively less friendly than most other microcomputer applications. Data usually can be entered from the keyboard or from disk data files; the latter method is an important feature when the data are voluminous. Typically, the data are entered as a flat table of multiple cases (rows), each containing several variables (columns). Data transformations can be made using mathematical operations to convert the input data into some other desired form (e.g., the logarithm of a variable, or the ratio of two variables).

Statistical programs are called packages because they usually comprise multiple modules or "routines" to which the data can be submitted (e.g., for descriptive statistics, analysis of variance, regression analysis, plotting). It is not always obvious how the data must be organized for submission to the modules, or what assumptions are made in the analysis. The modules sometimes seem like black boxes expecting input and expressing output in standard ways. They are certainly easier to use if you are very familiar with standard statistical approaches; they are not helpful if you are uncertain about how you want to apply statistics to your data.

Given their complexity and less friendly interface, statistical packages are not efficient substitutes for standard statistical tables when you are performing simple tests, and they are rarely the easiest way to get simple data plots. Used properly, they can quickly perform complex statistical analyses on large sets of data and can help you tremendously—if you know what you want to do and learn how to work the statistical package.

Word Processing and Desktop Publishing

Word processing needs little explanation at present—it is indispensable for producing revisable or repetitive documents efficiently. The researcher need not use word processing directly to gain benefit from it; many prefer to write by hand or to dictate, and leave the word processing to a professional secretary. Others would rather type than write by hand, because they find it helpful to see their words and be able to modify them to their satisfaction.

There are endless debates about which word processor is "best." People tend to be strongly biased toward whichever word processor they are using well and, although differences exist, most of the mainstream word processors sold today are of very high quality, with very competitive features. A more important selection factor is that a group of people planning to share documents should use the same word processor. Documents can be transferred between different word processors, but the process is awkward, and some fine details of format can be lost.

Modern word processors offer several new advantages after some effort to master the new functions. Documents can be written under an outline structure that can be collapsed or expanded on the screen, to permit review of the overall structure and flow. Graphs, charts, or equations can be incorporated into a document as figures alongside the text; these figures can be imported from a variety of other charting or drawing programs. Different fonts or typefaces can be printed in a variety of point sizes, with excellent bold or italic characters. Some word processors have been designed especially for technical or scientific use and have such unusual capabilities as drawing organic molecular structures. Nevertheless, top quality standard word processors have enough capabilities for most researchers.

Desktop publishing (DTP) is a field akin to word processing, but oriented more toward dramatic printed output suitable for newsletters, flyers, or brochures. In comparison to word processors, a desktop publishing package might offer less advanced word processing features, but much more typographical flexibility. Examples of DTP features are larger assortments of typefaces and sizes, shading, graphics, and text flowing in different shaped columns. For most professional research reports, desktop publishing is unnecessary, but it may have a future for high impact poster presentations at meetings.

Presentation Graphics and Slide Making

Most research uses of computers do not require extensive use of color. Color monitors clarify and add interest, but printing colors is very expensive and generally less practical for formal written research. If a research report is printed using colors for graphical data, the color scale information is lost as soon as a black and white copy is made. Since virtually all written reports need to be copied, it is preferable to use black and white from the outset and code data by different symbol shapes rather than by colors.

Color is more important for high-quality presentation graphics and slides. Many presentation graphics programs can produce high quality color overhead transparencies or slides. Such programs often use a standard on-screen data entry "form" into which data are typed, as text or numbers. Many graphics programs can import data directly as a file transfer and this is useful for large amounts of data coming from an acquisition process, spreadsheet, or other source. The graphics program can automatically format the data into a picture, as text lines, or as a plot. Page-size color originals can be produced on paper or plastic transparencies using a color plotter or printer.

Slides can be made by photographing a color original printed from the computer, or by using an "image recorder" that accepts electronic output from the computer and directly produces exposed slide film. The image recorder functions as a computer-driven color display screen integrated with a camera. Once the slide film has been exposed, it is processed by standard color slide film techniques. Image recorders are often superior for slides because, unlike photographed paper originals, the slide background does not have to be white. Resist the temptation to use too many colors; they can distract your audience's attention from the information you are presenting.

Image recorders are available over a broad range of quality and cost. The least expensive, around $2000 US, produce lower quality slides—with about 600–800 lines of resolution and some jagged edges on curved lines or text—that are acceptable for local informal presentations. More expensive image recorders cost $10,000 and upward, yield 4000 or more lines of resolution, and produce higher quality slides suitable for formal national or international presentations. A more reasonably priced high-resolution image recorder is often found in the medical illustrations department at research or educational institutions. If one is available, check it out before you acquire software, to make sure you get something compatible.

Some commercial services use image recorders to make slides from a mailed disk or files transmitted by modem over telephone lines. They usually produce top-quality slides that can be returned to you by mail within a few days. Such services are more costly, but not as expensive as having professional artwork created and made into slides. Compatibility of your software with the commercial company's is required. (See also Section IV, Chapter 48.)

Types of Computer

What types of computer are used in research? How do they differ? Are personal computers always the best answer?

Virtually everyone has some exposure to personal computers, and many researchers first think of computing as having their own "PC." Some needs are best met, however, by computers of other types that are larger than personal computers. Each has its own characteristics and particular uses, but the boundaries between the three different types are somewhat blurred.

Large Computers: Mainframes

Large "mainframes," the most expensive computers, are usually found in centralized computing facilities of universities or hospitals. They are staffed by professionals, such as engineers, programmers, and technicians, who provide maintenance and support for the users. These computers are designed to handle vast amounts of data with more power and speed than smaller ones, and to share programs and data among many different users simultaneously. Being a shared resource, they offer less flexibility for individuals to select their own programs. Most researchers using mainframes depend to some extent on the programmers to set up or manipulate their data.

Any large data set requiring access by multiple contributors or users (e.g., a multicenter experimental trial, a national tumor registry) should be handled in a mainframe facility or, at least, one organized like a mainframe. In mainframe facilities, the approach to data base management includes formal methods for controlling the creation, maintenance, and protection of data records. In these shared data base situations, controls at entry or by specific audit checks can catch such potential errors as inconsistencies or duplications, and can perform the important function of maintaining the integrity and quality of the data.

You might choose a mainframe or professional computing facility for one-time or infrequent use, especially when you need to have the work done for you. Programmers are experts who can contribute valuable services and free your time for potentially better investment elsewhere.

Medium-Size Computers: Minicomputers

Minicomputers are scaled-down versions of mainframes; their cost, speed, and capacity lie between those of mainframes and personal computers. They function as shared facilities for small groups of researchers (e.g., 5 to 20) and require small staffs (e.g., 1 to 4) for their operation. The staff of each shared facility is an important resource, and the users can have more say in selection and hiring. The researchers will also have to pay for an annual maintenance contract, usually purchased from the computer vendor.

Since the computer is under local control, the users generally have more influence over the types of program used, and the facility can work more directly for their specific goals. More friendly and "personal computer" type software is becoming available for minicomputers, and they may become a more practical solution for shared personal computing functions.

Small Computers: Microcomputers

What about microcomputers? When is it better to use your own personal computer?

Microcomputers have developed as "grass roots" tools to meet the computing needs of individuals and are often easier to use than larger computers. Nevertheless, their potential is great and they yield more to those who invest more effort. Although they have less speed and capacity than larger computers, microcomputers often provide better performance and flexibility for the individual because each machine is completely dedicated to one user.

Better microcomputer programs often provide excellent features not found in their minicomputer or mainframe counterparts. As personal computers rapidly become faster and more powerful, there is a trend to making their software more friendly and helpful to relieve the user of more burdensome tasks. An example is the capacity of word processors to maintain convenient lists of documents, or to automatically generate a table of contents and an index. The microcomputer marketplace is so

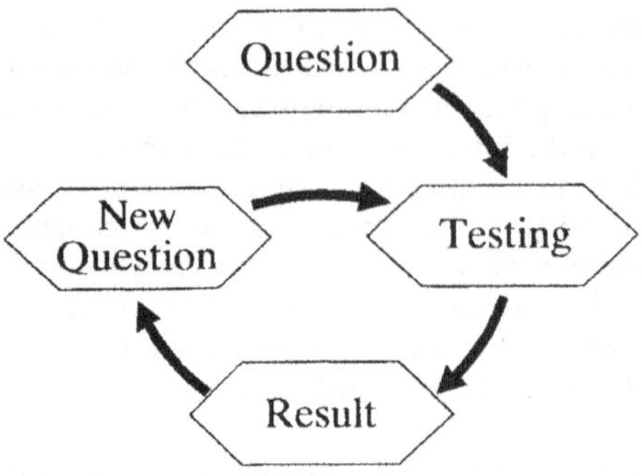

FIGURE 21.5. Reiterative cycle of question–trial–answer–new question.

TABLE 21.1. Summary of the advantages and disadvantages of larger vs personal computers.

Larger computers	Personal computers
More powerful resource	Better performance and responsiveness for individual tasks
Less direct access and personal control	More direct access and flexibility
Tighter control of shared data	More individual control over data and programs
Slower, indirect question-answer cycle	Rapid interactive question-answer cycle
Professional programmer can provide expert advice	User needs to know correct usage
Pooled maintenance efforts	Local responsibility for maintenance of data and system

dynamic and competitive that it continually offers more powerful products without a proportional increase in cost.

Along with their greater control and flexibility, microcomputers bring added responsibilities for operation and routine maintenance. You, or someone, must make the effort to install, customize, and preserve the integrity of your system and its data.

The benefits of microcomputers lie more in their capability, flexibility, and accessibility than in the idea that they will cost less. The start-up costs are smaller, but the continuing costs of time, effort, and system expansion can rise to equal or exceed the costs of providing each person with access to a shared facility. The point is that these costs may be justified by the additional flexibility provided.

One might liken computers to transportation. It is cheaper to buy a personal automobile than a bus, but individuals sharing a bus can travel more cheaply and the passengers don't have to perform the bus maintenance, personally. The automobile costs more in money and effort for the individual user, but it may be worth it if gets him somewhere in a time frame that the bus cannot match.

One specific advantage of personal computing in research is the "personal" aspect, that is, the direct interaction between you and your computer in getting what you are looking for: information. This interaction can be stimulating, and your expertise can improve the yield of information. This is particularly true when you are exploring any data, as in a literature search, or an evaluation of experimental results. Such exploration tends to be reiterative, a cycle of question–trial–answer–new question, like the scientific method. Your direct involvement in this cycle can accelerate the process, and provide changing direction according to the ongoing findings (see Figure 21.5).

Selecting the Computer Size Appropriate to Your Needs

What size of computer should you use? You can decide, on the basis of your specific needs, whether you want a larger or a personal computer. Their advantages and disadvantages are summarized in Table 21.1.

You might choose a larger shared computing facility if:

You require the special capabilities of a larger computer, or have infrequent need for computer services.
Multiple contributors need to submit and share the same data.
You have convenient access to a facility, or you have a group wishing to establish one.
You can identify an expert resource person who can help you achieve your goals.

You might take the personal computer approach if:

Your goals and intended uses are more compatible with microcomputer features and software.
You have the interest and willingness to learn microcomputing and to maintain your own system.
You wish to have the most direct control and fastest response time to your questions.
You have a friendly "local expert" who can assist you through your initiation into microcomputers.

If You Need a Larger Computer

If you have identified a need for mainframe or minicomputers, and are new to the business, seek the assistance of a resource person expert in the type of work you want to accomplish. He or she can provide valuable help in reviewing your plan before you implement it, advising you about its practicality and any potential pitfalls. You may need to hire a consultant, or someone may offer to help on a courtesy basis. In either case, you should define and express your goals as clearly and specifically as possible.

If you plan to use an existing mainframe, the easily identified experts are the professionals who operate the system. The services of a programmer may be necessary, or you may prefer to learn some techniques (e.g., data base entry and query) yourself. The estimated costs for services and computer time can be compared to your budget. Others who use the same system can offer the benefit of their experience in interacting with the mainframe facility, and can tell you how they have used its resources.

If you need to establish a minicomputer system, you should talk to others at your institution who have had experience with similar systems. Minicomputers are usually sold by regional manufacturers' representatives, and level of service is important. In general, buying mainstream hardware and software from a reliable representative, while possibly not the smallest initial cost, can save money in the long run when problems arise.

Larger computers and microcomputers are not mutually exclusive. People sometimes get microcomputers to communicate with mainframes in order to take advantage of such facilities as a centralized data base (e.g., MEDLINE).

Developing a Microcomputer System

After they have considered the different types of computers, many researchers will decide to develop or use their own microcomputer system. Because the microcomputer user may have fewer identifiable mechanisms for self education and support, some general perspectives and lessons gained from experience are offered to those just getting started.

Identify Local Experts and Support

In the world of microcomputers, experience has shown that most organizations tend to have "local experts"–users who have delved extensively into various types of application. Usually, these experts are willing to help others get started, and they are an excellent potential resource of support. Realize that most experts have some personal biases that may not reflect your needs; try to determine which specific factors they consider to be positive or negative features of different products or solutions.

Many institutions have formal organizations that provide microcomputer support. As part of their service, they may give suggestions about product selection, demonstrations, sales, instruction on software use, and maintenance service contracts. Because they know the microcomputer users at the institution, they can guide you to someone who may be using a specific product of potential interest to you. Their work usually involves trials of different software and hardware, and they can often comment on such specifics.

General institutional policies regarding hardware or software selection are often set by such organizations to maintain sharing of information and avoid the "Tower of Babel" syndrome. If one secretary who normally handles a manuscript becomes ill near the submission deadline, another will need to be able to work on it. Having many different hardware and software products is comparable to having a different keyboard pattern for each typewriter. When many people use the same products, everyone gains from sharing experience and expertise. Such standardization policies have merit up to the point at which they infringe on the needs of users; people do need some flexibility to use different products to solve their unique problems.

Decide Who Will Maintain Your System

Every microcomputer system, whether it consists of one personal computer or many, needs routine setup and maintenance, even when there is no hardware breakdown. The vendor will often provide initial setup, but the situation is rarely static. There are such continuing maintenance needs as new software installation, customizing individual software or hardware, problem shooting, testing new functions, and organizing backup methods for programs and data. If computers are communicating or being shared (e.g., on a local area network) operation of the network itself is required.

Although your friendly local experts may be willing to offer advice or demonstrate solutions, their guidance is a courtesy and they generally cannot set up and maintain your system for you completely. A decision has to be made about who will be the expert supporting your system.

You can become an expert yourself, if you choose to do so. All it takes is time, motivation, and effort to get experience; the skills required are generally within the reach of anyone doing research. Being your own expert is most advantageous in matters closely related to your own research, such as literature searching or interactive data analysis; it is less necessary in something less data intensive, like word processing. The advantage is that your closer contact with the literature or data enhances the professional direction, accuracy, or turnover time of the research process (see Fig. 21.5).

If you are a clinician or investigator, managing your own microcomputer system may not be worthwhile. Paid consultants are available to set up a system with complex applications, such as a data base, and they will maintain it for a fee. This route, which resembles a smaller version of the traditional mainframe approach, tends to be selected when your own time and the reliable operation of the system are more important priorities than keeping your expenditures low.

In some research situations, a professional colleague who is also a microcomputer expert might be interested in collaborating with you and others on a project utilizing microcomputers. Such a person may assume responsibility for operating and maintaining the microcomputer system on behalf of the group, especially if it involves direct acquisition, review, and analysis of the research data. In this case, the expert functions as a collaborator in the research project, not as a technician. Such an arrangement provides an opportunity to get the most from the microcomputer capabilities, because the system operator has direct and professional knowledge of the problem being researched.

Like any other machines, microcomputers and their peripherals can break down or develop problems. Support for maintenance and repair is necessary and should, preferably, be prearranged by service contract. The vendor, or your institution's microcomputer organization, can usually provide support contracts that cover maintenance and possibly the loan of parts during repairs.

Approach to Selecting Software and Hardware

When you decide to use a microcomputer, you are immediately confronted with choices of hardware and software. New products are coming out constantly. What do you need?

The first principle of selection is, the software works for you—the hardware just makes the software work. In other words, choose the software you need to accomplish what you want, first. Then be sure to get hardware that runs the software to its best advantage.

The two mainstream standards among microcomputers are those spawned by Apple and by IBM. Both have extensive software and hardware product lines, but they are fundamentally incompatible with each other. It is difficult to generalize fairly, but Apple has put somewhat more emphasis on graphics, drawing, desktop publishing, and pictorial ("icon") representation. The IBM world, which includes numerous compatibles or "clones," has been more oriented toward business uses, word processing, and the other scientific uses discussed in this chapter. Cross-fertilization and similarity between the two has been developing, gradually. It is generally simpler to use one type exclusively, or both separately. If you need to use both and have them communicate, network products to meet that need can be purchased.

The second principle of selection is to stay near mainstream or popular products, because of compatibility: software and hardware products are not all born compatible with each other, they must be made compatible by their producers. Development costs tend to make producers provide compatibility for other popular mainstream products, but not necessarily for more obscure products. One measure of the quality or usefulness of a given product is the number of other products it is compatible with.

Your investment is most effective, even potentiated, if your choice has extensive compatibility—either broadly with numerous other products, or deeply with intensive links to a single important product. For example, data acquisition, analysis, or statistical software should have broad compatibility to exchange data between different programs (i.e., standard data file import or export formats). Your word processor needs close enough compatibility with your printer to produce accurately such finer features as bold or italic text, tables, and graphics.

The most popular program or machine is not necessarily, however, the one for you. The most popular "best" products usually do have recognized quality and will meet most general needs, but every product has its tradeoffs and limitations. If you have very specific needs, and purchase the popular "best" without checking that it will meet them, you may be disappointed to find your needs are not met. You might find it helpful to investigate several of the top products of a given type to find which is more usable or specifically suitable to your requirements. If you are not too sure about what your specific needs are, or can't tell what suits you better, you need more experience; select a good general product, get the experience, and realize that you may need different products as your needs become clearer.

The newest computers with "hot new chips" are not always the best investments; despite their premium prices, the newest hardware often has features that cannot be utilized for several years because of a lag in the production of software to exploit them. Accordingly, "the best" is a moving target with steeply diminishing returns; many experts find it preferable to stay one hardware generation behind the leading edge, where the market breadth has matured to provide the most capabilities.

Specifics about IBM-type Microcomputers

General advice in the IBM-compatible market dictates avoidance of machines with the oldest processors, the 8088 or 8086, except in very lightweight portable computers. Equipment in the 80286 or the 80386 family is appropriate for lighter or heavier duty applications, respectively. In scientific work, a "math coprocessor" chip, such as an 80287 or 80387, is often helpful or necessary.

The VGA standard monitor provides a very satisfactory combination of color and resolution and is very broadly supported as a compatibility standard. The Hercules monochrome graphics adapter is also a good standard; it is less expensive and a good choice if your budget is more important than color capability.

Fixed disks, also called hard disks, have much more capacity and speed than floppy disks. Their prices are low enough, and their impact helpful enough, that virtually every machine should be using one. Whereas the first microcomputer hard disks came out with 10 megabyte capacity, something in the 30 to 40 megabyte range is a now reasonable minimum. If you plan to store large amounts of data, make a careful estimate of the storage volume needed and get a large enough disk at the start.

Some method of backup for hard disk data is required. Floppy disks can be used, but because they are relatively slow and tedious to use, they tend not to be chosen when reliable backups for larger hard disks are called for. Tape backup systems are most commonly used; other "removable hard disk" storage media, such as the Bernoulli disk, are more expensive, but they are very flexible and can double as hard disk storage space. The need for greater storage and backup capacity can also be met through the LAN approach, discussed in the next section.

Another question is whether to invest more in the top quality name manufacturers or spend less on cheaper "clones." This clearly depends on your resources and your vulnerability to breakdown problems. Breakdowns are rare but crippling, and other service may be needed to add future enhancements to your system. The less expensive brands can provide more power for a given price, but buying too cheaply, or without good service, can be more expensive in the long run—especially if you are stuck with data frozen inside a broken lump of electronics.

Select your vendor with an eye on support for maintenance and repair, especially for hardware. Because there is keen competition in microcomputer sales, you should expect to get good service after the sale. The vendor should be an authorized dealer buying through approved channels; you don't want machines from the gray market—they could be difficult to service. Check with others who have purchased from different sources and ask them if they have had good experience with their vendor's maintenance or repair services. Initial cost is not the only consideration in choosing what and where to buy; it may be worth paying a bit more to purchase from a source that provides better service after the sale.

Data Exchange and Microcomputer Communications

As your experience with microcomputers grows, you may wish to extend the breadth of your data communications. Different types of communication are possible, between programs on one machine or between different machines, and it is sometimes appealing to share such peripherals as expensive printers.

Data interchange between different application programs, even on one machine, reduces data entry effort and associated errors. For example, numeric data acquired by analog-to-digital conversion can be exported in electronic form to spreadsheet or statistical programs for analysis. The analyzed data can be transferred into graphics programs to produce publication-quality figures. Graphics, such as plots or figures, can be imported into word processing documents for reports or grant applications. Such transfers require standard data exchange formats that must be available in the sending and receiving packages. Several standard formats have arisen, such as ASCII, DIF, SYLK, Metafile, and Lotus Worksheet formats.

Communication between different microcomputers can also be accomplished by a variety of means. The least elaborate and cheapest method is by "asynchronous" communication, often called RS-232 or serial port communication. This method is useful for connecting two nearby machines (e.g., a desktop computer and a laptop portable) to transfer data. Asynchronous data can be transferred at different speeds measured in bits per second–commonly called "baud"–in a range of 300 to 19,200 baud. The faster transfer rates are naturally more desirable to reduce waiting time; both machines have to be set at the same baud and other asynchronous control parameters, such as parity, number of data bits, and stop bits. If the two machines are adjacent, one of several laptop linking programs can facilitate the transfer. Asynchronous communications are also used to communicate with other computers over telephone lines, but each computer requires a "modem" (MOdulator-DEModulator) device that transforms between computer digital signals and telephone sound signals. With a modem, you can connect to public information or telecommunication networks and access the MEDLINE data base. Since telephone network lines are prone to transmission errors when higher baud rates are used, most public networks use 1200 or 2400 baud. Data compression and error correction techniques, used in some specialized modems, provide effective transmission at speeds up to 9600 baud, even though they still transmit at 2400 bits per second. Unfortunately, there is no uniform standard, and different compression modems may not be able to communicate with each other. Specialized modems make sense only when you are communicating locally and the type of modem is standardized. For general communications with other modems of unknown type, the straight 1200 or 2400 baud is more compatible.

A different solution exists for individuals in a department who want to share data or resources among their microcomputers, very frequently. Local area networks (LANs) can provide this capability. Typically, one larger, faster microcomputer may act as a network "server" or common resource for disk space, programs, printers, backup facilities, etc. A group of users can share a word processing program on the server machine, keep their data files there, and have them backed up routinely with the rest of the server disk. These networks require a designated manager to maintain operation and provide services to the individual users. A microcomputer LAN can be structured to provide the best of individual flexibility and group efficiency; it may also allow more collaborative interaction and information sharing among coworkers.

Peripherals for Microcomputers

Microcomputers need different accessory devices, called peripherals, for different types of input and output, but they are not always compatible with all computers and programs. Many programs and peripherals interact through a small special program called a driver; each driver usually matches one particular computer or application program to one specific type of peripheral. When you select a peripheral, be sure a compatible driver is available for your specific computer or application software.

A printer is almost always a necessity, and you should usually buy one with the computer. Paper copies of records and data are indispensable as permanent archives and as backup copies in case of disk failure. Reviewing and editing manuscripts is often done with much better perspective on printed copy to appreciate the final impression. Most printers can handle simple text directly from the computer; but word processing programs need to print special text, such as underline, bold, italic, superscripts and subscripts. These more elaborate printing styles require that the printer have a matching driver in the specific word processing program used.

Laser printers have become an excellent standard for speed and output quality; they can even substitute for plotting devices and produce excellent graphics with appropriate software. The most common standard laser printer is probably the Hewlett-Packard Laserjet line. Laser printers do have drawbacks, including higher price, difficulty in feeding envelopes, blurring of heat-bonded inks, and inability to imprint through multiple copy forms; if none of these bother you, think first of getting a laser printer. Inkjet printers are a decent, quiet substitute at less cost. Impact printers are noisy but have been reliable for many years; they can print through on multipart forms. There are two types of impact printers: dot matrix and printwheel. Dot matrix types are more flexible for graphics, and the least expensive. Although their print quality is generally lower, there are very usable models that use more pins to produce "near letter quality." True letter quality (printwheel) printers provide excellent quality output but are slow, noisy, and lacking in graphics capabilities; they are often replaced by laser printers.

Modems are available as internal cards placed inside the microcomputer, or external boxes attached to the computer by cables. Both connect to one of the computer's serial ports and have connectors for attaching them to a telephone outlet. The internal boards are more convenient because they require fewer external cables; the external box is useful if the computer's internal board slots are full. They are used for asynchronous communication between computers or with outside communication networks. Compatibility is necessary between the modem and its controlling software; this is most likely when both products use the same standard, the most common being the Hayes command set.

Pointing peripherals can be used to manipulate a cursor around the computer display screen; the most common one is the hand-held mouse—a small plastic object shaped something like a bar of soap, that is moved around on a flat surface to draw or point the cursor, especially in graphics programs, because the keyboard cursor movement keys are too awkward. Mice are less helpful in text-oriented programs like word processors. They usually require drivers, and the most common compatibility standard is the Microsoft mouse.

Image scanners resemble copiers that input a flat image into the computer in electronic format, as a graphics file. They can be used to scan images, text, or even real objects placed on a scanning stage. Text interpretation is somewhat limited because it usually requires special typeface to be legible. Once they are internalized, the images can be manipulated with compatible graphics programs.

Try Before You Buy... But Don't Defer Starting

When you are considering implementation of a new microcomputer project, remember that the capabilities of particular software or hardware, may not be exactly as they appear or as you imagine them to be. Many optimistic users have invested in systems and later found that the capabilities were less than they expected. This is true even for experts, as compatibility problems between different software and hardware can produce unexpected results.

The best principle is to try to see and use a given system in operation, and test it for your purposes before you invest in it. This is not difficult for mainstream software and hardware, because most computer stores or vendors will allow you to try demonstration products on their premises. Less commonly used items may be more difficult to test, since demonstration samples may not be available. Ask around your organization to see if anyone is using the products in which you are interested. If your department or institution has a computing facility or information management office, see if it can obtain a product sample to test.

Ultimately, your productivity and expertise will be the result of the effort you invest and the experience you gain. Don't defer starting to wait for more advanced products or the perfect situation. The time you wait is lost experience. Make your best plan, do a prudent amount of testing to detect obvious flaws, then dive in to work with it and get your experience. The sooner you gain experience at the work you want to do, the more expert you will become and the more successful your efforts will be.

22

Ten Tips on Preparing Research Proposals*

W.O. Spitzer

New or potential investigators with good research ideas often fail to take even the first step in exploring or implementing them. This usually happens when the required resources do not appear to be available. Young investigators and even mature clinicians with strong track records in teaching and service become unduly discouraged at the thought of writing a study protocol, submitting to peer appraisal, and overcoming all the real and imaginary hurdles associated with the preparation of grant applications.

Unfortunately, clinicians who practice outside universities and colleges and whose ongoing contact with the "real world" makes their work particularly relevant to the needs of patients are among those who are most easily discouraged. They assume they do not have the ability or the credentials required to generate the financial support their project needs and merits, and they make no effort to seek it.

Although some skills are necessary, and there is a "right way" to do certain things, much of what is needed to prepare a research proposal is common sense. Seasoned investigators with long careers have learned most of what they need to know about writing grant applications from the comments, recommendations, and objections of the peer reviewers of their earlier proposals.

The suggestions that follow are not intended as a "checklist" that will guarantee your success in "shaking the money tree" of research foundations and other research funding agencies. They are simply some tips learned over the years from colleagues and passed on to the reader. Anybody venturing into research is certain to make mistakes at first; the suggestions that follow may help you to avoid some predictable pitfalls.

Before you consider each of the ten points, it is important that you realize that undertaking research without a protocol is irresponsible, at best, and unethical at worst. Doing so is just as reprehensible as embarking on the construction of a building without approved blueprints from an architect. As a general recommendation, avoid initiating or participating in "off the cuff" or "informal" research when no effort has been made to develop a plan, rationalize it, and commit it to writing in advance. Writing a grant proposal accomplishes these goals, whether it is funded on the first submission or not.

1. State Your Objective and Study Questions Clearly

When you come upon a good idea, an intriguing hypothesis, a burning question, or an important demonstration project, write your thoughts down, promptly. Then, preferably within days, carefully restate your project or study. Two important steps must now be taken; neglect of either will frequently jeopardize the quality of the rest of your work. First, write the broad objective of the study. Second, formulate the specific questions your research project seeks to answer.

Try to limit the questions to two or three; if you find yourself writing more than five or six, your objectives may be vague and your concepts woolly. Questions should be phrased to permit objective and preferably quantitative answers. Here are some examples:

Example I

Objective. To determine whether the introduction of a system in which a senior general surgery resident functions as a consultant in the emergency ward of a teaching hospital would expedite the handling of patients with surgical problems.

*Adapted with permission from Spitzer WO. Ten tips on preparing research proposals. Can Nurse 1973; 69(3): 30–33.

Related Study Questions

1. Is the span of time from the arrival of a patient in the triage station in the emergency ward to a disposition (i.e., discharge home or admission to hospital) reduced?
2. Are calls to other senior surgical residents and to surgical attending staff in the hospital to come to the emergency room reduced after introduction of the on-site surgical resident compared to the previous situation?
3. Does an assessment of the quality of surgical care for nonelective conditions, using a quantitative index developed specifically for surgical problems commonly seen in the emergency room, indicate any improvement following introduction of the new arrangement.

Example II

Objective. To determine whether a strategy of transporting trauma patients to hospitals that involves limiting intervention at the accident site or in transit to first aid and essential lifesaving maneuvers is preferable to deploying surgeons with sophisticated equipment to accident sites to initiate more immediate and definitive treatment.

Related Research Questions

1. What are the rates of mortality and of serious residual morbidity for cases treated with the first versus the second approach after adjustments have been made for case mix and severity?
2. What are the direct and indirect costs of the first compared with the second approach?
3. What are the barriers to the feasibility of each approach in urban and rural areas? ("Urban" and "rural" will have been operationally defined very carefully.)

Example III

Objective. To determine whether a specific preoperative bowel preparation in conjunction with intravenous administration of antibiotic *X* improves the results of aortofemoral grafting in patients with selected types of aortoiliac occlusive disease and abdominal aortic aneurysms.

Related Study Questions

1. What is the immediate postoperative morbidity (i.e., within 72 hours) of patients who receive the bowel preparation plus antibiotic *X* compared to those who receive antibiotic *X* alone?
2. What is the infection rate in the aortofemoral grafts within 30 days of the operation among patients in each of the arms of the study?
3. What are the 1-year and 5-year survival rates for patients in each arm of the study?
4. Do intervening dental procedures, minor operations, or viral or bacterial infections, such as pneumonia or gastroenteritis, affect the survival and morbidity rates for patients in each arm of the study?

When you have rewritten your objectives and study questions several times, review them with colleagues whose opinions you respect. They are likely to give you candid comments on the clarity of your objective, the feasibility of the project, and whether your research questions are sensible and amenable to research.

2. Study the Background Literature and Summarize It in Your Proposal

It is important to determine whether the kind of study or project you propose has already been done. Those who are asked to review grant applications are usually very knowledgeable in the appropriate field and are aware of related work reported in the literature or in progress. It is unlikely that you will be granted support for a project that is equivalent to seeking to "reinvent the typewriter." Expert advice on how to review the literature is provided above (Chapters 7 and 9).

When you have reviewed the literature, write it up briefly. If you are not breaking completely new ground, you should demonstrate how or why your project would shed new light on a problem already studied by others, how you will obtain new knowledge, or how you will test an innovative application of existing knowledge. If your emphasis is on application of existing techniques or knowledge, you should indicate the relevance of your work in such terms as "benefit to patients" or '"greater efficiency attained."

3. Decide on General Strategy

Before you consider the detailed tactics you might adopt (e.g., selection of comparison groups, delineation of criteria, selection of samples, scoring techniques), design your general strategy. Are you proposing a demonstration model? Will you be conducting a survey? Do you plan a true experiment? The nature of your objective and your research questions will usually suggest the proper strategy. When two or more approaches would be suitable your choice should be based on which is the most feasible and practical.

A common pitfall is to seek support from a research funding agency for a project that is clearly not research. If you are trying to establish a service or educational project, such as a counseling center for adolescents who have sustained serious skiing accidents, you should apply to granting agencies whose terms of reference include the provision of funds for service or educational programs on the basis of their merit rather than an agency whose primary focus is on research into the pathophysiology and treatment of trauma.

4. Identify the Most Appropriate Funding Agency

You should investigate whether accepted procedures or ethical considerations justify your applying to more than one funding agency for support for the same project. It is important to make a decision about possible sources of funds at this stage because the tactics you specify in your detailed research design may be influenced or even determined in part by the known policies of a funding agency. Most funding agencies publish their terms of reference and you should obtain and study them before proceeding.

5. Seek Expert Consultations

This is the time to consult some experts. Although you may have spoken with colleagues or other advisers when you formulated your objectives and study questions, you should now consult with resource persons, such as research methodologists, biostatisticians, or other experts in the field that concerns you. Too often, consultations are sought *after* a grant application has been rejected or the data have been gathered. By that time, it is usually too late for a consultation to be of much help to you. Consultation with the administration staff and with the director of the agency to which you are planning to apply is an invaluable but often neglected step. You can learn what is "fundable" under the agencies' present guidelines, and you can obtain many valuable suggestions about your application. For a major grant or contract, it is worthwhile to do this in person.

At most institutions, there are experienced investigators who have well-developed skills in the field of "grantsmanship." Do not hesitate to enlist their support in planning your grant. A critical review of the finished grant by such an adviser can be extremely valuable, even if the consultant is outside your field.

When you seek expert advice about your research design, it is wise to consider some ethical questions. Are there any risks to patients or other individuals who may become study subjects? If there are, do they outweigh the potential benefits to such individuals or to the population in general? Will the study subjects be free from invasion of their privacy or any form of personal assault? Are reasonable safeguards incorporated in the design to protect the confidentiality of personal or clinical information? Is it ethical in your particular study to withhold some treatment from a control group?

The following commitment, in these or equivalent terms, should be included in your grant application:

> The individuals and families involved in this investigation would enjoy freedom from assault: personal privacy, the ability to withdraw from the experiment at any time, and the confidentiality of all personal information obtained would be scrupulously protected. The applicants have carefully weighed the potential gains from the new knowledge that would be obtained from this investigation and have concluded that they vastly outweigh the risks to the individuals involved in this project. Consent to take part in this investigation will be requested only after full disclosure of the nature of the project and of any potential risks to the prospective participant associated with the delivery of health services in the proposed fashion.

Some agencies require a statement on ethics (i.e., approval of the project by a properly constituted ethics review committee) in each proposal, along with copies of the consent forms that will be used.

6. Specify the Criteria You Will Use to Evaluate the Answers to Your Study Questions and the Success of Your Project

Unless you indicate what kind of objective or quantitative answers to your research questions will constitute a particular verdict, your proposal may be regarded as a self-fulfilling prophecy. Specifying the criteria for judging the answers to research questions, *in advance*, usually distinguishes the disciplined and rigorous investigator from the wishful thinker who is out to prove a point. If we refer back to question 3 under Example I, the criterion for success might be:

Criterion. Bowel preparation plus antibiotic *X* will be judged to be better than antibiotic *X* alone if two of the following three outcomes are demonstrated:

1. The immediate postoperative morbidity in the combined approach is not only less than that with antibiotic alone, but is less than 2%.
2. The rate of infection of patients treated with the combined approach is 20% less than it is in those treated with antibiotic alone within 30 days of the operation.
3. The 1-year and 5-year survival rates for patients treated with the combined approach are at least 20% better than they are in those treated with antibiotic alone.

Although negative findings in a study tend to be viewed as evidence that it failed, it may really have been successful if it provided strong, irrefutable evidence that settled a question. *The success of a study or project is not determined by the verdict it yielded, but by the quality of the evidence it produced.* Consequently, it is wise to spell out the criteria that will determine the success of your project separately from the criteria to be used in evaluating the answers to your study question.

7. Be as Brief and Clear as Possible

Reviewers of grants are not particularly interested in reading countless typed pages. Most successful grant applications for clinical or health care research projects are not longer than 10 to 15 pages. Unnecessary verbiage reflects unfavorably on the applicant's ability to think clearly and communicate effectively. Brevity, however, should not be carried to the point of failure to communicate why your group is distinctive and able to make a significant contribution. If your proposal covers a large study involving several centers and a complex design, the detailed descriptions required may justify an application that is considerably longer.

Funding agencies take pride in identifying and supporting investigators who will be effective in solving problems. A helpful stratagem you can incorporate in the significance section of your grant application is to point out that your institution has already assembled most of the pieces of the puzzle. You can show, for example, with solid documentation, that you have access to all the patients needed for the study, most of the required laboratory equipment, and a well-developed plan with a proven record of productivity; *all you need* is support to obtain the few missing pieces of the puzzle. In other words, the granting agency can underwrite a solution to the problem very economically by supporting your research plan to provide the last few pieces of the puzzle.

Although the suggested outline for grant applications provided in Appendix I will require modification for each study and may have to be changed to conform with different requirements in various countries, it may be useful in getting your thinking started and in assembling the information you will need.

8. Keep Appendices and Supporting Documents to a Minimum

Lengthy appendices, supporting documents, and bibliographies will produce a cumbersome application. The reviewer will usually feel compelled to read them and may well be irritated when he has finished if the appendices do not contribute much. An appendix or supporting document should be included only if the proposal cannot be understood without it and it is clearly inappropriate to include the information (e.g., the precise format of an interview form) in the main body of the application. If you are in doubt, state what the document contains briefly in the text of your proposed and indicate that it is available on request. Do not attach it.

9. Be Realistic in Your Assessment of the Available and Required Resources

Do not propose to hire categories of professionals that are not available in your setting or community. If the execution of your project depends on nonexistent human or other resources, or on equipment you cannot maintain, you should not be applying for support. On the other hand, identifying *by name* the person who will perform a task strengthens the proposal by its concreteness.

Ascertain very carefully what funds you will need for salaries, equipment, supplies, specialized services, consultants, and other items. Underestimating what you require will cause you unnecessary difficulties when you come to carry out your study. Deliberately overestimating the cost of the required resources will undermine your credibility during the first review or when you submit your annual progress report.

The peers who will judge the merits of your proposal and assess its progress when you submit renewal requests are usually aware that errors of judgment can be made in estimating the requirements for a study; most of them have experienced such embarrassments and are sympathetic. Reviewers can be expected to be reasonable about applications for amendments of budgets when such requests are sensible and caused by unforeseeable contingencies. It is much better to submit supplementary requests, if the need arises, than to "pad" a submission at the outset.

10. Prepare and Justify Your Budget Carefully

Most granting agencies provide preprinted application forms that include the required breakdown of requested funding into budgeting categories. Nevertheless many research proposals are submitted without adequate justification of the expenditures included in the various categories or without enough detail about the budget as a whole to enable the appraiser to link listed items of expenditure with the activities described in the project.

Your justification of your budget should explain the need for each individual for whom a salary (or wages) is requested, for every item of equipment, for each category of supplies, for travel, and for any other special requirements.

It is wise to identify any major expenditure for which the estimates are not firm. Should budgetary difficulties concerning an uncertain estimate arise later, prior identification of the potential problem will have paved the way for approval of any necessary amendment.

Conclusion

Preparing a research proposal and applying for its support need not be dreaded as an unavoidable tournament that must precede any rewarding research activity. Designing a project, exploring feasible approaches to its implementation, identifying the resources needed, and communicating all this information in a grant application are integral components of investigative activity. If you don't win the award the first time, you have still organized your project. Seek a detailed critique from the reviewers, revise your application, and resubmit it. The whole process is intellectually challenging and can even be enjoyable.

Appendix I

Suggested Outline for a Research Protocol

A. Summary (300 words or less)
B. Main protocol

1. The objective and research question(s)
   a. Objective
   b. Question(s)—may be restated as a hypothesis or hypotheses if desired or appropriate
   c. Significance of the problem to health care or biomedical science
2. Review of pertinent literature
3. General strategy of the study, including a discussion of the rationale for the choice of method(s) (e.g., historical study, survey, experiment; use or not of comparison groups)
4. Laboratory and/or clinical facilities (if applicable)
5. Specific procedures or tactics
   a. Kinds of information to be collected
   b. Procedures to be used in the collection of information
   c. From whom the information will be collected
   d. By whom the information will be collected
   e. Where information will be collected
   f. Schedule for collection of information
   g. Copies of letters, recording forms, interview schedules, questionnaires, etc. should be included either in the text or appendices as deemed appropriate
6. Ethical considerations
7. Methods of data preparation
8. Method of analysis, including statistical techniques, if appropriate (for sections 6 and 7 justify any planned use of computers)
9. Dummy tables, charts, and graphs
10. Justification of budget
11. Criteria for success of the project

Summary of Ten Recommendations

1. State objective and research questions clearly.
2. Use the literature review to justify the need for the proposed project.
3. Be clear about your general strategy.
4. Identify the appropriate funding agency.
5. Seek early consultation with experts.
6. Declare criteria for evaluating answers to the research questions *and* the success of project.
7. Be brief.
8. Keep appendices and supporting documents to a minimum.
9. Assess the resources needed to implement your project realistically.
10. Justify your budget carefully.

Additional Reading

Apley AG. The Watson-Jones Lecture 1984: Surgeons and writers. J Bone Joint Surg (Br) 1985;67:140–144.

Dixon J. Developing the evaluation component of a grant application. J Nurs Outlook 1982;30:122–27.

Jagger J. How to write a research proposal. Grants Mag 1980;3(4):216–22.

Skodal HW. Research proposal: the practical imagination at work. J Nurs Admin 1985;15(2):5–7.

23

Writing Grant Applications for Laboratory Research*

R.E. Pollock, J.E. Niederhuber, and C.M. Balch

Purposes of a Grant Application

A research grant application serves a number of purposes. The most obvious is its potential as an entré to research funding, but it is also a critical planning document that can be used as a precise and detailed research "road map" for the ensuing project. By competing for a peer-reviewed research grant, the investigator receives a critique of his best efforts from other experts in the field. If the grant application is successful and funded, it becomes a very strong statement of peer approval and recognition of the quality of the applicant's research efforts.

Types of Grant

A number of organizations offer grants. Two major sources of medical research funding are the National Institutes of Heath (NIH) in the United States and, in Canada, the Medical Research Council (whose grants and review process are very similar to those of the NIH). Other sources of funding include national and regional grants sponsored by the American Cancer Society, the Kidney Foundation, the American Heart Association, etc. Surgical organizations such as the American College of Surgeons, the Association for Academic Surgery, and the Society of University Surgeons have also established training grant programs. Similar sources of support exist in many other countries (see Section V), and you should explore them fully if you are seeking funding.

Three basic types of grant are available to investigators or aspiring investigators. Training grants—for example, the NIH Clinician–Investigator Award (KO8 series) and institutional training grants—are targeted to physicians with 2 to 7 years of clinical training who are interested in academic careers but lack appropriate basic research training. Training grants usually require applicants to commit 75% or more of their time to their training effort over the course of 3 to 5 years. The goal is to train a clinical investigator capable of functioning independently at the end of the training period. The award is made to the trainee and the training institution.

The second type of grant funds investigator-initiated research projects (e.g., the NIH RO1 and R29 award series). These grants presuppose that the applicant is fully trained and capable of functioning independently; the surgeon–investigator has to compete with other fully trained autonomous scientists, both physicians and holders of doctorates in other disciplines. The award is made to the individual investigator in conjunction with his or institution; funds are transportable to other institutions if the investigator moves to a new department.

The third type of grant is for program projects (e.g., the NIH PO1 series). Applications for these grants are submitted by senior RO1-funded investigators with established research track records. A younger investigator may have the opportunity to participate as a coinvestigator in a project covered by a larger program grant. The program project is developed around a unified, defined research goal encompassing a number of sound individual complementary projects that will be strengthened by being part of the overall program. Such applications are reinforced by a convincing demonstration of the significant cost savings that will accrue from creating the facilities to support the POl-related projects. The strength and unity of the program

*Extensively adapted from Niederhuber JE. Writing a successful grant application. J Surg Res 1985;39:277–284 and Pollock RE, Balch CM. The NIH Clinician–Investigator Award: how to write a training grant application. J Surg Res 1989;46:1–3.

stem from the excellence of its component projects, the focus on a common goal, and collaboration among the project investigators.

Prewriting Phase

You must accurately assess your ability to function independently versus your need for additional training prior to becoming an autonomous investigator. A project (independent or program) grant application is required if you are capable of conducting independent research; if not, an application for a training grant is appropriate. Making this decision first, in the prewriting phase, is necessary because the applications are markedly different.

To write a successful training grant application, you will need to think carefully—during the prewriting phase—about the four essential elements of your application: you—as the applicant, your mentor (sponsor), the research environment in which you propose to pursue your training, and your research project.

The first component is you, because your *potential* to develop independent research capacities will be evaluated. You must demonstrate a serious intention to pursue an academic research career, because the granting agency is investing its money primarily in your potential to develop into an independent investigator rather than in your project, per se.

The second matter you must decide is who your mentor (sponsor) will be. It is important to select someone who is recognized as an accomplished investigator, as documented by the quality of his or her bibliography and track record in getting peer-reviewed support. The granting agency will also evaluate your mentor's ability and availability to guide and support you; that is, can he or she foster your development into an independent investigator? Evidence that your mentor has successfully trained one or more fellows, who were subsequently funded as independent investigators, is usually required.

The third element of your application is the quality of the research environment in which you wish to receive your training. The granting agency's reviewers are looking for proposals for training within strong, well-established, active research programs because such programs imply the presence of a critical mass of faculty members in the clinical and basic sciences. Your proposed research training center should have a reputation for helping young investigators develop independent research careers. An important factor in evaluating the research environment is evidence that the chairman of the department supports and protects trainees during and after their training period.

The fourth consideration is your research project. You will need to demonstrate the overall merit of a multiyear plan of research. The reviewers will examine how the project dovetails with your career plans and how likely it is that it will help you develop the skills you will need. That is, assuming you complete the project, will you be equipped to function as an independent investigator and will you have developed a research attitude that enables you to shift your focus of concentration from a project aimed at getting a single result to one that opens an area of investigation you can pursue in the future?

You must also obtain a departmental letter of support to accompany your application for a training grant. It is a binding guarantee from the chairman of your clinical department that the required percentage of your time and effort for basic research will be protected if your proposal is funded. A vague statement from a well-meaning, but naive chairman is insufficient; the chairman must state exactly how you will be protected and supported while you are executing the proposed research.

The prewriting phase of an independent research grant application is different. You will be evaluated on your established strengths as an independent investigator, not on your potential to become one; you will need to recruit coinvestigators, not select a mentor. Choosing coinvestigators will require as much careful deliberation as selecting a mentor does for a training grant. It may be particularly important that you, as a clinician, choose coinvestigators with strong bibliographies, their own peer-reviewed grant support, and the complementary scientific expertise needed to ensure the success of your project. Review committees are very aware of the demands on the time of clinicians, and of the buttressing value of basic science coinvestigators who need not apportion their time between clinical and investigative tasks.

Your research environment should have the space and equipment required to perform your proposed research. Your independent project application will be strengthened if you can show that other established investigators work in the same general vicinity and that cross-collaborations could develop during the project. It is essential to provide evidence that you have departmental support, especially with regard to projected time requirements.

Your project should be plausible, original, and significant; the quality of these parameters is more important than in a training grant application. The training grant project is a vehicle for the acquisition of independent investigative skills; the individual grant project must have inherent potential for significant scientific advance—its value as a training mechanism is not relevant to the review process.

Compiling the Grant Application

Although the format of an application is unique to each funding agency, the principles underlying most grant applications are sufficiently similar to warrant using the NIH as a generic example.

The detailed instructions in the booklet that usually accompanies the application form should be followed exactly; the requirements and format are frequently revised. If your institution has a grants administration office staffed by individuals who are knowledgeable about grant applications, be sure to identify them and make use of their experience. It would also be helpful to obtain a funded grant proposal from an established senior investigator and use it as a model. Respect *absolutely* all stated page limitations; applications exceeding the stipulations are frequently returned unread! Do not use photoreduction to gain space; if the proposal is not easy to read, it may not be read at all. Use a clear, concise scientific writing style; for the NIH, the official guidelines require the type size to be 12 pitch or greater.

An important first element is the budget. You must complete 12-month and multiyear budget statements, with justifications addressing both time and money parameters. Feel free to contact the granting agency staff to gain insight into grant program restrictions. You may be tempted to inflate your budget to offset anticipated cuts during its review, but resist doing this, because an unrealistic budget reflects poorly on you and can exert a detrimental influence.

You must provide justification for each budget item (e.g., personnel, supplies, travel, equipment). Do not treat this part of your application too lightly; you must formulate your justifications thoroughly, carefully, and skillfully to ensure maximum support for your project. Ask yourself: Is the budget completely justified? Is it in keeping with grant program restrictions? Does it show, specifically and credibly, how you propose to spend both your time and the granting agency's money?

Biographical sketches for you and any coinvestigators or mentors usually come next. Present the best possible, but accurate, image of yourself and any other participants. It is important to demonstrate the adequacy of your investigative training and its relevance to the research you propose to do. Your bibliography should support your qualifications by clearly delineating a common theme in your research efforts. For RO1 and First Awards, your bibliography should provide evidence of independent work; and for PO1 applications, evidence of existing collaborations.

Your application must document other grant support currently under your control as principal investigator, or under the control of your coinvestigator(s) or mentor, in sufficient detail to allow the reviewer to grasp your situation quickly and easily. One- or two-sentence outlines describing the objective and the distinctiveness of each listed project should make it evident that the grants are cohesive, nonoverlapping parts of an overall theme of investigation.

The granting agency's reviewers will usually be familiar with the various institutions and departments supporting your application, but you should describe in detail the laboratory resources available for your proposed project, and characterize your institution's environment in terms of laboratory space, animal facilities, core equipment, and access to needed patient materials.

When you are compiling a grant proposal, you must keep institutional and granting agency deadlines in mind. At the M.D. Anderson Cancer Center, five separate M.D. Anderson forms have to be completed before a grant proposal is allowed to leave the premises. The five forms require seven signatures from seven different offices. There are also 6-page animal care approval forms and equally lengthy human surveillance clearance forms. Completing these forms requires time, and the job must be done early enough to allow sufficient time for internal peer review before submission of the application to the granting agency!

The most important part of your grant proposal is your research plan, in four sections with a limit of 20 pages: specific aims, significance, preliminary studies, and experimental design and methods. Your research plan has a critical bearing on the final rating your proposal will receive and will gain or lose you the most points. Despite its importance, writing the research plan is often left until last.

A successful grant application is based on a significant idea or hypothesis that is not only interesting and exciting but entirely plausible and feasible. Once your research hypothesis/objective has been carefully defined, you will need to devise a series of specific aims that will provide answers to the questions raised by your hypothesis. You are allowed to devote one page to a succinct and feasible statement of the specific aims of your proposal. The challenge is to show that the aims are achievable and are based on a sound and important biologic hypothesis. An outline (Appendix I) is an excellent format for helping the reviewer understand your hypothesis and specific aims. List each aim separately, in the logical sequence you will follow when you implement the plan.

The statement of significance comes next. Your critical review of the pertinent peer-reviewed literature is limited to 3 pages. It allows you to show that you are aware of the most critical areas of current inquiry in your chosen area of research. You must demonstrate a thorough knowledge of the subject area and the relevant and current questions surrounding your proposal, and you must relate your project's specific aims to the critical questions being asked by other scientists working in the same area. The significance section should make it clear that successful completion of your proposed experiment(s) will make a meaningful contribution to the knowledge base of your subject.

The preliminary studies section follows the one on significance and must not exceed 8 pages. If your application is to be successful, you must describe enough completed preliminary work to convince the reviewer that your project has an excellent chance of being carried to a successful completion. This is also your opportunity to convince the reviewer that you have the requisite skills and experience. The reviewer's expectations regarding the extent and sophistication of your preliminary studies are greater for an independent research project grant than for a training grant.

Presenting the data obtained in your preliminary studies in the form of tables and graphs is a great help to the reviewer; these materials should be of publication quality, and it should be possible to photoreduce and insert them at appropriate places in the text to simplify the reviewer's job (Appendix II). This is better than attaching the figures and tables as appendices because it relieves the reviewer of the tedium of having to go back and forth between the text and the appendices. Each table and figure should be easily understood and should have appropriate legends. The topic sentence in each paragraph should be underlined or highlighted by boldface type; for easier review, the paragraphs should be displayed in a numerical, protocol-type format.

The experimental design and methods section is possibly the most important part of your entire application; the evaluation it receives will count most heavily in determining the priority score the review committee assigns to it. Consequently, devote at least two-thirds of your allotted writing time to this part of your application. Help the reviewer focus on the flow of your planned experiments and how they relate to each other by using a diagram showing the research you plan to do as the introduction to this section (Appendix III). The flow diagram will also demonstrate how each step will address the questions you posed under your specific aims. This format helps a busy reviewer under the pressure of reviewing a lengthy application. Note the 8-page limitation on this section.

When you are describing your methods, provide details without being diffuse; lack of focus is one of the most frequent criticisms of grant applications. Use the first portion of the experimental design and methods section to describe the routine methods to be used, in detail, and keep it separate from the research plan. The experimental techniques you will employ should be up to date and referenced, and you must demonstrate a thorough knowledge of their use. The reviewers will judge your experimental design by asking such questions as: Does the experimental design address a significant research question? Does the design build logically on the preliminary studies? Will the design satisfy the specific aims as they have been articulated? Will the design reveal underlying biologic mechanisms, or will it hover at the superficial level of phenomenology?

You must demonstrate a thorough understanding of the difficulties you may encounter when you conduct the proposed experiments and what alternative methods could be flexibly applied to correct or resolve such problems. The most common error is to be too descriptive; you must be able to distinguish coincidence and epiphenomena from true cause and effect.

Mechanism of Review

Some insight into the review process will help you understand why research applications are disapproved or rated poorly.[1] For example, NIH research grants are assigned to an appropriate panel of scientists—known as a study section—which is assisted by an executive secretary who assigns each application to a primary and a secondary reviewer. At the scheduled meetings of the study section, the assigned reviewers lead a discussion of the scientific merit of the proposal. The committee will be composed of investigators of national stature who are engaged in basic research and multiple professional activities that leave them very little time to devote to voluntarily reviewing grant applications. The review committee may, or may not, include a surgical investigator.

Accordingly you must examine your application very skeptically to see whether it could be adequately digested by a primary reviewer in as little as 2 hours. Bear in mind that your primary reviewer will take 15 minutes, at most, to present your application to the entire review committee of 7 to 16 members. The success or failure of your application will depend on the primary reviewer's ability to digest its salient features quickly, and present your ideas in a favorable light to the review committee. Anything you can do to make the reviewer's job easier can only help you; brevity, clarity, and logical organization are essential.

Members of the committee vote to approve or disapprove the application; if it is approved, the review committee will then vote on a priority score. A summary statement of the critique, referred to as the "pink sheet," is prepared by the executive secretary and is sent to you, the applicant.

Your application and its initial review results are then presented to the appropriate NIH advisory council responsible for program review. The council determines how well your proposed research would advance the institute's mission and what funds are available to support external applications. The council relies heavily on study section reviews and their priority scores in determining which applications will be funded. The most critical determinant of success is the initial review by the primary reviewers and the panel of scientists serving as members of the study section.

If you are a new faculty member making your first application for external research funding, seek help from your more experienced and senior colleagues, especially those who members of grant study sections. Remember that one of the major and oft-cited weaknesses of grant applications is lack of focus, especially in the presentation of research plans. Allow enough time to complete the application and have it reviewed internally, by colleagues who are thoroughly knowledgeable in your particular area. It is preferable to miss an application deadline than to submit a proposal that has not received an internal review, because an unreviewed proposal has a much higher likelihood of being rejected.

Commonly recurring reasons for grant disapproval, identified by the NIH, are outlined below.

Reasons for NIH Grant Disapproval[2]

1. Lack of new or original ideas; weak or trivial hypothesis.
2. Diffuse, superficial, or unfocused research plan.
3. Lack of knowledge of published relevant work.
4. Lack of expertise in the essential methodology.
5. Uncertainty concerning future research directions.
6. Questionable reasoning in experimental design.
7. Absence of an acceptable scientific rationale.
8. Unrealistically large amount of work.
9. Lack of sufficient experimental detail.
10. Uncritical approach to current knowledge.

If the application is not successful, you can obtain this information and the critique, usually a few weeks after the study section meeting. If you rewrite your application, address the comments of the critique very carefully. A rewritten grant application taking adequate account of the reviewers' comments may achieve an improved priority score that will warrant funding after resubmission and review.

If your grant application is funded, you may want to apply for additional funding in subsequent years. Competitive renewal has its own set of challenges, but it is an opportunity to show that the initial funds allocated to you by the granting agency were well spent, your specific aims were met, your time and money budgets were not exceeded, you kept abreast of and integrated changes in your field of research and, most pertinent, you contributed to progress by presenting and publishing your work in peer-reviewed forums.

In conclusion, a training grant represents an investment in the possibility that, with the proper training, you can emerge as an independent investigator. In contrast, a research project grant is an investment in the quality and potential of the project itself. An awareness of these distinctions will help you to select a mentor, coinvestigator(s), or project, astutely, and to formulate a grant application in accord with its underlying purpose. (See also Chapter 22.)

References

1. Pollock RE, Balch CM. The NIH Clinician-Investigator Award: how to write a training grant application. J Surg Res 1989;46:1–3.
2. Niederhuber JE. Writing a successful grant application. J Surg Res 1985;39:277–84.

Additional Reading

NIH peer review of research grant applications. Washington, DC: Department of Health and Human Services, 1988.

Appendix I

Outline of specific aims that derive from underlying biological principles. Each specific aim is addressed by studies described in the experimental methods and design section of the research plan (see Appendix III).

In small animal models, the application of surgical stress can be shown to reproducibly increase the success rate of tumor implantation, the rate of growth and the size of primary tumor, and the rate, size, and incidence of subsequent metastases. Surgical stress-induced metastases may be related to impaired bloodstream clearance and increased pulmonary localization of circulating tumor emboli, as has been noted in the rat as early as 1 hr after surgery. Among the many host responses that are important in the control of circulating tumor emboli, the natural killer (NK) cell may be particularly critical because of its emerging role as a first line of defense against the intravascular route of metastasis. Because tumor emboli are generated in humans undergoing tumor resection, and because murine and human studies conducted by ourselves and others demonstrate a profound and acute impairment of perioperative NK cytotoxicity, we would like to elucidate the underlying mechanism of this human perioperative NK cell impairment and develop in vitro preclinical therapy for this impairment process. This proposal shall address the following specific aims:

1. Determine the mechanism of surgical stress impairment of human NK cytotoxicity in the immediate perioperative period.
   a. Cells that suppress NK cells.
   b. Depletion of NK cells.
   c. Direct toxic effects on NK cells.
2. Determine the perioperative consequences of this surgical NK cell cytotoxic impairment.
   a. Impaired NK cell tumor target binding.
   b. Impaired NK cell tumor target lysis.
   c. Impaired NK cell recycling.
3. Examine the perioperative role of NK cells in killing autologous tumor.
4. Develop preclinical in vitro therapy using biologic response modifiers to treat the perioperatively impaired NK cell cytotoxicity.

Appendix II

Preliminary results incorporate publication quality figures for ease of review. Note that each experiment is numbered and the topic sentence is underlined in protocol fashion.

1. *Time Kinetics of Human NK Cell Cytotoxicity Impairment by Surgical Stress*

Three patients undergoing cancer-related surgical procedures had NK cytotoxicity examined preoperatively and on the first, third, fifth, and seventh postoperative days. The assay system was a 3 hr ^{51}Cr release assay using Ficoll Hypaque passed mononuclear cells and cultured K562 human erythroleukemia targets at 6 effector:target ratios (200:1-6:1). Data is expressed as either percent NK cytotoxicity or as lytic units per 107 peripheral blood mononuclear cells, where one lytic unit represents the number of effector cells needed to cause 20% target cell lysis (calculated using the Von Krogh equation as per Pross; 54). Each patient was paired with a different individual cryopreserved normal donor who was simultaneously assayed at the same time points using the same target cell aliquots throughout the perioperative period. Marked impairment of NK cytotoxicity was noted as early as 24 hr after surgery. This NK cell impairment persisted throughout the perioperative period during the time points studied. Cryopreserved normal donors assayed simultaneously against the same target cell aliquots showed minimal NK cytotoxicity variability over time, and so the impairment in patient NK cytotoxicity could be attributed to the effect of surgery rather than any change in target cell sensitivity to lysis.

continued

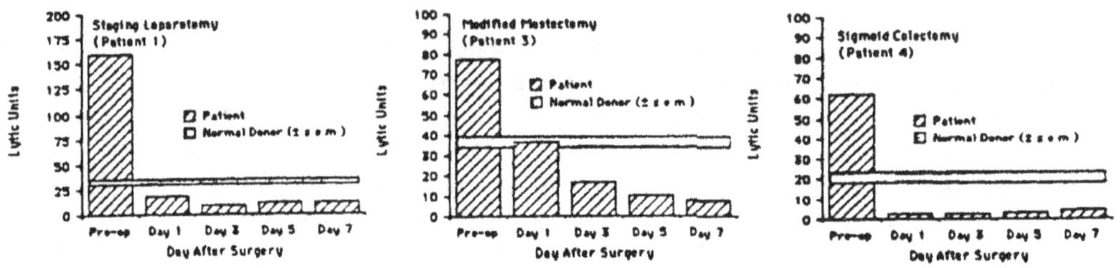

2. *Impairment of Human NK Cytotoxicity in the Immediate Perioperative Period*

Seven additional tumor-bearing patients underwent a variety of cancer resections. Because of our interest in the possible perioperative discharge of circulating tumor emboli, NK cytotoxicity was studied immediately before and 24 hr after surgery. Cryopreserved normal donor controls were used as controls with minimal NK cytotoxic variability (cryopreserved data not shown). All 10 patients demonstrated significantly impaired NK cytotoxicity immediately after surgery. Even at very low effector:target ratios (6:1), significant differences were observed between the pre- and 24 hr postoperative NK cytotoxicity values ($p < 0.001$ for all effector:target ratios). The decreased NK cytotoxicity is thought not due to NK cell depletion because, at least by morphologic criteria, the percent large granular lymphocyte in preoperative and postoperative cytospin differentials was not significantly different (preoperative %LGL: 8.30 $\pm$1.91 vs postoperative %LGL:5.50$\pm$1.14).

No clear correlation between epidemiologic factors (age, sex, extent of surgery, amount of blood loss, type of anesthesia, tumor size, histology, etc.) and the postoperative decline in NK cytotoxicity could be made, although the sample size studied to date is too small for that purpose.

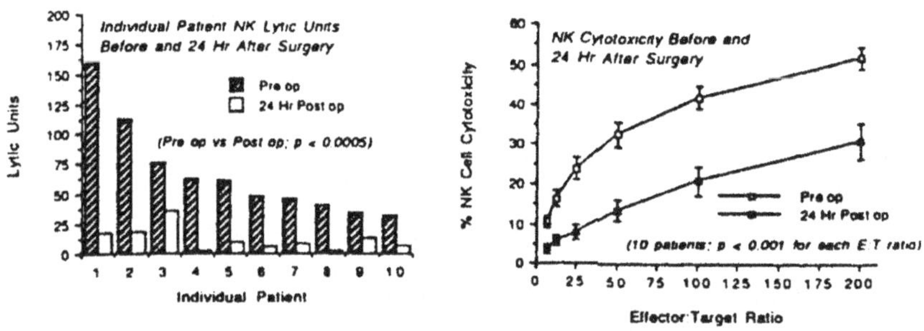

Appendix III

An experimental design flow sheet provides a guide for the reviewer. The sequence, relevance, and rationale of each experiment can be determined at a glance. Their connections to specific aims are clear (Appendix I), as are the descriptions of specific experimental methods following immediately after this flow sheet.

I. Mechanism of Perioperative NK Cell Cytotoxicity Suppression

1. *Distinguish between NK cell cytotoxicity suppression due to surgical generation of suppressor cells, surgical depletion of NK cells, or surgical "poisoning" of NK cells.* Make this distinction in mixing studies where the postoperative PBMC are NK cell purged by Leu 11b + C treatment prior to mixing with preoperative PBMC ("unmasking" possible suppressor cells). Confirm NK cell purge with FACS and ^{51}Cr release assay (phenotypic and functional confirmation).

Suppressor Cell

2. *T suppressor cell*
Create T cell purified and depleted postoperative subpopulations using FACS. Use these populations in mixing studies to detect the presence of suppressor cells. Confirm depletion/enrichment: functionally by testing proliferative response to PHA, and phenotypically with FACS.

3. Deplete *monocyte/MO suppressors* using nylon wool adherence followed by plastic adherence. Enrich for monocyte/MO using same techniques. Confirm enrichment using flow cytometry, cytospin diffs, latex phagocytosis. Do mixing studies with these populations. If monocyte/MO suppressor detected in mixing studies, treat in vitro with indomethacin to see if this relieves suppression.

4. *Granulocyte suppressors* not likely; confirm their removal with Ficoll-Hypaque by examining cytospin differentials.

(Note: If the presence of a suppressor cell is demonstrated, the studies outlined in experiments 7-10 will be done in postoperative PBMCs with and without depletion of that suppressor cell population in order to specify the mechanism of that specific suppression.)

"Poisoned" or depleted NK cells

5. Examine for *NK cell depletion* using FACS to tabulate % of cells that are Leu 11+, Leu 19+ pre and post operatively.

6. Examine for *NK cell "poisoning".* Enrich for LGL using pre- and postoperative PBMC Percoll/sRBC rosette purified. Compare resultant cells for NK cytotoxicity. Confirm results by comparing cytotoxicity of FACS purified Leu 11+, Leu 19+ pre- and postoperative PBMC. "Poisoned" NK cells, even after purification, should still be less cytotoxic than dose-equivalent numbers of "unpoisoned" NK cells.

7. Single cell assay: possible *problems with target binding, target lysis, percent active NK cell, or NK cell recycling.*
   a. If *problem with target binding*; see if related to *LFA-1 surface antigen expression.*
   b. If *problem with target lysis*; see if defect is in *programming for lysis vs killer cell independent lysis (KCIL).*

8. *Inhibition of NK cell migration.*

9. *Inhibition of NKCF, cytolysin production.*

10. *Decreased responsiveness to IL-2*; lack of autocrine circuit inducibility.

II. In Vitro Therapy of Surgical Stress Impairment of NK Cell Cytotoxicity

11. *Autologous targets*
Use preoperative and postoperative effectors after percoll enrichment and sRBC rosetting. Study their cytotoxicity at population and single cell level using K562 and autologous tumor in ^{51}Cr release assays, single cell assays, and two target conjugate assays (K562-FITC and autologous targets). Show that the specific defect identified in Part I also occurs when using autologous targets. Confirm using flow cytometric effector:target conjugation/lysis assay.

12. *Treatment*
IL-2, gamma IFN, OK432 alone and in combination. Use preoperative and postoperative cells before and after treatment against K562 and autologous tumor. Show that treatment corrects specific defect identified in Part I above.

Appendix IV

Some Agencies Granting Awards to Surgical Investigators

American Academy of Orthopedics
(Apply to secretary)

American Association for the Surgery of Trauma
Trauma Fellowships available annually
(Apply to secretary of AAST)

American Association for Thoracic Surgery
AATS Research Scholarship
(Apply to secretary of AATS)

American Burn Association
(Apply to Secretary)

American Cancer Society
American Cancer Society Clinical Oncology
Career Development Award
Clinical Awards Program Director
American Cancer Society, Inc.
3340 Peachtree Road
Atlanta, GA 30026

American College of Surgeons
American College of Surgeons Scholarships
Scholarships Division
American College of Surgeons
55 Erie Street
Chicago, IL 60611

American Heart Association
American Heart Association
Clinical Scientific Award
American Heart Association
National Center Research Department
7320 Greenville Avenue
Dallas, TX 75231

American Society of Clinical Oncology
American Society of Clinical Oncology
Young Investigators Award
American Society of Clinical Oncology
435 North Michigan Avenue
Suite 1717
Chicago, IL 60611

American Surgical Association
American Surgical Association
Foundation Fellowship Award Program
(Consult secretary of ASA)

National Cancer Institute
Program Director, Clinical Investigator
Awards Cancer Training Branch
Division of Cancer Prevention and Control
National Cancer Institute
Blair Building, Room 424
Bethesda, MD 20205-4200

Society for Surgical Infection
(Apply to Secretary)

Foundations

The Foundation Grants Index, 18th ed., Ruth Kovacs, ed. New York: Foundation Center, 1989.

Section III

Implementation of Research

No textbook could cover all the research strategies useful to an academic clinician. This text considers selective strategies. We emphasize research of clinical scientists who care for patients, and care enough that they wish to do *more* than is possible given the current state of our knowledge. We focus particularly on strategies that enable a clinician to have direct involvement in a research investigation without abandoning the operating theater or the wards.

We, the editors, are all clinicians responsible for the care of patients. If there is an imbalance in this book, it is toward too much patient-oriented research. Yet the principles of research are universal; they are as applicable to animal research as to clinical investigation. They work as well in the chemistry and physiology laboratories as in the ward.

Clinicians, and particularly action-oriented surgeons, have a tendency to underestimate the importance of small gains in therapy or in knowledge. Nevertheless, small gains are the norm, and demonstrating them with scientific rigor so that they compound into an aggregate benefit of even a few percentage points of improved outcome for thousands or millions of people is central to both clinical and laboratory research today. Remember that economists and bankers rest all their strategies on gaining a few percentage points, which become significant when compounded over time and applied to large populations.

Despite the limitation on the inferences that can be drawn from case reports, descriptions of what happens or what exists are frequently indispensable precursors of good controlled research. Observations and descriptions of a side effect or an unexpected benefit usually come to our attention through case studies. Much progress in research is attributable to the alert clinician who is skillful enough as an observer and sophisticated enough as a consumer of research information to recognize the germ of a hypothesis and to write it up. Career scientists depend on career clinicians for pointers to a better future in medicine.

The laboratory is our workshop; its location and the tools employed in it are extraordinarily diverse. Consider the difference between the workplaces of Pasteur and Lister, although both worked on basically the same problem. Today, the broad scope of research is manifest by studies that range from those initiated in the operating room to others using the tools of molecular biology or engaging the power of computers to model complex biologic relationships. No single textbook could possibly capture the panoply of color, texture, and quiet drama that characterizes modern science; we can only display selected vignettes that portray some of its richness.

Complex laboratory techniques demand highly focused, intensive knowledge for their proper application to problem solving and hypothesis testing. Gastrointestinal physiologists have made an odyssey—from observing the digestive process through a war-injury stoma—to hormonal control of gastrointestinal function—to cell receptor identification—to genetic control of effector expression. The range of inquiry in vascular disease extends from the intricacies of the blood–biomaterial interface to the genetic control of thrombolytic enzymes and endothelial cells. To develop techniques that avoid myocardial injury in the operating room and accelerate patient recovery, cardiac surgeons are seeking new insights into the mechanisms of protein regulation in the pre- and postoperative interval. Patients' complex reactions to trauma range from neuroendocrine responses to elaboration of new protein moieties in circulating cells that modify tissue tolerance to hypoxia.

The chapters in this section are offered as stimulants to your imagination and creativity as you formulate new hypotheses for investigation.

24

Why Clinical Research?

B.C. Walters and D.L. Sackett

This chapter and the several that follow are about real clinical research: posing and answering questions about the causes, diagnosis, prognosis, and management of disease in collaboration with human subjects. Let us begin by considering why clinicians should and do devote time and energy to clinical research.

First, why "clinical"? Because we must answer clinical questions. No matter how complete our knowledge of anatomy, physiology, pharmacology, and the like, our thinking must go beyond these basic sciences each time we see a patient, as we decide whether to apply this or that diagnostic test; to recommend operation A, operation B, or no operation at all; or to prescribe drug X, drug Y, or nothing. Although potential answers to these questions can originate in the laboratory, they will stand or fall on the basis of whether they do more good than harm to patients. The measurement of this good and harm, under circumstances that limit error, is a prerequisite to progress in patient care. Clinical research must be carried out if clinical care is to improve, rather than simply change.

In this chapter, we focus on clinical questions of two sorts:

1. Can we find a better treatment for this specific clinical problem?
2. Can we prevent or minimize the iatrogenic complications of a treatment already known to be efficacious?

To make our discussion of these questions easier to follow and more enjoyable, we shall employ a specific running example of each: "Is superficial temporal–middle cerebral artery anastomosis good for patients with symptomatic, surgically inaccessible atherosclerosis of their internal carotid or middle cerebral arteries? and "Can prophylactic antibiotics prevent iatrogenic cerebrospinal fluid shunt infections?

But why carry out "research" to answer clinical questions? Can't we simply apply the operations and treatments our individual or combined experiences have shown us to be efficacious?

The problem is that it has been repeatedly shown that our uncontrolled experiences, however, we may combine them, lead us into error. Those who doubt this should review the history of surgery for organ ptosis or constipation, the gastric freeze, and internal mammary ligation.[1] Three of the reasons for ever falling into such error stand out.[2]

1. Clinicians are more likely to recognize and remember favorable treatment responses in patients who comply with treatments and keep follow-up appointments. There are, however, five documented instances in which compliant patients in the placebo groups of randomized trials exhibited far more favorable outcomes, including survival, than their noncompliant companions.[3-7] This demonstration of high compliance being a marker for better outcomes, even when a treatment is useless, illustrates how our uncontrolled clinical experiences can often cause us to conclude that compliant patients must have been on efficacious therapy.
2. Unusual patterns of symptoms (e.g., transient ischemic attacks) or signs (e.g., high blood pressure levels), and extreme laboratory test results tend to return toward the more usual normal result when they are reassessed even a short time later.[8] Given this universal tendency for "regression toward the mean," any treatment initiated in the interim will appear to be efficacious, regardless of its real efficacy.
3. Routine clinical practice is never "blind"; patients and their clinicians know when active

treatment is underway. The "placebo effect," which has shown that angina pectoris can be relieved by the skin incision of a mock internal mammary ligation,[9] and the desire of patients and their clinicians to have treatments succeed, can cause both parties to overestimate efficacy.

For the foregoing reasons, the "consensus" approach, based on uncontrolled clinical experience, risks precipitating the widespread application of treatments that are useless or may even do more harm than good. The same treatments are much less likely to be judged efficacious in double-blind, randomized trials than in uncontrolled case-series or unblinded "open" comparisons with contemporaneous or historical series of patients. This fact of life is embodied in the maxim: "Therapeutic reports with controls have no enthusiasm, and reports with enthusiasm have no controls."

We must, therefore, answer our clinical questions in a manner that limits error and permits us to draw conclusions that will not vary about biologic and clinical phenomena that do vary. We use two methods to accomplish this:

1. **Design:** the way we assemble, manipulate, and make measurements on our patients. Proper design—inclusion criteria, random allocation, complete follow-up, objective outcome criteria, blinding, etc.—enables us to avoid systematic error or "bias."
2. **Statistics:** the way we manipulate the data that arise from our clinical research. Proper statistics help us to limit nonsystematic error or "noise" (see Chapters 15 and 16).

Design is the primary focus of this chapter: statistics will be discussed only when necessary. The emphasis throughout the chapter will be on thinking "How might your answer be wrong?" and "How can you safeguard against this?" rather than on such mindless cookbookery as lists of do's and don't's (see also Chapters 13 and 14.)

Finally, why should surgeons carry out clinical research on surgical problems rather than leaving this task to some other group of clinicians or methodologists? There are at least three reasons. First, by reason of their training and experience, surgeons understand the questions that need to be asked about surgical conditions better than any other group of clinicians or methodologists. Second, surgeons can fuse clinical sense with good research design in a way that will generate results that are clinically credible as well as scientifically valid. Third, surgeons who seek academic careers face the difficult task of dividing their time between research and clinical surgery. When research takes place at a laboratory bench, it may be far removed from clinical practice; it may demand laboratory skills and basic science knowledge that are foreign to the practicing surgeon; and it may involve competition with full-time laboratory scientists with Ph.D.'s. Surgical scholars risk losing their grants if they spend too little time in the lab, and their surgical skills and credibility if they spend too much.

Clinical research is generated, executed, and applied in the front lines of clinical practice; clinical research and clinical practice do not compete, they reinforce each other. This synergistic relationship has major implications for efficiency, productivity, and career satisfaction; the academic clinician who wishes to live, as well as survive, should keep it in mind.

Translating a Clinical Problem into a Research Question

To translate a clinical problem into a research question, you must understand the biology and pathophysiology underlying the problem, define the clinical question you wish to pose, and transform the clinical question into a scientific question that can be answered by "yes," "no," or a number.

Although the clinical care and outcome of many diseases have undergone major improvements in the absence of any profound understanding of their biology and pathophysiology, there is a consensus among biologists and clinicians that we are more likely to make advances in care if these benefits arise as logical extrapolations based on the fundamental mechanisms of health and disease.

If your investigation is to be focused on an issue in therapy, the formulation of your clinical question will be influenced by the intended purpose of the answer, since the questions posed can be of two different sorts.[10,11] The first deals with explanation and asks such questions as "Can operation A reduce overnight acid secretion by the stomach?" The second deals with management and asks such questions as "Does offering operation A to patients with peptic ulcer do more good than harm?"

The two types of trial that result from the two types of question have contrasting attributes. The explanatory or efficacy trial seeks to describe how a treatment produces its effects and to determine whether it can work under what are often ideal or restricted circumstances. The management trial, sometimes called pragmatic trial, seeks to determine all the consequences, both good and bad, of treating an illness in a certain way and to ascertain whether the therapy works under clinical circumstances that are as close as possible to those usually encountered in practice. For sound scientific reason, the two types of trial may recruit study patients in quite different fashions. The explanatory trial may justifiably restrict admission to the patients who are most likely to consent to the particular operation and to respond to it. The management trial may, also justifiably, accept all comers, including patients with comorbid conditions or poor compliance, to obtain a better estimate of the usefulness of starting down a particular treatment path. (Some patients should be excluded from both sorts of trials: e.g., patients incorrectly diagnosed or subsequently shown, on blind adjudication, to violate the inclusion/exclusion criteria.)

The experimental procedure may with good reason be applied quite differently in the two sorts of trial. If an explanatory trial is an attempt to find out whether the operation can work in the best hands, the protocol may restrict it to the most experienced and gifted surgeons and may call for frequent follow-up examinations and other procedures that violate contemporaneous practice. The management trial, in contrast, usually strives to replicate current practice.

Finally, these two types of trial differ in the eligibility of the events used to determine the outcomes. The explanatory trial focuses on a restricted range of events and often seeks to exclude from analysis events that befall both experimental patients, who have not received the experimental operation, and control ("crossover") patients, who have. In contrast, the management trial tends to encompass a wide range of events and usually includes all events that occur after randomization in order to assess the results of a decision to offer a particular operation.

When the question that is the essence of the trial is posed from the investigator's perspective, the issue of primary interest may be either explanation or management; when it is posed from the patient's perspective, the primary issue is management. In the latter case, for example, the fact and mode of dying are far more important than its cause, and all events are of interest.

For all the foregoing reasons, the specification of the clinical question deserves considerable thought, and always benefits from discussion and debate with one's colleagues.

The crucial third step is the conversion of the clinical question to a scientific one that can be answered by "yes," "no," or a number. The final product usually combines designation of the clinical condition, the intervention, and key clinical outcome. Your clinical question might be: "What is the role of extracranial–intracranial bypass in cerebrovascular disease?", but its lack of specificity is obvious. Such a clinical question must be converted into a scientific one before you can proceed to fashion the detailed protocol in an unambiguous way: for example, "Among patients with symptomatic, surgically inaccessible atherosclerosis of the internal carotid or middle cerebral arteries, will the performance of superficial temporal–middle cerebral artery anastomosis reduce the risk of subsequent fatal and nonfatal stroke?" Your colleagues can argue that the latter question is not the right one to ask, but they cannot say it is not specific.

Once your scientific question has been formulated, you can begin to fashion the study protocol, the document that describes the architecture of the investigation and details which patients will be assembled or excluded; who will do what to them and when and how; what measurements will be made on them, by whom, when, and how; how the resulting data will be analyzed and interpreted; and what will be done about missing patients and data. Throughout the development of your protocol, you must repeatedly ask yourself the question that lies at the root of sound science: "How might my answer be wrong, and what can I do to protect against this?"

The next two sections describe the development of the protocols generated in response to the clinical questions presented at the beginning of this chapter. These are presented to illustrate key elements of proper study design, not as a set of knee-jerk reflexes to be mindlessly acted out for every study, but as a set of problem-solving responses to specific threats to the validity of the clinical investigations we were undertaking at the time. These sections are only an introduction to the development of study protocols; they should be supplemented by selective readings from the score of recent textbooks on clinical trials and, most important, from your personal experience in struggling to develop your own protocols.

Can We Find a Better Operation for This Clinical Problem?

Entire books have been devoted to the design of therapeutic trials. The information provided here will not suffice as a base from which to carry one out. However, it will accordingly raise, and hint at the answers to, the questions that will arise as you attempt such research. If you wish to proceed further, you must follow the questions and hints into the longer, more formal expositions of experimental research methods. Several of them are cited at the end of this chapter. (See also Chapters 14, above, and 29, in Section III).

The trial we shall use for our example is the International Cooperative Study of Extracranial/Intracranial (EC/IC) Bypass,[12,13] in which one of us (D.L.S.) was a coinvestigator. It was designed and executed to answer the question, "Will anastomosis of the superficial temporal artery to the middle cerebral artery decrease the rate of stroke and stroke-related death among patients with symptomatic disease of the internal carotid and middle cerebral arteries?"

Which Patients Should Be Entered into the Trial?

Four issues have to be considered. The first is the establishment of a detailed description of the sort of patient who should be entered into the trial. Clearly, since we are testing the efficacy of an operation, we should enter patients who are likely to benefit from the procedure. Moreover, the description, or "eligibility criteria," must be stated so clearly that clinicians who read the report of the trial will be able to tell whether its results apply to specific patients in their practices. The description of EC/IC Bypass Trial patients read as follows (all subsequent excerpts are taken from reference 12, the published protocol). To be eligible for the trial, patients have had to satisfy clinical, radiologic, and inclusion criteria.

Clinical Inclusion Criteria

Patients had to have experienced, within 3 months prior to entry, one or both of the following: (i) transient ischemic attack(s) (TIA) in the carotid distribution [one or more episodes of distinct focal neurological dysfunction or monocular blindness (amaurosis fugax), the symptoms and signs of which cleared completely in less than 24 hours]; (ii) minor completed stroke(s) in the carotid distribution (one or more events of distinct focal neurologic dysfunction or amaurosis fugax, the signs of which persisted for more than 24 hours). Patients without useful residual function in the affected territory have not been entered.

Radiologic Inclusion Criteria

An angiogram demonstrating an atherosclerotic lesion in the appropriate territory has had to be submitted for central confirmation and adjudication by the principal neuroradiologist; bilateral common carotid arteriograms have been requested on all patients, and angiography of the vertebrobasilar circulation has been optional.

One or more of the following atherosclerotic lesions must have been demonstrated in vessels appropriate to the patient's symptoms: (i) stenosis or occlusion of the middle cerebral artery trunk; (ii) stenosis of the internal carotid artery at or above the C2 vertebral body (i.e., inaccessible to carotid artery operation).

For radiologic eligibility, stenosis has been defined as "any recognizable atherosclerotic lesion of the surgically inaccessible portion of the internal carotid artery or middle cerebral artery which, in the opinion of the attending neurosurgeon, might reasonably be expected to benefit from bypass surgery."

Exclusion Criteria

The second issue is the recurring question, "How could my answer be wrong?" In this step of the study, we would risk generating the wrong answer if we entered patients of the wrong sorts, specifically those who, because they are too ill or are suffering from comorbid conditions, would not reasonably be expected to respond to, and benefit from, the operation. Such patients would have to be analyzed as treatment failures, and any attempts to remove them from analysis "after the fact" would damage the credibility of the study. It is far better to exclude them from the outset, and this is the purpose of "exclusion criteria."

Patients have been excluded from the study if they were unable to meet at least the following functional standards: (i) capability of self-care for most activities of daily living (may require some assistance); (ii) retention of some useful residual function in the affected arm or leg; (iii) comprehension intact, with no evidence of Wernicke's receptive aphasia; (iv) no, or only mild, motor (expressive, Broca's) aphasia; (v) ability to handle their own oropharyngeal secretions.

Patients also have been excluded from the trial if any of the following pertained: inability to provide informed consent; evidence that the original stroke was due to cerebral hemorrhage; within 8 weeks of an acute cerebral ischemic event; exhibition of nonatherosclerotic conditions causing or likely to cause cerebral dysfunction (fibromuscular dysplasia, arteritis, blood dyscrasias, a cardiac source of cerebral emboli, chronic atrial fibrillation, complete heart block, significant valvular heart disease, cardiomyopathy, or nonatherosclerotic dissection); the presence of any morbid condition(s) likely to lead to death within 5 years [cancer, renal failure (BUN > 50 mg%], cardiomegaly [cardiothoracic ratio of exceeding 0.50 (> 0.55 in Japanese patients)[14-16] or any hepatic or pulmonary disease constituting an unacceptable anesthetic risk], the occurrence of ischemic symptoms isolated to the vertebrobasilar circulation; prior participation in the study (regardless of the occurrence of new ischemic events or success or failure of previous therapy); myocardial infarction within the preceding 6 months; a fasting blood sugar of 300 mg% or more on the most recent assessment despite appropriate therapy; and diastolic blood pressure exceeding 110 mm Hg (using disappearance of sounds for diastolic pressure) despite appropriate medical therapy. Once uncontrolled diabetes or hypertension had been corrected, otherwise eligible patients could be entered.

The third issue is the inevitability that a mistake will be made in entering patients, regardless of good will and hard work. How should inappropriately entered patients be handled? Their removal at the end of the study, even though justified on scientific grounds, leaves the investigators open to criticism and damages the credibility of the result. It is far better to have the eligibility of all patients adjudicated shortly after entry by clinicians who are not only "blind" to the patient's treatment allocation, but also are not even entering patients into the study.

Every entry form has been reviewed by both the Central Office and the Methods Center. All angiograms have been reviewed (without knowledge of the treatment group to which the patient had been randomized) by the principal neuroradiologist at the Central Office. When this review has suggested that an ineligible patient had been entered, an external group of adjudicators (who were not real participants and were "blind" to the patient's allocation) has reviewed the entry data and angiograms and decided whether the patient should be excluded from the trial.

The fourth and final issue is the establishment and publication of explicit rules for dealing with the specific clinical situations that call for interpretation of, rather than mere adherence to, the study protocol.

Because cerebrovascular disease often involves multiple sites, guidelines for managing, and arbitrary rules for analyzing, specific clinical situations have been established. When "tandem lesions" (two lesions in the same vessel or sequence of vessels, one proximal to the other) have existed, and both lesions have fulfilled the entry criteria, the patient has been entered for the more distal lesion. If the proximal lesion has been amenable to endarterectomy, the decisions of whether to perform endarterectomy, and the selection of the initial site for surgery (i.e., endarterectomy or EC/IC bypass) have been left to the participating surgeon. In patients judged to require external carotid endarterectomy as a preparation for bypass, it has been recommended that this be performed only after the patient has been randomized to the surgical group. If external carotid endarterectomy had been performed prior to randomization, then 30 days have had to elapse following endarterectomy before the patient could have been entered.

When contralateral carotid disease has existed and has been accessible to endarterectomy, the decision of whether and when to perform contralateral endarterectomy has again been left to the participating neurosurgeon. Once again, if contralateral endarterectomy has been carried out first, 30 days have had to elapse following contralateral endarterectomy before the patient could have been entered.

When eligible patients have had appropriate symptoms and angiographic lesions in both carotid distributions, the patient has been entered for the most recent clinically eligible event. If more than one TIA or stroke has occurred prior to entry, the most recent has served as the basis for enrollment.

In all the circumstances above, if a 30-day waiting period has applied, the patient was still eligible for randomization, despite the passage of more than 3 months since the last episode of cerebral ischemia.

What Baseline Investigations Should Be Carried out on Study Patients?

The study patients have already undergone several investigations to determine their eligibility for the trial. Why carry out any more? There are three reasons. First, when the clinical measure that will be used to determine whether surgery does more good than harm goes beyond mere mortality and involves the determination of symptoms, signs, or some level of function, it is important to make the initial measurement at the start of the trial. This ensures that the measurement process is working properly (i.e., you can identify and correct problems in observer variation in making and interpreting the measurement) provides a baseline against which to identify differences within and between patients as the study proceeds and provides key data for determining the comparability of the experimental and control groups at the start of the trial. The second reason for carrying out additional baseline measurements is to guide any ancillary therapy for disorders in either group during the study. The third reason is to obtain information for "prognostic stratification," as in the next section.

At entry, detailed neurological and medical histories and examinations have been carried out and recorded on standardized forms. The examination has included a 12-item functional status assessment in which the patient's ability to perform activities of daily living, such as eating, toileting, and ambulation, have been rated on a three-point scale:

1. Able to perform task without difficulty,
2. Able to perform task with difficulty.
3. Unable to perform without mechanical or personal assistance.

Additional historical data have been gathered about employment status, as well as history of diabetes mellitus, hypertension, angina pectoris, myocardial infarction, intermittent claudication, cardiac surgery or other serious illness, current medications, and smoking habits. The patient's blood pressure, heart rate and rhythm, cardiac murmurs, and neck bruits have been recorded. Finally, the following baseline investigations have been carried out: hemoglobin; platelet count, prothrombin time, random blood glucose, blood urea nitrogen, cholesterol, electrocardiogram (for left ventricular hypertrophy, new or old myocardial infarction and rhythm), chest x-ray to estimate the cardiothoracic ratio, and, if available, a computerized tomographic (CT) scan of the head.

How Should Patients Be Allocated to Treatments?

How should we decide which patients will receive the experimental operation? The quick answer is randomize. The reasons for giving so unequivocal an answer are both historic (we have made such fools of ourselves when we have used other methods of determining efficacy) and scientific. The latter will be summarized with an example.

Suppose that a surgeon developed a new vascular bypass procedure until it was ready for testing in humans. Because it was a lengthy procedure and not without risk, it was understandable that the surgeon carried out the first few bypasses on patients who were, for the most part, free of hypertension (even if it were controlled) or other extraneous disorders that increased their surgical risk. Suppose that the initial results were encouraging: all patients survived the procedure and their symptoms remained stable or even improved. In contrast, many of the poor-risk patients, who were rejected for surgery because of coexisting hypertension, either died or experienced progression of their symptoms. When the results are reported, a substantial segment of the profession might conclude that the bypass procedure is of obvious efficacy and ought to be performed on all good-risk, and even some poor-risk, patients. The canny reader will have identified three properties of hypertension in this hypothetical example.

1. It is extraneous to the question posed. The efficacy of the bypass surgery is at issue, not the biology of hypertension.
2. It is a determinant of the outcomes of interest. Hypertensives are more likely than normotensives to experience progressive arterial disease and to die.
3. It is unequally distributed among the treatment groups being compared and the inequality is marked. Very few hypertensives were bypassed; almost all were rejected for surgery.

In the technical jargon of causation, hypertension is a confounder, and the presence of such confounders has complicated the evaluation of the efficacy of almost all preventive, therapeutic, and rehabilitative maneuvers. Confounding leads to bias—the arrival at a conclusion that differs systematically from the truth—and examples abound in human research, whether experimental, where allocation to the maneuvers under comparison occurs by random allocation, or subexperimental, where allocation occurs by any other process.[17]

If confounding hampers the valid demonstration of efficacy and effectiveness, how can it be avoided? Briefly, seven strategies exist for preventing confounding; all of them attack the property of unequal distribution among treatment groups, but one is clearly superior to the rest. First, you could prevent confounding by restricting the criteria for inclusion; that is, you could simply exclude hypertensives from either the operated or nonoperated patient groups. Second, you could individually match, in both the sampling and analysis stages, operated and nonoperated patients for their hypertension status. Third, you could carry out stratified sampling (i.e., create cohorts of operated and nonoperated normotensives). Fifth, you could apply an adjustment or standardization procedure, analogous to age standardization, in the analysis. Sixth, you could establish a model for the risk of the outcome of interest that would include a correction factor for hypertension or could be expanded to include other possible confounders, such as symptomatic coronary heart disease and diabetes. Seventh and finally, you could randomly allocate appropriate patients to undergo or not undergo the new microvascular surgical techniques.

The final strategy, random allocation, has a profound advantage over the other six. Because random allocation prevents distortion by unknown as well as known confounders, it reduces bias from known confounders and from undiscovered potential confounders. This boon to validity places the true experiment, in which assignment to the maneuvers under comparison occurs by random allocation, above the subexperiment, in which allocation occurs by any other process, in determining the efficacy or effectiveness of any clinical maneuver or new technology.

The true experiment is now the standard approach for determining the efficacy and effectiveness of chemotherapeutic agents and most other drugs and is increasingly used in evaluating surgical technology. The strategies can also be combined. For example, many trials involve randomization within prognostic strata, followed by adjustments for residual differences in the analysis. Such prognostic stratification ensures the baseline similarity of experimental and control groups for key attributes and contributes to the clinical credibility of the results: If the patient has been judged eligible on clinical and radiographic grounds, informed consent has been requested. If obtained, a tentative date for surgery has been booked (to minimize the time interval between randomization and surgery) and the Methods Center has been contacted by telephone for registration and random allocation (for logistic reasons, a separate randomization center has been set up in Kyoto, Japan, for patients from Japan and Taiwan).

To ensure balance between the medical and surgical limbs of this trial, a stratified randomization has been carried out. The strata have been defined by the underlying vascular lesion (stenosis or occlusion of the middle cerebral or internal carotid artery), the presence or absence of a related neurologic deficit and, in the case of patients with internal carotid occlusion, whether related symptoms have occurred since its angiographic demonstration (some centers have joined the trial with a commitment to exclude patients with no symptoms since the internal carotid occlusions were demonstrated). Then, based on a computer-generated randomization scheme established at the Methods Center for each participating center and stratum, the patient has been assigned to either the medical or the surgical limb of the trial.

A final remark on the timing of randomization is required. Because most methodologic purists, and journal editors, will insist on charging all events, including those occurring between randomization and operation, to their respective treatment groups, it may be wise to have an early operative date already scheduled for a patient before he or she is randomized, to cover the possibility of his or her being randomized to surgery.

How Should the Treatments Be Specified?

The experimental operation must be described in sufficient detail to accomplish two things. First, participating surgeons must have discussed and debated it in sufficient detail to have generated the precise operating room protocol that will be followed. Second, if the operation is found to do more good than harm, those who read the trial report must be able to replicate it precisely on their own patients.

Surgical trials must also take another issue into consideration at this stage of design. Which surgeons should do the experimental operations or, more precisely, how skilled and experienced should participating surgeons be? The answer depends on the question being posed. If an explanatory trial is planned (i.e., Can the operation work, under ideal circumstances?), only the best surgeons, with substantial experience and documented success in performing the operation, should participate, and the quality of their work should be documented and assessed before and during the trial, as was done in the EC/IC Bypass Trial. If a management trial is planned (i.e., Does the operation do more good than harm when performed under the circumstances of routine practice?), an equally sound case is made for having surgeons with average skill and experience take part.

Even random allocation and attention to the foregoing will not exclude all sources of bias, nor will it ensure the validity and generalizability of the results of an experiment. First, the performance of additional therapeutic procedures on the experimental group should be avoided unless the same procedures are performed with equal vigor on the comparison group.[17] For example, if experimental patients are seen more frequently than control patients, the additional opportunities for clinical evaluation and management may spuriously inflate the estimate of the benefit of the test therapy, or, by promoting the recognition of mild or transient side effects, inflate the estimate of harm.

This problem is exaggerated in surgical trials, where it is usually impossible to use a major strategy for preventing cointervention (i.e., the blinding of study patients and their clinicians to the experimental therapy through the use of placebo drugs and maneuvers). Second, the trial that is most efficient ensures that all experimental, but no control, subjects receive the test therapy. When members of the control group receive the test therapy—a major potential problem when "medical" patients "cross over" and undergo the experimental surgery—the resulting contamination tends to systematically reduce any difference in outcomes between experimental and control subjects. The study architecture must recognize this danger and, if possible, participating clinicians must agree to protect against it, at least for some negotiated period of follow-up.

Patients randomized to the surgical limb have undergone microsurgical, end to side anastomosis of the superficial temporal or occipital artery to a cortical branch of the middle cerebral artery. All participating surgeons have agreed to follow an identical procedure in the performance of the EC/IC bypass, but minor variations in the surgical technique have been permitted and left to the individual surgeon's discretion.

Surgical patients have undergone postoperative angiography; the recommended timing has been 3 to 6 months following bypass. All the postoperative angiograms have been reviewed by the principal neuroradiologist at the Central Office. The success of the anastomosis has been assessed by the following features: the comparative size (smaller, same, or larger) of the superficial temporal artery proximal to the anastomosis on preoperative and postoperative angiograms; the degree of retrograde flow in the middle cerebral artery filled. Overall flow through the bypass has been estimated as none, slight, moderate, good, or excellent. Further follow-up angiograms have been recommended when the first postoperative angiogram has suggested poor bypass function.

A random sample of 20 postoperative angiograms have been reviewed a second time by the principal neuroradiologist (who had been blinded to his original report) to assess intraobserver agreement. Because previous randomized trials have established the efficacy of aspirin in patients with TIA and minor stroke,[18] all patients (both medical and surgical) have been prescribed acetylsalicylic acid 325 mg, q.i.d., throughout the trial, unless contraindicated or not tolerated. Furthermore, the control of hypertension has been stressed and monitored in both medical and surgical patients; the treatment of other risk factors has been left to individual clinical judgment.

Patients who initially accepted their randomization to medical therapy but later underwent EC/IC bypass on the randomized side, or patients who accepted randomization to surgical therapy and then declined the operation were labeled "crossovers." Strokes occurring to such patients before their crossover are to be charged to the medical limb and the surgical limb, respectively, in the primary analysis. Those who had no events prior to the crossover were judged to have been randomized improperly and to have failed to give proper informed consent. They were placed in one of the exclusion categories.

What Sort of Follow-up Should Be Carried Out?

Follow-up should be carried out with sufficient frequency and intensity to accomplish three things: to identify important events, to identify important side effects, and to keep track of the entire group of patients so that none are lost.

All patients, both medical and surgical, have been examined by a participating neurologist 6 weeks after randomization and at 3-month intervals thereafter; surgical patients have received an additional review approximately 30 days following surgery. At each visit, an interim history has been obtained and a detailed neurologic examination has been performed, including the functional status assessment. In addition, repeat assessments have been made of the patient's employment status, medical and smoking history, medications, blood pressure, and cardiac status.

Other medical problems, medications, and perioperative complications have been monitored to detect unexpected adverse effects of any medical and/or surgical treatment that patients have undergone during the trial.

What Should Be Done About Withdrawals?

The simple solution to the problem of withdrawals, to be pursued assiduously, but never achieved, is never to have any. Withdrawals are the bane of all prospective clinical research because they bedevil the analysis. Should they be counted or not? What if we don't know what has become of them? Two rules of thumb may help. First, because a refusal to participate at entry to a trial, prior to randomization, can detract only from the generalizability of the result, whereas a refusal to continue to participate (i.e., a withdrawal) after randomization can also detract from the validity of the result, the former is always preferable. Consequently, it is wise to inform prospective subjects of all features of the study that might discourage their continuing cooperation. Second, withdrawal is a time for negotiation, not farewell. Attempts should be made to retain cooperation for at least certain portions of follow-up—if only by mail or telephone or through the patient's primary physician – so that it is at least possible to state whether withdrawn patients are alive at the conclusion of a trial.

Only patients who refused to continue under observation were to have been withdrawn from the trial; others were to be retained. EC/IC surgery on the side opposite to the qualifying lesion and internal carotid endarterectomy on either side have been discouraged; however, patients who have undergone these additional procedures have not been withdrawn from the trial. A second EC/IC bypass on the same side has been omitted in a small number of surgical patients in whom it has appeared likely to improve bypass function; however, these surgical procedures have not, by themselves, constituted events, and such patients have not been withdrawn.

What Events Should Be Measured in the Trial, and How?

The events to be measured will follow from the question posed by the trial. They should be clinically important, highly reproducible measures of the success or failure of the experimental operation, including its complications. We will focus more on how to measure than on what is measured, and will once again consider "How might the answer be wrong?"

Because many efficacious operations trade an immediate, small risk of death for later, larger benefits, it is important to measure the former and to continue long enough to capture the latter. Patients in the nonoperated limb should receive equally vigorous follow-up to render their events just as likely to be recognized and reported.

Surgical trials do not lend themselves to the bias-avoiding strategy of double-blindness. They can, nevertheless, use another strategy for limiting error. The clinical criteria for events can be made so "hard" and objective that they can be measured, and this adjudication can sometimes be carried out on clinical records that have been "purged" of any mention of whether the study patient was in the operated group.

The main study events are the occurrence of fatal or nonfatal stroke following randomization. However, to include any excess perioperative risk, deaths from all causes have been included if they occurred between randomization and 30 days following EC/IC bypass among surgical patients and for a comparable duration among patients in the medical group.

Events have been identified and classified in one or more of three ways. First, participating neurologists have identified and reported them during routine patient follow-up. Second, the principal investigators at the Central Office have identified events during their weekly clinical reviews of the follow-up data, supplemented when necessary by further communication with the participating neurologist. Third, a computer program at the Methods Center has identified possible events by comparing the functional status, signs, and symptoms on each follow-up with those recorded on previous follow-up assessments.

The best current means for diagnosis (including CT scan where available) have been used to differentiate strokes due to infarction from those due to hemorrhage. The severity of the stroke, in terms of the impairment of functional status, has been rated on a 10-point scale, using information derived from the neurologic follow-up forms.

Transient ischemic attacks, other major cardiovascular morbidity, and deaths from noncerebrovascular causes have also been recorded but have not constituted main events. Thorough documentation (including autopsy findings; emergency room, operative, and hospital discharge reports; death certificates; and the observations of any witnesses) has been sought for every death from any cause.

Adjudication of the cause of death and the occurrence and severity of strokes has been performed independently by a neurologist and a neurosurgeon who have not cared for patients in the study and have been blind both to the patients' treatments and to each other's judgments. Disagreements between the two adjudicators have been resolved by consensus. Disagreements between the adjudicators' consensus and the results of the Central Office's weekly clinical reviews have been resolved through discussion with the principal clinical investigators.

How Should the Data Be Analyzed?

Neither the length nor the intent of this chapter permits a comprehensive discussion of the analysis of randomized trials. All we can do is state a few maxims.

1. Patient-centered research that is badly designed or badly analyzed is unethical, because it exposes humans to risks without guarding against bias and imprecision. The only solution is to involve competent biostatisticians as full collaborators from the very beginning of protocol development.
2. A clinical trial, like any other experiment, can answer only one or two questions, not more. Although the results of a trial should undergo as

much subgroup and exploratory analysis, or "data-dredging," as time, budget, and energy allow, these explorations must be recognized as exercises in hypothesis forming, not hypothesis testing.

3. A trial should be stopped as soon as the better treatment is identified. This calls for interim analysis of the emerging results and is another reason for obtaining biostatistical collaboration from the outset.

To discharge the ethical responsibility of stopping the trial as soon as a clear-cut conclusion is evident, the accumulating data have been analyzed at 6-month intervals. An "alerting" procedure has been developed and adopted that calls for the early stopping of the study to have been considered if two consecutive interim analyses have shown either that the surgically treated group are faring significantly better (at the $p = .02$ level) or that it has become very unlikely that any surgical benefit could have been demonstrated.[19] The results of these interim analyses, known only to the principal epidemiologic investigator and chief biostatistician at the Methods Center, have been summarized and reported to the monitoring committee.

Appropriate allowance has been made for the statistical effect of these interim challenges of the data; if the trial has not been terminated early, a p value of .04 or less would have constituted statistically significance in the final analysis.

How Many Patients Do We Need?

If the foregoing section failed to convince you of the need for early collaboration with a biostatistician, this one should. Investigators are unlikely to obtain clinical collaborators, and can almost never obtain outside research funds, without being able to explain how many patients they need to answer their study question.

Briefly, the four elements of any trial that, when specified, will determine the number of patients required for the study, are:

1. The expected rate of events in the control group.
2. The degree of reduction in the risk of these events that, if it occurred in the experimental group, would indicate that the operation was efficacious.
3. The risk the investigator is willing to run of drawing the false-positive conclusion that the operation is efficacious when, in truth, it is not.
4. The risk the investigator is willing to run of drawing the false-negative conclusion that the operation is not efficacious when, in truth, it is.

The required sample size and duration of follow-up initially had been determined on the basis of data available when the protocol was designed (February 1977). The following estimates and specifications have been employed.

1. For medically treated patients: an expected combined stroke and stroke-death rate of 23.6% over 5 years.[20-26]
2. For surgically treated patients: an estimated 30-day perioperative stroke and death rate of 4%[21,24] followed by a 50% reduction in the subsequent rate of fatal and nonfatal stroke compared with medically treated patients, for a net surgical benefit of 33% reduction in the 5-year risk of fatal and nonfatal stroke. It has been agreed that this degree of risk reduction constituted a clinically important surgical benefit which, if achieved in the trial, would justify advocating the EC/IC bypass procedure.
3. A risk of 5% of drawing the false-positive conclusion that surgery is better than medical therapy when, in truth, surgery results in the clinically important benefit stated above ($\alpha = .05$).
4. A risk of 10% of drawing the false-negative conclusion that surgery is no better than medical therapy alone, when, in truth is ($\beta = .10$).

These considerations had required a sample size of 442 patients per treatment group, followed for an average of 5 years. Allowing for dropouts, an initial total sample size target of 1000 patients had been established.

By February 1981, 35% of trial patients had been entered with internal carotid artery occlusion without further ischemic symptoms since angiography. Because this group had been thought to be at a lower risk of subsequent stroke, it had been feared that large numbers of such cases might have obscured a surgical benefit to other patients. This situation was discussed by executive committee members who were blind with respect to events in both treatment groups, and they proposed to increase the total sample size target to 1400 patients. This proposal was accepted by the monitoring committee and was implemented.

Adjustments to sample size calculations are available[25] for dropouts, crossovers, and withdrawals. More important than these considerations, however, is the need to recognize that it is not enough simply to project estimates of the prevalence of the trial condition to the local population. Affected individuals must not only be around. They, and their referring clinicians, must be willing to participate; the experimental therapy and follow-up procedures must be acceptable to them; and they must satisfy the specific inclusion/exclusion criteria. Even when viewed through jaundiced eyes, the availability of suitable patients may still be overestimated, and safety margins of 100% to 400% have been suggested by scarred investigators.

When realistic estimates suggest that the required numbers of study patients may be hard to find, a number of strategies can be considered. First, you can rethink the issues of risk and responsiveness raised earlier and possibly increase the trial's efficiency. Second, you may wish to rethink the risks of false-positive and false-negative errors you are willing to take; when the restrictions are relaxed, the sample size requirements falls.

Third, you can attempt to reduce the noise in the measurement of events and outcomes by improving the precision of the measurements. The result will be higher values for the test statistic at any level of between-group differences. Where it is sensible, although impossible in most surgical trials, you can also benefit from the paired examination of treatment effects within individual study patients by performing crossover trials—this solution should have been explored when the basic architecture of your study was first considered. Finally, the local sample size problem can be solved by converting to a multicenter design, but this will incur substantial costs in administrative complexity and investigator effort (see below, Chapter 29).

Can We Prevent or Minimize the Iatrogenic Complications of a Surgical Procedure Already Accepted as Useful?

In the previous example of a surgical study, we explored some important aspects of a trial designed to answer a question about the value of a particular surgical therapy. Other questions of interest to clinicians revolve around preventing complications associated with well-established surgical procedures. Examples of this include prevention of deep vein thrombosis and pulmonary embolus following surgical procedures, and infections of various kinds, including those associated with the use of indwelling foreign bodies such as hip prostheses, vascular grafts, and cerebrospinal fluid (CSF) shunts. The example we shall use for this type of trial is the randomized controlled trial of perioperative antibiotics in the prevention of CSF shunt infection designed for the Hospital for Sick Children (HSC) in Toronto, in which one of us (B.C.W.) is the principal investigator. In addition, we will show how this same clinical question can be addressed by another study design: a case-control analytic design carried out by one of us (B.C.W.).

Cerebrospinal fluid shunts were first widely used as a treatment for congenital hydrocephalus in the 1950s, when various technical problems that had plagued neurosurgeons since the turn of the century were ironed out. A randomized controlled trial carried out in England in 1958 demonstrated the obvious value of cerebrospinal fluid shunts in the treatment of this condition.[26] Early on, however, it was discovered that a major complication of the procedure was infection. Since it was clear that the source of infection was usually the surgical event, various efforts were made to prevent the infections by the use of perioperative antibiotics. Reports began to appear in the literature in the 1960s claiming the usefulness of "prophylactic" antibiotics in the prevention of shunt infection. However, these reports were only a series of cases with no control or comparison group, and were therefore of questionable scientific value. It was not until 1975 that a randomized clinical trial of prophylactic antibiotics in shunt surgery was published,[27] and it showed that there was no difference between the experimental and control groups in rate of infection.

Two other trials that supported these findings were subsequently published.[28,29] However, all these trials had the same major flaw; namely, insufficient numbers of patients to find a clinically significant difference, if one existed. This is the failure of study design called the beta error; that is, the risk of missing a clinically significant difference in groups (or therapies) due to insufficient numbers. As mentioned in the section on patient numbers needed for the EC/IC bypass trial, it is one of the four design elements that must be calculated in advance of a study's being undertaken. The *power* of the study, then, is a reflection of the study's ability to minimize the beta error ($1 - \beta$). Table 24.1 compares the beta error (and power) of these randomized controlled trials of perioperative antibiotics in shunt surgery referred to above. It is easy to see why these studies were at risk for finding a negative outcome with such small numbers of patients.

But How Many Patients Should We Have in a Well-Designed Study?

As we have seen, there is no one set answer, because the number of patients needed to test the hypothesis adequately depends on the frequency of the outcome event (i.e., infection), and on the magnitude of the difference between experimental

TABLE 24.1. Beta and power calculations ($1 - \beta$) on randomized trials of perioperative antibiotics in CSF shunt.

Study	Ref.	Number of patients	Power	Risk of missing a 50% difference	Number of infections
Haines and Taylor: 1982	28	74	.20	80%	7
Wang et al: 1984	29	120	.27	73%	9
Bayston: 1975	27	132	.28	72%	3

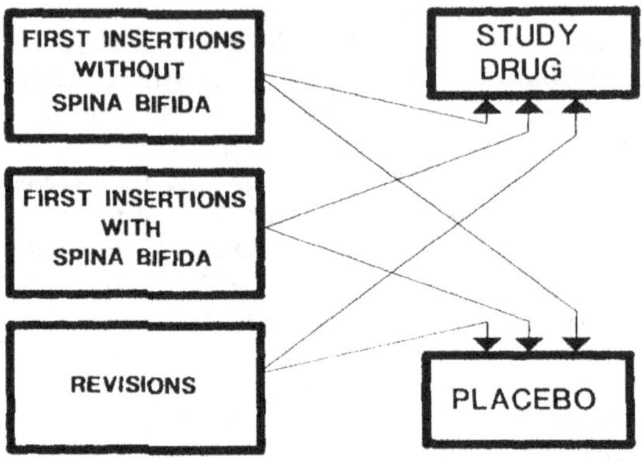

FIGURE 24.1. Stratified randomization in a trial of perioperative antibiotics in cerebrospinal fluid shunt surgery.

and control groups that we consider to be clinically significant. For example, in CSF shunt infection, the usual shunt infection rate quoted is around 10% (although the literature range is 1% to 30%). If we think that a reduction in infection to 7.5% would be clinically significant, and yet would want to keep low our risks of being wrong in either direction (i.e., saying there's a difference when there isn't, or saying there isn't a difference when there is), we would need so many patients to detect this difference that such a trial would be virtually prohibitive. This, then, is where the numbers game begins, and frequent visits to your friendly local biostatistician are in order. As pointed out earlier, you will have to balance fastidiousness in designing your study with pragmatism in its execution. But early on you will realize that the smaller the study is, the greater the risk in being wrong in one direction or the other. In the HSC study, we chose the following parameters:

.05 = α, or risk of claiming a difference which, in truth, does not exist
.20 = β, or risk of missing a clinically significant difference between treatment and control groups
.10 = infection rate in the placebo group
.05 = infection rate in the treatment group

Using these design parameters and a standard formula, we calculated that we would need 690 patients for the study. This is only an estimate, but it is clearly a far cry from the patient numbers of the other studies previously reported, and is likely to minimize the opportunities for error.

What Other Design Issues Arise in an Effort to Diminish the Threats to Validity in This Type of Study?

In the preceding section, we saw how one aspect of study design, when ignored, can threaten the integrity of a study design, causing its conclusions to be drawn into question. Let us consider other aspects, as well. First of all, what are some of the sources of systematic error (also called "bias") that might influence the conclusions of the trial and threaten its validity?

There are really two major sources of bias in clinical studies; one involves inherent differences between treatment and control groups with respect to disease state or some other relevant variable; the other has to do with differences in management of the two groups, in addition to the experimental maneuver that forms the basis of the study. Applying this to the example of cerebrospinal fluid shunt infection and perioperative antibiotic therapy, we asked ourselves the question "In what ways might patients differ inherently that might cause them to have a variable response to the study maneuver or be more likely to become infected?" This caused us to think about the etiologies of hydrocephalus and to divide patients into those who had spina bifida and those who did not. The literature is divided on whether the presence of a myelomeningocele increases the risk of infection, but there is good biological reason to assume that it might. In addition, it seemed reasonable to believe that the more operations (or revisions) a patient had, the more opportunity there might be for infection. We, therefore, divided patients into those having their first shunt ever and those whose shunt equipment was being revised in some way (usually because of malfunction). Taking all these factors into consideration, we thus divided patients into those with and without myelomeningocele, and those having revision procedures, as illustrated in Figure 24.1. Clearly, the division of patients was carried out *prior* to randomization into treatment and placebo groups. This process, called *stratification*, is an attempt to assure an even distribution or balance of patients between treatments, thus eliminating these factors as possible explanations for the findings of the study.

As explained above, we were able to think of two large factors that might influence the outcome of our study; but as every clinician knows, there are many subtle and invisible differences between patients that might also influence the trial's outcome but cannot be determined or specifically protected against by stratification. These differences will most likely not influence the study findings, however, because of the randomization process itself. There is no guarantee that this will be so, and a poststudy analysis (referred to previously as data-dredging) may be able to detect the effects of these other variables.

Who Should Be Blinded in the Study?

The whole issue of blinding is often misunderstood until it is related to our old outlook of trying to protect ourselves from being wrong in the conclusions we reach as a result of the study findings. In the issue of shunt infection, the patients who did not receive antibiotics might receive closer observation and more careful medical and nursing care if there were a belief that somehow they were being placed at greater risk by their not having received the perioperative antibiotics. Blinding, along with a standard protocol of follow-up and assessment, would obviously prevent this inequality from occurring. In addition, firm, objective outcome measures by assessors uninformed of previous exposure to perioperative antibiotics would reinforce this. Our protocol for dealing with shunted patients was standardized, and we chose two outcome measures that could not be influenced by knowledge of therapeutic modality: one year of trouble-free clinical status and presence or absence of bacteria on culture of the shunt apparatus submitted at the time of revision for malfunction. We, therefore, achieved a "triple-blind" design: neither the surgeon, nor the patient (or the patient's parents or guardians), nor the microbiologist who cultured the removed shunt apparatus was aware of which patients had received drug or placebo.

Other design issues such as the exact drug that will be given the experimental group (and the rationale for choosing it), ethical issues (including informed consent), realistic expectations for time necessary to accrue appropriate study candidates, inclusion and exclusion criteria, and other such crucial details have been carefully built into the study protocol but are not discussed further here. Suffice it to say that without the careful consideration of all these details by all the participants in the study *prior* to its implementation, the trial may not be protected against the threats to validity to which it may fall prey.

What Other Study Design Might Be Used to Answer This Clinical Question?

Although it is unquestionable that the randomized controlled trial is the study design of choice for the production of conclusions of the highest scientific merit, certain problems associated with randomized controlled trials may limit their use. For example, in the two cases discussed above, only large institutions or several institutions banding together could provide the number of patients necessary for implementation of the trial. Other problems such as compliance with sometimes unwieldy study protocols or lack of funds can also inhibit the undertaking of a large-scale trial. It has, therefore, been suggested that other study designs, such as the case-control analytic design, be used to test hypotheses in clinical medicine.[30-32] Although most commonly used to demonstrate association between an outcome and a risk factor (see above, Chapter 13), this type of subexperimental design can be strengthened so that many of its potential flaws can be protected against. Positive attributes of the case-control analytic design include the following.

1. As a retrospective study, it is based on data already generated in the everyday practice of clinical medicine.
2. Because of the nature of the sample size calculation, fewer patients are required to reach statistical significance.
3. Fewer personnel are required to carry out the study, since it is primarily a medical record review.
4. The cost of executing the study is minimal.

It is easy to see why a case-control analytic design is attractive, but it should be obvious that its big danger is *retrospectivity*, with the "experimental" maneuver out of the hands of the investigator and having been applied in an uncontrolled fashion to a group of selected patients, who may or may not qualify for a randomized controlled trial. This type of study design is therefore open to many biases and other threats to validity. It is clearly not the study design of choice, but there may be situations in which it may be of value.

At the Hospital for Sick Children in Toronto, we were contemplating implementing the randomized controlled trial of perioperative antibiotics as prophylaxis against cerebrospinal fluid shunt infection, as described earlier. As already mentioned, the trials that had been done did not show any significant difference in the rate of shunt infection in the antibiotic group compared to the placebo group. And, as we have said, we felt that this failure to reject the null hypothesis could be explained by the inadequate numbers of patients studied. However, one could also argue that there was truly no difference. We, therefore, decided to carry out a case-control analytic study to determine whether there was any stronger evidence to support the use of prophylactic antibiotics than the weak case series designs that had been published previously.

Notwithstanding our desire not to produce a flawed study, we were attracted to the idea of a case-control design because we felt we might be able to build into the design various protections against the threats to validity that might be identified. This had already been carried out in the literature in at least one study.[26] If we could build a strong study design whose conclusions could be trusted, this would convince us to invest the time, energy, effort, and funds into a more formalized randomized controlled trial.

In brief, a case-control study of therapy is different from a randomized controlled trial in that it is a retrospective study, usually without a formalized protocol, without blinding, and (usually) without inclusion and exclusion criteria. The research question is posed differently, too, although the clinical question is obviously the same. For example, as clinical neurosurgeons we want to know whether we should be using prophylactic antibiotics in cerebrospinal fluid shunt surgery to help prevent infections. In the randomized controlled trial, the research question is, "When treatment X is given to group A, but not to group B, is there a difference in the rate of infection between the two groups?" In the case-control situation, we ask, "When a group of infected patients are compared to a group of similar, but not infected patients, was there a greater percentage of antibiotic use among the noninfected versus the infected patients?" From this, we can derive a "relative odds" between the groups, which indicates which group has more risk of becoming infected. If the noninfected group had more patients in it who had been given perioperative antibiotics, then we infer that the antibiotics may be of some benefit.

With this background, we set out to explore this avenue of clinical study.[33] The following details are from this study.

1. **Eligibility criteria.** All children who required shunting for hydrocephalus, whatever the cause, were included, with the exception of any patients allergic to antibiotics used commonly as prophylaxis (e.g., cloxacillin, clindamycin, cephalosporins), those with known systemic infection, or those being treated for recent infections. The sample population was assembled from the cohort of patients shunted at the Hospital for Sick Children from 1972–1977. Only the initial operation for shunting was studied.

   It can be seen from this that these patients could have participated in a randomized controlled trial, had one been underway, and this feature allows a more refined analysis than if we included all patients treated. We chose the cohort of 1972–1977 so that we could have a lengthy follow-up, and we limited the study to those having only the first insertion of a shunt to eliminate the influence of multiple procedures on the outcome.
2. **Outcome criteria.** Cases were defined as any patient developing a shunt infection (a positive culture of cerebroshunt fluid or shunt tubing in a ventriculoperitoneal shunt and/or blood in a ventriculoatrial shunt). Controls were defined as those patients whose shunt apparatus was negative for culture of bacteria at first revision or who had asymptomatic follow-up for five years or longer. Absence of infection at insertion was ascertained by negative cultures of cerebroshunt fluid.

   We, therefore, nailed down ahead of time the criteria we felt would provide convincing evidence regarding the outcome of importance (i.e., infection).
3. **Definition of exposure.** "Antibiotic prophylaxis" was defined as any antibiotic regimen given perioperatively and intended to prevent shunt infection. Usually this meant pre- and postoperative administration of antibiotics for a limited time, but occasionally included antibiotics beginning immediately postoperatively. Drug regimens were checked for adequate dosage. Individual antibiotics were not controlled for, since the research question is dealing with the policy of antibiotic use and not the use of any specific antibiotic preparation.

   This lack of uniformity of therapy is the bugbear of retrospective studies, but by choosing the "accepted therapy" of the time, we hoped to fairly evaluate the policy of using of antibiotics.
4. **Sample size estimation.** The parameters used to calculate sample size included a significance level of .05, a power of .80, estimated proportion of patients receiving "prophylactic" antibi-

otics of 30%, and an overall infection rate of 10%. Using a standard formula,[34] we ascertained that a total of 32 cases and an equal number of controls would allow us to detect a difference in risk of infection of 6.5 times or greater between the groups.

As can be seen from this outline, we demanded the same rigor of this study that we demanded from our randomized controlled trial, in terms of power and significance. The sample size formula for calculating groups for a case-control study differs from an randomized controlled trial in that one tries to estimate relative odds (in this case, 6.5 times). One notices immediately that the number of patients needed is well below that calculated for our randomized controlled trial. This is more easily understood when one realizes that the group with the outcome of interest (infection) is equal to the number without, whereas these patients represent only a small proportion of treated patients in a randomized controlled trial.

5. **Data collection.** Using the data set generated by the computerized data storage and retrieval system in the Division of Neurosurgery at HSC, a search was made for cases and controls with a random sampling of patients by year of shunt insertion, age, and etiology of hydrocephalus. The patients' charts were then examined and their suitability for designation as either "case" or "control" was verified, using the above criteria. At a separate inspection, the use of antibiotic prophylaxis was determined from the doctors' orders sheets.

   By determining the suitability of potential cases and controls in a blinded fashion, we were able to avoid the bias of choosing the patients with the treatment favoring our hypothesis. Once the patients had been chosen, we looked at their "exposure" to antibiotics.

6. **Data analysis.** Significance testing was carried out using Fisher's exact test (α = .05, two-tailed). Relative risk of infection with and without antibiotics was estimated using an odds ratio . . . , and a stratified analysis was carried out using the Mantel-Haenszel Chi-square.

   After the data were collected, we exposed them to rigorous statistical testing in an appropriate method. This sort of test is different from what would be used for a randomized controlled trial, because the numbers are different, and the study question is posed in a different way.

In summary then, we attempted to design a case-control study to answer a clinical question of therapeutic effectiveness, imposing on it as much of the same protection against error that we used in our randomized controlled trial. We, therefore, hoped to generate support for our hypothesis that perioperative antibiotic therapy could reduce the rate of infection. Our results were encouraging in that there was a much higher rate of "exposure" to antibiotic use among the noninfected patients than among the infected patients.

Because of this preliminary study, we were encouraged to go ahead with the randomized controlled trial described earlier. Thus, we demonstrated that this sort of study design could be used in the present context, and perhaps even in the circumstance of a rare disease in which an randomized controlled trials would never be done.

TABLE 24.2. Results of a case-control study of risk of infection with and without antibiotics in CSF shunt surgery.

	Cases	Controls	Total
No antibiotics[a]	28	18	46
Antibiotics	4	14	18
Total	32	32	64

p = .01 (Fisher's exact test, two tailed)
Summary odds ratio = 3.27 (Mantel-Haenszel)[b]

[a] The risk factor in this analysis is "no antibiotics."
[b] Greater than three times more likely to become infected after surgery without antibiotics.

Prerequisites for a Successful Surgical Research Project

The protocol for a clinical research study must not only be attractive to potential collaborators but must also set minimal performance criteria for continuing or abandoning the trial. Five elements of a protocol influence its attractiveness. First, there must be a convincing statement of the need for the trial. This statement must provide the basis on which clinicians can justify, to themselves, their colleagues, and their patients, the special conditions and efforts required to ensure the success of the trial. Second, the experimental maneuver not only must be clinically sensible and applicable, but also it must be able to withstand close scrutiny so that the clinicians can defend it against its critics. For example, if a surgical operation is involved, the expertise with which it is executed may vary considerably, and a biologically valuable maneuver maybe made to appear useless or even harmful when it is performed with less than adequate skill. The credibility of the trial can be protected by invoking current specifications on clinical competency (e.g., surgical mortality and graft patency) as criteria that must be met prior to joining a trial, in addition to a pledge to monitor performance during the trial. If, despite these precautions, the level of expertise is expected to change with time, this circumstance should be taken into account by balancing treatment allocations at several points during the trial and by using calendar time as a covariate in planning the analysis.

The third element in the attractiveness of the protocol to potential clinical collaborators is the specification of the minimum appropriate requirements for the documentation and follow-up of study patients. Clinical trials often gather far more data than are required to answer the question at hand. Investigators who feel burdened with excessive documentation of overly frequent follow-up visits may falter in their entry of new study patients. Fourth, the principal investigators must be perceived by their potential clinical collaborators as individuals who know what they are doing. Consequently, they must either possess or quickly establish their credibility in the relevant areas of clinical medicine, human biology, and research methods. Finally, each potential collaborator must be shown how participation in the trial will bring personal rewards, such as further education, additions to one's prestige and bibliography, and recognition as someone who has made a significant contribution to the generation of useful new knowledge.

The ultimate test of the feasibility of a trial protocol is often provided by a brief pilot run involving only a small number of patients. When you are considering whether to carry out a pilot study, you ought to bear its advantages and disadvantages in mind. A pilot study certainly can help you to identify and solve problems with definitions, data forms, and data flow and to "debug" the application of the study protocol. When study events are early and frequent, a pilot study can test and possibly confirm your earlier sample size estimates. Finally, a pilot trial can, on rare occasions, provide definitive answers of efficacy when the test therapy is very, very good or very, very bad.

Against these potential advantages, you must consider the drawbacks and difficulties of such a pilot study. First, it will "consume" patients who would otherwise be in the formal trial. This happens because pilot studies are often executed in an unblinded mode and because they often lead to substantive changes in the protocol that make it impossible or inappropriate to include the subjects in later analysis. If study patients are in short supply, a pilot study could scuttle your trial. When study events are rare or late, a pilot study cannot provide a helpful commentary on your sample size requirements, and it may be difficult to interest potential clinical collaborators or funding agencies in committing themselves to a task with such meager short-term benefits. Finally, if your pilot study results are not going to be included in later analyses for efficacy, the ethics of including human subjects in it raises an additional problem.

Instead of adopting an all-or-none position on the need for a pilot study, you should define what you need to know prior to the formal execution of your protocol, and then consider alternative strategies for gaining this knowledge. For example, if the adequacy of forms, data flow, and definitions is at issue, these features can be tested on "gram samples" of patients who, although they have the disorder of interest, are otherwise ineligible for the trial. Such patients can also be used to test the documentation and handling of events, to telescope the long latent period that may occur in the trial proper. In this way, you can save eligible patients for the later, definitive trial and still do a pilot study by inviting ineligible patients to help you with the debugging of the study protocol.

When McFate Smith corresponded with the investigators in 12 large hypertension trials and asked them to identify their five worst problems, administrative problems led scientific problems by more than 2 to 1.[35] Although some were organizational problems of special pertinence to multicenter trials, most were problems in the everyday management of the trial that could, if mishandled, destroy the credibility and validity of the trial. Accordingly, attention to administrative issues is the sixth and final prerequisite for a successful clinical trial.

The trial protocol, when translated into the working document for the trial (hereafter referred to as the study manual), should include all the study forms and the rules for their completion and submission. In addition, it is vitally important to include in the study manual unambiguous rules for following and reporting on study patients who refuse therapy, withdraw, fail to comply, suffer side effects, drop out, or otherwise fail to adhere to the protocol, as well as precise and objective criteria for eligibility and events. The responsibilities for executing and documenting each step in the protocol need to be assigned, even to the point of writing job specifications where necessary.

Other key issues in the organization and administration of your trial may not appear in your study manual but they are, nonetheless, key factors in the success of your trial. Chief among these is the specification of the authority and responsibility of the clinical and methodologic investigators: who is to do what to whom, and "where the buck stops." Publication policies, especially those related to authorship, should be stated at the outset and should be accompanied by a pledge to present the results to your clinical collaborators first. The rules for monitoring trends in the data, often accomplished by forming a committee of respected investigators who are outside the trial, and for halting the trial as soon as an unambiguous answer is apparent, should be spelled out in advance.

The financial resources for the trial must be sufficient to support the staff and facilities required for the assessment and follow-up of both the study patients and the study data. A key requirement is the provision of sufficient funds for thoughtful secondary data analyses, which can, in certain circumstances, provide important clues to the presentation, course, and prognosis of the disorder under study.

References

1. Bunker UP, Barnes BA, Mosteller F. Costs, Risks and Benefits of Surgery. New York: Oxford University Press, 1977.
2. Sackett DL, Haynes RB, Tugwell P. Clinical Epidemiology; A Basic Science for Clinical Medicine. Boston: Little, Brown, 1985.
3. Coronary Drug Project Research Group. Influence of adherence to treatment and response of cholesterol on mortality in the Coronary Drug Project. N Engl J Med 1980;303:1038–41.
4. Asher WL, Harper HW. Effect of human chorionic gonadotropin on weight loss, hunger, and feeling of well-being. Am J Clin Nutr 1973;26:211–18.
5. Hogarty GE, Goldberg SC. Drug and sociotherapy in the aftercare of schizophrenic patients. Arch Gen Psychiatr 1973;28:54–64.
6. Fuller R, Roth H, Long S. Compliance with disulfiram treatment of alcoholism. J. Chronic Dis 1983; 36:161–70.
7. Pizzo PA, Robichaud KJ, Edwards BK, Schumaker C, Kramer BS, Johnson A. Oral antibiotic prophylaxis in patients with cancer; a double-blind randomized placebo-controlled trial. J Pediatr 1983; 102:125–33.
8. Sackett DL. Rules of evidence and clinical recommendations on the use of antithrombotic agents. Chest 1986;89(2 Suppl):25–35.
9. Cobb LA, Thomas GI, Dillard DH, Merendino KA, Bruce RA. An evaluation of internal-mammary-artery ligation by a double-blind technique. N Engl J Med 1959;260:1115–18.
10. Schwartz D, Lellouch J. Explanatory and pragmatic attitudes in therapeutic trials. J Chronic Dis 1967; 20:637–48.
11. Sackett DL, Gent M. Controversy in counting and attributing events in clinical trials. N Engl J Med 1979;301:1410–12.
12. EC/IC Bypass Study Group. International cooperative study of extracranial/intracranial arterial anastomosis (EC/IC) bypass study; methodology and entry characteristics. Stroke 1985;16:397–406.
13. EC/IC Bypass Study Group. Failure of extracranial/intracranial arterial bypass to reduce the risk of ischemic stroke. M Engl J Med 1985;313:1191–1200.
14. Oberman A, Myers AR, Karunas, TM, Epstein FH. Heart size of adults in a natural population—Tecumseh, Michigan: variation by sex, age, height, and weight. Circulation 1967;35:724.
15. Shibata H, Matsuzaki T, Shiohida K, Saito N. Study on usefulness of cardiothoracic ratio in the aged. Jpn J Geriatr 1976;13:406.
16. Yano K, Ueda S. Coronary heart disease in Hiroshima, Japan: analysis of the data at the initial examination, 1958–1960. Yale J Biol Med 1962–63;35: 504.
17. Sackett DL. Bias in analytic research. J Chronic Dis 1979;32:51–63.
18. Canadian Cooperative Study Group. A randomized trial of aspirin and sulfinpyrazone in threatened stroke. N Engl J Med 1978;299:53–9.
19. Taylor DW, Haynes RB, Sackett DL. Stopping rules for long-term clinical trials (abstr). Controlled Clin Trials 1980;1:170.
20. Toole JF, Janeway R, Choi K, et al. Transient ischemic attacks due to atherosclerosis: a prospective study of 160 patients. Arch Neurol 1975;32: 5–12.
21. Heyman A, Levitan A, Millikan CH, et al. Transient focal cerebral ischemia: epidemiologic and clinical aspects. Stroke 1974;5:277–87.
22. Matsumoto N, Whisnant JP, Kurland LT, Okazaki H. Natural history of stroke in Rochester, Minnesota, 1955 through 1969. Stroke 1973;4:20–29.
23. Fields WS, Maslenikov V, Meyer JS, Hass WK, Remington RD, MacDonald M. Joint study of extracranial arterial occlusion. V. Progress report of prognosis following surgery or nonsurgical treatment of transient cerebral ischemic attacks and cervical carotid artery lesions. JAMA 1970;211:1993–2003.
24. Delong WB. Microsurgical revascularization for cerebrovascular insufficiency. Stroke 1976;9:15–20.
25. Halperin M, Rogot E, Gurian J, Edener F. Sample sizes for medical trials with special reference to long-term therapy. J Chronic Dis 1968;21:123–24.
26. Lorber J, Zachary RB: Primary congenital hydrocephalus. Long- term results of controlled therapeutic trial. Arch Dis Child 1968;43:516–27.
27. Bayston R. Antibiotic prophylaxis in shunt surgery. Dev Med Child Neurol 1975;17(Suppl 35):99–103.
28. Haines SJ, Taylor F. Prophylactic methicillin for shunt operations: effects on incidence of shunt malfunction and infection. Child's Brain 1982;9:10–22.
29. Wang EL, et al. Prophylactic sulfamethoxazole and trimethoprim in ventriculoperitoneal shunt surgery. A double-blind, randomized, placebo-controlled trial. JAMA 1984;251(9):1174–77.
30. Horowitz RI, Feinstein AR. The application of therapeutic trial principles to improve the design of

epidemiologic research: a case-control study suggesting that anticoagulants reduce mortality in patients with myocardial infarction. J Chronic Dis 1981;34:575–83.

31. Morgan PP. Clinical trials on trial: Must we always do a randomized trial? Can Med Assoc J 1981;125: 1309–11.

32. Hayden GF, Kramer MS, Horwitz RI. The case-control study. A practical review for the clinician. JAMA 1982;247(3);326–31.

33. Walters BC, et al. Decreased risk of infection in cerebrospinal fluid shunt surgery using prophylactic antibiotics: a case-control study. Z Kinderchir 1985; 40(Suppl I):15–18.

34. Cornfield J. A method of estimating comparative rates for clinical data. J Natl Cancer Inst 1950–1951;11:1269–75.

35. Smith WM. Problems in long-term trials. In: Mild Hypertension: Natural History and Management, Gross F, Strasser T. eds. London: Pitman, 1979;244–53.

25

Organizing a Clinical Study

L. Del Greco, J.I. Williams, and D.S. Mulder

Each year, a particular surgeon performs about 70 operations for aortofemoral bypass grafting to restore blood supply to the extremities. Initially, he judged the success of the surgery in terms of survival and the saving of limbs. As methods for assessing blood flow in peripheral vessels improved, as well as diagnostic and surgical techniques, the proportion of patients under the age of 65 years increased. In the course of following his patients, particularly those under 65 years of age, questions arose in the surgeon's mind about the impact of this surgery on patients' return to work and sexual functioning.

Concern arises from the possibility that current surgical procedures damage the pelvic and autonomic nervous system. Alternative operations are more invasive, but the question still arises: "Do sexual dysfunction and nonresumption of principal activities, whether related to work or retirement, indicate that a comparative trial should be considered?" The surgeon, who has been gathering data on the patients, wants to know "How can a clinical research project be organized to address this question?"

The First Step: Establish the Scope of Study

The surgeon presented data on the clinical findings at several meetings,[1] and colleagues raised a number of questions and issues. In response to the issues so raised, the surgeon changed the data collection procedures; Table 25.1 summarizes the information gathered so far.

Initially, the surgeon relied on the patient interview, a physical examination, and clinical judgments formed about the responses of the patients to the bypass. Later, he introduced noninvasive laboratory studies and employed the Ankle–Brachial Index, routinely.[2] As blood supply in the pelvic region became an issue, the surgeon began to ask the patients a series of questions suggested by a urologist. Still later, he experimented with the use of the Penile–Brachial Index.[3] At this point, he is uncertain about the clinical usefulness of the data gathered for assessing outcomes.

When the surgeon reviewed the foregoing information with a research consultant, it was agreed that the scope of the study had to be established by defining the research questions as hypotheses, specifying the data gathering instruments for putting key concepts into operation, and planning the collection and editing of data to ensure the reliability and validity of measurements. The task is to restrict the scope of the study to the patients and period of time required to answer the research questions and hypotheses.

Definition of the Basic Terms of the Research Question

The basic terms of the research questions or hypotheses may include diagnosis, prognostic indicators, type of surgical intervention, complications, pain, physical functioning, and quality of life. Each term requires two types of definition, conceptual and operational. A conceptual definition specifies the phenomena to be studied in theoretical or clinical terms that are consistent with the accepted usage of the terms in medical science. The operational definition is the set of rules for assigning numbers, henceforth called scores, to the phenomena to be observed and recorded. The scoring system should follow logically from the conceptual definition, so that the numbers assigned make sense and convey a meaning to the investigator.

TABLE 25.1. Clinical data gathered on aortofemoral bypass patients preopoeratively, postoperatively, and after one year.

Data gathered	Preoperatively	Postoperatively	One year
Survival	National Institute on Aging	Hospital records	Hospital records
Blood supply in limbs	Physical exam; Ankle-Brachial Index	Hospital records	Hospital records
Levels of principal activities	Doctor-patient interview	Clinical observation	Doctor-patient interview
Significant prognostic indicators (age, smoking, comorbidity)	Doctor-patient interviews; information from referring physician	Clinical observation	Doctor-patient interview
Medications	Doctor-patient interview	Medical record	Doctor-patient interview
Sexual dysfunction	Doctor-patient interview; urologic tests; Penile-Brachial Index	Medical record	Doctor-patient interview; urologic test; Penile-Brachial Index
Diagnosis and treatment plan	Arteriogram		
Complications (sepsis, wound infection)	Doctor-patient interview	Clinical observation	Doctor-patient interview; physical exam
Pain, discomfort	Doctor-patient interview	Clinical observation	Doctor-patient interview
Quality of life	Assessed indirectly	Assessed indirectly	Patient reports

It is common to have two or more measures for the same concept. Scores can be compared in terms of how well they fit the theoretical concept, their reliability and validity, and the time and cost of data collection.

In this case, the primary outcome of interest is the restoration of the blood supply to the legs to assure physical functioning and minimize the likelihood of amputation or death. The clinical efficacy of aortofemoral bypass grafting is beyond dispute.

During further discussions between the surgeon and the research consultant, it became clear that the surgeon could focus the research on changes in the patients' principal everyday activities, sexual functioning, and quality of life. He could focus on the physical capacity for activities or sexual functioning, or the actual levels of functioning and the patients' satisfaction with them.

Since age, comorbidity, medications, and smoking are prognostic indicators of outcome, the surgeon could establish a hypothesis on the likelihood of particular outcomes, given the presence or absence of the prognostic factors.

With respect to sexual functioning, impotence may be the result of inadequate blood supply to the pelvic region, operative injury to the parasympathetic nerves, urologic problems, reactions to medication, other health problems, or psychological or other problems in sexual relationships. One approach is to classify patients, at the time of diagnosis, in terms of sexual activity. For those sexually active preoperatively, reduction in sexual function postoperatively could be related to possible nerve damage; if the preoperative sexual dysfunction appeared to be related to reduced blood supply, the capacity for erection and ejaculation should increase following surgery. In those with impotence-related physiological problems, the surgery should have a minimal impact apart from any improvement in the blood supply. Accordingly, a research question can be asked about the level of sexual functioning in each of these groups following surgery, assuming that appropriate measures are available for each *key term*.

Separate research questions can also be formulated for principal activities, quality of life, and satisfaction with the surgery.

Limiting the Data To Be Gathered

As interest in the findings of the surgeon increased, colleagues posed more questions and suggested the gathering of interesting information on the clinical, personal, and social characteristics of the patients. Their specific suggestions included the use of new clinical measures, such as the Ankle-Brachial Index or a Penile-Brachial Index. As a consequence, considerable new information accumulated.

The term "data gathering instrument" is used to signify any and all types of data collection aids, such as questionnaires, indexes, and observation forms, and such mechanical devices as calipers, blood pressure cuffs, and thermometers.

When you are planning a study, you may be tempted to collect interesting information above and beyond what is required to answer your research question or hypothesis. But data are costly, not only in terms of the time and money required to produce them, but in terms of the problems of data management and analysis, which increase with the volume of information you have to process. If you collect data without a specific purpose or question in mind, you will probably leave them unanalyzed.

The three general guidelines for limiting the urge to collect too many data are brevity, clarity and precoding.

1. **Brevity.** Restrict data collection to the information you need to answer your research questions or hypotheses and collect in the most efficient manner possible.
2. **Clarity.** Keep data collection as simple and straightforward as possible. Make your instructions for obtaining the information explicit so that there is no ambiguity about where the data are to be found or how they are to be recorded. The more judgments the data collector has to make, the greater the likelihood of error.
3. **Precoding.** Establish rules for the classification, scoring, and coding of data before collection so that the data gathering forms can be precoded. If you leave such decisions to the end you run the risk of ending up with information that is incomplete.

Reliability and Validity

The surgeon recognizes that much of the data obtained from patient interviews and physical examinations reflected the questions he asked and the clinical judgments he made regarding the responses. He had a set of questions to ask, but he had not set them down in a standard form. He could have anticipated or assumed the answers to some of the questions. He also used the patients' responses to determine their levels of physical functioning, and did not employ exercise tests. He asked the questions the urologist had suggested but he wasn't always clear about their purpose.

The surgeon noted the strength of the peripheral pulse on a four-point scale devised for the purpose, but he didn't check the reliability of the scoring. After the vascular laboratory tests were introduced 3 or 4 years ago, readings for the Ankle–Brachial and Penile–Brachial indices were taken for a large series of patients with vascular disease, but he didn't test their sensitivity and specificity as measuring instruments. He now gathers data for these indices for all patients, preoperatively and at the one-year follow-up. As a part of another research project, he will compare the preoperative data for the two indices with arteriograms to test their diagnostic accuracy.

The surgeon recognizes the limits of the approach he adopted for gathering data. Many of the data have been coded and entered into computer files, but he has not yet explored the potential for using them to answer any of his research questions.

To be scientifically acceptable, an instrument must be reliable and valid. It is reliable when it performs consistently for the same person in different applications when the phenomena being recorded have not changed, and for different observers during simultaneous applications. The validity of an instrument is defined in terms of its accuracy. An instrument must be reliable to be valid, but a reliable measure may not be valid because the observers may simply be consistently reproducing errors. Chapter 17 discusses research strategies for testing the reliability and validity of instruments. The key point is that you, as the researcher, are responsible for assuring the reliability and validity of the data collected in each of your projects.

The first task for the research adviser and the surgeon is to agree on which research questions and hypotheses are of central importance. The impact of surgery on sexual functioning, given the level of sexual functioning preoperatively, is a researchable question. It could be the focal point for a single study. A study may include two or more hypotheses, but it is generally advisable to have no more than three or four in a given study.

The operational measures could include physiological tests, scales or indices that are appropriate for the outcomes, and clinical judgments. Clinical investigators in the field of sexual therapy and counseling could be consulted about other possible measures. The reliability and validity of the measures should be established, and the investigators should satisfy themselves that the measures are sufficiently precise to detect clinically important changes in available sample sizes of patients. These steps define the boundaries of the study. The next stage is the specification of plans for collecting and managing the data.

Advantages and Disadvantages of Different Methods of Data Collection

Basically, four different data collection strategies are available for clinical research. They are the medical record, the self-administered questionnaire, the interviewer-administered questionnaire, and observation.

The Medical Record

The medical record of each patient contains the results of history taking, physical examination, laboratory tests, diagnostic consideration, interventions, and follow-up. Health professionals are accustomed to making medical records, and a large number of records can be abstracted inexpensively over a relatively short period of time. However, if the medical record is entirely in narrative form, the reliability and validity of the clinical judgments it contains may not be known. Reports of particular laboratory or diagnostic tests may not be included in all the charts; that is, they are incomplete for research purposes.

Researchers often introduce forms designed specifically for research purposes. The research medical record assumes that data will be recorded on a standardized form so that missing information can be quickly identified. Because clinicians often find it difficult to adapt to new forms and may be reluctant to complete research charts as well as existing medical records, some teams employ research nurses to gather the necessary information for all eligible patients. This requires the finding of research funds to pay their salaries.

Self-Administered Questionnaires

Patients and their partners could be asked to complete a questionnaire on background characteristics, past and present levels of physical functioning and activity, and structured questions on levels of sexual functioning and satisfaction.

The main advantages of this strategy are that many questionnaires can be filled out in a very short period and fewer field workers need to be employed. The main disadvantages are that the researcher can never be sure that each questionnaire was completed by the intended person; also, the response rate tends to be low, particularly if the questionnaire is administered by mail. A low response rate could bias the study's results, and the completeness of responses has to be carefully monitored.

Interviewer-Administered Questionnaires

The surgeon, another health professional, or a trained interviewer can obtain additional information by interviewing the patient or a significant other person in each patient's life. The main advantages of the interviewer-administered strategy are that it yields a better response rate and allows the greatest flexibility in questionnaire construction and length. Its main disadvantage is its cost. Quality interviewers are usually paid well, and travel expenses will be incurred if the interviews are conducted in the homes of interviewees spread over a large geographic area. Another problem is that interviewees may not be as honest in their answers as they would be on a self-administered questionnaire because of interactions with the interviewer that cause them to give socially acceptable responses.

Observation

If the researcher wishes to know whether the patient can perform certain basic physical activities, such as walking two blocks or climbing a flight of stairs without pain or discomfort, the patient can be asked to perform these activities in the presence of the observer, who then records the responses.

The advantage of the observational or measurement technique is that the problem of eliciting socially desirable answers is eliminated. There is, however, a problem in ensuring consistent results from the same rater, over time, and between raters. A further disadvantage is that the rater's presence may alter the subject's behavior, and the results may indicate what the patient *can do* rather than what he or she usually does.

Multiple Methods of Data Collection

Researchers may strive to include all the outcomes or variables considered important, and to rely on multiple sources for the required data. If you use multiple methods to gather data, you may have to rank-order the methods according to the relative importance of the information they are intended to produce. Should problems arise in employing all the methods equally well, you should focus your time and attention on those of primary importance in the testing of the research question or hypothesis.

Repeated Measures

You can gather the same data at two, or more, different times to monitor the patients' progress. The problem of maintaining high-quality data increases each time you repeat a measure. Scheduled appointments may be missed, your commitment and that of your subjects may falter, and a pattern of fixed responses may systematically bias the results. Monitor the administration of repeated measures carefully, to reduce the number of problems.

Data gathering procedures must be acceptable to clinicians and health professionals, cause minimal disruption of patient care activities, and collect only information that is essential to the answering of the research question(s).

The problems of maintaining complete files of reliable and valid data increase exponentially with the complexity of your study. High-quality data depend, to a great extent, on the vigor of the members of your research team and your clinical partners in intervention trials.

Multicenter Trials

The surgeon performing the aortofemoral bypass grafts wants to know whether the prophylactic use of antibiotics would reduce the subsequent requirement for their therapeutic use. Since the sepsis rate in such cases is less than 5%, 1000 patients would be needed in each treatment and control group to do a trial. Such a study would require the participation of a number of centers to obtain sample sizes large enough to make the statistical test of differences in outcomes reliable.

Since the surgeons and clinical staff in each center have their own techniques, considerable time, effort, and fiscal resources would have to be expended to assure uniform data collection in all the centers. Usually, at least one center drops out of a multicenter trial, or is asked to withdraw by the coordinating committee responsible for monitoring the research procedures. The ratio of the resources required for data management to those needed for data collection tends to increase as more centers are included. The design, organization, and management of multicenter trials are discussed in greater depth and detail in Chapters 26 and 14.

Recruiting and Deploying an Effective Research Team

All persons associated with a research project can be described as being either core or staff members. The core team comprises the investigator(s) and coinvestigator(s) who are responsible for the designing, funding, quality, and completion of the study; they do not necessarily engage in the day-to-day execution of the study. The research staff frequently consists of a research associate or coordinator who runs the study on a day-to-day basis, and research assistants who organize and deal with the field workers responsible for gathering and coding the data. Each research assistant's tasks also include the editing and supervision of the coding of data sheets. Finally, a data manager is responsible for preparing the data for analysis. The actual analysis is usually carried out or supervised closely by a statistician, who may be a core or staff member or a consultant. Core members can also play an active role in data gathering and management. Inputs from health professionals, such as surgeons, radiologists, pathologists, internists, physical therapists, or nurses may be required on a core or staff level or both.

Training the Research Staff

Regardless of the level of professional expertise or experience of the persons involved in recording data, training personnel to behave in a standardized manner enhances reliability and validity. The goal is to have the phenomena under study recorded with minimal distortion arising from the expectations and subjective impressions of the research personnel. Ideally, the data gatherers should be unaware of the research questions and hypotheses, and blind to the groups to which subjects have been assigned, when applicable. Subjective judgments on the part of the coders should also be minimized. The key to achieving this is to have explicit rules for data reduction that eliminate as completely as possible the need for subjective judgments.

Data must be not only reliable and valid, but complete. Missing information can be a major problem, and alternate sources should be sought when required. All persons providing information for the project must appreciate the importance of its being complete and be trained accordingly.

Evaluation of the Research Staff

During training sessions, you can use simulated exercises and practice runs to evaluate the data collection process. This evaluation has two parts: the assessment and correction of the performance of the members of the research staff, when necessary, and the modification of procedures for collecting data to make them acceptable, straightforward, unambiguous, and easy for field workers to use. Comments and suggestions regarding forms and procedures from the team members can be used to improve data collection and management.

Pretesting the Study Procedures

To verify that the research study will proceed as planned, and that the data gathering instruments will perform as intended, always conduct a pretest, or dress rehearsal, of the study in the field. The pretest is a critical step because it is impossible to anticipate all the potential detrimental factors that may come into play. The pretest trial offers you the opportunity not only to identify but to correct for such factors. During the pretest, you can examine the three main components of the study: the data gathering instruments, the logistics, and the personnel. When you are examining the logistics, note whether the data can be gathered with few losses; that is, can charts be retrieved, subjects accrued, and measures taken? When you examine the data gathering instruments, determine whether they work in the field. For questionnaires, examine the vocabulary to make sure it is understandable by the subjects; find out whether the subjects are compliant and appear to be giving honest answers to all questions; and determine the length of the interview. You should also check the precoding schema for the questionnaire and determine the adequacy of its format and skip patterns. A 10.0% verification will indicate the quality of the work performance of personnel. Research personnel have to respect the dignity and rights of patients at all times; betrayal of the confidentiality of patients is sufficient reason for dismissal from the project.

There is no formula for determining the number of pretest subjects, but the accepted number seems to be between 30 and 50 regardless of the intended sample size. Since the pretest subjects are drawn from the same pool as the actual study subjects, a major consideration in determining the number of pretest subjects is their availability. You will want to avoid depleting a large proportion of the population on the pretest trial. Establishing the size of the pretest sample is, therefore, a subjective decision influenced by the availability of potential study subjects. To avoid contaminating the sample population, draw your pretest subjects from a hospital or region at some distance from your intended study area. There is no predetermined number of pretest trials; any number may be needed to convince you that the study can be conducted.

Preparing the Data for Analysis

Cleaning the Data

The editing of questionnaires or clinical data sheets is the first step in cleaning the data. The field worker checks the questionnaire or data sheet line by line, to ensure that all the appropriate items have been correctly completed. If there are any errors, the questionnaires or data sheets must be sent back to the data gatherer for correction. This helps to eliminate the problem of missing data.

The next step is coding, the process of converting written answers into numbers suitable for analysis by computer. The codes for precoded items are transferred to the coding boxes first; open-ended items are coded next. Each open-ended item is read and given a code number that corresponds to the answer. Make sure that special care is taken to code what is written and to avoid interpreting the answers. Each distinct response is given a new number; identical responses share the same code. This process is repeated for each item until all the open-ended items have been coded. To ensure quality, a 10% sample of the questionnaires or data sheets is recoded blindly—a process commonly referred to as double coding. By examining the accuracy with which the codes are assigned during the first and second codings, you can estimate the error rate for each item and for the entire data gathering instrument.

Keypunching

The advent of the personal computers and database programs allows for direct control of data entry and management. In using mainframe computers, coding forms are taken to a data entry service where data are key punched and verified. The magnetic file is then transferred to the computing centre for processing. The managers of the computer centres dictate the rules and policies for managing files and the analysis of data.

There are a number of database programs for personal computers that permit the users to design data entry screens and build in editing routines and checks that minimize errors while entering the data into a file. The database programs have programming languages that permit modifications and transformations of data, and the linking and relating of data across two or more data files. The programs are relatively easy to learn and use so that a research assistant can enter and edit data for a project. Well designed data entry programs and screens permit entries that are within a specified range and logically possible, and the data need only be entered once. If questions arise while the data are being entered, the research assistant can check with the persons recording the information to sort out errors and problems. The research staff can also review the data files to make sure they are logically ordered and structured.

Software is now available that will translate a given file between the major database, spreadsheet, and statistical packages. This permits the investigator or research unit to use the software of their choice, and yet produce data files that can be moved freely amongst programs of choice. Data files can be managed and analyzed with the statistical packages available for use on personal computers.

A major issue in structuring a data file is the coding of missing values. There are items that are not applicable to all subjects (e.g. follow-information for persons who had specific procedures), and there are questions which the subject may not be able to answer (e.g. questions on family medical history). There is a tendency to leave the field blank for incomplete data. There are databases and statistical packages that interpret a blank as a zero, and this is a problem when the zero is a valid response (e.g. how many times have you had pain in the chest in the past week). The best approach is to give a specific code that specifies the reasons for incomplete data. For example, we assign the following values as follows, 7 for 'not applicable', 8 for 'unknown' and 9 for 'missing' data. If the field is two columns wide, we double the digits so that the codes become 77, 88, and 99 respectively. For a variable such as age where 77, 88, and 99 are valid response, we define age as a three column field and use the codes 777, 888, and 999 to designate the reason for incomplete data. Regardless of the system used, the key is to have special codes to designate the reasons for incomplete data, codes that will not be interpreted as real values.

The first step in data analysis is to produce frequency distributions of the responses for each variable. The investigator can make sure that the data are free of errors and make sense. The investigator may decide to work with the raw data or to recode or transform the data into codes suitable for analysis. If an index score is to be constructed from several items of data, these and the calculations should be recorded so that it is possible to check that the index scores were accurately computed. Once the data have been checked and the responses have been recoded or transformed, and scores have been computed, the data file is ready for analysis.

Budget Concerns

The collection and management of data are expensive undertakings, and there are numerous ways to cover the costs. Some physician–investigators collect and analyze data in their own small research projects, and the principal cost is the time they spend on the project.

Diagnostic tests, laboratory work, and clinical examinations performed solely for research purposes represent the most expensive data to collect. In some jurisdictions, the cost of such procedures can be charged against health insurance plans or be absorbed by the hospital or clinic; in others, research procedures must be covered by a research budget.

Data collected from individuals will include the responses to self-administered questionnaires, and face-to-face and telephone interviews. If you use rigorous follow-up procedures to assure a high response rate, self-administered questionnaires and telephone interviews usually cost about the same, whereas face-to-face interviews cost about twice as much.

Data gathering may include the collection of laboratory and other test results and the abstraction of data from clinical records. Research personnel can be salaried or paid for each piece of work completed. For example, a data collector could be paid a specified amount for each *complete* set of data for a given subject. This arrangement provides an incentive to make certain that all the required information is collected, and it fits well with the strategy of paying nurses, residents, and others to collect data in the course of their regular patient care duties. The data manager must be certain that the data forms are complete and that the data are of high quality. If you use this approach, the data collectors should be assured that if they work for a week at a reasonable pace, they can complete enough forms to earn a reasonable wage.

There will always be a certain number of subjects for whom data cannot be completed, because the information is missing or the subjects have been lost to follow-up. Do not penalize data collectors for any loss of information that is beyond their control. Adjust the work schedule or rate of pay to allow for the expected percentage of their time they will have to spend on incomplete data.

Security and Confidentiality

The completed research record is the primary product of the research project. Its monetary value is related, in part, to the time and costs required to complete it, and to the confidentiality of the information. Keep the "hard copies" of the research file in locked cabinets in locked rooms to which only one designated research worker has access. Once the data have been entered into the computer, store the hard copies safely, as a general rule, for one year following data analysis. Destroy them then if appropriate.

Use identification numbers to collate the information on subjects and to protect confidentiality. A master list of personal identifiers and identification numbers for each subject is recommended. Record the identification numbers, but not the individual identifiers, on the data forms. If a person who is collecting information needs a name to find information, it can be included on a cover sheet, which should be destroyed when the information is collected.

Enter data onto a computer disk, or diskettes. Because such data processing files can be accidentally altered or destroyed, create master files and store them separately from the working file.

Once the data have been edited and "cleaned," you can modify the data files as variables are recorded, transformed, and created. Document every change made on the data file and keep one copy with the coding manual so that you can determine, at any time, how any score has been derived or modified. Keep backup copies of the working files and update them as changes are made. Ensure the security of the data at each stage of data analysis.

You can store computer data files in archives indefinitely, but if you have not used them within 5 years following the completion of your project, you probably never will. When your data are no longer used to answer questions, your project is complete. Ethical guidelines governing the confidentiality of personal information in research records justify destruction of all hard copies and computer files in the archives at this time.

References

1. Chiu RC-J, Lidstone D, Blundell PE. Predictive power of penile/brachial index (P.B.I.) in diagnosing male sexual impotence. Vasc Surg 1986;4:251–256.
2. Barnes RW. Hemodynamics for the vascular surgeon. Arch Surg 1980;115:216–223.
3. Barnes RW. Noninvasive diagnostic techniques in peripheral vascular disease. Am Heart J 1979;97(2): 241–258.

26

Using the Operating Room as a Laboratory

G.T. Christakis and R.D. Weisel

Collection and documentation of data from patients during surgical procedures are highly useful but seldom used methods of surgical research. Intraoperative clinical research provides important information, whether the reports are descriptive or randomized controlled interventional trials. Clinical application of surgical techniques has increased dramatically following perioperative documentation of their benefits. At the University of Toronto, the use of blood cardioplegia in cardiac surgery increased from approximately 10% in 1980 to 98% in 1989, following identification of its beneficial effects on myocardial metabolism, ventricular function, morbidity, and mortality. Although the benefits of a surgical technique evaluated in the laboratory may influence many surgeons, improved clinical results have a greater impact on clinical practice. Extended tracheal resections were performed in dogs for many years, but Grillo and Pearson's validation of the techniques in humans permitted their widespread clinical use.

The relative paucity of intraoperative experimentation compared with laboratory reports may be due, in part, to the extraordinary organizational efforts required for intraoperative experimentation. A clinical research program must progress through the steps of identifying the clinical problem requiring study, evaluating the contributing mechanisms, enumerating the hypotheses, and constructing the protocol to test the hypotheses. In addition, careful consideration must be given to human experimentation ethics and the concerns of colleagues, other health professionals, and referring physicians.

Identification of Clinical Problems

Clinical research begins with the identification of a problem of sufficient clinical or scientific significance to warrant the interest of other surgeons and scientists, and an investigation that may improve understanding of the disease process or patient problem. Ventricular dysfunction following aortocoronary bypass surgery is an example. If different intraoperative techniques could reduce the incidence and impact of postoperative ventricular dysfunction, intraoperative experimentation would be more readily accepted by colleagues and other health professionals.

For an interventional trial, the clinical problem must occur frequently enough to allow completion of a study in a reasonable period of time. If other surgeons are to identify and appreciate the clinical problem, it must be clearly defined. For example, a surgeon studying ventricular dysfunction following aortocoronary bypass surgery should not include all patients with blood pressure less than 90 mm Hg without further clarification, because this would result in the inclusion of less hypovolemic patients and those with a high cardiac output and low systemic resistance; modification of intraoperative techniques of myocardial protection would benefit the latter group, but not the former. The clinical problem must also have measurable endpoints that the researcher has the resources to measure.

Intraoperative experimentation that examines physiological principles or abnormalities, rather than clinical problems, can be justified if the interventions can be performed with minimal risk to the patient.

Evaluation of Mechanisms and Formulation of Hypotheses

Once a clinical problem has been selected, a hypothesis to explain how intraoperative events are related to the outcome must be formulated. For example, it could be hypothesized that poor myocardial cooling during cold cardioplegic arrest accounts for impaired ventricular function after cardiac surgery. A hypothesis can be based on laboratory or clinical literature, known physiological or biological principles, or observed correlations between clinical outcome and the hypothesized mechanism. Although elucidation of the mechanisms of a clinical problem is not a prerequisite for testing a hypothesis with an intraoperative trial, it greatly enhances the study's scientific validity and its acceptance by the academic community.

Descriptive studies can also be of help in evaluating possible mechanisms and hypotheses. For example, a descriptive study correlating temperatures with the incidence of postoperative ventricular dysfunction would enhance the hypothesis that colder temperatures prevent postoperative dysfunction. When a hypothesis has been previously tested, descriptive studies may elucidate the mechanism of injury by identifying intraoperative clinical, biochemical, or pathological processes. Correlation of myocardial anaerobic metabolism, reduced high-energy phosphates, and histological evidence of injury during cardioplegia, with poor postoperative ventricular performance, provides important information and generates new hypotheses.

Unfortunately, descriptive studies can only generate hypotheses. Clinical problems are usually multifactorial, and confounding factors abound. Interventional trials, especially prospective randomized controlled trials, may be more effective in studying mechanisms and evaluating clinical benefit than descriptive studies. If patients are randomized to colder or warmer myocardial temperatures by different cardioplegic techniques, most other confounding factors affecting postoperative outcome could be controlled, the study would provide stronger evidence of the effect of the intervention, and intraoperative measurements could elucidate possible mechanisms for any change in postoperative clinical outcome. Cooling the heart will decrease myocardial metabolic demand and may reduce anaerobic metabolism and preserve high-energy phosphates. Additional intraoperative measurements during a randomized trial would provide further evidence to validate the effect of the intraoperative intervention.

Constructing a Protocol

To conduct a successful clinical experiment, you must have a detailed protocol containing the following sections: introduction, rationale, methods, anticipated results, sample size calculations, risks and benefits to the patient, and consent form.

Introduction

The clinical problem must be defined precisely, and its importance to patient care must be stated. For example:

> Ventricular dysfunction after aortocoronary bypass surgery results in a 30% mortality; any intervention that elucidates the mechanism or lowers the incidence of postoperative low-output syndrome may save lives.

Rationale

The hypothesized mechanism by which an intraoperative intervention would improve a clinical outcome should be described in logical sequence. An adequate literature review is required to provide compelling support for intraoperative experimentation.

Methods

Criteria for patient selection, inclusion and exclusion, and the method of randomization – if the trial is randomized – must be stated. The surgical procedure should be standardized, and any deviations from the usual practice, such as additional measurements, insertion of additional catheters, withdrawal of additional blood specimens, and procurement of tissue for the study should be specified

Risks and Benefits to Patients

Intraoperative experimentation provides information that may dramatically improve patient care, but any associated risks must be minimal because any complications from the experimentation are unacceptable. An experimental intervention must be employed only after the potential risks have been considered carefully and the investigator is confident that they are low.

The best way to develop intraoperative experimentation is to introduce simple, low-risk interventions and demonstrate to yourself and your colleagues that the procedures can be accomplished without risk to the patient; subsequently, the complexity of the intervention can be slowly increased with careful documentation. A consistent approach to a clinical problem through a progressive intraoperative research program increases its scientific validity and the institutional acceptability of such experimentation.

Between 1979 and 1989, we conducted intraoperative research in 590 patients undergoing elective aortocoronary bypass surgery. We evaluated the risks and benefits of coronary sinus catheters first, and then arterial and ventricular catheters, to assure ourselves that they are safe and clinically beneficial. These catheters permit sensitive measurements of intraoperative and postoperative myocardial metabolism and ventricular function for comparison when alternative techniques of myocardial protection, diltiazem cardioplegia, blood cardioplegia, and glutamate- and aspartate-enriched blood cardioplegia are employed.

Next, we performed transmural left ventricular biopsies for assessment of the myocardial high energy phosphates and their precursors – creatine phosphate, lactate, and glycogen. The first 50 patients were carefully compared with 50 matched patients not subjected to biopsy, and the ventricular function in the region of the biopsy site was examined by nuclear ventriculography 4 months after surgery. The results confirmed our belief that our study protocol is safe and that our intraoperative experimentation was ethical.

The protocol requires an estimation of the number and volume of all proposed blood samples and precise, detailed descriptions of all measurements to be made on them. A program that slowly increases the number of blood samples will prevent excessive sampling.

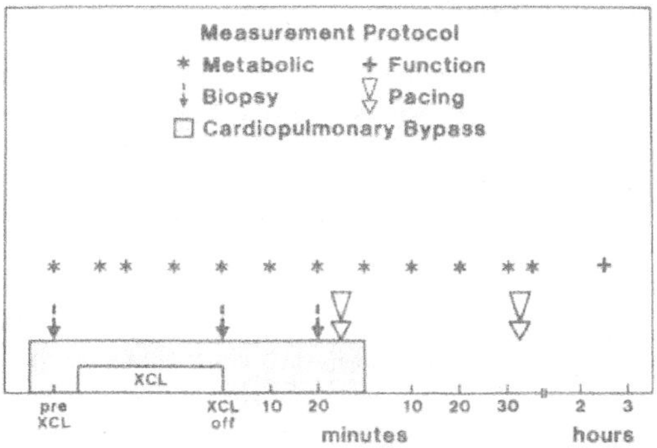

FIGURE 26.1. The protocol employed for intraoperative experimentation is displayed. Myocardial metabolism was assessed by obtaining blood and biopsy samples at various time intervals. Cardiac function was evaluated postoperatively. (XCL = Crossclamp.) Reprinted with permission from Teoh KH, Mickle DAG, Weisel RD, Madonik MM, Ivanov J, Harding RD, Romaschin AD, Mullen JC. Improving mycardial metabolic and functional recovery after cardioplegic arrest. J. Thoracic and Cardiovascular Surgery, The C.V. Mosby Company, St. Louis, Missouri, USA, May 1988;95:788–798.

Anticipated Results and Sample Size Calculations

You should carefully evaluate each outcome measurement and estimate its value in the control group and its variation on the basis of previous laboratory or human experience. Next, you should estimate a clinically relevant improvement with the proposed intervention based on the rationale of your study. You should then make a sample size calculation to determine how many patients will be required to detect the clinically relevant difference. At this point, you must outline the experimental study and show that enough patients could be studied to meet the sample size requirement. Intraoperative experimental protocols that are not feasible, or will not recruit sufficient patients, are unethical because they put the patient at risk without benefit.

Administration

Establishing intraoperative experimentation in a university-affiliated hospital creates such administrative problems as increases in surgical costs, nursing hours, operating room time, and equipment usage (catheters, solutions, tubing, needles, etc.), which must be addressed before a research project can be initiated. Using patients in experimentation may influence referral practices and the confidence of referring physicians, anesthetists, nurses, and other health professionals.

Intraoperative research is not possible without the cooperation and support of the hospital and university administration, and the heads of departments and divisions. To get approval for the increased costs, you must convince administrators that a clinical problem exists, that your research goals are valid, and that the results of intraoperative research may contribute to improved patient care and reduced perioperative morbidity and mortality; extensive discussions will be required to accomplish this. For example, patients who require urgent coronary bypass surgery for unstable angina face a 5% to 10% risk of operative mortality that may be reduced with improved methods of myocardial protection. Referring physicians, nurses, and other health professionals must be convinced that the clinical problem is important, that it may be improved by intraoperative experimentation, that the intraoperative research will not be harmful, and that the experimental interventions are simple, safe, and logical modifications of existing surgical techniques.

Collaboration and cooperation are essential. Collaboration with anesthesia staff can improve their academic productivity as well as your own, and it can facilitate intraoperative experimentation. The cooperation of residents and nurses is essential, and new surgical techniques and measurements that prolong operating time should be introduced slowly. Nurses and other health professionals must have knowledge of the protocols so that additional equipment, catheters, tubing, and special sutures will be made available routinely. The intraoperative study of blood cardioplegia at our institution required a new system of cardioplegia delivery that was enthusiastically supported by our perfusionists.

Intraoperative research should begin with simple, uncomplicated measurements and be built slowly by adding more measurements and interventions. Once a routine has been established and accepted by the operating room personnel, additions and modifications to the protocol can be made with ease. Because additional time will be required for each surgical procedure, surgical schedules must be revised to guarantee that the operating room personnel are not unduly inconvenienced.

Ethics and Intraoperative Experimentation

All intraoperative experimentation requires approval by the Human Experimentation Committee. The committee must be convinced that the research is important, that it will result in improved patient care, that risks to the patient are minimal, that the investigator can effectively treat complications, and that the benefits to the patient and society outweigh the risks.

Intraoperative experimentation must be designed with the philosophy that no complications can be tolerated. Complications can be prevented by strict adherence to the protocol; extensive measurements can be made in low-risk patients, but few can be made in high-risk patients. In low-risk patients, minor complications are easily tolerated and blood sampling is unlikely to increase any clinically significant problems.

Clinically relevant improvements can be expected only in high-risk patients. To avoid complications, patients who become unstable during anesthesia induction or who develop technical problems during surgery are immediately withdrawn from further involvement in the research project; only 2% of patients have been removed from our studies because of intraoperative complications. All patients involved in surgical research must be closely observed for complications by the surgeon, a research physician, and the research personnel, intraoperatively and postoperatively. Patient sedation, comfort, and care supersede all research-related activities.

In our cardiac surgery research program, bleeding and postoperative arrhythmias are the most mportant complications. In more than 1500 transmural left ventricular myocardial biopsies, we have had only one episode of surgical bleeding related to the site of myocardial biopsy; no significant bleeding has been attributable to the insertion or removal of coronary sinus or intraventricular pressure catheters. Our surgical techniques to avoid postoperative bleeding were developed and perfected in laboratory animals before being applied to humans. The nature of the experimental studies is explained to patients and their family members and repeated again in the hospital; all potential risks, no matter how small, are clearly stated, and patients are reassured that their refusal to participate in a study will in no way prejudice the quality of their care. In our experimental studies, 95% of all the patients we approached agreed to participate and gave preoperative informed consent.

Collaboration and Consultation

Surgical research cannot be accomplished by the concerted efforts of a single individual; close collaboration and consultation with other colleagues and health-related professionals is mandatory. Over a period of 10 years, we have performed more than 40,000 assays of blood samples, including thousands of assays employing high performance liquid chromatography for high-energy phosphates, creatine phosphate, glycogen, and lactate. This was achievable only with the collaboration of interested individuals in the Department of Biochemistry and constant communication with them to ascertain the feasibility of assays, the logistics of delivery, preparation, and storage of specimens, and the interpretation of the results. This close and extensive collaboration has produced innovations in assay methodology, more sensitive assays, better measurements, and more sensitive indices of the mechanisms of clinically relevant problems.

Cooperation with anesthetists, perfusionists, residents, and operating room and ICU nurses is critically important in the successful conduct of research. You must give all these individuals copies of your experimental protocol and include them in discussions of patient care and research strategies. Make anesthetists and nurses aware of the reason, timing, and goals of blood sampling before you interpose research personnel between them and the patient. Cooperation from coworkers in the operating room is essential, because experimental study patients require longer periods of surgery as a result of the instrumentation used and the measurements performed.

Additional Reading

Christakis GT, Fremes SE, Weisel RD, Tittley JG, Mickle DAG, Ivanov J, Madonik MM, Benak AM, McLaughlin PR, Baird RJ. Diltiazem cardioplegia: A balance of risk and benefit. J Thoracic and Cardiovascular Surgery, 1986;91:647–661.

Dr. Christakis performed this prospective randomized trial as a surgical trainee. He wrote the protocol, performed the study and wrote the paper.

Fremes SE, Christakis GT, Weisel RD, Mickle DAG, Madonik MM, Ivanov J, Harding R, Seawright SJ, Houle S, McLaughlin PR, Baird RJ. A clinical trial of blood and crystalloid cardioplegia. J Thoracic and Cardiovascular Surgery, 1984;88:726–41.

Dr. Fremes performed this prospective clinical trial as a surgical resident. He wrote the protocol, performed the study and wrote the paper.

Teoh KH, Christakis GT, Weisel RD, Wong PY, Mee AV, Ivanov J, Madonik MM, Levitt D, Reilly P, Rosenfeld J, Glynn MFX. Dipyridamole preserved platelets and reduced blood loss following cardiopulmonary bypass. J Thoracic and Cardiovascular Surgery, 1988;96: 332–341.

Dr. Teoh performed perspective randomized trial evaluating preoperative oral and intravenous dipyridamole on postoperative bleeding. As a result of this trial, oral dipyridamole is given to all patients prior to cardiac surgery at the University of Toronto.

Teoh KH, Mickle DAG, Weisel RD, Madonik MM, Ivanov J, Harding RD, Romaschin AD, Mullen JC. Improving myocardial metabolic and functional recovery after cardioplegic arrest. J. Thoracic and Cardiovascular Surgery, 1988;95:788–798.

Dr. Teoh evaluated the effects of increasing arterial lactate concentrations on intraoperative myocardial metabolism as a surgical trainee. He found that lactate infusion was beneficial and, the University of Toronto uses Ringer's lactate exclusively.

27

Research in the ICU

H.D. Reines and L. Oxley-Droter

Introduction

All medical research involving human subjects has a single goal: "to improve diagnostic, therapeutic and prophylactic procedures, and understanding of the etiology and pathogenesis of disease."[1] Dramatic advances in the prevention of poliomyelitis, smallpox, and measles have been made with vaccines, but therapeutic advances among the critically ill have been slower, partly because of the difficulty of establishing studies in a heterogeneous population.

Intensive care units (ICUs) have developed over the past 30 years, to provide physical places where critically ill patients can obtain special care and monitoring by readily available nurses and physicians. Invasive and noninvasive monitoring devices allow easy access to the vascular and respiratory systems with an acceptable risk/benefit ratio. The patient is integrated with the monitoring systems to provide physiological data constantly. The investigator needs only proper methodology to study problems in the care of critically ill patients.

The ICU patient and environment need to be studied for a number of reasons. As third-party payers push for shorter hospital stays and more outpatient procedures, a growing proportion of patients admitted to hospitals requires special care. The nursing shortage directly affects care at a time when the population is aging and technology is expanding at a rate outdistancing our ability to keep up with it. The ICUs consume 15% to 25% of hospitals' financial resources. Since medical care costs 10% of the gross national product (GNP) of the United States, ICU expenditures represent 0.75% to 1.0% of the GNP.

Limited critical care resources must be used in an efficient and efficacious manner that maintains human dignity and preserves life. This goal can be achieved only by knowing the benefits and risks of intensive care, and developing therapies and techniques that provide maximum benefit to patients. Commitment to research in critical care and utilization of the ICU as a laboratory are essential factors in the improvement of patient care.

As a microcosm of the hospital environment, the ICU offers numerous opportunities for research. Everything done to patients in the ICU environment needs justification, from the new specialty beds costing $20,000 to 30,000 each to the use of new monitoring devices. The ICU is the only place where inotropic drugs and therapies for adult respiratory distress syndrome (ARDS), sepsis, and cardiogenic shock can be studied closely, and over time. Now that life can be prolonged, even in hopeless situations, ethical considerations need to be addressed and studied to determine whether medicine is truly making a difference by applying everything that modern technology and therapy can muster to all critically ill patients.

In a 1966 article in the *New England Journal of Medicine*, Henry Beecher reiterated the National Research Act of 1964.[2] This document required human research to be scientifically sound and the risks to be minimized and reasonable for the benefits. The Belmont report of 1978 expanded these principles to a bill of rights in human research based on three principles[3]:

1. Respect for persons.
2. Beneficence.
3. Justice.

Respect for persons means that the individual should be treated as an autonomous agent capable of making his or her own choices. Furthermore, subjects must be dealt with fairly—if the patient is incapacitated and unable to choose, a surrogate must voluntarily decide whether to give informed consent on the patient's behalf, after being given adequate information and reaching a sufficient degree of understanding to make the choice valid.

The principle of beneficence means "do no harm." The risk/benefit ratio must be assessed by an independent institutional review board (IRB).

Justice dictates that the benefits of the study be equitably distributed to prevent poor, elderly, or imprisoned persons from being singled out, or taken advantage of, as study patients. Consequently, studies should be randomized, prospective, and diversified in terms of patient demographics.

Scientific advances must be made without compromising the dignity of research subjects. How one decides when to use critically ill human subjects to prove a hypothesis is a complicated process that weighs real and potential risks and benefits to the patient against animal data and potential societal and financial benefits.[4]

The physician preparing for clinical ICU research must have a sound knowledge of physiological principles and the most up-to-date concepts in the area to be studied. He or she will be accountable not only to the patient and the patient's family, but also to medical peers, nurses, and ancillary personnel. To obtain the necessary level of cooperation and assistance, the investigator should be aware of the practical, logistical, and theoretical aspects of patient care in the ICU and should be attuned to the needs of everyone involved. The researcher should have specialized skill in interpreting cardiopulmonary parameters and in recognizing and treating the diverse clinical problems that may arise during a study.

Collaboration

Collaboration is essential. The surgeon exploring basic concepts of human sepsis can benefit from other clinical disciplines such as pulmonary medicine to assess bronchoalveolar lavage in the study of pulmonary macrophages. Basic scientists, especially physiologists and biochemists, are usually anxious to collaborate in a study that can bring their basic research discipline to the clinical arena. A core unit, such as a "shock group" or a "reperfusion group," comprising a number of disciplines, can promote the exchange of ideas and make usually inaccessible laboratory tests available to the clinician.

The seven major collaborative interdisciplinary groups that must be coordinated, before you conduct clinical research in the ICU, are the institutional review board, the sponsoring agency, the ICU staff, the laboratory staff, the medical records department, the pharmacy, and the clinical research coordinators.

Institutional Review Board (IRB)

The IRB is the legally designated protector of patient rights and safety to ensure that the risk/benefits aspects of a study are reasonable. It must approve the informed consent statement and protocol prior to any enrollment of patients in any study. A standard consent is required for all investigational studies and must meet federal and local guidelines. Obtaining final approval of the protocol and informed consent statement can require up to 4 months, depending on how often the IRB meets. This time must be taken into consideration before you set a starting date for patient enrollment.

Sponsoring Agency

The investigator should contact a funding agency—for example, a pharmaceutical company or the National Institutes of Health (NIH)—with a protocol of the study. Investigators may also be approached by a company to perform a study on the basis of referral or past experience. Clinical research studies sponsored by industry require detailed perusal of the protocol by the company and negotiation prior to the initiation of the study and during its implementation. Once the study has received final IRB approval, the clinical research associate (CRA) in charge of the study will review its goals and objectives with the research team. After the patient enrollment process has begun, the sponsoring agency's monitor will make site visits to audit data collection and record keeping. The investigator must realize that private funding is frequently provided to obtain U.S. Food and Drug Administration (FDA) approval for a process or drug. This is the pharmaceutical company's primary reason for sponsoring clinical trials, and science may not be as important to the funding agent as meeting FDA requirements. Budgets should be fair and include salary, laboratory, and travel support.

ICU Staff and Doctors

It must be constantly remembered that the hospital staff's primary responsibility is to protect and assure quality patient care. To execute and fulfill study protocol requirements, researchers must win the confidence and cooperation of the hospital staff and of the attending physicians whose support is necessary to permit enrollment of their patients.

The ICU nurses' cooperation is essential to document patients' vital signs, medications given, hemodynamic monitoring, and laboratory values. Researchers should ask for as little of their time as possible and should provide a research nurse who has an understanding of the ICU settings, equipment, monitoring, policies and procedures.

A research nurse will have optimal cooperation if she can communicate a feeling of respect and demonstrate ability and sound clinical knowledge. Nurses can be very protective of their patients and may be hesitant to cooperate; resistance to change must be anticipated.[5] The level of resistance is usually minimized by establishing a working rapport between the primary investigator, the research nurses, and the ICU staff. To help reduce anxieties, the staff must be clearly informed of their responsibilities prior to the enrollment and monitoring of study patients. An additional measure that may be used to facilitate the identification of potentially eligible patients is an educational or financial incentive to reward staff for referrals and cooperation with study. A combination of in-service, supplemental updates; frequent interaction among the research nurses, primary investigator, and ICU staff; and positive reinforcement is very beneficial to teamwork.[6]

Laboratory

All medication-related studies performed on ICU patients require monitoring of laboratory values. Infection-related studies require cultures and special disc sensitivities. The research grant is billed for all services rendered, including laboratory charges. A method for retrieving results is essential. Meetings with the accounting department, the microbiology director, and the hematology and chemistry director are arranged to keep them informed about the study protocol requirements relevant to their departments. Special payments and discounts may be negotiated prior to study enrollment.

Medical Records

Strict documentation of all procedures must be recorded in every patient's medical record, and a copy of the signed informed consent must be placed in the chart.

Pharmacy

The pharmacy is a key factor in implementing random trials of an investigational drug. An orientation session with the pharmacy supervisors prior to study initiation is essential. A system for dispensing medication on short notice during nights, weekends, and holidays must be addressed in accordance with hospital policy.

Clinical Research Coordinators

A research nurse/data coordinator is vital to any study. The research nurse/coordinator is responsible for coordinating and maintaining harmonious relations with the ancillary departments, as well as patient enrollment and data collection and documentation. A registered nurse with ICU experience is an advantage because she or he can assist in patient care, data translation, monitoring procedures and definition of the ICU nurses' responsibilities.[6]

Study Design

The problems inherent in all human studies are frequently compounded in the ICU because of the lack of a homogeneous population, the small numbers of patients, and the existence of multiple confounding disease processes. Several populations are exceptions to these constraints and are well-suited to clinical trials—for example, patients with uncomplicated myocardial infarction, and coronary artery bypass patients.

Designing any study requires that the hypothesis be testable and answerable in the population being studied. This implies an adequate number of patients who meet strict criteria and demonstrate changes that can be monitored and documented. Prior to initiating any study, it is important to establish the sample size necessary to achieve statistical significance. It is better to overestimate than to have too few patients. A periodic examination of the data may be necessary to ensure that one study group is not being harmed by the experimental therapy or control.

A retrospective review of demographics requiring only a chart review may be worthwhile to determine what the mortality rate is in a given ICU. Such a review requires minimal risk and resources, but it also produces minimal benefits. A prospective study on the effects of steroids on ARDS requires enormous resources, personnel, money, and commitment, as well as a multicenter approach to accrue sufficient patients over a reasonable time. The problems with numbers are compounded by the following conditions.

1. Identification of patient populations may be difficult.
2. The population must be identified before alternate therapy is instituted.

3. Informed consent must be obtained from a population that may not be able to speak for itself.
4. After the patient has been identified and deemed eligible, and consent has been obtained, a study nurse or physician must be present to administer the drug or therapy. This frequently happens at 11:00 P.M. on a holiday weekend.
5. Investigators must be vigilant to ensure that the protocol is followed over the course of therapy. This becomes extremely important if the course of therapy is prolonged.
6. Immediate access to clinical and experimental laboratories must be available for processing.
7. Unexpected complications or needs may arise, such as hyperkalemia requiring dialysis that may alter kinetics, or a CT scan altering schedules and making evaluation of a particular therapy difficult.
8. Data collection, retrospectively, may lose important information while concurrent collection may be impractical.
9. Long-term effects of therapy may be difficult to quantify.

Patient Selection

Ideally, all patients admitted to an ICU would be eligible for admission to a study, but numerous difficulties confront the prospective investigator. Obtaining informed consent can be a time-consuming and frustrating experience. Many patients in the ICU are intubated or receiving drugs that render them incompetent. Even patients who appear to be competent are difficult to evaluate because the stress of the ICU situation may cloud their judgment. In some states and institutions, only patients may grant informed consent, and this eliminates a large portion of the population, for example, as in the Veterans Administration (VA) study on steroids.[7] Families may be divided or difficult to collect together for consensus on whether their loved ones can enroll. Wives often will not consent without their children's agreement. The use of a placebo worries families who feel that their relation is not receiving all the benefits medicine can provide.

Deciding who meets the criteria can be difficult. Numerous medications, such as cimetidine or aspirin, interact with study drugs and need to be discontinued. Requirements for invasive monitoring subject the patient to further risks that may or may not improve care but are necessary to assess the experimental therapy adequately. Studies involving sepsis may require initiation of therapy prior to its confirmation, since early and prompt treatment needs to be initiated before culture results are available. Patient accrual demands that some patients enrolled will not be eligible for inclusion in the final data presentation. Originally, many sepsis studies required positive blood cultures. It became evident that waiting for blood cultures, which were positive only in 40% of the population at risk, was not reasonable; most studies now require only the presence of a source of infection and evidence of a systemic sepsis response.[7]

The majority of critical care units are not administratively organized to perform clinical research. ICU nurses have numerous tasks and cannot be expected to participate actively in studies that add a large time commitment to their patient load. A nurse–clinician with ICU experience who can deal with the staff, be available 24 hours a day to assist in the study, and administer phase 2 or phase 3 drugs is essential. The nurse–clinician is also responsible for gathering the appropriate data and sorting the meaningful numbers from the "garbage." This role becomes even more important when the experimental therapy may interfere with the routine ICU care. Pain medication will alter mental and hemodynamic status; dressing changes and bathing will increase metabolic demands and change hemodynamic parameters. The nurse–clinician helps to reschedule these activities to provide optimal data for research without affecting patient care. Unless the physician can be present for the entire study, the nurse–clinician must ensure that drugs are given on time. Laboratory tests such as thromboxane levels need special handling. Plasma for Thromboxane B_2 (TXB_2) requires collection in iced plastic syringes and immediate transfer into iced test tubes containing 0.1 ml of indomethacin heparin solution.[8] The blood then requires refrigerated centrifugation and the plasma aliquot must be stored at −20°C until extraction and assay. This cannot be performed by an ICU nurse because of the diversion of time involved.

Few ICU populations are homogeneous. Each patient population yields a totally different study group. Penetrating trauma patients frequently are young and healthy; coronary care patients are older and have intercurrent diseases. Postoperative cardiac surgical patients are among the easiest to study because mortality is low, the population is large, and the therapy can be relatively standardized. Studies related to modes of ventilation, vasoactive drugs, or new blood substitutes are all easily studied in this population. Septic patients, however, are a heterogeneous group with wide variations in age, underlying disease, and disease etiology.

Comparing patient groups is difficult. Several attempts have been made to classify patients according to disease process, severity of illness, and prognosis. Systems that describe these variables, such as Apache II, Medicus, and Lemshew-Terres, have flaws that make interpretation of data difficult. Dissecting out the parameters before beginning to compare patients is a time-consuming, arduous task.

What kind of study needs to be performed in ICU? Are double-blinded placebos necessary, or are open label studies acceptable? Must all studies be randomized, or can patients be told they will be given the experimental therapy after they have been randomized? Zelen proposed a new method of planned randomization in which patients are first allocated to best standard or experimental therapy, and those in the latter group are then asked if they will accept the experimental therapy.[9] This methodology could eliminate many of the exclusionary factors now present in clinical research. Guyatt et al. described a method for performing randomized controlled trials on individual patients ($n = 1$).[10] It is impossible to "blind" a study of ventilator technique or specialty beds. Is it justifiable to administer a placebo down the nasogastric tube if the study is an evaluation of an experimental acid blocking agent for the prevention of stress ulcers? "Deferred consent" is a possibility and is ethically justifiable.[11]

The large amount of data available may create problems. Blood pressure can be obtained constantly from an arterial cannula and pressure transducer, every 5 minutes from a noninvasive cuff, or every hour by the nurse; which the clinician chooses to report is vital. Does an arterial line systolic blood pressure of 70 torr mean anything, or did the patient bend his wrist? Is the cuff pressure or the arterial line pressure the number you believe? Does the infiltrate on chest x-ray represent pneumonia or atelectasis? It becomes essential for the researcher to decide, carefully, what data will be acceptable and what parameters will be utilized—prior to enrolling patients. With thousands of data points available, it is easy to skew the data depending on which information is recorded on the data sheet.

Financing clinical ICU studies is very difficult. The NIH finances molecular biology and basic science, not clinical trials. Industry wants studies of drugs that will profit them, but they have budgetary constraints that may cripple the pure science of the study, especially a study of new technology. Because they are poorly regulated, technological advances made by industry are not driven by the need to prove themselves to the extent that new drugs are. There is no randomized prospective study of the benefit of the Swan Ganz catheter because it has become accepted as "routine"; nor is there proof that new advances in ventilator therapy, such as pressure support, have any advantages over other technologies. The result is that many studies have to be performed on a small patient population.

Occasionally industry is willing to fund a major scientific effort at enormous cost in money, time, and personnel. A study was sponsored by Upjohn Company to answer the question of the usefulness of methylprednisolone in the treatment of septic shock.[12] The study was conducted at 19 centers from November 1982 to December 31, 1985. During this time, only 382 patients were enrolled despite the use of numerous large teaching centers with interested faculties. The total cost of such a study exceeds several million dollars. The Veterans Administration funded a similar major effort which screened 2568 patients in 10 VA hospitals, but randomized only 223 (9%) over 31 months.[7]

Numerous clinical studies have been performed over the past several decades, despite these difficulties. An example of the problems and rewards of ICU research is the study of arachidonic acid metabolites in critically ill patients in the ICU. Sepsis has been estimated to occur in 15 per 1000 hospital admissions[13]; circulatory shock develops in 20% of these patients, with a mortality of 30% to 60%.[14] A frequent sequela of gram-negative sepsis is ARDS, the acute form of noncardiogenic pulmonary edema resulting in acute respiratory failure.

The activation of inflammatory mediators, especially the arachidonic acid cascade, appears to contribute to the development of ARDS. One metabolite, thromboxane A_2, has been implicated in the pathogenesis of endotoxic shock and ARDS in numerous animal experiments since 1980.[15] Thromboxane synthetase inhibitors have been shown to increase survival in septic animals by decreasing severity of the thrombocytopenia and ameliorating pulmonary artery hypertension, although they did not prevent pulmonary capillary leakage associated with ARDS.[16] Ibuprofen, a cyclooxygenase inhibitor, has also been demonstrated to improve survival in oleic acid induced ARDS in animals.[17]

The first thromboxane B_2 clinical study was performed to determine if levels were elevated in human sepsis. Reines et al. demonstrated markedly increased levels of TXB_2 in patients dying of sepsis and noted that this group had significantly worse parameters for ARDS than the control group.[8] Given these clinical and experimental data, a pilot clinical trial of TX synthetase inhibitors was designed. Patients meeting criteria of sepsis syndrome were randomized in a single-blind manner to receive Dazoxiben, a TX synthetase inhibitor, or placebo.[18] Patients were required to have pulmonary artery and arterial catheters in place, and were entered into this study less than 8 hours after the diagnosis of sepsis was made. Full hepatic and renal laboratory screening was performed, and the patient then received the drug every 4 hours, for 72 hours. Because of the potential effect of shifting arachidonic acid production to another pathway, especially prostacyclin, the study nurse administered all the doses, and one of the investigators stayed at the bedside during most of the study. This constant attendance requirement made it impossible to enter more than one patient a week into the study.

Although thromboxane levels fell significantly following the administration of the first dose of the drug, no significant improvement in any of the parameters of the pulmonary function were noted.[18] This and other papers suggested that selective thromboxane blockade alone was not beneficial in the management of patients with established ARDS and sepsis.

These studies exemplify the trends in modern clinical ICU mediator research. The hypothesis is tested in animal models first; elevated levels of the mediator then need to be found in the selected patient population; and finally, clinical trials of a single mediator stimulator/blocker are attempted. Because of the myriad of mediators involved in the septic response, including tumor necrosis factor interleukins, the eicosanoids, platelet activating factor, complement, and superoxide radicals, it is doubtful that a study of any single agent will ever be successful in significantly altering mortality. Eventually, a multicenter, multiarmed study will be necessary to solve this difficult problem.

The use of steroids in the critically ill is an example of how the field of ICU investigation is progressing. Glucocorticoids have been reported to disaggregate clumps of granulocytes, stabilize cell membranes, prevent the activation of the alternate complement pathway, and block the release of phospholipase A_2.[19] In 1975 Sladen reported an uncontrolled, nonrandomized study of 10 patients with shock lung treated with methylprednisolone in high dose (30 mg per kg of body weight given every 6 hours) that resulted in only 1 death.[20] The following year, Schumer conducted a large prospective study that demonstrated that the same dose of methylprednisolone (30 mg per kg) reduced mortality from 38.4% to 10.5%.[21] This became the standard of care for critically ill septic patients. It was not until Sprung repeated a similar study, in 1984, and showed no difference in mortality with the use of steroids, that the Schumer study was successfully challenged.[22] Finally, two collaborative studies – one sponsored by a pharmaceutical company and the other by the VA – with a combined total of 605 patients, concluded that steroids produced no benefit in sepsis and ARDS.[7,12] The Severe Sepsis Study Group reported that methylprednisolone not only did not improve mortality in ARDS but increased the mortality to 52% in a subpopulation of the treatment group.

Numerous problems were enumerated in these studies. In the VA study a large number of patients had to be screened before adequate numbers were obtained. The entry criteria were so strict that a bias may have been built into the study. Because the presence of abnormal mental status prevented many VA patients from signing a consent, a whole population was left out. The VA investigators wanted to continue the study, but the sponsors ended it when the statistical evidence did not show efficacy of the steroid solution. The other multicenter study began to identify a subgroup with renal failure, who were at risk, and this prompted the company to issue a warning that steroids may be harmful in this group. Once again, there may have been subgroups in this study who might have benefited from steroids, but they were not statistically identified.

Although these two studies were exquisitely planned, meticulously executed, and well funded, the question will remain – "How could 100 animal studies and numerous human studies consistently yield data that did not hold up under sufficiently controlled human conditions?" These two studies are excellent examples of why human studies are essential and why they are so difficult to perform.

An example of a clinical investigation examining methodologies was the comparison of assist control/T-piece versus intermittent mandatory ventilation (IMV) for weaning patients from the ventilator.[23] Since the advent of positive pressure breathing, the best methodology for electively removing ventilatory support has been controversial. This study asked the question "Which of the two most commonly used weaning techniques is better?" The protocol was established by a committee of the senior authors (each of whom had initial prejudices regarding technique), a respiratory therapist to give technical input, and a biostatistician to determine the number of patients necessary to answer the questions and determine the validity of the methodology.

Randomizing prospectively was felt to be impractical, and blinding was impossible because the availability of the same type of ventilator could not be guaranteed and because of the difficulties of alerting all therapists, nurses, and house staff to the randomization. Blanket permission was therefore obtained from all attending physicians admitting patients to the various intensive care units. Randomization was undertaken according to the month; during odd months, patients were assigned to assist control; during even months, IMV was used. Practicality overcame purity of science. Patients had to be clinically stable and meet four weaning criteria prior to entering the study.

The study was divided into three groups—the easy wean group (< 72 hours), the long-term wean group (> 72 hours), and a group that had been on ventilation for more than a week, or had failed three weaning attempts.

It took several months to convince physicians that patient care would not suffer. Because the early period revealed a preponderance of coronary artery bypass graft patients, the study was expanded to two other hospitals and took 16 months. To avoid the bias of work of breathing, it was felt that a single ventilator, the Puritan Bennett MA-1, equipped with an H-valve, would be required on all patients in the study.

Two hundred patients were enrolled, and 165 (82%) began the protocol. Of the patients withdrawn, two-thirds were removed because the attending physician requested termination of the study.

Because patient accrual can be difficult for numerous reasons and cooperation of attending physicians is imperative, all protocols should be written with the approval and knowledge of the individuals whose patients will be enrolled.

Extremely sick patients who are difficult to wean are relatively rare, even in a busy ICU. Accordingly, it is important to have a mechanism to capture all patients. Even though the respiratory therapist saw every patient on ventilator and listed all of them, only small numbers of critically ill patients requiring prolonged ventilation were entered. The answer to the original study question is in doubt in this population. In the future, such studies will require a multicenter approach, even though it is expensive and can lead to wide variations in techniques by individuals.

An example of in vivo observation leading to an in vitro study is well illustrated by the elucidation of myocardial depressant substances in patients with septic shock.[24] A clinical study to characterize cardiac function was performed on 20 patients with documented septic shock using serial radionucleotide cineangiography. ECG-gated cardiac scintigraphic examination was performed using a portable scanner at the bedside to determine left ventricular ejection fraction simultaneously with hemodynamic monitoring of ventricular function. Despite supranormal cardiac indices, 10 patients demonstrated ejection fractions (EF) of less than 40%. Both index and EF returned to normal among survivors.

To evaluate the mechanism of severe reversible myocardial suppression, plasma from the septic patients was compared to three control populations including normals, patients with chronic cardiovascular disease, and patients admitted without evidence of sepsis.[25] A myocardial cell suspension of contractile newborn rat muscle was devised, and the beating myocardial cells were placed in petri dishes on a microscope stage monitored by a high-resolution video camera. Myocardial contractility was measured by plotting the percentage of the video area occupied by the cells over time at rest and following incubation with the test sera. The derivation of extent of shortening provided the velocity of the myocardial cell contraction. The study confirmed the study impression that septic shock patients' serum significantly inhibit myocardial contractility in a dose-related manner.

The serum was then dialyzed against a phosphate buffer and the myocardial depressant substance (MDS) was dialyzable. Gel filtration with a G-25 Sephadex column revealed MDS as a polypeptide of approximately 2000 daltons. These studies confirmed earlier animal studies that MDS exists and may play a role in the cardiac performance of septic shock.

Despite the difficulties, studies of critically ill patients are essential if we are to improve outcomes and decrease morbidity within this costly and resource-consuming group.[26] Multiple aspects of critical care are currently under study, including stress ulcers, ethical problems, outcome predictors, ventilatory methodology, and the efficacy of invasive monitoring. More clinical work needs to be performed. Of what value is the expenditure of billions of dollars in basic mechanisms in molecular biology if the results cannot be transformed into practical applications to improve life? Clinical research needs support, not only from private industry, which can benefit financially from the research, but also from federal sources, to ensure that objectivity is preserved. NIH and other agencies need to recognize critical care as a subspecialty and offer it the resources necessary to improve quality of life and maximize utilization of our limited resources. Investigators need to persevere in the pursuit of questions basic to improving survival from critical illness.

References

1. Declaration of Helsinki. Adopted by the 18th World Medical Assembly, Helsinki, Finland, June 1964.
2. Beecher HK. Ethics and clinical research. N Engl J Med 1955;274:1354–60.
3. National Commission for the Protection of Human Subjects of Biomedical and Behavioral Research.

The Belmont report: Ethical principles and guidelines for the protection of human subjects of research. Publication (OS) 78-0012, U.S. Department of Health, Education and Welfare, 1978.
4. Laupacis A, Jackett D, Roberts RG. An assessment of clinically useful measures of the consequences of treatment. N Engl J Med 1988;318:1728–33.
5. Breu C, Dracup K. Implementing nursing research in a critical care setting. J Nurs Admin December 1976:14–17.
6. Loanzon P, Weissman C, Askanazi J. Clinical research and nursing in the intensive care unit. Heart Lung 1983;12:480–84.
7. VA Systemic Sepsis Co-operative Study Group. The effect of high-dose glucocorticoid therapy on mortality in patients with clinical signs of systemic sepsis. N Engl J. Med 1987;317:659–65.
8. Reines HD, Halushka PV, Cook JA, et al. Plasma thromboxane concentrations are raised in patients dying with septic shock. Lancet 1982;1:174–75.
9. Zelen M. A new design for randomized clinical trials. N Engl J Med 1979;300:1242–45.
10. Guyatt G, Sackett D, Taylor W, et al. Determining optimal therapy—randomized trials in individual patients. N Engl J Med 1980;314:889–92.
11. Kopelman L. Consent and randomized trials: are they moral or design problems? J Med Philos 1986; 11:317–45.
12. Bone RC, Fisher CJ, Clemmer TP, et al. A controlled trial of high dose methylprednisolone in the treatment of severe sepsis and septic shock. N Engl J Med 1987;317:653–58.
13. Berringer R, Harwood-Nuss AL. Septic shock (Part I). Emery Med Rev 1985;3:75-82.
14. Kreger BE, Craveb DE, Carling PC, et al. Gram negative bacteria: III. Reassessment of etiology epidemiology and ecology in 612 patients. Am J Med 1980;68:332–40.
15. Cook JA, Wise WC, Halushka PV. Elevated thromboxane levels in the rat during endotoxic shock; protective effects of Imidazole, 13-Azaprostanoic acid or essential fatty acid deficiency. J Clin Invest 1980;65:227–30.
16. Demling RH, Smith M, Gunther R, et al. Pulmonary injury and prostaglandin production during endotoxemia in conscious sheep. Am J Physiol 1981;240:348–53.
17. Fuhrman TM, Hollon MF, Reines HD, et al. Beneficial effects of Ibuprofen in oleic acid induced lung injury. J Surg Res 1987;42:248–89.
18. Reines HD, Halushka PV, Olanoff LS. Dazoxiben in human sepsis and adult respiratory distress syndrome. Clin Pharm Ther 1985;37:391–95.
19. Hammerschmidt DE, White JG, Craddock PR, et al. Corticosteroids inhibit complement-induced granulocyte aggregation: four possible mechanisms for their efficacy in shock states. J Clin Invest 1979;63: 798–803.
20. Sladen A. Methylprednisolone pharmacological doses in shock lung syndrome. J Thorac Cardiovasc Surg 1976;71:800–6.
21. Schumer W. Steroids in the treatment of clinical septic shock. Ann Surg 1976;184:333–41.
22. Sprung CL, Caralis PV, Marcial EH, et al. The effects of high-dose corticosteroids in patients with septic shock. N Engl J Med 1984;311:1137–43.
23. Tomlinson JR, Sahn SA, Reines HD, et al. A prospective comparison of IMV and T-piece weaning mechanical ventilation. Chest 1989;96:348–52.
24. Parker MM, Shelhamer JH, Bacharach SL, et al. Profound but reversible myocardial depression in patients with septic shock. Ann Intern Med 1984; 100:483–90.
25. Parillo JE, Burch C, Shelhamer JH, et al. Circulating myocardial depressant substance in humans with septic shock. J Clin Invest 1985;76:1539–53.
26. Knauss, WA. The science of prediction and its implications for the clinician today. Theor Surg 1988;3: 93–101.

28

Experiments in Human Volunteers

M.F. Brennan

The proper study of mankind is man.
Alexander Pope

Francis D. Moore or George F. Cahill made me aware of the above maxim, early in 1970. Where would human body composition[1] or the physiology of starvation[2] be without the studies performed in man by these two investigators? [Cahill's classic monograph[2] describes how a simple study of normal man can translate into meaningful understanding of human physiology. It is a prototype for other clinical investigations.]

In the 1950s, and possibly until 1970, clinician investigators were physicians at the bedside, identifying clinical and patient care problems, biological contradictions, and areas of misunderstanding; then, with care and focused deliberation, they set about understanding them. Such noble pursuits were often the province of the young academician, but they were always carried out in a context of superb clinical training. On occasion, the investigator may have taken 2 or 3 years to gain the additional skills required to pursue such investigations, but not to the exclusion of clinical activity.

The situation today is very different. The entire concept of clinical research is under scrutiny. Many believe that clinical research, as it was 40 or even 20 years ago, is dead. An understanding of molecular biology now requires a full-time commitment. New techniques, new technology, and the dramatic explosion in biological knowledge have led the physician–investigator away from the patient and into the laboratories of basic science. This has had two major effects: the atrophy of clinical skills in physician–investigators and the reduction of applied clinical research by clinicians. Clinical care combined with clinical research has become academically undesirable. How many academic departments have active programs in clinical research being performed by respected clinicians? Academic promotion is *no longer* related to clinical care. Given that practical skill is paramount to good clinical care in the discipline of surgery, departments of surgery have been slow to adopt the same criteria for academic advancement. But they are doing so, and they will. "Academic department" has already become synonymous with poor clinical care, inactive clinical programs, and derogatory comments about the "rat doctors." This situation serves only to divide and further estrange the clinicians who do not understand the concepts of molecular biology from the research-oriented clinician–scientists who, frustrated by their clinical colleagues' lack of knowledge, turn further inward to techniques of basic investigation and ever further from the patient in their struggle to stay with their basic science colleagues.

How similar these thoughts are to those expressed by Relman,[3] in 1961! [This now historical piece documents the fact that problems in applied research are not new, and indeed are constantly evolving. This careful and erudite description should be read by all investigators or investigators-in-training.] I believe, however, that these observations increase the opportunity for a renewed interest in clinical research. We have no choice: "The proper study of mankind is man." Man is not a solitary circuit, but an integrated complex of checks and balances, actions and reactions, which can be studied only intact!

Clinical Research

Clinical research in man covers clinical trials, studies in normal volunteers, and patient studies in nontrial situations. Clinical trials are complicated and are covered elsewhere in this book (see Chapter 14, in Section II; Chapter 24, above, offers a more comprehensive description of the ways in which young surgeons can be involved in clinical investigation.) That they are essential is not in dispute; as physicians we remember what works and not what fails. The successful pancreaticoduodenectomy for carcinoma of the pancreas is shown to the staff when the patient returns disease-free at 5 years. The perioperative death is soon forgotten.

I want to focus on what I consider to be the most difficult of all human studies—pharmacologic, physiologic, and metabolic studies of hospitalized patients. Doing this in no way denigrates the importance of volunteer studies. They provide a unique approach in which the participant, for financial gain or from personal conviction, willingly and knowingly enters into a study whose goal is the advancement of knowledge. The study of normal volunteers is more of an ethical than a medical problem and this is discussed in Section II (Chapter 12). In contrast, hospitalized patients are vulnerable, concerned, frightened, and potentially terrified of their disease or its outcome if they are afflicted with malignancies.

Metabolic, pharmacologic, and physiologic studies in hospitalized patients are of two kinds: those that are of potential benefit to the patients involved and those that are not.

In the first kind of study, the patient is undergoing treatment and the purpose of the study is to examine the metabolic/physiologic consequences of the treatment or the disposal or disposition of an administered agent. Since I wish to focus on my own area of expertise, I shall comment on and then dismiss the pharmacologic studies. Benefit may *potentially* accrue to a patient participating in such studies, whether he or she is receiving an antibiotic or an antineoplastic agent, and even though the study may be concerned with the pharmokinetics or toxicity of the agent.

A metabolic/physiologic study might examine fat turnover on metabolism in a patient to whom tumor necrosis factor (TNF) is being administered for evaluation of the therapeutic impact of TNF on patients with malignancy.[4-6] The patient is a potential benefactor of the investigational treatment, and the biological and metabolic consequences of the administration of a cytokine can be elucidated at the same time. The metabolic study is relatively easily to justify on much the same basis as the pharmokinetic study during the course of a therapeutic trial, but there is a difference. In the pharmokinetic study, there is an intimate relation between therapeutic benefit and drug disposal, whereas in the metabolic study, the data obtained in parallel are not related to the examination of potential therapeutic benefit. It is possible, indeed probable, that knowledge of the rate of disposal of a drug will subsequently allow better therapeutic application of that drug in terms of dose-timing. No such claim can be made for the determination of glucose kinetics in response to TNF! Nevertheless, such studies, if carefully designed and adapted to the primary study, may be accomplished with little inconvenience to the patient. If blood sampling can be integrated with that required for the monitoring of the primary therapy, no significant disadvantage accrues to the patient.

Patient Compliance

Such exact integration is unlikely: the gathering of the information needed for the secondary study rarely runs so parallel to what is required for the primary investigation. Although the extra demands may be very small and the risks minimal, the patient may hardly be a willing participant! Already distraught by the failure of conventional therapy and looking to an investigational agent or research treatment as the only source of hope, can such a patient really give informed consent to any secondary or associated study? Consequently, considerable care must be exercised to ensure that there is no coercion, or even worse, cause for the patient to feel "If I don't agree to participate in the research study, I won't get treated." Fortunately, with frankness and empathy, the goals of both patient and doctor can be fulfilled.

My research colleagues and I have been interested in fat metabolism in the septic cancer patient in intensive care. The examination of fat turnover in such patients, under the influence of a euglycemic clamp, can provide a large amount of information that is difficult to obtain by any other means.[7,8] The likelihood that any individual patient will benefit significantly from such an investigation is low. One might argue that we are providing presumably beneficial exogenous nutrients and that monitoring and maintaining the patient's blood glucose within a tight normal range may, in theory at least, benefit the patient. Nevertheless, such arguments become specious if pushed too far. While the letter of the law may be maintained, the intent is circumvented. Such studies are justifiable, however, because the question being asked is of basic therapeutic relevance to the patient, although not necessarily beneficial. It is valuable to know whether "obligatory" host catabolism can be turned off in the septic patient by whatever means. The therapeutic event, the euglycemic clamp, is related to the question "Can exogenous nutrient and insulin arrest the accelerated fat catabolism?"

The second kind of study is the metabolic/physiologic study that has no potential for direct patient benefit. An examination of glucose intolerance when a new cardiotoxic beta-blocking drug is used to improve cardiac performance would be such a study. Its primary function would not be to examine the consequences of beta blockade in cardiac function, but the peripheral issue of the effect of such treatment on a different physiological process.

Another example is the determination of peripheral amino acid flux in hospitalized patients.[9,10] While such a study is invasive and has no chance of benefiting the individual participating patient, it does have very significant potential for subsequent benefit for other patients. In contrast, the determination of blood flow by noninvasive methods[1] may be easily justified on the grounds that the only inconvenience to the patient is the time required to make the measurement.

Studies with Limited Potential Benefit to the Patient

But, how do we justify such purely investigational studies as the examination of hyperinsulinemia, with a euglycemic clamp, in a patient with malignancy? The legal and moral requirements vary from country to country. In some, the approval of an institutional review board is not required or is almost perfunctory; informed consent may mean nothing more than informing patients that they are part of a study. In the United States, however, it is difficult to obtain permission to do experimentation in humans; moreover, the process is extremely expensive and is controlled by institutional review boards (IRBs) with almost religious zeal.

The risk associated with small doses of radiation from radiolabeled tracers is inconsequential if the patient is to receive therapeutic external beam radiation, but the issue has to be readdressed if radiation is not part of the therapy. What is the life expectancy of the patient? Is it more acceptable to conduct such a study in a patient whose life expectancy is short than in one whose life expectancy is long? This is a difficult and emotionally charged subject. If the answer to the question is yes, how do we approach the control for such a patient? It is extraordinarily frustrating to have reviewers roundly criticize manuscripts reporting studies in humans because of the absence of controls, when ethical review boards would find such an experiment in control patients difficult or impossible to accept! Often, the reviewers might accept the study if it were done in volunteers. This would be acceptable to an IRB, but the reviewers would then demand that the study be done in a patient population without the disease entity being examined! How can we resolve these dilemmas? What of the patient in the intensive care unit—intubated, ventilated, sedated, and certainly unable to give informed consent? How emotionally valid is the consent of a relative?

The practical issue for investigators proposing such a study is whether they, or members of their families, would feel comfortable participating in the study. This is not to minimize the essential importance of patient protection. I believe that such studies, designed and performed appropriately, can be conscientiously, ethically, and morally completed with minimum risk to the patient. This issue, in the context of a clinical trial, has serious consequences. A brief piece in *The Lancet*[12] raises the issue of ethics and morality in clinical trials. It focuses, provocatively, on issues that must be addressed and is a good and simple introduction to them.

Human Experimentation: The Practical Issues

The first requirement of any study involving human experimentation is scientific validity.

Study design is similar to that of any other experiment: the hypothesis to be tested must be formulated and testable. If we think the question out carefully, we *may* get an answer. If the question is an unfocused "What happens if . . .?", we will often describe, but rarely learn. The question must be important, the likelihood of an answer real, and the results of some importance in long-term management or understanding that can lead to improved care.

Are there other ways of getting the information? Preferably, the desired information should be unobtainable by any other means or, if obtainable in animals, should require validation of its transferability to humans.

Once the scientific validity of the question has been established, all potential risks must be clearly elucidated and weighed against the value of the information. This is not an easy task. It is extremely difficult to make value judgments about the potential value of information versus the discomfiture due to the invasive procedures required to get it. Information obtained from a simple venous sample may be easily justified, but more aggressive tests, such as right heart catheterization, may be totally unjustifiable unless the information is extremely important. Making a decision to carry out such an experiment requires considerable introspective thought, because what may be acceptable to one investigator, or to one patient, will not be acceptable to another.

When the question has been designed and the risks justified, usually for a directed population, the next step is to identify the appropriate population sample. Earlier, we broached the problem of "captive" cancer-afflicted or hospitalized patients who are fearful that failure to participate in the physician's research investigation may compromise the care they will receive. Every effort must be made to avoid any semblance of such coercion. It is not incorrect, however, to ask a patient to assist the physician in learning something. Such conversations can often weld a physician–patient bond that not only transcends the need for obtaining the information but allows the physician to provide more emotive and empathetic care. Nevertheless, inclusion criteria still have to encompass more than the appropriateness of the subject and must address the issues of potential coercion, particularly in patients with advanced disease of any kind.

A clear definition of the population, and an equally clear definition of the number of participating patients required to obtain meaningful information must be carefully prepared for the IRB. In metabolic studies, the issue is not large numbers of patients but large amounts of information, and the number of patients needed may be quite small. Whenever possible, patients should serve as their own controls to avoid the very difficult issue of obtaining an appropriate control population. A good IRB will examine the ethical and moral questions. If these matters have been addressed in a forthright manner within the context of the protocol, they should almost certainly be accepted.

The most damaging IRB criticism of any human experimentation will be provoked by a protocol that is less than forthright or indulges in obfuscation. If the protocol induces any perception that the investigator is trying to hide or minimize the consequences of an experiment or maximize the need for its performance, the ethics of the investigator and the morality of the protocol will be called into question. No benefit can ever be obtained from trying to "get something by the IRB." Conversely, investigators should not be overwhelmed by a rigid and narrow IRB, and the problem often can be solved by the investigator's appearance before the IRB to argue the merits of the protocol. Unfortunately, some institutional review boards prefer to carry out their deliberations and adjudications "in camera" and do not allow the investigator to appear before them. This is totally inappropriate, in my opinion; it serves neither the needs of the investigator nor of the institution. Whenever such discussions are held in closed session, they carry the implication that there is something to hide.

When the IRB approves the protocol, the investigator must obtain the informed consent of the patients who will participate. This should be done in a frank and open way. Often, the best approach is to have the primary care physician convey his or her willingness to have the patient participate directly to the patient. Patients will rarely participate, nor should they, if primary care physicians are unaware of the protocol or unwilling to have their patients involved. Nothing is more damaging to the patient–physician relationship than the appearance of some unknown physician at the patient's bedside to introduce a protocol of which the patient is totally unaware. Conversely, it is neither necessary nor appropriate that the primary attending physician obtain consent. What is required is the attending physician's stamp of approval and willingness to gain a clear understanding of any question raised, to be able to explain the answer to the patient, if necessary. The issue of consent can be difficult. An extraordinarily complicated consent form, several pages long and documenting every conceivable risk, has no advantage. Failing to give the patient a clear and frank understanding of what the investigator is trying to learn is even less rewarding.

The format of current consent forms is daunting. Any semblance of simplicity disappears as institutional legal counsels reword the content so that patients cannot possibly understand that they are abrogating all potential future claims against the institution. Blame is dismissed! It must be frightening to realize that, if something does go wrong in any treatment or investigative protocol, it will be the patient/subject's fault! The trust that medical care requires is a reciprocal affair, patient to doctor, subject to investigator. Failure to maintain such trust, whichever side is responsible, should doom an investigative protocol, regardless of its merit.

The investigator is responsible for close personal monitoring of the experiment in terms of its design, accuracy of completion, and value as a source of useful information. This responsibility cannot be delegated to junior research fellows and technicians while weeks or months pass before the data are analyzed and their value is thoughtfully weighed. The investigator must examine and study the data from each individual experiment, usually before going on to any next stage of the investigation. If any complication arises, the investigator must notify the IRB and redesign the experiment to avoid it, if at all possible. Meticulous records, including a daily log book recording every event and every observation, are imperative in all human research. Such records allow retrospective analysis in case any laboratory determination is unexpected or some unappreciated event is forgotten. It is so much easier to understand an apparently erroneous or inconsistent value if an incident of fever, catheter blockage, or unintended food intake has been recorded. Such meticulous records protect both the investigator and the patient from charges of malfeasance or inappropriate criticism.

On rare occasions, complications or unexpected side effects will indicate that termination of the experiment is the only appropriate behavior. This should be seen not as failure, but as evidence of the clinical conscience of the investigator.

Additional risk to the patient–physician relationship occurs in studies performed on patients in intensive care units or otherwise unable to sign the consent form. An additional burden is placed on families when they are asked for permission to include loved ones in an investigational protocol at a time of deepest concern. If such studies are not carefully monitored and thought through, the potential for implied, though unintended, indifference is great. We are all familiar with the institutional mentality that perceives a patient as simply a "client" in a great assembly-line endeavor. The investigator must always appreciate that no matter how simple the ultimate outcome may appear, the potential collaborators in the study are being asked to participate when they and their families are struggling with the intense emotional and physical stress imposed by the possibility of impending death. Honesty, forthrightness, sensitivity, and empathy are mandatory.

Finally, the investigator has a moral and ethical obligation to perform the experiment in as thoughtful, careful, and diligent a way as is humanly possible. Performing a study in patients in an inefficient, crass, or incompetent manner is a flagrant demonstration of indifference to the concerns surrounding human experimentation.

Training of the Clinical Investigator Interested in Applied Studies in Man

Experimental studies, such as those just outlined, require an integrated, committed interval of research of rarely less than 2 years' duration and occasionally more. Young investigators need to be in clinical investigation units or in clinical research settings, where their initial experience is participating in already-defined ongoing projects with other investigators.

I believe that the investigator's laboratory is integral to the adequate performance of clinical investigations in humans; a mere conglomeration of collaborators is insufficient. While collaboration in individual assays is often important, the young investigator can rarely be fully educated unless he or she participates in a study that entails basic laboratory involvement. This means that the investigator-in-training must participate not only in such management aspects of a study as appropriate documentation, sample preparation, infusion monitoring, and data recording, but also in assay determinations. My research colleagues and I have adopted the practice of requiring each investigator to become completely familiar with at least one of the basic assays employed in a given study. This promotes better understanding of the difficulties inherent in any biological assay and, more importantly, enables the investigator to dissect problems when specific assays do not function properly, given the vagaries of their limitations, calculation, interpretation, and understanding.

Conversely, the young investigator's entire time must not be devoted merely to providing technical service support for a senior investigator's study. Although young investigators initially learn many of the techniques that parallel clinical investigation, two further stages in their development are essential. They involve, as they do in surgical residency, the progressive assumption of increasing responsibility.

The developing investigator must actively participate in the design, documentation, and presentation of a second study to the institutional review board. The primary objective of this study will not necessarily be chosen by the young investigator, but rather by the focused laboratory head. The opportunity to shepherd it through the IRB has a value that should not be underestimated, just as the importance of subsequent assumption of responsibility for the study's performance, completion, and documentation cannot be overemphasized.

Such a process exposes young investigators to the ethical and moral aspects of human experimentation and often stimulates their interest in further basic training courses in biostatistics or ethics. I do not believe that formal rotations through such secondary educational processes are necessary. It is preferable that young investigators seek out the help they need to resolve the specific problems they have encountered. This ensures focused, efficient learning. It must be assumed that, at this stage of their development, young investigators are mature enough to perceive what they need to know to improve their ability to carry out good research. Indeed, the development of an understanding of just what is involved in the design of experimental studies in humans is probably more important than any specific formal training.

The information explosion in biomedical science will make more and more young investigators spend at least some period of time in nonsurgical laboratories, focusing on "single" areas of molecular biology to equip themselves to carry out subsequent clinical studies. Those committed to clinical investigation should not forget, however, that "the proper study of mankind is man," and that molecular biological techniques should be utilized only when they make it possible to answer a question relating to the whole person. This is not a criticism of any other research discipline; it is a pragmatic choice for those interested in applied human experimentation.

Young investigators *must* make frequent presentations of their data, no matter how preliminary or few in number the data may be, before their small laboratory groups. This should be done in a collegial atmosphere, so that early unexpected results, errors, or new insights can be picked up and developed before large quantities of time, effort, and resources are needed for the retrospective examination of uninterpretable results.

Finally, "work not written up is work not done." Young investigators must be given opportunities to present their work formally before a critical audiences and to prepare it for publication. Such learning experiences will have relevance throughout the remainder of the each investigator's career.

Future Developments

Applied clinical investigation has never been more needed and never more difficult to perform. The competing attractions of participating in the explosive growth in molecular biology and being able to delve into fundamental molecular processes must be balanced against the need to translate the understanding gained by such endeavors into applied developments and improved treatments for human disabilities and disease processes.

The protection of individuals from unnecessary invasions of their rights competes, similarly, with our desperate need to understand disease processes and their impact on humans. Our success or failure in addressing and resolving these apparently conflicting imperatives will pace and determine our progress in understanding and dealing with human disease.

References

1. Moore FD, Olesen KH, McMurrey JD, Parker HV, Hall MR, Boyden CM. The Body Cell Mass and Its Supporting Environment: Body Composition in Health and Disease. Philadelphia: Saunders, 1963.
2. Cahill FG Jr. Starvation in man. N Engl J Med 1970;282:668-75.
3. Relman AS. What is clinical research? Clin Res 1961;9:516-18.
4. Starnes HF Jr, Larchian EA, McHugh NE, Gabrilove JL, Brennan MF. Metabolic effects of tumor necrosis factor and gamma-interferon are not abrogated by indomethacin. Surg Forum 1988;39:1-3.
5. Starnes HF Jr, Warren RS, Gabrilove J, Larchian W, McHugh N, Jeevanandam M, Oettgen HF, Brennan MF. Tumor necrosis factor and the acute metabolic response to tissue injury in man. J Clin Invest 1988; 82:1321-25.
6. Warren RS, Donner DB, Starnes HF Jr, Brennan MF. Modulation of endogenous hormone action by recombinant human tumor necrosis factor. Proc Natl Acad Sci 1987;84:8619-22.
7. Levinson MR, Groeger JS, Jeevanandam M, Brennan MF. Free fatty acid turnover and lipolysis in septic mechanically ventilated cancer bearing man. Metabolism 1988;37:618-25.
8. Sauerwein HP, Pesola GR, Groeger JS, Jeevanandam M, Brennan MF. Relationship between glucose oxidation and FFA concentration in septic cancer-bearing patients. Metabolism 1988;37:1045-50.
9. Daly JM, Mihranian M, Kehoe J, Brennan MF. Effects of postoperative infusion of branched-chain amino acids on nitrogen balance and forearm muscle substrate flux. Surgery 1983;94:151-58.
10. Bennegard K, Eden E, Ekman L, Schersten T, Lundholm KG. Metabolic balance across the leg in weight-losing cancer patients compared to depleted patients without cancer. Cancer Res 1982;42:4293.
11. Dresler CM, Jeevanandam M, Brennan MF. Extremity blood flow in man: comparison between strain-gauge and capacitance plethysmography. Surgery 1987;101:35-39.
12. Tunkel V. Drug trials: who takes the risk? Lancet 1989;2:609-11.

29

Multicenter Collaborative Clinical Trials

R.G. Margolese and C.M. Balch

The controlled clinical trial is the most rigorous method we have to evaluate and compare alternative treatments. During the past two or three decades, this procedure has almost replaced historical reviews or extensive personal experience as the basis for choosing treatment strategies.

Multicenter clinical trials have played a major role in advancing surgical knowledge and treatment approaches over a range of diseases (e.g., antrectomy vs. highly selective vagotomy for duodenal ulcer, duodenal ulcer surgery vs. acid inhibitor treatment, coronary or carotid surgery vs. medical treatment, cyclosporin in organ transplantation, etc.). Such studies have been performed by groups of clinicians banding together, for a single study or a series of clinical protocols, through such formal cooperative group mechanisms as the National Surgical Adjuvant Breast and Bowel Project (NSABP), the Trauma Cooperative Group, the Veterans Administration Cooperative Group, and the World Health Organization Melanoma Group.

We will describe some basic principles and organizational structures that we consider to be necessary to ensure high quality, reproducible results in multicenter studies. Although many of the examples arise from extensive experience with cancer cooperative groups, the principles also apply broadly to other surgical disease.

Types of Trial

Phases of Trials

Clinical investigations of a new treatment are usually classified according to three sequential stages: phases I, II, and III.

Phase I

Trials in the first phase cover the introduction of a new treatment concept or drug. Examples are surgical adjuvant studies in immunotherapy (e.g., vaccine treatments) or new chemotherapies that usually involve a small number of patients and test primarily for safety and complications. When the studies focus on drugs, dose limiting toxicities are sought by beginning with a low dose and increasing it until toxic levels are reached. Demonstration of a therapeutic gain is not necessarily a goal in this phase.

Phase II

Phase II trials are conducted as single arm studies involving a limited number of patients treated consecutively within each disease category. The aim is to establish some degree of treatment efficacy. If responses are seen, the feasibility of a phase III trial is explored to see if the benefits can be extended and clarified.

Phase III

In the third phase, the new treatment or drug is compared to known, effective, standard treatments in a prospective, randomized fashion. The new therapy or drug may be evaluated by itself or in combination with other standard treatments as a new combined modality. Phase III trials require large numbers of patients and frequently have to employ the multicenter collaborative group mechanism.

Sometimes, clinical investigators stop at phase II without sufficiently proving that the new treatment is effective. The converse is also true; phase III trials have been started before optimization of the treatment approach and minimization of any associated morbidity. Many clinical research endeavors should take the form of a logical series of different investigations over time.

Randomized Controlled Clinical Trials

The most exacting and widely accepted design for clinical trials is the randomized controlled trial. Participating patients are assigned to treatments by random selection, rather than by any conscious decision, to ensure the formation of a control group that differs from the treatment group only in the treatment being studied—and in no other respect. Even though randomized trials can lead to important information of lasting value, *a poorly designed or inappropriately analyzed randomized trial can lead to just as much confusion and conflict* as the biases in nonrandomized studies with historical controls.

Without careful evaluation and confirmation by phase III trials, expensive or dangerous treatments can be widely applied with little chance for benefit. The immediate acceptance of postoperative radiation therapy for breast cancer in the years following World War II is a good example. Improvement in equipment had made safe and effective radiation therapy available, and it was widely assumed that supplementing the then standard operation of radical mastectomy with radiation would improve the rates of control and cure. This assumption went unquestioned for a long time and radiation, although unproven as an adjunctive therapy, became standard treatment throughout North America. By the late 1960s, the biology of cancer was better understood, and randomized controlled clinical trials to evaluate the postoperative use of radiotherapy were finally undertaken. The eventual result[1,2] was discontinuance of routine adjunctive radiation and a consequent reduction in morbidity and costs, without impairment of survival.

Evaluation of a widely established therapy is often difficult, because the need for a "no treatment" control arm suggests the withholding of a putatively useful treatment. The evaluation of a new therapy is preferably made before its use becomes widely established, so that it can be compared to "standard therapy." The difficulty in entering patients in a trial in which treatment is determined by random selection has prompted a long search by investigators for other methods of choosing control groups, but a better method than randomization has yet to be found.

Historical Control Trials

Historical controls remain a popular alternative to randomized controls. This approach uses a selected group of patients treated in the past as a control for a group currently receiving a new treatment; the patients can be matched for such factors as age, sex, and extent of disease. Although this method sounds useful, it has many limitations, including the following.

1. Criteria for patient selection are difficult to define.
2. Changes occur in the natural history of the disease.
3. Changes occur in the pathological definitions or staging of the disease.
4. Changes occur in patient referral patterns.
5. Investigators may be more selective than past physicians in choosing patients for a new treatment.
6. Recorded data may be of inferior quality.
7. Criteria for response may be difficult to ascertain consistently in the records.
8. Improvements in patient care may improve new treatments.

Nonrandomized trials with concurrent controls also introduce bias that may cause incorrect interpretation of the results. Nevertheless, because some types of nonrandomized study provide important information needed for the better design of randomized clinical trials, they do have their place in the sequential scheme of research. For example, a retrospective review of 294 melanoma patients treated at the University of Alabama at Birmingham[3] led directly to the design (including stratification criteria) for a multicenter randomized clinical trial involving various surgical treatment options.[4]

There is clear evidence that uncontrolled studies are much more likely than controlled trials to lead to falsely enthusiastic recommendations for a treatment.[5,6] A study by Gilbert and colleagues[7] showed that only 50% of the surgical innovations tested by randomized clinical trials were associated with significant improvements, even though all of them tested treatments already shown to be efficacious by historical or noncontrolled comparisons.

Advantages and Disadvantages of Multicenter Trials

Advantages

Consider a multicenter trial under six conditions, outlined below.

1. *When a large number of patients is required.*

Many types of clinical questions can be addressed only in clinical trials involving a large sample size. For example, in a 10-year period, the NSABP entered 10,000 patients into randomized clinical trials to assess the comparative value of using one, two, or three drugs and multimodality combinations of chemotherapy and hormonal therapy. Without the resources of a large collaborative group, it would have been exceedingly difficult to allocate a smaller number of patients to so many drug choices and combinations. The collaborative group mechanism has enabled us to gain much more knowledge of the biology of breast cancer than we could have obtained within a single institution.

2. *When rapid accrual of patients is needed.*
If it takes too long to recruit the required number of patients, other findings or treatment advances can make a study obsolete before it is completed. A recent NSABP trial (adjuvant colon carcinoma NSABP-C03) entered 830 patients and closed to patient accrual within a 16-month period.

3. *When studying rare events.*
Multi-institutional protocols make it possible to study uncommon diseases or specific subgroups of patients rarely seen at tertiary medical centers. Studies of surgical and adjuvant therapy for childhood cancers (e.g., rhabdomyosarcoma and Wilms' tumor) were feasible only with a series of national trials. The Intergroup Melanoma Surgical Trial made it possible to study a specific subgroup of melanoma patients with intermediate tumor thickness to ascertain the optimal surgical management of the primary melanoma and the regional lymph nodes.[4] This protocol has accrued more than 700 patients treated at more than 200 institutions; it could not have been conducted in any single institution.

4. *When more precisely defined subject groups are needed.*
Large numbers of patients for each protocol make it possible to stratify for important patient characteristics. In an NSABP protocol for evaluating the efficacy of adding tamoxifen to the standard two-drug regimen, estrogen receptors (ER) and progesterone receptors (PR) were measured and recorded for all patients. A good response to tamoxifen was seen in patients with high ER and PR levels and in older age groups. In subsequent studies, pretreatment determinations of ER and PR levels were used as the basis for assigning patients to different treatment groups to explore research questions related to differences in ER status.

If studies like those just described were attempted with only 150 patients in each arm, much of the needed information could not be obtained. Splitting trial participants into groups that are large enough to be meaningful may require a total of 2000 patients. Since a busy urban hospital may average only about 100 new cases of primary breast cancer each year, it is impractical to attempt a study requiring 2000 cases without some form of multicenter collaboration.

5. *When improved generalizability is important.*
Many collaborative groups comprise a combination of university, large urban, and smaller community hospitals that affords access to a more representative mix of patients than would be found in any one type of institution. As a result, their findings are more readily generalizable to broad clinical practice. The necessity of having all participating hospitals comply with such special protocol requirements as immunochemical staining or high-energy radiotherapeutic treatments may, however, exclude some institutions that wish to be involved. Such obstacles can often be surmounted by making referral arrangements within the group.

6. *When rapid technology transfer is needed.*
Involving community clinicians in routine clinical trial group meetings is an excellent way to promote the rapid transfer of ideas, techniques, and knowledge. Discussing new protocols and hypotheses, participating in clinical research, and using good clinical trial methodology are valuable learning experiences that lead to better clinical care for participating patients.

Disadvantages

Multicenter trials are both expensive and complex.

First, the cost of supporting a trial group's central operations, travel to group meetings, and research personnel within member institutions usually ranges from $1500 to $3000 (US) per patient entered. The National Cancer Institute in the United States spends more than $60 million per year to support multi-institutional clinical trials. Allocations of funds for these clinical research studies are approved through an extensive and rigorous peer review process.

Moreover, as the number of investigators participating in a study increases, there must be a parallel increase in quality control efforts to minimize variability among patients, treatments, assessment, investigators, and institutions. This is only a relative disadvantage, however, because the results are generally more representative and achievable only by a diverse group of institutions and physicians.

Multicenter Surgical Trials in Oncology

Completed multicenter clinical trials in breast cancer and melanoma exemplify the principles, rationale, and value of using this approach to address significant issues in clinical research.

TABLE 29.1. Two divergent hypotheses of tumor biology.

Halstedian	Fisher
Tumors spread in an orderly defined manner based on mechanical considerations.	There is no orderly pattern of tumor cell dissemination.
Tumor cells traverse lymphatics to lymph nodes by direct extension supporting en block dissection.	Tumor cells traverse lymphatics by embolization, challenging the merit of en block dissection.
The positive lymph node is an indicator of tumor spread and is the source of further spread.	The positive lymph node is an indicator of a host–tumor relationship that permits development of metastases rather than the instigator of distant diseases.
Regional lymph nodes (RLNs) are barriers to the passage of tumor cells.	RLNs are ineffective as barriers to tumor cell spread.
RLNs are of anatomical importance.	RLNs are of biological importance.
The bloodstream is of little significance as a route of tumor dissemination.	The bloodstream is of considerable importance in tumor dissemination
A tumor is autonomous of its host.	Complex host–tumor interrelationships affect every facet of the disease.
Operable breast cancer is a local–regional disease.	Operable breast cancer is a systemic disease.
The extent and nuances of operation are the dominant factors influencing patient outcome.	Variations in local–regional therapy are unlikely to substantially affect survival.

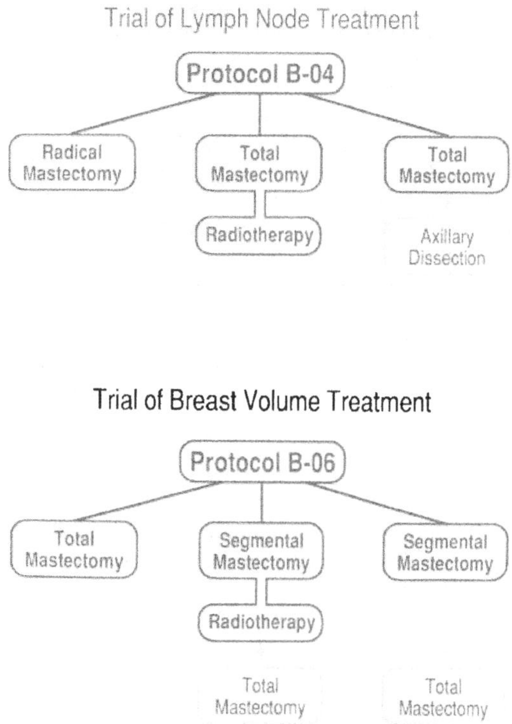

FIGURE 29.1. The clinical design of two NSABP trials that illustrate how a systemic analysis of breast cancer treatments can be evaluated by a series of prospective, randomized multicenter trials.

Breast Cancer

The first major surgical multicenter trial ended 70 years of controversy about primary breast surgery.

The Halsted radical mastectomy, developed at the turn of the century, was based on the widely held view that cancer was a local and regional problem that could be addressed by a surgical solution. From the 1930s to the 1960s, reports describing variations on the Halsted mastectomy were published, but none resulted in a substantial or widely accepted change in surgical practice. All the studies suffered from such methodological weaknesses as lack of appropriate control groups, poor patient selection methods, and improper or absent randomization techniques; their net effect was the promotion of further controversy. The nonacceptance of these studies is a powerful demonstration of why studies must be designed and executed in a manner that gives credibility to their findings.

Fisher[8] conceived a new hypothesis on the nature of breast cancer that was tested through a succession of cooperative clinical trials under the NSABP. Table 29.1 compares the features of these two hypotheses.

The first NSABP protocol, B-04, tested the effect of regional therapy—the impact of treatment on lymph nodes; the second, B-06, tested local therapy—the impact of treatment on the remaining breast. The schema (Fig. 29.1) shows how the designs were similar for both studies: surgical versus radiation treatment versus a control group. The results support the hypothesis that variations in local and regional treatment have little or no effect on outcome if the disease is systemic, and adequate local treatment suffices if it is not.[8] The protocols addressed questions about the biology of multicentric carcinoma, the importance of local recurrence, and the role of lymph nodes in cancer dissemination.

These trials had a successful impact because they tested a specific hypothesis in a defined way. Many of the procedural points illustrate the key elements described in this chapter. In 3 years, 1765 patients were enrolled in the NSABP trial. Patient eligibility in terms of age, tumor stage, clinical axillary stage, and medical history were all clearly defined. The specifics of the operations were described, and workshops were held to instruct participating surgeons on how to execute operative procedures as uniformly as possible. Similar processes were followed to ensure uniform treatment of pathology specimens and uniform radiation therapy.

Quality control was constantly maintained. Radiotherapy machine calibrations and techniques of treatment were examined and verified at each institution. To ensure performance of the operations, as intended, similar controls on operative reports and pathology techniques were maintained. The average number of nodes found by pathological examination of radical mastectomy specimens was 15; in typical total mastectomy specimens it was zero. This result answers any criticism about the purity of the operative groups. All the factors that could possibly influence prognosis (age, race, endocrine history, childbirth history, taking of contraceptive pills, etc.) were considered and compared to verify that the randomization process had distributed these covariates equally throughout the treatment arms.

The total patient enrollment goal was predetermined from statistical analyses that indicated the sample size necessary to justify confidence in the results. Careful monitoring of the scientific methods was maintained from conception of the trial to analysis of the results to ensure scrupulous adherence to the protocol.

The methods of analysis used were discussed in detail in the study reports; life table actuarial analyses were used extensively. The 5- and 10-year reports[9,10] confirmed the hypothesis that treatment of axillary lymph nodes does not influence the outcome and provided information on the biology of cancer.

The NASBP study illustrates why the scientific problem under review must be understood and soundly defined. Posing a surgical question to compare treatments A and B and having a statistician suggest an appropriate sample size is easy, but selecting the individual treatments requires a great deal of thought and clinical judgment if the results are to be meaningful. A comparison of two minor surgical variants of a standard operation might meet all the statistical guidelines for a good study, but it would hardly be worth doing because the question is unimportant.

Protocol R-04 was designed to confirm a fundamental change in biologic theory. Although surgical removal was compared to irradiation of lymph nodes, a third arm of the study for negative node patients who were given no additional treatments provides better insight into the biologic relevance of lymph nodes and the cancer process. A simple comparison of surgical versus radiotherapy treatment of lymph nodes would have met the general methodologic guidelines, but would not have been as illuminating. If treating the lymph nodes does not improve prognosis, they are clearly not an intermediate station in the dissemination of cancer, but merely one of the places to which cancer spreads when dissemination takes place. Positive nodes imply dissemination; treatment of nodes alone cannot be useful. The study results made the need for systemic treatments clear and prompted the immediate generation of adjuvant chemotherapy studies.

The findings of the Cooperative Surgical Trial of the 1970s brought a new perspective to biologic theories and surgical practices that had generated controversy for more than 50 years, in contrast to the conclusions of nonrandomized clinical studies that were not widely accepted[11-13] and contributed little to advancing our understanding and treatment of breast cancer. When the study based on protocol B-04 was begun, radical mastectomy accounted for 85% of the therapeutic procedures performed for primary breast cancer in the United States and Canada; it now accounts for less than 15%.[14]

Although a number of investigators in North America, England, France, and Finland pioneered the partial mastectomy approach and presented useful data,[13,15-17] only randomized controlled studies could generate sufficiently believable data to assure that partial mastectomy is an adequate operation for breast cancer patients.

Melanoma

The Intergroup Melanoma Surgical Trial is another example of the value of multicenter surgical trials and the importance of quality control criteria.

For decades, surgeons have debated the timing of lymph node dissection in patients with cutaneous melanomas. Some surgeons prefer to excise only clinically demonstrable metastatic nodes—termed therapeutic lymph node dissection; others choose to excise apparently normal nodes because of the risk of occult or microscopic metastases—termed elective lymph node dissection (ELND).

Because opinion is unanimous that all melanoma patients do not need an ELND, debate has centered around two issues:

1. Is it possible to accurately identify a subgroup of melanoma patients with a high risk for microscopic regional node metastases, but a low risk for distant micrometastases?
2. What is the optimal timing of the operation—immediate versus delayed—even if such a high-risk group can be delineated?

The potential benefit of ELND is based on the hypothesis that microscopic metastases may disseminate sequentially, from the primary melanoma to the regional lymph nodes and then to dis-

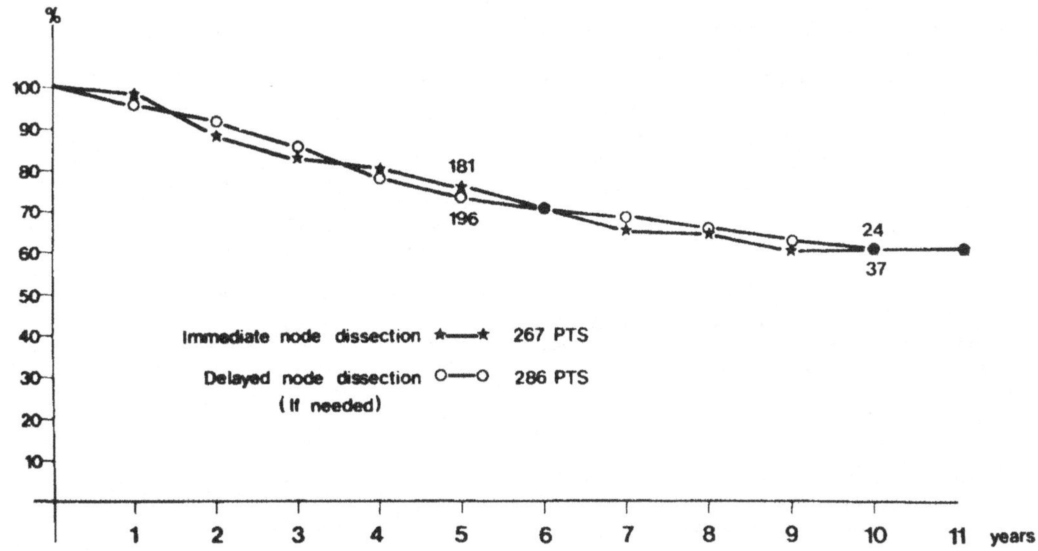

FIGURE 29.2. Results of randomized prospective study involving extremity melanoma patients (all thickness) conducted by the WHO Melanoma Group. Survival of 553 patients with stage I melanoma showed no benefit from elective lymph node dissection. Reprinted with permission from Veronesi U, Adamus J, Bandiera DC et al. Delayed regional lymph node dissection in stage I melanoma of the skin of the lower extremities. *Cancer.* 1982; 49(11):2420–2430.

tant sites. Accordingly, survival will be increased if the nodal micrometastases are surgically excised before they disseminate further to distant sites. Conversely, patients with clinically palpable nodal metastases will most likely have distant micrometastases by that time and a consequently lower probability of cure from a regional operation.

Combinations of prognostic factors can accurately predict the risk of occult lymph node metastases. The primary criterion is tumor thickness; melanomas of intermediate thickness (1.4 to 0.4 mm) have an increased risk (up to 60%) of occult regional metastasis, but a relatively low risk (< 20%) of distant metastasis.[18] Ulceration and anatomic site of the primary melanoma are also important parameters to include in the design and interpretation of clinical trials concerning this issue. In addition, a radionuclide cutaneous scan has been developed to identify lymph nodes at risk for harboring micrometastases, especially in anatomic sites such as the trunk, which may have ambiguous lymphatic drainage by clinical criteria.[19]

The controversy about the surgical issue arises from discrepancies in the results of four retrospective studies and two randomized prospective studies. The results of the retrospective studies demonstrated improved surgical success rates in patients with intermediate thickness melanomas, ranging from 0.7 to 4.0 mm, who underwent ELND compared to those who did not; more than 3000 patients with melanomas in all anatomic sites, from four melanoma treatment centers, were followed from 10 to 20 years.[4]

Two prospective randomized trials have been performed: one by the World Health Organization Melanoma Group (Fig. 29.2), the other by surgeons at the Mayo Clinic[20,21]. These excellent studies, performed by competent investigators, clearly demonstrated that not all patients with melanoma benefited from ELND, but they had some limitations that make it difficult to interpret the results for the intermediate thickness subgroup. The sources of the difficulty included the following.

1. The studies were confined largely to women who are not likely to be representative of the natural history of melanomas at all anatomic sites; namely, women with lower extremity melanomas.
2. The WHO Melanoma Group trials begun in the 1960s were not stratified for such important prognostic factors as tumor thickness and ulceration, because their significance was not known at that time; analysis of the trial data revealed a serious maldistribution of patients with ulcerative lesions, and it may have influenced the results.
3. There appeared to be differences in staging criteria and surgical treatment results among the participating countries.

TABLE 29.2. Protocol design used by the Intergroup Melanoma Study for patients with intermediate-thickness melanomas (1–4 mm).

Randomized treatment arm	Primary excision margin (cm)[a]	Elective (immediate) lymphadenectomy
1	2	No
2	2	Yes
3	4	No
4	4	Yes

[a] All the major cooperative groups in the United States and the National Cancer Institute of Canada are participating in the study. Patients with melanomas of the head and distal extremities will have a 2 cm primary excision and then will be randomized into treatment arm 1 or 2.

TABLE 29.3. Basic outline for a clinical research protocol.

1. Objectives
2. Background and rationale
3. Criteria for patient selection
4. Surgical guidelines
5. Pathology guidelines and procedures
6. Studies to be done
7. Randomization procedure
8. Reporting procedures and follow-up
9. Patient evaluation criteria
10. Quality control and evaluation
11. Statistical requirements
12. Forms and records to be submitted
13. Patient consent
14. Bibliography

4. The Mayo Clinic Surgical Trial included so few patients in the intermediate thickness subgroup that no conclusions could be made about it.

A patterns of care study conducted by the Commission on Cancer in the United States and a separate survey of surgeons in Canada clearly demonstrated there was no standard approach to selecting patients to have, or not have, ELND.[22,23]

The retrospective studies suggested some benefit from ELND, but they may have contained unrecognized biases that influenced the interpretation of the data. The two prospective studies had some methodologic flaws, or limited sample size in the specific subgroup of patients with intermediate thickness melanomas, that made it impossible to draw a firm conclusion even though both trials were randomized.

The conflicting data and lack of a clear consensus prompted the design of a prospective randomized trial with current stratification criteria,[4] but melanoma is an uncommon disease, and the study was targeted to a subgroup of patients that included only 40% of the total. As a consequence, it was impossible for a single institution to accrue enough cases to answer the questions, given the necessity of applying several stratification criteria to permit proper interpretation of the results. Besides the ELND question, there were no objective data about the appropriate margins of excision for the primary melanoma. A multicenter trial was, therefore, initiated in 1983. It involves all the cancer cooperative groups in the United States, Canada, and Denmark (Table 29.2), has accrued more than 700 patients, and is one of the largest studies to address specifically the optimal surgical treatment of cancer. This study will be closed to patient accrual in the near future, but the results will not be known for several years.

The Organization and Management of Multicenter Clinical Trials

The best time to build a collaborative group is during the design phase of a trial. Early in the planning stage, all the possible participants should be invited to a meeting to consider a clearly stated study question accompanied by relevant background material and the rationale for the proposed study. The enclosed concept paper should not be longer than 3 pages.

If you are participating in the organization of a multicenter trial, give consideration to establishing the following committees if they are in accord with the scope of the project and the planned duration of the group.

A *protocol committee* is a suitable way to create the actual trial. Circulate the concept paper to interested people who have experience in the subject area to be studied, and ask them to discuss the pros and cons of various aspects of the proposed protocol.

Writing the protocol is one of the most important components of a study and it serves two purposes. The first is to describe the scientific design, which is always built best around a biological hypothesis; if it is, your results are more likely to be publishable—whatever answer you obtain. The second purpose is to create an operations manual that will enable all the participating investigators to perform in a uniform, systematic way. A basic outline of a clinical research protocol and a list of data forms to be generated are provided in Tables 29.3 and 29.4, respectively. Some examples of the issues and questions that should be addressed in the development of a protocol are as follows.

1. The surgery, or other intervention, to be performed must be defined. (A standard version of

the operation is necessary. Any variations considered important or unimportant must be specified.)
2. What are the inclusion/exclusion criteria?
3. What preliminary studies need to be performed before a patient is entered (e.g., kidney function tests if a renal-toxic drug is involved)?
4. What special procedures need to be performed on the surgical specimen or the patient (e.g., receptor or immunofluorescent studies)?
5. What pathology controls will be performed?
6. What follow-up intervals will be used, and what observations will be made and recorded?
7. What records are to be kept?

A *study chairman* (or cochairmen) should be designated for each protocol. This person (or persons) has responsibility for the ongoing conduct of the study. He or she can respond, on an ad hoc basis, to unanticipated questions about patient eligibility for entry or about the conduct of the study. The chairman assumes responsibility for ensuring that data reports come in on time, that eligibility requirements are met, and that no deviation occurs.

A *principal investigator* should be identified at each participating institution. The principal investigator has overall responsibility for the conduct of the studies and the maintenance of the institution's level and quality of activity. He or she is the focal point for disseminating information about progress or changes in ongoing studies and the institution's representative in the collaborating group, especially for the administrative and organizational aspects of the study.

A *surgical monitoring committee* is necessary for any surgical clinical investigation. The surgical operation should be clearly defined, and a description of how it is to be performed should be provided in the protocol. The anatomic limits of the dissection and the anatomic structures to be preserved or removed should be clearly specified. For example, in NSABP colon studies, each type of segmental colon resection is clearly described, the vasculature to be divided is identified, and the scope of the operative report is specified and compared to the check-off data form to ensure that the surgical requirements are being met. Similarly, the Intergroup Melanoma Committee developed surgical guidelines and check-off forms for lymph node dissections at each anatomic site.

A *pathology monitoring committee* is required to formulate guidelines for examining all surgical specimens, delineating criteria for the diagnostic and prognostic features of the pathology, and developing forms for reporting pathology results in a standardized fashion. Many pathological features are difficult to quantify because they require personal interpretation (e.g., histological grading). A pathology reference center is the best way to ensure standard diagnoses. A data form should be created to prompt the pathologist to provide answers to all relevant questions and ensure good data control.

A *radiotherapy monitoring committee* should be created whenever radiotherapy is employed. If the effects of radiotherapy are being tested in a protocol, very careful attention to the planning and monitoring of the treatment is mandatory. All the collaborating institutions should have their radiation therapy units calibrated, their methodology standardized, and their dose calculations reviewed centrally. Complications and toxicity should be

TABLE 29.4. Data forms that might be necessary for a multicenter clinical trial.

Form	Function
On-study form	All vital information about the patient and the diagnosis. When a patient enters the study, the names and addresses of three relatives, who will know the patient's whereabouts in the event he or she moves, should always be obtained. This information can be invaluable after several years of follow-up when a patient suddenly relocates without leaving a forwarding address.
Progress forms	For recording data about the patient status during the conduct of the study, including such study parameters as drug dose received, toxicities encountered, and the status of the patient (e.g., free of relapses or site of relapse).
Follow-up forms	May include results of physical exam and laboratory and x-ray results.
Off-study form	Completed when a patient goes off study because of one of the following quality control reasons: intercurrent illness (e.g., a second type of serious cancer), or death from unrelated cause (e.g., auto accident).
Surgery checklist	Created for reviewing operative reports; can be a part of the protocol documentation and should be filled out by the operating surgeon following each operation. A second data form, for such complications as an anastomotic leak or a seroma, should also be created so that a good statistical analysis can be performed at a later date.

monitored and recorded on data forms designed for the purpose.

A *drug monitoring committee* is needed to control adherence to the protocol, to monitor for drug toxicities, and to develop specific criteria and schedules for adjusting drug doses for defined levels of toxicity. A data form should be designed for easy supervision of any departure from the stipulated schedules or doses and for recording toxicities and unanticipated problems.

All these monitoring committees have a double function. One is to ensure conformity to the protocol and the recording and evaluation of any deviations; the other is to monitor and document toxicity and alert investigators to serious problems requiring changes in the protocol when a patient's safety is concerned.

An *executive committee* should he created to make decisions and to oversee the continued functioning of the collaborating groups and their protocols. Ideally, this committee should comprise representatives from the various monitoring committees and the principal investigators at each participating institution. The committee should have guidelines for the probation and suspension of any individuals or institutions failing to participate or violating protocol guidelines. Because inadequate performance by an individual or an institution will sometimes make it necessary to invoke one of these unpleasant actions, appropriate rules and regulations should be agreed on prospectively, when the group is organized, to facilitate the handling of problems if the need arises. The existence of the monitoring process and rules for dropping a center may help to prevent its occurrence.

Decisions to close or abort a study, or any portion of it, should follow guidelines laid down in the protocol. The monitoring process, maintained by the executive committee, should provide information on when to close or abandon one arm of a study that is jeopardizing an otherwise good program. For example, in some aggressive chemotherapy programs, unexpected life-threatening toxicities may occur; careful monitoring and evaluation will allow the study to be closed before too many patients are exposed to danger.

Group Meetings

Information dissemination increases in importance as the group grows and gains experience. Annual or semiannual group meetings with a backup system of mailings and updatings is one way to keep group communications current. Group meetings provide opportunities to disseminate information on the status of various studies, to discuss any problems, to explain any changes or clarifications in the conduct of the study, and to keep participants abreast of what has been learned. Results will not be published until accrual targets are met, but toxicities can be discussed, and findings and correlations in ancillary areas can be presented. Group meetings also provide a forum for the exchange of information between participants and are an ideal way to stimulate and maintain interest in the study.

Headquarters

One institution should act as the headquarters from which a full-time director and data manager(s) will supervise the day-to-day conduct of the trial.

Authorship

If a publication committee does not exist, a clear decision about who will be responsible for writing the report should be made at the outset. This ensures the completion of this task and helps in the assignment of appropriate credits for authorship and for participation in the study. A committee can also help to choose the journal for publication or the scientific meeting at which the report will be presented.

Ethics

It is imperative that a clinical trial follow ethical guidelines. A carefully written consent form, counseling about the trial's investigational nature, and full disclosure of its risks and uncertainties are inherent ethical components of any clinical trial. In North America, the law requires the creation of review boards composed of scientists not involved in the project, physicians who are not necessarily investigators, representatives of the nonmedical community, such as lawyers and members of the clergy. The board's role is to determine whether the proposed research is scientifically and ethically appropriate and whether provision has been made to ensure the patients will receive adequate information about the choices presented to them. It is important that investigators cooperate with review boards to assure the proper conduct of the trial.

Finances

Each participating institution needs money to maintain one or more secretarial data managers and to cover travel expenses for group meetings. The headquarters for a large project will need data managers, supervisors, biostatisticians, computer experts, and adequate computer resources. In addition, large studies may require salaries for investigators. Even though the total outlay of funds for such an entire apparatus may be large, a demonstration of the usefulness of some treatments and the desirability of abandoning others that are not will result in reductions in morbidity and health care costs.

Statistical and Data Management

A *quality control data management program* should be instituted at the group headquarters. It is one thing to specify the data to be collected, the forms to be used, and the records to be kept, but another to ensure that they are accurate, complete, and punctual. Some form of audit will be needed to ensure that the data collected are correct. This is usually best done by a spot check method in which the original hospital charts of randomly selected patients and certain predetermined data (e.g., the accuracy of eligibility criteria and the consistency of drug administration) are examined. Pharmacology logs should also be examined and nursing notes correlated to make sure that the chemotherapy was given according to the protocol, and that the dose actually given corresponded with what was reported on the data forms.

A *data manager* should be appointed for each institution accruing cases, to be responsible for maintaining and submitting accurately completed data forms on schedule. The data manager becomes involved with each patient at the time of consideration for entry into the protocol – to verify eligibility, perform the randomization, contact trial headquarters to register the patient, and transmit the treatment assignment to the investigator. The data manager immediately assembles a dossier containing the required study forms, and eventually keeps a parallel protocol chart for each patient containing all the paperwork required by the protocol. A copy of every document sent to headquarters should be kept in the patient's protocol chart so that verification can be easily done on a moment's notice.

The data manager is also responsible for scheduling return visits for treatment or follow-up and for maintaining records on long-term scheduling. As patient numbers increase, it is very important to maintain complete follow-up and to ensure that no patient is lost to the process.

Data manager seminars at group meetings are an invaluable way of exchanging information and teaching the newer members of the organization the techniques of data management.

As the number of patients being followed increases, difficulties in tracking and scheduling

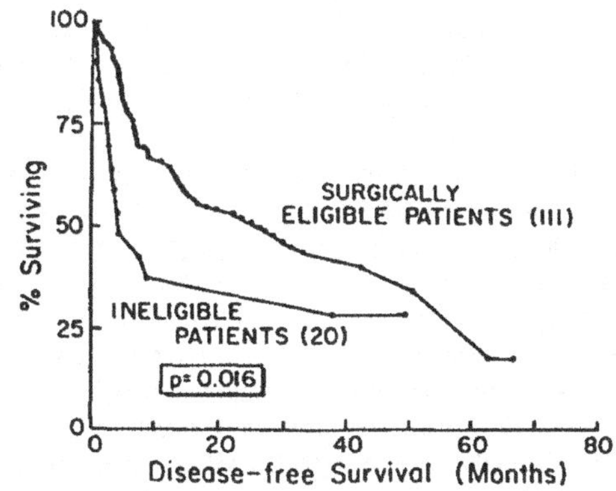

FIGURE 29.3. Disease-free survival of surgically eligible and ineligible melanoma patients entered into the SEG Cooperative Group protocol for adjuvant immunotherapy. The surgically ineligible had a lower disease-free survival rate ($p = .01$) and a lower absolute survival (data not shown, $p = .07$). This illustrates the importance of having surgical quality control criteria and monitoring in multicenter clinical trials.

can occur. The Institutes at McGill University have designed a computer-aided scheduling system, the McGill Protocol System, which contains master or template schedules for each protocol. Patients can be matched to a specific treatment program and a schedule can be generated at any time to show the data manager which patients are due for which treatments or tests in which time period. As dividends, patients can be given copies of their schedules for the next time frame, and each participating laboratory can have advance lists of all the patients it will have to schedule in the coming weeks. This kind of system minimizes mistakes and assures the flow of good quality data.

Quality Control Criteria and Monitoring

Results of one multicenter adjuvant therapy trial for melanoma have proven that surgically ineligible patients can introduce significant bias into the results of adjuvant therapy trials, without regard to the cancer treatment being studied[24] (Fig. 29.3). Consequently, considerable effort must be devoted to establishing quality control guidelines for each adjuvant therapy protocol. Quality control review mechanisms must be established within each member institution and centrally at the operations or statistics office. In oncology protocols, for example, quality control measures are used to monitor drug dose schedules (including adjustments for toxicity), radiation therapy (including dosimetry and port planning), and surgery, to ensure the surgical procedure was conducted according to written guidelines.

Surgical guidelines must be written for each adjuvant therapy protocol to describe the minimum amount of surgical dissection required for different anatomical settings. The melanoma surgical protocol specified that a parotid dissection was essential for patients with metastatic melanoma from a primary site in the anterior scalp, temple, or face. Precise definitions of regional node dissections were described for cervical, axillary, and inguinal lymphadenectomies.

In NSABP protocol B-06, the segmental mastectomy operation was new to most surgeons in North America, and early experience revealed unanticipated problems in its performance with respect to tumor control and cosmetic outcome. Several NSABP investigators who had extensive experience with the operation proposed solutions that were discussed and refined in workshops of participating surgeons. The workshop concept was so successful that it was continued over the 8-year period of accrual to the protocol, to ensure that surgeons joining later did not have to learn the operation by repeating the same initial errors.

Pathology guidelines must also be defined. For example, all lymph nodes must be examined, and the pathologist must report the total number of nodes examined and the number that contained metastases. A minimum number of nodes must be examined to maintain quality control; in our studies, it was 5 for superficial inguinal dissections, 10 for axillary dissections, and 20 for cervical dissections. Outside pathology slides had to be reviewed by a pathologist at the member institution or by the pathology committee of the entire group.

A surgeon at each member institution should review the operative note and pathology report, and sign the on-study form certifying that the minimum surgical guidelines were adhered to before the patient was randomized into the protocol. The operative record and pathology report are forwarded to the statistics office for central review by the surgical investigator assigned to each adjuvant therapy protocol.

Communicating the Results of Multicenter Trials

After the clinical trial has been closed to patient accrual, the investigators must decide when to analyze the results, how to interpret them, and when to publish.

It is important to "let the data speak for themselves" and not to overinterpret results, especially before the information on follow-up has become sufficiently mature. Because there is a natural tendency for others to overinterpret, distort, or amplify the results, it is vitally important that the authors frame their interpretations of the results carefully and realistically; premature publication and overinterpretation of results still in a state of flux must be avoided.

Even large randomized clinical trials may not yield absolute conclusions; but the results and the interpretation of data may increase the level of confidence that the treatment under study should be adopted as standard treatment in defined subsets of patients, at least. It is important to publish the results, even when they are negative.

The following questions or issues should be addressed when investigators are deciding when to publish and what to say.

1. Is the follow-up of the patients long enough to permit the drawing of valid conclusions?
2. In studies with survival endpoints, especially oncology studies, is the difference in relapse-free survivals great enough to permit a definite prediction that they will also translate into significant differences in overall survival rate?
3. In patient studies with very large sample size, small differences may be statistically significant, but the investigators will have to ask whether these statistically significant differences are also clinically significant—especially in settings where toxicity, cost, or morbidity might be involved.
4. Are the patients entered into the trial representative of the entire universe of similarly staged patients?
5. Are there any subsets of patients in which different results occurred? Caution must be exercised in interpreting results in subsets of patients defined by criteria not used in the original design of the trial.
6. Are the results internally consistent using different statistical approaches, and consistent with existing knowledge of the biology of the disease under study?

Conclusion

If you are considering a multicenter trial clinical trial, all the points discussed in this chapter should be taken into account although some will be more important in some studies than in others. In practical terms, you should always design the ideal study and then make the compromises necessary for feasibility. Setting down rules and guidelines at the beginning is the best way to proceed, but unrealistic rigidity can be self-defeating. All rules or compromises should be considered in the light of how to anticipate and prevent adverse criticism about the conduct of the study or its outcome. The objective is to do good clinical science and contribute to meaningful progress.

The randomized controlled clinical trial is the most reliable and useful investigative tool in clinical medicine. Despite its imperfections, it produces the most credible and generalizable results and has justifiably become—and is likely to remain—the mainstay of clinical research. It is doubtful that any clinical research program can be developed without a good understanding of how randomized controlled trials are designed and implemented. A collaborative multicenter randomized controlled trial is expensive, but the return on investment is worthwhile if the question it seeks to answer is clinically and socially important.

References

1. Butcher HR, Seaman WB. Eckert C, et al. Assessment of radical mastectomy and postoperative irradiation therapy in treatment of mammary cancer. Cancer 1964;17:480–85.
2. Paterson R, Russel MH. Clinical trials in malignant disease: III. Breast cancer: evaluation of postoperative radiotherapy. J Fac Radiol 1959;10:175–80.
3. Balch CM, Murad TM, Soong S-j, Ingalls AL, Halpern NB, Maddox WA. A multifactorial analysis of melanoma: prognostic histopathological features comparing Clark's and Breslow's staging methods. Ann Surg 1978;188:732–42.
4. Balch CM. The role of elective lymph node dissection in melanoma: rationale, results, and controversies. J Clin Oncol 1988;6:163–72.
5. Chalmers TC, Block JB, Lee S. Controlled studies in clinical cancer research. N Engl J Med 1972;287: 75–78.
6. Moertel CG. Improving the efficiency of clinical trials: a medical perspective. Stat Med 1984;3:455–68.
7. Gilbert JP, McPeek B, Mosteller F. Statistics and ethics in surgery and anesthesia. Science 1977;198: 684–89.
8. Fisher B, Redmond C, Fisher E, et al. The contribution of recent NSABP clinical trials of primary breast cancer therapy to an understanding of tumor biology—an overview of findings. Cancer 1980;46: 1009–25.
9. Fisher B, Montague E, Redmond C, et al. Comparison of radical mastectomy with alternative treatments for primary breast cancer. Cancer 1977;39: 2827–39.
10. Fisher B, Redmond C, Fisher E, et al. Ten-year results of a randomized clinical trial comparing radical mastectomy and total mastectomy with or without radiation. N Engl J Med 1985;312:674–81.
11. Kaae S, Johansen H. Breast cancer: comparison of results of simple mastectomy with postoperative roentgen irradiation by McWhirter method with those of extended radical mastectomy. Acta Radiol (Stockholm) 1959 (Suppl);188:155–61.
12. McWhirter R. Simple mastectomy and radiotherapy in treatment of breast cancer. Br J Radiol 1955;28: 128–39.
13. Peters MD. Cutting the "Gordian knot" in early breast cancer. Ann R Coll Phys Surg Can 1975;8: 186–91.
14. Nemoto T, Vana J, Bedwani RN, Baker HW, McGregor FH, Murphy GP. Management and survival of female breast cancer: results of a national survey by the American College of Surgeons. Cancer 1975:35:2917–24.
15. Crile G. Results of conservative treatment of breast cancer at 10 and 15 years. Ann Surg 1975;181:26–30.
16. Mustakallio S. Conservative treatment of breast carcinoma—review of 25 year follow-up. Clin Radiol 1972;23:110–16.
17. Calle R, Pilleron JP, Schlienger P, et al. Conservative management of operable breast cancer: 10 years experience at the Foundation Curie. Cancer 1978; 42:2045–53.
18. Urist MM, Balch CM, Soong S-j, Milton GW, Shaw HM, McGovern VJ, Murad TM, McCarthy WH, Maddox WA. Head and neck melanoma in 534 clinical stage I patients: a prognostic factors analysis and results of surgical treatment. Ann Surg 1984;200: 769–75.
19. Logic JR, Balch CM. Defining lymphatic drainage pattern with cutaneous lymphoscintigraphy. In: Cutaneous Melanoma: Clinical Management and Treatment Results Worldwide, Balch CM, Milton GE, eds. Philadelphia, Lippincott, 1985:159–70.
20. Veronesi U, Adamus J, Bandiera DC, et al. Delayed regional lymph node dissection in stage I melanoma of the skin of the lower extremities. Cancer 1982; 49:2420–30.
21. Sim FH, Taylor WF, Pritchard DJ, et al. Lymphadenectomy in management of stage I malignant melanoma: a prospective randomized study. Mayo Clin Proc 1986;61:697–705.
22. Balch CM, Karakousis C, Mettlin C, et al. Management of cutaneous melanoma in the United States. Surg Gynecol Obstet 1984;158:311–18.
23. Shelley W, Kersey P, Quirt I, Pater J. Survey of surgical management of malignant melanoma in Canada: optimal margins of excision and lymph-node dissection. Can J Surg 1984;27:190–92.
24. Balch CM, Durant JR, Bartolucci AA, Southeastern Cancer Study Group. The impact of surgical quality control in multi-institutional group trials involving adjuvant cancer treatments. Ann Surg 1983;198: 164–67.

Appendix to Chapter 29*

NSABP OPERATIVE REPORT FORM (PROTOCOL C-04) **FORM OR**

INSTRUCTIONS: This form is to be completed by the surgeon. Answer all questions in the boxes and spaces provided. Submit this form within 30 days of patient entry along with the dictated operative report.

STUDY NUMBER (1-9) | Patient's Last Name First M.I.

1st 3 letters of Patient's Last Name (10-12) | INSTITUTION | Initials of Person Completing Form:

OPERATIVE PROCEDURE Mo. Day Yr.

Date performed: (13-18)

Type of Procedure (19)
1. Total Colectomy
2. Hemicolectomy
3. Segmental Resection
4. Anterior Resection
5. A-P Resection
6. Other Specify

Colostomy at Resection (20)
1 = Yes 2 = No

If yes, specify whether (21)
1. Temporary
2. Permanent

Was a preliminary colostomy performed? (22)
1 = Yes 2 = No

If yes, Date performed: Mo. Day Yr. (23-28)

Was colostomy for decompression of obstruction prior to resection? (29)
1 = Yes 2 = No

Tumor obstructing Bowel? (30)
1 = Yes 2 = No

Was there perforation of the tumor? (31)
1 = Yes 2 = No

If yes was it: (32)
1. Free (as manifested by free air in the abdomen)
2. Walled off
3. Other: Explain

Omentum Resected (33)
1 = Yes 2 = No

Spleen Removed (34)
1 = Yes 2 = No

LOCATION OF TUMOR (When multiple tumors are present indicate all sites)

Site 1 (35-36)
Site 2 (37-38)
Site 3 (39-40)

01 Appendix
02 Cecum
03 Ascending Colon
04 Hepatic Flexture
05 Transverse Colon
06 Splenic Flexture
07 Descending Colon
08 Sigmoid
09 Rectosigmoid
10 Rectum
11 Anal Canal
Others ______

Site of proximal transection of Bowel? (41-42)

Site of distal transection of Bowel? (43-44)

01 Ileum
02 Ascending Colon
03 Transverse Colon
04 Descending Colon
05 Sigmoid
06 Recto-Sigmoid
07 Rectum
08 Perianal (A-P Resection)
09 Unknown
10 Other Specify ______

1 = Yes 2 = No

Abdominal wall involved? (45)

If yes, was it resected? (46)

Other Viscera Involved? (47)

If yes, specify ______ (48-49)

Was it removed enbloc? (50)

COMMENTS:

*Reproduced with kind permission from National Surgical Adjuvant Breast and Bowel Project, Dr. Bernard Fisher, chairman.

Anastomosis

1 = Yes 2 = No (51) [ ]

Resection margin grossly free of tumor? 1 = Yes 2 = No (52) [ ]

Reason for Procedure
1 = Cure
2 = Palliation (53) [ ]

Were polyps removed?

1 = Yes 2 = No (54) [ ]

Was it necessary to open the pelvic peritoneum in order to define the distal extent of the tumor? (55) [ ]
1 = Yes 2 = No

Was there isolated, distant, or noncontiguous intra-abdominal metastases (other than regional lymph node involvement? (56) [ ]
1 = Yes 2 = No

POST OPERATIVE COMPLICATIONS
1 = Yes 2 = No

Wound infection (57) [ ]

Wound Dehiscence (58) [ ]

Anastomotic Dehiscence/Fistula (59) [ ]

Intra-Abdominal Abscess (60) [ ]

Death (61) [ ]

Other ______________ (62) [ ]

OPERATIVE DIAGRAM

Please indicate the exact location of primary tumor(s) as well as the relative margins of resection depicting all vessels ligated. Also indicate the number and location of other lesions, if any.

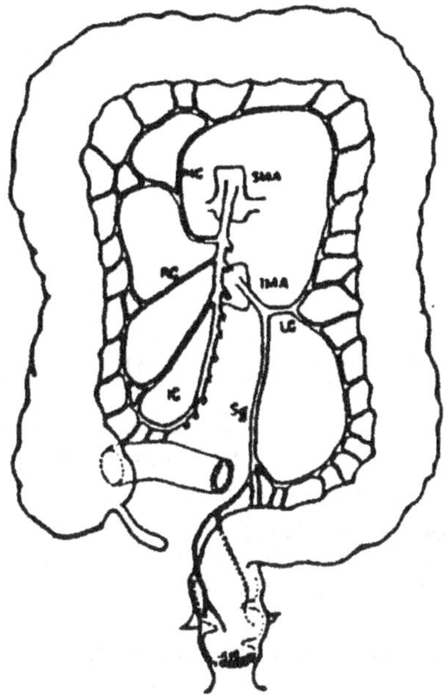

Supply any details on Post-op complications: (attach documentation if available).

BLOOD TRANSFUSION - Did the patient receive blood transfusion for this episode?
1 = Yes 2 = No (63) [ ]

Type:
1. Whole Blood
2. Packed Cells
3. Leukocyte-poor
4. Frozen Red
5. Leukocyte-rich

IF YES:	Principal Date No.	Day	Yr.	Autologous 1=Yes 2=No	No. Units of Blood	Type	1 = Washed 2 = Unwashed	
☐ Yes, within 30 days pre-operative	[ ][ ]	[ ][ ]	[ ][ ]	[ ]	[ ][ ]	[ ]	[ ]	(64-74)
☐ Yes, intraoperative	[ ][ ]	[ ][ ]	[ ][ ]	[ ]	[ ][ ]	[ ]	[ ]	(75-85)
☐ Yes, within 30 days post-operative	[ ][ ]	[ ][ ]	[ ][ ]	[ ]	[ ][ ]	[ ]	[ ]	(86-96)

Method of preparation of leukocyte poor blood: ______________ (97) [ ]

30

Health Services Research

J.I. Williams

Toward a Definition of the Field

Health services research is a field of study rather than a discipline. Investigators come from health sciences (biostatistics, epidemiology, medicine, and other health disciplines), management sciences (finance, management, marketing, organizational theory, and operations research), and the social sciences (anthropology, demography, economics, history, political science, psychology, and sociology). The mix of disciplines has shifted over time to meet changes in health policy, advances in research methods and technology, the availability of research funds, and the priorities of funding bodies.

A review of the literature reveals no one widely-accepted definition. Spitzer, Feinstein, and Sackett[1] have defined health services research as the scientific investigation of alternate modes of service. As Battista and his colleagues note,[2] the definition can be restricted to the organization, programs, and policies governing health services. In the broader sense of the term, it can encompass practice patterns of the health professional, quality assurance, appropriateness of care, and the efficacy and effectiveness of medical and surgical interventions, areas of study usually included in the discipline of clinical epidemiology.

Classical epidemiologists have noted that the epidemiologic perspective should serve as the basic framework for health services research.[3,4] At some point, we try to relate health services to the numbers of individuals at risk, the incidence or prevalence of disease, the determinants of disease, and the natural history of the resulting health problems. While the cited definition includes the epidemiologic perspective, health services research requires data on the political context, organization, and functioning of services; the sociopersonal characteristics of individuals that determine the use of services; and the measures of functional status and quality of life used to assess the impact of health services. Health sciences research seeks this information in addition to the demographic and clinical data traditionally employed in epidemiologic research.

The Study on Surgical Services for the United States (SOSSUS),[5] undertaken by the American College of Surgeons and the American Surgical Association, focused on factors influencing patients, surgeons, and facilities. The factors influencing patients include patterns of disease, attitudes, socioeconomic status, and the availability and quality of care. With respect to surgeons, the study group focused on manpower supply, distribution, organization of practices, prevailing practices, workloads, and methods of remuneration. Ambulatory and inpatient facilities were related to patterns of payment, utilization, and various other factors that are internal and external to surgical services.

Health service is to provide efficacious care to persons who can benefit from it in a manner acceptable to the providers, yet at an acceptable cost to the public at large. Health services research tries to determine whether the goal has been achieved, in whole or in part, and to identify factors that enhance or diminish the possibility of achieving it. Schieber[6] compared the financing and delivery of health care for the 24 countries in the Organization for Economic Co-operation and Development (OECD) in the 1970s and the 1980s. In 1984 the health costs per capita ranged from \$275 in Portugal to \$1637 in the United States, a sixfold variation. The average expenditure per capita for the 24 OECD countries was \$917. These variations were only marginally related to differences in mortality rates for these countries.

From 1960 to 1984, the real growth in health expenditures, after adjusting for the effects of inflation, was 60% greater than the real growth of the gross domestic product per capita. The increases were due to increased utilization and intensity of services, and, to a lesser extent, to population growth. Schieber noted that little is known at a cross-national level about the linkages between the implementation of technology, utilization, and the intensity of services, outcomes and costs.[6] He questioned whether it is possible to measure health outcomes or to evaluate the effectiveness and efficiency of health care policy. This is the challenge of health services research.

The Development of Health Services Research

Two major conferences have been held on health services research. The Health Services Research Study Section of the U.S. Public Health Service commissioned the first one, and a series of meetings were held, beginning in 1965. The *Milbank Memorial Fund Quarterly* published the proceedings in 1966. The U.S. Center for Health Services Research sponsored the second conference in 1984; *Medical Care* published the results in 1985.

The Institute of Medicine of the National Academy of Sciences reviewed health services projects funded by the federal government in the United States and published its report in 1979.[7] Georgopoulos[8] reviewed 1303 studies of hospital organization published between 1960 and 1969; Flook and Sanazaro[9] reviewed 1293 studies through 1972. Culyer et al.[10] compiled a bibliography of articles on health economics, written in English; Griffiths[11] noted articles from Western European sources; and Van Eimeren and Kopcke[12] abstracted nearly 5000 health research studies from 27 countries. More recently, Warner and Luce,[13] completed a major review of studies of cost-benefit analysis of health interventions.

Four new major foci of health services research have emerged over the past decade: technology assessment, outcomes, quality of care, and quality of life. Technology assessment involves the evaluation of drugs, devices, and procedures, together with the organizational and support systems through which they are delivered.[14] Offices of technology assessment have emerged in North America and Europe, and in the World Health Organization. One finds such offices in government agencies and professional associations, as well as in the private sector. The *International Journal of Technology Assessment in Health Care* began publication in 1985. In the United States, the Institute of Medicine formed a committee to undertake a critical review of the methods for assessing medical technologies, and the comprehensive report was published in 1985.[15]

Researchers have worked over the past two decades to develop measures of outcome that will reduce the distance between the clinical endpoints of survival, remission of symptoms, and recurrence of disease, and the methods used to ascertain the health status of individuals in community and national surveys. Health status measures commonly used in health services research include the Health Status Measures developed by Rand, the Health Insurance Experiment,[16,17] the Sickness Impact Profile,[18] the Nottingham Health Profile,[19] the Index of Well-Being, and the Quality of Well-Being Index developed by researchers in San Diego.[20,21] Researchers[22] at Rand and the New England Medical Center have developed a short form of the Rand measures for use in the Major Outcome Study of medical services.

The study of appropriateness of care for specific diseases and procedures requires disease specific measures of outcome. Rand developed some disease specific criteria. InterStudy, a research group in Minnesota, is developing an outcome management system for evaluation of hospital and medical services that includes the Short Form-36 item survey and a series of disease specific measures. The system is being adopted for use in hospitals in the United States and Canada.

There is little question that improvements in medical and surgical care have contributed to increases in life expectancy observed in industrialized nations, even though it may be difficult to specify direct connections between specific procedures and management systems and years of life gained. Age-standardized mortality rates for all diseases except cancer have declined since the 1960s. Even though some dispute the point, evidence is reasonably clear that some of the years of increased life are lived in worsened health; that is, there may well be a tradeoff between death and disability.[23] In the United States and Canada, age-specific disability rates have increased at all ages over the past 20 years. The management of chronic and disabling conditions, particularly among the elderly, has become a major issue in health care.

As the result, researchers are studying the impact of disease and its management on quality of life. While researchers have long used a variety of measures of disability, health status, mood, affect, and psychological well-being, generic and disease-specific measures are a more recent development.[24] The first widespread use of such measures occurred in cancer and cardiovascular research, but the measures are now widely used in all fields of health services research. Major conferences on quality of life research have been held in Portugal and Italy, and the Institute of Medicine has recently sponsored a monograph on the use of quality of life measures for the assessment of technology.[25]

While health services research projects take place around the world, most of the research is carried out by investigators in the United States. In addition to research funds provided by the Agency for Health Care Policy and Research, the National Institutes of Health give grants for research and training. Major private foundations such as the Robert Wood Johnson Foundation, the Kaiser Health Foundation, and the Kellogg Foundation provide major grants for national studies. A large number of university and private research firms compete for research awards and contracts.

Schaffarzick and Bunker[26] report that 45 organizations in the United States perform technology assessments. The government offices include the Congressional Office of Technology Assessment, the Agency for Health Care Policy and Research, the Food and Drug Administration, the National Institutes of Health, and the Centers for Disease Control. Private agencies such as the Clinical Efficacy Assessment Program of the American College of Physicians, the Diagnostic and Therapeutic Technology Assessment Panel of the American Medical Association, and the Technology Evaluation and Coverage Department of the Blue Cross and Blue Shield Association also sponsor technology assessment. In 1985 the Institute of Medicine of the National Academy of Sciences founded a Council on Health Care Technology to promote the development and application of technology assessment in health care and the review of medical technologies for their appropriate use.

In Canada, the federal and provincial governments have commissioned major inquiries, both before and after the introduction of universal, public medical care insurance. A working group of federal and provincial health officials meets periodically and has sponsored national conferences on technology assessment, prevention services, and quality care assurance. Quebec has created a council on technology assessment. In Ontario Ministry of Health and the Ontario Medical Association jointly formed the Task Force on the Provision of Medical Services, and the task force undertakes a number of studies on the uses of medical services. The federal and provincial governments have also established foundations or government organizations to fund research proposed by health service researchers.

In Great Britain, the Medical Research Council funds major studies medical and surgical intervention. The Department of Health and Social Services commissions research projects on health services as well.

Governments show increasing concern about the public expenditures for health services, and seek new strategies for the containment of costs and the management of health services. They commission studies and sponsor conferences to learn about the experiences of other countries in the search for new models of health care.

Research studies reflect shifts in health policy over the past two decades. Twenty years ago, the major issues were the availability of and access to health resources and financial coverage of costs of health services. The most striking change, noted by Neuhauser,[27] is a shift in focus from the internal dynamics of medical care to its costs and effects.

Relatively few health services studies focus on surgery and related fields. In this chapter, we highlight the major research issues that have emerged in relation to surgical services. The terms encountered most commonly in published articles are organization of health services, financing of health services, availability, accessibility, utilization, health manpower, health status, need, demand, supply, mode of practice, method of payment, patient–provider relationships, health beliefs, health promotion, information systems, technology assessment, clinical decision making, outcomes, appropriateness of care, monitoring, quality assurance, risk management, efficacy, effectiveness, utility analysis, benefits, and evaluation.

One can note the recent publications of two major edited works of surgical services, *Socioeconomics of Surgery*, edited by Rutkow,[28] and *Surgical Care in the United States: A Policy Perspective*, edited by Finkel.[29] The reader may wish to turn to both these books for additional information on surgical services research.

Availability, Accessibility, and Acceptability of Surgical Services

There is a surplus of physicians in North America. Governments are cutting the number of approved postgraduate training positions, and some states and provinces are reducing the size of classes entering medical schools. Countries in Europe are exercising the same options, and they no longer can guarantee that graduates will obtain postgraduate training posts or licenses to practice. Health policy analysts raise concern about the total number of physicians, their distribution by region, and their types of practice. They focus on the availability and accessibility of physicians, as well as on patterns of utilization.

Availability

Availability relates to the *supply* of health resources. Inventories of health manpower, hospitals, and other services show the numbers of physicians and hospital beds by specialty and region, the number of physicians or hospital beds per 10,000 or 100,000 population, or the number of persons per physician. These data show marked variations in resource-to-population ratios between and within countries, particularly for surgical specialties.[30,31]

We do not know the optimal surgeon-to-population ratio. One of the most extensive investigation of the question was the Study on Surgical Services for the United States, previously cited. After studying the surgery performed in four diverse geographical areas, the SOSSUS group concluded in 1976 that there were too many surgeons, low workloads, and marked variations in the distribution of surgeons across the country.[32] The SOSSUS researchers weighted surgical services in terms of time and complexity, using California Relative Values, and derived workload estimates for the physicians performing surgery in the areas studied. They recommended that the numbers of programs, the numbers persons entering the programs, and the number of surgeons entering practice be reduced. Williams[33] used the same procedures to study surgical services in Rhode Island in 1977, and compared his results to the earlier findings. He found that the trends had continued in spite of the recommendations from SOSSUS.

Physician manpower continues to increase. Because of these and other concerns, the Graduate Medical Education National Advisory Committee (GMENAC) was created by the U.S. government in 1976. In its 1980 report, GMENAC estimated that by 1990 there would be a surplus of 38,600 surgeons in the United States. The report recommended reductions in places for students in medical schools, in the number of first-year trainees in surgery, and in the number of surgeons entering practice. The American College of Surgeons conducted their own study[34] and argued that the numbers of trainees in the programs was not as large as estimated. As in their response to the SOSSUS, they denied that a surplus of surgeons existed.

Rutkow argues that the number of surgeons relative to the number of operations performed is so large that some surgeons may not be able to maintain technical proficiency because of their relatively low workloads. He predicts that the quality of surgical care will decline as the increased numbers of surgeons will perform inappropriate or unnecessary surgery, and their skills will decline.[35]

In most industrialized countries, the rural and remote regions have less favorable physician-to-population ratios, even in communities with hospitals equipped to provide surgical services. Provincial governments in Canada have used a range of incentives and disincentives to coax doctors into rural and remote areas, largely without success. The spread of physicians into smaller communities has occurred as an increased number of doctors go into practice, but most physicians locate in or near metropolitan areas.

The availability of health resources should relate to changes in the population as well. A large post-war baby boom in the United States and Canada lasted from the end of the 1940s into the 1960s. As with other industrialized countries, the birthrates have now reached record lows, and the population is aging, in terms of both the numbers of persons reaching the age of 65 years and the life expectancies for persons of that age. The percentage of the population aged 65 years and older will continue to increase into the 2020s, when the last of the "baby boomers" pass into retirement.

Not only does the use of health services increase with age, but in Canada, the utilization rates for persons over 75 years appear to be increasing more rapidly than for any other age.[36,37] Governments must now address the costs of providing care for the elderly.

In Canada, Lefebvre, Zsigmond, and Devereaux[38] studied the potential impact of an aging population on hospital beds. By applying the 1975 rates of hospital admissions and average lengths of stay to various projections of the age–sex composition of Canadian society, they estimated that demand would outstrip the availability of hospital beds in the 1990s. Using similar projections, a task force in Ontario[39] has projected that the demand for physicians' services will outstrip the supply by 2001.

Detsky[40] has outlined the mechanisms used by the state to regulate the supply of physicians:

1. Funds for medical schools based on the number of students.
2. Financial aid to students.
3. Control of the number of residency training positions.
4. Setting of size and composition of the medical student body.
5. Regulating the flow of foreign medical graduates.

Governments vary in the extent to which they regulate physician supply, in toto or by specialty. One can anticipate that governments will monitor the supply of health resources and projected levels of demand, and search for less costly ways of meeting the requirements.

Accessibility

In the 1960s and 1970s, investigators studied inequities in access to health care related to age, place of residence, race, and ability to pay. Respondents selected in large probability samples were used to study the determinants of health services accessibility to the population at large. The major health surveys conducted in the home included those by the U.S. National Center for Health Studies, the Center for Health Administration Studies at the University of Chicago,[41,42] the Internal Comparison of Medical Care Utilization of the World Health Organization[43] conducted in eight countries, and Cartwright and others in England.[44,45]

Kars-Marshall, Spronk-Boon, and Pollemans[46] reviewed the experiences of the nine countries with national health surveys. They found that the topics covered in the survey included sociodemographic characteristics, health status, life style and risk factors, health knowledge, attitudes and opinions, health care utilization, health care experiences, and health-related expenses and insurance.

By comparing the self-reports of symptoms, disability, and other health problems with those of health services used by respondents, investigators have attempted to measure unmet need.[47] There is now a consensus that perceived needs are the principal reason for using health services, and that inequities in access have been reduced over time. The changes are related to increases in the health insurance coverage of the surveyed.

Although the surveys ask about outpatient and hospitals surveys, surgical services have not been a major focus of any of the studies. Andersen, Lion, and Anderson[41] noted an increase in the use of surgical services over two decades in the United States. They report an increase in rates of 5 surgical services per 100 person-years in 1963 to 6 per 100 person-years in 1970.

Since 1965 the National Center for Health Statistics in the United States has monitored the number of operations performed annually through its National Hospital Discharge Survey. They survey between 5% and 8% of acute care general hospitals, exclusive of military and Veterans Administration facilities. They monitor an extensive array of operations, but minor procedures such as the abortion, vasectomy, angioplasty, cystoscopy, and cardiac catheterization are not included in the reports.

The estimated numbers of operations, surgeons, and residents in training for the years 1970, 1974, 1979, and 1985 are as follows:

Year	Operations	Surgeons	Residents
1970	11,984,000	58,378	13,979
1974	14,949,000	62,801	16,164
1979	16,223,000	85,136	17,727
1985	16,050,000	106,324	18,657

In 1985 the data base was expanded to include outpatient procedures. During the 1970s the number of operations increased by one-third and then declined slightly over the next 5 years. The numbers of surgeons increased by 82% during the same time period, and the number of residents in training increased by 34%.

Schwartz and Mendelson[48] have studied patient visits, hours of patient care, and weeks of work of physicians between 1982 and 1987 as reported in the Socioeconomic Characteristics of Medical Practice by the American Medical Association. They report that the demand for medical care indicates that increases of patient visits and patient hours of care have more than kept pace with the numbers of physicians. Changes in technology, growth and aging of the population, and the likely extension of insurance coverage should result in an annual growth rate of 2.2%. Accordingly, Schwartz and Mendelson[48] argue that the demand for services justifies the supply of medical manpower.

Surgery aims at correcting specific health problems, referred to surgeons by other physicians. Consumers may have a perception of the availability of surgeons in their areas, but it is unlikely that they identify their unmet needs and the required level of access to relevant surgical services.

Acceptability

Beyond the study of availability and accessibility of health services, researchers have focused on acceptability as it is expressed in terms of patient satisfaction. Patients are asked questions about the timing involved in obtaining primary care, the facilities, the costs, the competence of the clinician, and the quality of doctor–patient relationships. The articles by Ware and Associates[49] and Linder-Pelz[50] are the best summaries of the literature that have been written.

Most of the measures were developed for studies of community-based ambulatory care. Research on doctor–patient communication and compliance focuses on medical care and regimes that require doctor–patient interactions over a period of time. Because the surgeon–patient relationship usually ends relatively soon after treatment, it may differ in character and quality from that of a physician who provides comprehensive and continuous care.

Patients' complaints, claims of damage, and malpractice suits concern surgeons. In some jurisdictions, an increase in medical liability insurance fees has become large enough to force changes in the ways surgeons practice. Manuel[51] reports that the average medical malpractice jury award in the United States increased from $228,818 in 1975 to $1,017,716 in 1985. He provides a review of a flurry of activities in search of a solution, including the Medical Liability Project of the American Medical Association. There are hopes that the United States can move to no-fault medical insurance plans such as those implemented in New Zealand and Sweden.

Few studies have examined which patients are most likely to initiate legal action or the characteristics of the physicians against whom the action is taken. Some evidence suggests that patients are more likely to sue if their physicians have not taken time to communicate and establish an adequate therapeutic relationship with the patient.

When dissatisfaction leads to a formal complaint and legal action, the insurance industry and the legal sector play key roles in the process; but health service researchers have been slow to initiate studies in these areas.

Utilization

Data forms for the administration and financial reimbursement of health services rendered offer major sources of information on those who provide and consume health services. Hospital discharge summaries, such as those submitted to Professional Activity Survey in the United States or the Hospital Management Rresearch Institute in Canada, and billing statements of physicians, provide basic information about the specialties of physicians, diagnoses, and services rendered, as well as the age, sex, and residence of patients. Hospital discharge summaries tend to be more complete and more readily available for secondary analysis than outpatient data.

Depending on the political jurisdiction, data on inpatient services may be more readily available and more informative than those on outpatient services. Outpatient data are collected only if third-party payment occurs. The lack of information on outpatient surgical services becomes more important as the proportion of surgical services performed on an outpatient basis increases.

Most comparisons of surgical services focus on in-hospital procedures. Studies have looked at surgical utilization rates over time, or at national or international variations occurring at the same time. While variations occur in all surgical procedures, most of the studies focus on elective procedures, such as tonsillectomy/adenoidectomy (T/A), hysterectomy, excision of varicose veins, and coronary bypass. Given the lack of agreement in defining need, diagnosis, and clinical decision making, nonmedical factors may play a major role in determining how many elective surgical services are performed.

McCarthy, Finkel and Ruchlin[52] have noted that, in the United States, the rates of surgical services remained relatively constant between 1940 and 1970, but rose 24% between 1970 and 1978. While some surgical services, such as operations on the knee, cataracts, and prostate, increased 70.3%, 46.9%, and 43.5%, respectively, appendectomies and T/As declined by 6% and 43.3%, respectively. More recently, we find a steady increase in the number of coronary bypass procedures. Although it was not introduced until the early 1970s, by 1981 coronary bypass artery grafting had become the most commonly performed major surgical procedure (160,000 procedures) in the United States.[53]

Health economists, such as Evans[54] in Canada, believe that physicians hold a monopoly over medical services and can create a demand for them. These economists suggest that the increase in surgical procedures is a direct reflection of the increasing number of surgeons available to perform them.

McCarthy and Finkel[55] considered other reasons, such as changes in diagnostic coding procedures, improvements in technology, and increased consumer demand arising from coverage of costs by health insurance. Improvements in technology have improved the benefits of surgery while reducing the risks. Some increase in demand also arises from the increased coverage of the population by health insurance. The research question now is what is the relative importance of the various factors in explaining variations and changes in the rates of surgical services?

McPherson, Wennberg, Hovind, and Clifford[31] studied variations in surgical rates in New England, England, and Norway; McPherson, Strong, Epstein, and Jones[30] studied variations in England and Wales, Canada, and the United States; and Stockwell and Vayda[56] made earlier comparisons between Canada, England, and Wales. At the risk of overgeneralization, we draw two sets of conclusions from these studies. The utilization rates of surgical services are highest in the United States and Canada, lowest in England and Wales, and midway in Norway. Second, the within-country variations were greatest in Canada, followed by the United States, Norway, and England and Wales, in that order. The differences relate, in part, to variations in the availability of surgical services.

Some studies, such as those by Wennberg[57] in New England, Vayda and his associates in Ontario,[58] and Roos et al.[59] in Manitoba have focused on variations within countries. Essentially, they all found large variations in the rates for elective surgery that cannot be explained by differences in demographic characteristics, indicators of health status, or other characteristics. Depending on the elective procedure under review, the variations seem to depend on the availability of surgical resources, be they hospital services or surgeons.

Wennberg and Gittelson[60] and Wennberg[61] are proponents of the use of small areas – discrete hospital market areas of between 10,000 and 200,000 residents, for utilization analysis. In their supply-side model, analysis focuses on the relation between hospital beds, personnel, modes of practice, and utilization rates. They use census data on demographic and economic characteristics to describe the population; utilization rates can be adjusted for age, sex, and other confounding variables. Special-purpose household health interviews may define patterns of consumer behavior in the areas.

The surveys conducted to assess access, availability, and satisfaction with service have been based on a model developed by Andersen.[62] This epidemiologic model of consumer behavior describes predisposing factors, enabling factors, and need as the primary determinants of utilization, with need as the most important.[63]

Wennberg[61] favors the supply model over the needs model, for two reasons. First, Roos and Roos[64] have demonstrated that, for the aged in Manitoba, variations in surgical rates are not related to the health needs or status of the elderly; rather, rates of surgical use were higher among the more highly educated elderly, and this suggests that the difference may be due to demand. Wennberg's study[61] confirmed the lack of relation between variations in surgical rates and apparent need. Second, Wennberg prefers to focus on factors amenable to change by way of modifications in health policy.

The government of Alberta asked Halliday and Le Riche[65] to examine small-area variations across the 103 geographically defined general hospital districts in that province. The investigators selected 14 surgical procedures and linked the characteristics of the patient, the surgeon performing the surgery, and the hospital into one data set. The rates across the province were compared to the rates for the Edmonton General Hospital District, (Edmonton is the largest city in the province and the location of university health sciences center). Relative to this standard, the rates in most regions were lower for specialized procedures and higher for commonly performed operations. The key determinants of the variations were the teaching status of the hospital, the number of doctors performing surgery, and the general hospital district in which the patients resided.

Chassin and his colleagues[66] studied variations in utilization of the Medicare population in eight states for the year 1981. They studied 123 medical and surgical procedures and found threefold variations between the sites with the highest and lowest rates. The variations in rates across procedures were not consistent.

Two general assumptions arise in the studies of small-area variations. As the variations do not make "clinical sense," the first assumption is that the procedures are being used inappropriately. The second assumption is that reductions in the variations would improve the quality of care and serve to contain costs of health care.

Using the data from the study of Medicare patients,[66] Leape and his colleagues[67] studied the variations in the use of coronary angiography, carotid endarterectomy, and upper gastrointestinal tract endoscopy across 23 adjacent counties in one state. Using explicit criteria set by an expert panel, they audited the hospital charts and rated the appropriateness of the procedures. The variations in rates per 10,000 Medicare enrollees ranged from 13 to 158 for coronary angiography, from 5 to 41 for carotid endarterectomy, and from 42 to 164 upper gastrointestinal tract endoscopy. The rates of inappropriate use per county ranged from 8% to 75% for coronary angiography, from 0% to 67% for carotid endarterectomy, and from 0% to 25% for endoscopy. The variations in utilization rates could not be explained by variations in appropriate use.

The results confirm an earlier study of tonsillectomy rates in Manitoba.[68] The most important implication of these studies is that *overuse* or inappropriate use of procedures occurs in low-use areas and high-use areas alike. There is no direct relation between variations in use and appropriateness of care for the procedures studied.

Roos and her associates[69] have extended their studies to look at patterns of hospital admission and readmission for patients of family practitioners, internists, general surgeons, and obstetrician–gynecologists, when these physicians were the unique providers of hospital care. Again there were marked variations in hospital admissions and readmissions that could not be explained by the health or sociodemographic characteristics of the patients. Physicians who were high users had 27% of the patients, and they accounted for 42% of the hospital days. The high users tended to be rural physicians in areas with high bed-to-population ratios and hospitals with low occupancy rates. The patterns did not vary significantly by the specialty of the physician providing hospital care.

Utilization review and studies of local hospital markets have their problems. Such studies have focused on elective procedures for conditions in which medical uncertainty is supposedly high and the role of nonmedical factors can be assessed. It would be interesting to see whether the same patterns hold for surgery driven by demand, such as plastic surgery for cosmetic purposes, and for required or urgent surgery. For example, there are large elements of uncertainty in cardiovascular or even breast surgery for cancer, and nonmedical factors may play an important role in decision making.

Secondary or tertiary hospitals in other regions or areas may also serve local hospital markets. When patients in one area go to another area for a specific procedure, how important are factors in the local hospital market?

Measures of functioning, disease, and disability suitable for household interviews or drawing epidemiologic profiles may be measures of need so crude that important variations in the requirements for surgical services are missed. Since we lack research models to demonstrate how changes in modes of practice or clinical decision making relative to supply factors, it is not clear how health policy could affect the desired changes in surgeons' clinical decisions.

The marked variations are not characterized in terms of "over-" or "under"-utilization. Appropriate utilization can be judged only by relating the expected benefits to specific needs. Beyond need, one must consider demand. At some point, consumer demands and preferences must be taken into account, but this has not been done yet in surgical services research.

There is little question that surgeons are influenced by nonmedical factors when they make clinical decisions. Eisenberg[70] includes among these factors physicians' personal desires and interests, motives when acting for patients, and concerns for social good. Personal desires include income, style of practice, practice setting, and a desired role in clinical leadership. Physicians also take account of patients' ability to pay, desire for quality clinical care in the face of uncertainty, and other demands, including defensive medicine and convenience. The tradeoffs in decision making become more complex when the constraints of societal resources are added to the balance between the physician's personal desires and the patient's well-being.

Outcomes

Since physicians seek to provide health services to those who may benefit from them, researchers have studied the impact of medical and surgical care on the lives of patients and have developed measures for determining the effects of interventions on health status. The highest priority outcome is avoidance of death, the second is prevention of disability, and the third is reduction of morbidity from disease and interventions. Functional status and quality of life are related, but independent, concerns. Ideally, if the first three goals are achieved, the last two will follow; but this is not necessarily so. Interventions may be made when death or disability is inescapable, and the health professional is striving to improve the functional status or the quality of the life that remains. For a discussion of specific measures of outcome, see Chapters 17 and 20, above.

Surgeons introduce technical innovations or change surgical procedures at will; and they need not demonstrate the efficacy or effectiveness of such modifications. Once styles of practice have been established, surgeons have no reason to change unless they are the subjects of disciplinary reviews or legal proceedings.

If surgeons deem certain innovations or changes in procedures to be beneficial, they may report them as case studies or as outcomes in a cohort of patients over time. In teaching and research institutions, the experiences of patients receiving new surgical services can be compared with those of patients receiving conventional therapy (see Chapter 14).

Ideally, a given surgical intervention takes place only after its efficacy and effectiveness have been established in well-designed studies. A treatment's efficacy is defined as the outcome observed in a specific population of patients who receive a defined treatment—usually in the context of a controlled trial of the treatment. In the real world, surgeons vary in skill and techniques, hospitals vary in quality of care, and patients vary in compliance.

Effectiveness is defined as the outcomes likely to be achieved when a treatment is introduced into clinical practice. In general, a treatment found to be efficacious in the relatively artificial conditions of a controlled trial may prove relatively less effective when introduced into widespread clinical practice.

In summary, efficacy deals with the question "*Can* an intervention work under ideal circumstances?" Effectiveness, in contrast, answers "*Does* it work in the real world?"

Although controversies about the efficacy of various surgical procedures abound, there have been relatively few clinical trials. Gray, Hewitt, and Chalmers[71] reviewed the literature to identify surgical trials with control groups and identified 270 published studies. Half of these were randomized clinical trials. Two-thirds of studies compared one surgical procedure with another, and half of these studies were randomized. The proportion of randomized trials was highest among evaluations of cardiovascular procedures and for the treatment of cancer.

The number of trials is increasing, and there are noteworthy studies, such as those undertaken since 1971 by the National Surgical Adjuvant Breast Project Group to assess alternative forms of surgical, chemical, radiation treatments for cancer of the breast (see Chapter 29).

Randomized controlled trials by the Veterans Administration,[72] the European Coronary Surgery Study Group,[73] and the Coronary Artery Surgery Study (CASS)[74,75] have established the short term efficacy and long-term effectiveness of coronary artery bypass surgery for patients with impaired left ventricular function in terms of survival and quality of life. The improvements have not extended to employment or recreational activities. The same studies have established that medical management is preferable for patients with angina or clogged vessels who do have impaired left ventricular function. In the latter groups, surgical treatment reduces angina and pain, and improves the quality of life, but it does not reduce mortality.

Although these results have been accepted scientifically, appropriate changes in surgical practice for cancer of the breast[76] and coronary artery disease in the United States[53] have been slow to follow. Each year, thousands of patients who are inappropriate candidates according to the criteria established by the three cited studies, have coronary bypass operations.

Critics argue that the CASS study is out of date, that the patients are not representative of those seen in current practices, and that surgical and medical treatments have improved. Proponents of coronary artery bypass grafts for managing coronary heart disease in the elderly, angina of varying degrees, and postmyocardial infarction are extending the use of the procedure.

Holloway and Schocken[34] reviewed the CASS findings and information from the follow-up of patients in the trial and the registry of patients undergoing coronary arteriography at the participating centers to correct misinterpretations of the study that have arisen. They argue that the conclusions from the study continue to be valid after 8 years of follow-up, and they contend that the guidelines for operating continue to be appropriate. They recognize that calcium channel blockers, multiple drug regimens, and coronary angioplasty may result in even larger numbers of candidates for surgical management. They call for investigators to exercise care in analyzing the use of the newer modalities in managing coronary artery disease.

A major randomized trial reported most recently is the one on extracranial–intracranial (EC/IC) arterial bypass by the EC/IC Bypass Study Group.[77,78] Patients with symptomatic atherosclerotic disease of the internal carotid artery were randomly assigned to the best medical care currently possible or to medical care with bypass surgery. During the period of follow-up, which averaged 56 months, the bypass patients demonstrated a lack of benefits with respect to mortality, morbidity, and disability, when compared to the medically treated patients. No subgroup of patients benefited specifically from the procedures.

Sundt[79] challenged the results of the study after he surveyed neurosurgeons participating in the trial and discovered that most of the eligible patients had been neither entered in the trial nor followed by the research team. He claimed that the results could not be generalized to surgical practice because most of the patients who received the procedure were excluded from the study. A committee of the Association of Neurological Surgeons investigated the study, and they were similarly critical of the findings.[80] While the trial was well designed and executed, the committee noted that investigators failed to follow the large numbers of eligible patients who were surgically treated outside the trial, as proposed by the EC/IC group. The committee did not believe that the results of the trial could be generalized beyond the patients who had participated in it. More specifically, they said that decisions about insurance coverage for the procedure could not be based on the trial. The investigators responded,[81] but the response did not resolve the controversy, as evidenced in the debate that followed.

It is harder to evaluate surgical procedures than medical care by means of randomized clinical trials. In medical care, specifically drug trials, patients who meet the eligibility criteria can be randomly assigned to a therapy and be placed on standard protocols while keeping both the physicians and patients blind to the assignments.

In surgical care, the surgeon and patient are unavoidably aware of the assigned treatment arm. Moreover, since surgeons vary in skill and make minor modifications in their techniques, the treatment itself can never be completely standardized. Surgeons have confidence in their professional skills, and patients have faith that the procedure selected by their surgeon is the best one for them. Since neither the surgeons nor the patients are blind to the procedures used, the assessments of outcomes by either groups may be biased.[82]

"Crossovers" are another major problem plaguing trials. Patients or doctors may decide that the patients should change treatments after group assignments have been made. While there are methods of analysis for handling the problem, crossovers undermine the trial.[71]

The scientific and ethical issues of randomized trials are intensified if the effects of the experimental therapeutic maneuver cannot be reversed. Generally speaking, the risk of this occurring is greater for trials for surgical interventions than medical interventions. The randomized, controlled trial is unquestionably the optimal design for the evaluation of clinical interventions. As Rudicel and Esdaile[82] suggest, there are times when scientific and ethical issues dictate that other designs should be employed in surgical trials. Finding the best design for a trial is a constant challenge to the clinician and methodologist alike.

Trials of modes of delivering and paying for health services can be organized.[83] In patient care trials like those just cited, the goal is to assess the effect of a specific treatment intervention on clinical outcomes. In health services trials, the goal may be the assessment of (a) different modes of payment and insurance (e.g., the Health Insurance Experiment Study by the Rand Corporation[16]), (b) a new type of health professional (e.g., the Burlington randomized trial of nurse practitioners),[83] facility, or practice (e.g., outpatient surgery versus inpatient surgery), or (c) the introduction of new arrangements for health care (e.g., reorganization of emergency medical services and introduction of paramedic services into Kings County, Washington[84]).

Depending on the kind of health service under study, the experimental unit may comprise providers, practices, hospitals, geographical areas, or insurance plans. Ideally, the unit of analysis should be the same as the unit of assignment; if it is not (e.g., if community or neighborhoods are assigned to a new or a conventional organization of services, but the responses of individuals in the community are used as the unit of analysis), difficulties will be encountered in the design of the trial.

Trials of new services present a number of problems. While you may randomly assign experimental units to different modes of delivering health services, everyone concerned will be aware of what the assignments are and will react accordingly. For example, once a trial has been set, those involved in providing service in a traditional mode may strive to show that their services are as good or better than the new ones, and may succeed in doing so. Another problem arises if the new model is evaluated during the introductory period, when organizational problems are common and those delivering the service have not had a chance to achieve an operating level of efficiency. Last, if the new mode is perceived as a threat, individuals involved in the conventional mode of delivering services may lobby or maneuver to protect their interest. The health services trial must be carefully designed and implemented if the new mode of delivery is to receive a fair and objective testing.

Cost Analysis

Given the current emphasis on cost containment and the rationing of health services, it is not surprising that economic analysis of medical care is a major part of health services research. The cost of health care includes service costs, out-of-pocket expenses paid by patients and their families, and indirect costs. The service costs include the fees or salaries of the health care providers, the cost of technical services, and the fraction of overhead and administrative costs allocated to each service. Patients and their families may pay supplemental amount for drugs, appliances, travel expenses, and other goods and services directly related to treatment. Service costs and out-of-pocket expenses can be referred to as direct costs.

Indirect costs include time lost from work and the burden imposed by uncertainty, pain, and suffering on patients and their families, but the assignment of dollar values to the indirect costs is controversial.[54] More detailed information on this topic is provided in the literature.[85-88]

The four types of cost analysis are cost–efficiency, cost–effectiveness, cost–benefit, and cost–utility.[89] Cost–efficiency analysis is the simplest. It focuses on the cost per unit of service produced, without regard to the effects. Generally, it is assumed that the effects of the two modes of health service delivery (e.g., surgical care in an outpatient center vs. in hospital) are equivalent and acceptable. Costs are analyzed, usually from the perspective of the provider, and a judgment is made concerning the relative efficiency of the two modes of health service delivery.

Cost–effectiveness analysis involves relating marginal difference in cost per unit of service to marginal differences in effects or outcomes. Pineault and his associates[90] compared costs, clinical outcomes, and patient satisfaction for patients who received tubal ligations, hernia repairs, or meniscectomies on an inpatient versus on outpatient basis. The clinical outcomes were comparable, but the efficiency of outpatient surgery produced savings of \$86 for each tubal ligation and \$115 for each hernia repair. The outpatient cost of each meniscectomy was $173 higher for outpatients than for inpatients. Aside from the costs, the outpatients thought that the length of care they received was too short and clearly preferred inpatient care, particularly the meniscectomy patients. Although the indirect costs identified by the consumers were not put into dollar terms, it is clear that they have to be taken into account.

A major problem in cost-effectiveness analyses is deciding how to equate the different clinical outcomes that were judged to be equivalent. In the example above, the consumers preferred inpatient services, but it is not clear how these preferences should be weighted in interpreting the results.

Cost-benefit analysis tries to translate all the effects or outcomes of importance into economic terms (i.e., dollars or other monetary units). The calculations include the costs of treatment over time, lifetime earnings, and external costs and benefits encountered by patients and their families, such as the impact on family life and opportunities foregone by one or more family members. Money loses value over time through inflation, and interest or dividends could be earned by making investments rather than expenditures on health care. Consequently, the costs saved over time, or the benefits gained in the future, have to be discounted and expressed in terms of their monetary value when the medical care is delivered. A number of assumptions and value judgments have to be made about the economic values to be attached to the effects of care over time and the discount rate to be applied.[54]

For example, patients with stable angina may undergo coronary bypass surgery and experience symptomatic relief, but the other effects and benefits would be the same if they received medical care, instead. Hemenway and associates[91] estimate that the cost of care over 3 years is four times higher for surgical than for medical patients. The challenge is how to state the benefits of relief from angina and other complaints in monetary terms so that the reduction is psychic costs achieved by surgery can be compared to the increase in the cost of care incurred by surgery.

Boyle and Torrance[92] recommend cost-utility analysis as an alternative to cost-benefit analysis. When the effects of health care are known, the health status of the individual can be described in terms of the key dimensions of functioning. Respondents are then asked to rate each discrete health state on a continuum of 0 (the same as death) to 1 (normal health and functioning). The mean utility value for a given health state is then used to estimate the value of the care. It takes the place of benefits expressed in economic terms in the analysis.

In an economic evaluation of a neonatal intensive care unit, Boyle, Torrance, et al.[93,94] used cost-effectiveness, cost-benefit analyses, and cost-utility analysis, to assess the impact of intensive care on very low birthweight infants. Some health states were given negative utility values; that is, severe mental or physical disability was rated as being worse than death. Although some infants weighing less than 1000 grams survived, their health states were such that the value of intensive care for them could be questioned in terms of cost-utility or cost-benefit. This is a new approach to economic analysis, and clinicians and researchers, alike, are debating its merit.

Warner and Luce[13] reviewed cost-benefit and cost-effectiveness studies and found that relatively few economic evaluations of surgical services were published prior to 1980. Most are included in a book on the costs, risks, and benefits of surgery, edited by Bunker, Barnes, and Mosteller.[95]

Organization and Financing of Medical Care

Alternate strategies for rationing health care[96] and for cost containment are controversial topics. In the United States and England, and to a lesser extent in Canada, the relative merits of private and public control of health resources[97] are debated, and considerable attention is now devoted to the effects of alternative modes of payment and organization on the costs and quality of health care. This section is limited to brief discussions of a second opinion for elective surgery, alternative organizations for surgical centers, and modes of payment for health care.

Second Opinion for Elective Surgery

Various states in the United States have set up programs that require patients receiving public assistance for medical expenses to obtain a second medical opinion before payment can be authorized for designated elective surgical procedures. The goal is to contain costs by curtailing unnecessary surgery.

Leap[98] reviewed the major studies on the second-opinion programs. Upon second opinion, the nonconfirmation rates of the original opinion ranged from 7.5% to 18.7%; for patients with confirmations, the surgical rates varied from a low of 67.8% to a high of 93.1%. Between one-third and two-fifths of patients whose cases were not confirmed had surgery.

The overall reduction of surgery rates of about 25% in regions with second-opinion programs is greater than can be accounted for by nonconfirmation on second opinion. The programs do result in cost savings, partly because surgeons are more likely to be cautious in recommending operations. However the reductions may be indiscriminate as both needed and unneeded operations are likely reduced. The impact of the programs on the health of the patients is unknown. The studies lack proper controls, and the criteria for judgment are based on clinical judgment rather than widely recognized explicit standards. Consequently one cannot judge the impact of the second-opinion programs on unnecessary surgery.[98]

Alternative Organization of Surgical Centers

In the United States, profit and not for profit corporations, such as health maintenance organizations, large groups of physicians in practice, and multihospital systems are reorganizing health services. One of the most dramatic changes has been the development of free-standing surgical centers in the United States since the introduction of the first one in 1970.[99] In 1983, more than 370,000 operations were performed in about 260 such centers, and by 1986 the numbers had increased to 592 facilities and slightly over a million procedures. Seventy percent of the facilities were independently owned, 23% were part of corporate chains, and 7% were hospital owned. Detmer and Buchanan-Davidson[99] estimate that by 1990 there will be more than 800 facilities and 1.9 million procedures.

The Joint Commission for Accreditation of Health Care Organizations and the Accreditation Association for Ambulatory Health Care accredit free-standing surgical centers. Third-party payers pay for outpatient surgery, and the Health Care Financing Association is expanding the number of procedures that Medicare will cover from 150 to 950.

Although it is easy to understand how substantial cost savings can be achieved, the case mix and severity of cases may not be the same in free-standing centers as it is in hospitals, and so-called cost savings may relate only to the costs of providing care, without considering the direct and indirect costs paid by patients. The few studies of outcomes in free standing surgical centers reveal small numbers of surgically related deaths and postoperative complications, but this may be the result of careful screening of patients prior to surgery.[100]

So far, no data system in the United States has uniform information on all surgical patients. Davis[101] has recommended that such a system be established and that the following classification be used to define the levels of surgical care provided:

Level 1. Minor ambulatory surgery—surgery on patients who are neither hospitalized nor held for observation following surgery.
Level 2. Minor ambulatory surgery—outpatient surgery for which a period of postoperative care is provided.
Level 3. In-hospital surgery.

If hospitals provide care for patients with more serious surgical and other health problems, and free-standing surgical centers provide care for young, healthy patients, free-standing surgical centers may appear to be more efficient if only operating costs are compared. Any research study must control for the differences in case mix, and then compare the free-standing surgical centers with hospitals in a complete cost-effectiveness analysis.

Mode of Payment

Payments for surgical services in the United States are controlled to some extent by the type of organization through which services are contracted and now by the use of diagnosis related groups (DRGs) for prospective payment. Health services research on the modes of organization and DRGs will be briefly reviewed.

Health maintenance organizations (HMOs) provide a set range of services for a fixed premium or capitation payment. Physicians who sign HMO contracts agree to an organization's policies for compensation, utilization control mechanisms, use of contracting hospitals, and reporting policies. The HMOs started in the 1970s. By 1987 there were 662 HMOs, and they have enrolled more than 28 million people, or about 12% of the population. The most popular form of HMO is one that contracts directly with physicians in private practice. The control of utilization is the key to operation of the HMOs.

HMOs offer a wide range of ambulatory services and practice less intensive hospital care. They deliver care with about 40% fewer hospital admissions and a 75% reduction in costs, compared to fee-for-service practices. LoGerfo and his colleagues[102] have found surgical care to be comparable to, or better than, that found in fee-for-service settings.

The Rand Health Insurance Experiment included a comparison of an HMO with a fee-for-service practice. In the reports, the investigators concluded that the HMO saved money by reducing hospital use but that HMO patients were less satisfied with their care.[103] There were indications, as well, that low-income HMO members ended the experiment with worse health than fee-for-service patients.[104] Wagner and Bledsoe[105] believe that the conclusion about worsened health among low-income HMO members can be questioned because of a lack of consistency in the data.

There is concern that the cost containment push in the United States and elsewhere could lead to a lowering of the quality of, and access to, health care for the poor.[106] Ermann and Gabel[107] recommend that studies on the impact of service reorganization address the issues of quality and access as well as cost.

Researchers at Yale University sought a way to group patients into homogeneous diagnostic categories with respect to resource consumption. They collapsed the 10,000 diseases and procedures in the International Classification of Diseases, ninth revision, Clinical Modification (ICD-9-CM) into 468 diagnosis related groups (DRGs). Each DRG has its own weighted index value to show the level of resources consumed. The DRGs have been adopted by several state governments and by Medicare in the United States for determining the payments the hospitals receive for providing care. In 1986 the U.S. Congress created the Prospective Payment Commission to maintain and upgrade the DRG system.[108] DRGs, or other adaptations of them, are being considered for use in other countries as well.

The DRGs are adjusted to take into consideration the severity of illness and other health problems the patients may have. Even so, there is concern about the heterogeneity of case mix, and surgeons have complained that the funding based on DRG has not covered the costs for particular problems and procedures. Trauma surgeons, in particular, have complained about the deficits they encounter under DRG reimbursement systems. Horn has demonstrated that the DRGs have not been adequately adjusted for severity of illness, and she has developed a Computerized Severity Index for making adjustments.[109] Apache II, the Acute Physiologic and Chronic Health Evaluation, has been considered for the same purpose.

As Munoz[108] notes, issues of cost containment and surgical economics assume major importance as constraints are placed on health care. In addition to studying issues of costs, access, quality of care, and outcomes, surgeons must justify the costs of marginal improvements in outcome they obtain with surgical procedures and therapies.

Monitoring, Quality Assurance, and Information Systems

Studies of interventions follow a pattern. The development of the intervention occurs first and clinical trials take place later. Ideally, the efficacy and effectiveness of an intervention are established through well-controlled trials, and its marginal effects and benefits yield acceptable cost ratios vis à vis other interventions. Next we have the quality assurance step–making sure that, in a large-scale implementation, the intervention is effectively and efficiently provided to needful patients in the community. The last steps are to assess the impact of the intervention in terms of the public good, and to determine what changes, if any, should be made.

Monitoring, quality assurance, and information systems are required to determine whether efficacious and effective surgical services are being efficiently provided to the patients who can benefit from them. Monitoring can be simply a review of the rates of delivery of specific surgical services to detect outliers. For example, Luft[110,111] studied the relation between hospital size and case mortality rates. The hospital discharge summaries of more than 800,000 surgical patients taken from the PAS files for 1974 and 1975 were grouped by patients' age and sex and the presence of single or multiple diagnoses. For each of the 20 patient groups so established, Luft compared the specific surgical case fatality rates for hospitals grouped according to the frequency with which they provided the same specific surgical services. For open heart, coronary artery bypass, vascular, and transurethral prostatic surgery, case fatality rates consistently dropped as the number of such operations increased in any given hospital. For a second set of operations, the case fatality rates were highest in hospitals in which the operations were performed relatively infrequently and lower in hospitals where they were performed a basic number of times each year. No further decline in fatality rates occurred in hospitals in which more than the same basic number of operations were performed. Case fatality rates for a third set of surgical procedures were not related to the surgical activity levels of the hospitals. On the basis of these results, Luft suggested that specific sets of operations be regionalized, to permit the hospitals providing them to do so often enough to minimize case mortality rates by more frequent use of the procedures.

Luft and Hunt[112] have reported on a study of cardiac catheterization procedures for 70,348 patients performed in 151 hospitals in 1982. They observed 738 deaths. The ratio of observed deaths to expected deaths ranged from 1.54 in hospitals with less than 200 procedures per year to 0.74 in hospitals with high volumes (i.e., >750 procedures/year). While there were some low-volume hospitals with good outcomes, Luft and Hunt note that their data support the concept of regionalization of care to ensure the best possible results.

Farber, Kaiser, and Wenzel[113] reviewed 25,000 surgical operations in the state of Virginia and came to similar conclusions about the frequency of operations and infection rates. Infection rates in appendectomy, herniorrhaphy, cholecystectomy, colon resection, and abdominal hysterectomy cases were inversely related to the logarithm of the number of such operations.

The provincial government of Saskatchewan expressed its concern about the increasing number of hysterectomies being performed by appointing a professional monitoring commission. The subsequent dramatic drop in the number of hysterectomies was attributed to this surveillance.[114] A similar experiment with a medical care review organization did not alter patterns of medical care in New Mexico.[115]

Quality assurance systems go one step further. They review the entire spectrum of providers' practice activities to identify questionable areas and to pinpoint specific providers whose practices require change. In the United States and Canada, hospitals must have active quality assurance programs to maintain their accreditation.

Donabedian[116,117] and Williamson et al.[118,119] have written definitive treatises on the design and implementation of quality assurance programs. Such programs should include measures of structure, process, and outcome, and their standards and criteria should reflect the findings of evaluative studies in health care. However, it is not yet possible to describe the systems currently being put into place, nor to discern what cost-effective improvements if any they have produced in the provision of health care.

The lack of appropriate information constrains and impedes the current activities of health service researchers and clinical investigators. The revolutions in computer design and data management systems offer some hope that adequate informational data bases will eventually become realities.

Conclusion

Health services research has developed very rapidly during the past 20 years, and the issues that dominate the field relate to cost containment, outcomes, and quality of care. There is, however, no direct relation between health services management, health policy decision making, and the availability of information from health services research. Because studies have to be focused on specific places, persons, and events within a given time period, the results may not be applicable to other settings. Even studies in the same area may yield findings that are contradicting, in whole or in part. Decision makers are understandably slow to adopt controversial findings, unless they are predisposed to believe them. When the information obtained is consistent over a series of studies, it can be persuasive enough to induce providers, the public, and policy makers to pay attention. Health services research is most likely to have its greatest impact in such instances.

Despite the contemporary limitations of health services research, some issues require systematic study to assess the impact of health services on society. For example, millions of dollars and extensive efforts by the health professions, hospitals, and government have been directed into the establishment of regional trauma programs in the United States. The Emergency Medical Services System legislation of 1973 and 1976 mandated the formation of 303 nationally-designed, geographic EMS areas with the following characteristics.[120]

1. Rapid notification of injury (one emergency telephone number, 911, and coordinated communication between police, fire, and ambulance services).
2. Immediate provision of basic and advanced life support by ambulance services.
3. Designated regional hospitals with trauma teams and definitive trauma services.
4. Triage protocols and transfer agreements between hospitals.

The respective roles and responsibilities of ambulance personnel and physicians in the emergency room, the organization of hospital services for trauma victims, and what technologies to employ (at the accident or injury site, in the ambulance, in the emergency room, and in the hospital) have been topics of considerable debate.

Surgeons in the United States have established the American Trauma Association as a forum for debates about the organization of emergency medical services and a stimulator of research on the impact of such services. Surgeons are also involved in such related associations as the American Association of Automotive Medicine. Numerous clinical and some regional studies have evaluated the outcomes of trauma care. Measures of the severity of different injuries have been developed to estimate the expected mortality and morbidity; their precision and predictive power are being evaluated in clinical and methodological studies. Attempts are also being made to establish a national trauma registry.

Although widespread improvements have occurred in emergency services, the shape and character of trauma services varies from region to region. In Canada, provinces are being pressed to upgrade emergency medical services and to introduce regional trauma programs, but there is considerable controversy about which policies should be pursued.

Given the improvements made in the health sector during the past 20 years, it is not clear what potential effects or benefits can be expected from specific recommendations or changes. Because most of the innovations and changes in the United States were not evaluated in well-controlled studies, the relative contributions made by various components of the emergency medical services cannot be specified. Well-designed studies in clinical and health services research could provide important information. The active participation of surgeons in research on surgical services is essential.

References

1. Spitzer WO, Feinstein AR, Sackett DL. What is a health care trial? JAMA 1975;233:161–63.
2. Battista RN, Contandriopoulous A-P, Champagne F, Williams JI, Pineault R, Boyle P. An integrative framework for health-related research. J Clin Epidemiol 1989;42:1155–60.
3. Morris JN. Uses of Epidemiology, 2nd ed. London: E & S Livingstone, 1964.
4. Buck C. The role of epidemiology in health care research. In: Health Care Research: A Symposium, Larsen DE, Love EJ, eds. Calgary: University of Calgary, 1974:37–43.
5. Study of Surgical Services for the United States. Surgery in the United States. American College of Surgeons and American Surgical Association: 1976.
6. Schieber GJ. Financing and Delivering Health Care: A Comparative Analysis of OECD Countries. Paris: Organization for Economic Co-operation and Development, 1987.
7. Institute of Medicine. Report of a Study, Health Services Research. National Academy of Sciences, Washington, DC: 1979:1–102.
8. Georgopoulos B. Hospital Organization Research: Review and Source Book. Philadelphia: Saunders, 1975.
9. Flook EE, Sanazaro PJ. Health Services Research and R&D in Perspective. Ann Arbor, MI: Health Administration Press, 1973.
10. Culyer AJ, Wiseman J, Walker A. An Annotated Bibliography of Health Economics: English Language Sources. New York: St. Martin's Press, 1977.
11. Griffiths DAT, Rigoni R, Tacier P, et al. An Annotated Bibliography of Health Economics: Western European Sources, New York: St. Martin's Press, 1980.
12. Van Eimeren W, Kopcke W. Bestandsaufnahime: Gesundheitsystemforschung (State of the Art Report: Health Services Research). Munich: Institut für medizinische Informationrerarbeitung, Statistik und Beomathematik, 1979.
13. Warner KE, Luce BR. Cost-Benefit and Cost-Effectiveness Analysis in Health Care: Principles, Practice, and Potential. Ann Arbor, MI: Health Administration Press, 1982.
14. Sisk JE, Ruby G. The federal assessment of surgical procedures. In: Surgical Care in the United States: A Policy Perspective, Finkel ML, ed. Baltimore: Johns Hopkins University Press, 1988:159–74.
15. Mosteller F, ed. Assessing Medical Technologies: Institute of Medicine. Washington, DC: National Academy of Sciences, 1985.
16. Brook RH, Ware JE Jr, Rogers WH, et al. Does free care improve adults' health? Results from a randomized controlled trial. N Engl J Med 1983; 309: 1426–1434.
17. Ware JE Jr. Standards for validating health measures: definition and content. J Chronic Dis 1987; 40:473–80.
18. Bergner M, Bobbit RA, Carter WB, Gilson BS. The Sickness Impact Profile: development and final revision of a health status measure. Med Care 1981;19:787–805.
19. Hunt SM, McEwen J, McKenna SP. Measuring health status: a tool for clinicians and epidemiologists. J Roy Coll Gen Pract 1985;35:185–88.
20. Kaplan RW, Bush JW. Health related quality of life measurement for evaluation research and policy analysis. Health Psychol 1982:61–80.
21. Kaplan RM, Atkins CJ, Times R. Validity of Quality of Well-Being Scale as an outcome measure in chronic obstructive pulmonary disease. J Chronic Dis 1984;37:85–95.
22. Stewart AL, Hays RD, Ware JE Jr. The MOS short form general health survey: reliability and validity in a patient population. Med Care 1988;26:724–35.
23. Verbugge LM. Longer life but worsening health? Trends in health and mortality of middle aged and older persons. Milbank Mem Fund Q Health Soc 1984;62:475–516.
24. Williams JI, Wood-Dauphinée S. Assessing quality of life: measures and utility. In: Quality of Life and Technology Assessment, Mosteller F, Falotico-Taylor J, eds. Washington, DC: National Academy Press, 1989:65–115.
25. Mosteller F, Falotico-Taylor J, eds. Quality of Life and Technology Assessment. Washington, DC: National Academy Press, 1989.
26. Schaffarzick RW, Bunker JP. Regionalized surgical health care. In: Socioeconomics of Surgery, Rutkow IM, ed. Toronto: Mosby, 1989:154–63.
27. Neuhauser, D. Health services research, 1984. Med Care 1985;23:739–42.
28. Rutkow IM, ed. Socioeconomics of Surgery. Toronto: Mosby, 1989.
29. Finkel ML, ed. Surgical Care in the United States: A Policy Perspective. Baltimore: Johns Hopkins University Press, 1988.
30. McPherson K, Strong PM, Epstein A, et al. Regional variations in the use of common surgical procedures: within and between England and Wales, Canada and the United States of America. Soc Sci Med 1981;15:273–88.
31. McPherson K, Wennberg JE, Hovind OB, Clifford

P. Small area variations in use of common surgical procedures. An interactive comparison of New England, England and Norway. N Engl J Med 1982;307:1310–14.
32. Nickerson RJ, Colton T, Peterson OL, Bloom BS, Hauch WW Jr. Doctors who perform operations. A study on hospital surgery in 4 diverse geographic areas: Parts I and II. N Engl J Med 1976;295: 921–26, 982–89.
33. Williams DC. Surgeons and surgery in Rhode Island, 1970 and 1977. N Engl J Med 1982;305: 1319–23.
34. Holloway JD, Schocken DD. CASS in retrospect: lessons from the randomized cohort and registry. Am J Med Sci 1988;295:424–32.
35. Rutkow IM. Surgical operations and manpower: can technical proficiency be maintained? In: Socioeconomics of Surgery, Rutkow IM, ed. Toronto: Mosby, 1989:3–14.
36. Barer ML, Pulcins IR, Evans RG, Hertzman C, Lomas J, Anderson GM. Trends in use of medical services by the elderly in British Columbia. Can Med Assoc J 1989;141:39–45.
37. Barer ML, Evans RG, Hertzman C, Lomas J. Aging and health care utilization: new evidence on old fallacies. Soc Sci Med 1987;24:851–62.
38. Lefebvre LA, Zsigmond Z, Devereaux MS. A Prognosis for Hospitals: The Effects of Population Change on the Need for Hospital Space. Ottawa: Statistics Canada, 1979.
39. Medical Manpower for Ontario. Toronto: Ontario Council of Health, 1983.
40. Detsky AS. The Economic Foundations of National Health Policy. Cambridge, MA: Ballinger, 1978.
41. Andersen R, Lion J, Anderson OW. Two Decades of Health Services: Social Survey Trends in Use and Expenditure. Cambridge, MA: Ballinger, 1976.
42. Aday LA, Andersen R, Fleming GV. Health Care in the U.S. Equitable for Whom? Beverly Hills, CA: Sage, 1980.
43. Kohn R, White KL, eds. Health Care: An International Study. New York: Oxford University Press, 1976.
44. Cartwright A. Patients and Their Doctors: A Study of General Practice. London: Routledge & Kegan Paul, 1967.
45. Hannay DR. The Symptom Iceberg: A Study of Community Health. London: Routledge & Kegan Paul, 1979.
46. Kars-Marshall C, Spronk-Boon YW, Pollemans MC. National health interview surveys for health care policy. Soc Sci Med 1988;26:223–33.
47. Aday LA, Andersen R. Development of Indices of Access to Medical Care. Ann Arbor, MI: Health Administration Press, 1975.
48. Schwartz WB, Mendelson DN. No evidence of an emerging physician surplus: an analysis of change in physicians' work load and income. JAMA 1990;263:557–60.
49. Ware JE Jr, et al. The measurement and meaning of patient satisfaction. Health Med Care Serv Rev 1978;1:1–16.
50. Linder-Pelz S. Toward a theory of patient satisfaction. Soc Sci Med 1982;16:577–82.
51. Manuel BM. The malpractice crisis and the surgeon. In: Socioeconomics of Surgery, Rutkow IM, ed. Toronto: Mosby, 1989:368–85.
52. McCarthy EG, Kinkel EC, Ruchlin HS. Second Opinion Elective Surgery. Boston: Auburn House, 1981.
53. Braunwald E. Effects of coronary-artery bypass grafting on survival: implications of the randomized Coronary-Artery Surgery Study. N Engl J Med 1983;309:1181–84.
54. Evans RG. Strained Mercy: The Economics of Canadian Health Care. Toronto: Butterworth, 1984.
55. McCarthy EG, Finkel ML. Second opinion elective surgery programs: outcome, status, over time. Med Care 1978;16:984–94.
56. Stockwell H, Vayda E. Variations in surgery in Ontario. Med Care 1979;17:390–95.
57. Wennberg JE. Factors governing utilization of hospital services. Hosp Pract 1979;14:110–27.
58. Vayda E, Mindell WR. Variations in operative rates, what do they mean? Surg Clin N Am 1982; 62:627–39.
59. Roos LL Jr, Roos NP. What are we learning about surgery? An update on the Manitoba study of common surgical procedures. In: Proceedings of the Second Canadian Conference on Health Economics, Boan JA, ed. Regina: University of Regina, 1984:341–65.
60. Wennberg J, Gittlesohn A. Variations in medical care among small areas. Sci Am 1982;246(4): 120–34.
61. Wennberg JE. On patient need, equity, supplier-induced demand, and the need to assess the outcome of common medical practices. Med Care 1985;23(5):512–20.
62. Andersen R. A Behavioral Model of Families' Use of Health Services. Chicago: University of Chicago Center for Health Administration Studies No. 25, 1968.
63. Hulka BS, Wheat JR. Patterns of utilization: the patient perspective. Med Care 1985;23:438–60.
64. Roos NP, Roos LL Jr. Surgical rate variations: do they reflect health or socioeconomic characteristics of the population? Med Care 1982;20:945.
65. Halliday ML, LeRiche WH. Regional variation in surgical rates, Alberta, 1978, and the relationship to characteristics of patients, doctors performing surgery and hospitals where the surgery was performed. Can J Public Health 1987;78:193–200.
66. Chassin MR, Brook RH, Park RE, Keesey J, Fink A, Kosecoff J, Kahn K, Merrick N, Solomon DH. Variations in the use of medical and surgical services by the Medicare population. N Engl J Med 1986;314:285–90.
67. Leape LL, Park RE, Solomon DH, Chassin MR, Kosecoff J, Brook RH. Does inappropriate use

explain small-area variations in the use of health care services? JAMA 1990;263:669–72.
68. Roos NP, Roos LL, Henteleff PD. Elective surgical rates: do high rates mean lower standards? N Engl J Med 1977;297:360–65.
69. Roos NP, Flowerdew G, Wajda A. Variations in hospital practices: a population based study in Manitoba, Canada. Am J Public Health 1986;76: 45–51.
70. Eisenberg JM. Physician utilization: the state of research about physicians' practice patterns. Med Care 1985;23(5):461–83.
71. Gray DT, Hewitt P, Chalmers TC. The evaluation of surgical therapies. In: Socioeconomics of Surgery, Rutkow IM, ed. Toronto: Mosby, 1989:229–55.
72. Murphy ML, Hultgren HN, Detre K, et al. Treatment of chronic stable angina: a preliminary report of survival data of the randomized Veterans Administration Cooperative Study. N Eng J Med 1977; 297:621–27.
73. European Coronary Study Group. Long-term results of prospective randomized trial of coronary artery bypass surgery in stable angina pectoris. Lancet 1982;2:1173–80.
74. CASS Principal Investigators. Coronary Artery Surgery Study Group (CASS): A randomized trial of coronary bypass surgery: quality of life in randomized subjects. Circulation 1983;68:951–60.
75. CASS Principal Investigators. Coronary Artery Surgery Study Group (CASS): A randomized trial of coronary artery surgery: survival data. Circulation 1983;68:939–50.
76. Kleinman JC, Machlin SR, Modaris J, Makuc D, Feldman JJ. Changing practice in the surgical treatment of breast cancer. Med Care 1983;21:1232–42.
77. EC/IC Bypass Study Group. The international study of extracranial/intracranial arterial anastomosis (EC/IC Bypass Study): methodology and entry characteristics. Stroke 1985;16:397–406.
78. EC/IC Bypass Study Group. Failure of extracranial–intracranial arterial bypass to reduce the risk of ischemic stroke: results of a randomized trial. N Engl J Med 1985;313:1191–1200.
79. Sundt TM Jr. Was the international randomized trial of extracranial–intracranial arterial bypass representative of the population at risk? N Engl J Med 1987;316:814–16.
80. Goldring S, Zervas N, Langfitt T. The extracranial–intracranial bypass study. N Engl J Med 1987; 316:817–20.
81. Barnett HJ, Sackett D, Haynes B, Peerless SJ, Meissner I, Hachinski V, Fox A. Are the results of the extracranial–intracranial bypass generalizable? N Eng J Med 1987;316:820–24.
82. Rudicel S, Esdaile J. The randomized trial on orthopaedics: obligation or option? Bone Joint Surg 1985; 67A:1284–93.
83. Spitzer WO, Sackett DL, Sibley JC, et al. Burlington randomized trial of the nurse practitioner. N Engl J Med 1974;290:251–56.
84. Eisenberg MS, Hallstrom AP, Copass MK, et al. Treatment of ventricular fibrillation emergency medical technician defibrillation and paramedic services. JAMA 1984;251:1723–26.
85. Drummond MF, Stoddart GL, Torrance GW. Methods for the Economic Evaluation of Health Care Programs. New York: Oxford University Press, 1987.
86. Drummond MF. Principles of Economic Appraisal in Health Care. New York: Oxford Unviersity Press, 1980.
87. Stoddard GL, Drummond MF. How to read clinical journals; VIIA. To understand an economic evaluation. Can Med Assoc J 1984;130:1428–33.
88. Stoddard GL, Drummond MF. How to read clinical journals: VIIB. To understand an economic evaluation. Can Med Assoc J 1984;130:1542–49.
89. Soloniuk L, McPeek B. Do the pluses outweigh the minuses? Theor Surg 1988;2:209–14.
90. Pineault R, Contandriopoulous AP, Valois M, et al. Randomized clinical trial of one-day surgery: patient satisfaction, clinical outcomes, and costs. Med Care 1985;(23)2:171–82.
91. Hemenway D, Sherman H, Mudge GH Jr, et al. Comparative costs versus symptomatic and employment benefits of medical and surgical treatment of stable angina pectoris. Med Care, 1985;23:133–41.
92. Boyle MH, Torrance GW. Developing multiattribute health indexes. Med Care 1984;22:1045–57.
93. Boyle MH, Torrance GW, Sinclair JC, Horwood SP. Economic evaluation of neonatal intensive care of very-low birth-weight infants. N Engl J Med 1983;308:1330–37.
94. Harwood SP, Boyle MH, Torrance GW, Sinclair JC. Mortality and morbidity of 500–1499-gram birth weight infants live-born to residents of a defined geographic region before and after neonatal intensive care. Pediatrics 1982;69:613–20.
95. Bunker JP, Barnes BA, Mosteller F, eds. Costs, Risks and Benefits of Surgery. New York: Oxford University Press, 1977.
96. Aaron HJ, Schwartz WB. The Painful Prescription. Washington DC: Brookings Institute, 1984.
97. McLachlin G, Maynard A, eds. The Public/Private Mix for Health: The Relevance and Effects of Change. London: Nuffield Provincial Hospital Trust, 1982.
98. Leape LL. Unnecessary surgery. Health Serv Res 1989;24:351–407.
99. Detmer DE, Buchanan-Davidson DJ. Ambulatory surgery. In: Socioeconomics of Surgery, Rutkow, IM, ed. Toronto: Mosby, 1989:31–50.
100. Natof H. Complications associated with ambulatory surgical centers. JAMA 1980;244:92.
101. Davis JE. The need to redefine levels of surgical care. JAMA 1984;251:2527–28.
102. LoGerfo J. Organizational and financial influences on patterns of care. Surg Clin N Am 1982;62: 677–83.
103. Davies AR, Ware JE Jr, Brook RH, Peterson JR, Newhouse JP. Consumer acceptance of prepaid and fee-for-service medical care: results from a ran-

domized controlled trial. Health Serv Res 1986; 21:429.
104. Ware JE Jr, Brook RH, Rogers WH, et al. Comparison of health outcomes at a health maintenance organization with those of fee-for-service care. Lancet 1986;1:1017.
105. Wagner EH, Bledscoe T. The Rand Health Insurance Experiment and HMOs. Med Care 1990;28: 191-200.
106. Mechanic D. Cost containment and the quality of medical care: rationing strategies in an era of constrained resources. Milbank Mem Fund Q Health Soc 1985;63:453-75.
107. Ermann D, Gabel J. The changing face of American health care: multihospital systems, emergency centers, and surgery centers. Med Care 1985;23: 401-20.
108. Munoz E. Impact of Diagnosis Related Groups and the Prospective Payment Assessment Commission. In: Socioeconomics of Surgery, Rutkow IM, ed. Toronto: Mosby, 1989:109-31.
109. Horn SD, Ashworth MA. Adjusting DRGs for severity of illness. In: Socioeconomics of Surgery, Rutkow IM, ed. Toronto: Mosby, 1989:133-41.
110. Luft HS, Bunker JP, Enthoven AC. Should operations be regionalized? The empirical relationship between surgical volume and mortality. N Engl J Med 1979;301:1364-69.
111. Luft HS. The relationship between surgical volume and mortality. An exploration of causal factors and alternative models. Med Care 1980;18:940-59.
112. Luft HS, Hunt SS. Identifying hospitals for the regionalization of care. In: Surgical Care in the United States: A Policy Perspective, Finkel ML, ed. Baltimore: Johns Hopkins University Press, 1988:144-58.
113. Farber BF, Kaiser DL, Wenzel RP. Relation between surgical volume and incidence of post-operative wound infection. N Engl J Med 1981;305:200-4.
114. Dyck FJ, Murphy FA, Murphy JK, et al. Effect of surveillance on the number of hysterectomies in the province of Saskatchewan. N Engl J Med 1977; 296:1326-28.
115. Brook RH, Williams KA, Rolph JE. Controlling the use and cost of medical service. The New Mexico Experimental Care Review Organization: a four year case study. Med Care 1978;16(Suppl) 9:1-76.
116. Donabedian A. Explorations in Quality Assurance and Monitoring, Vol I. The Definition of Quality and Approaches to its Assessment. Ann Arbor, MI: Health Administration Press, 1980.
117. Donabedian A. Explorations in Quality Assurance and Monitoring, Vol II. The Criteria and Standards of Quality. Ann Arbor, MI: Health Administration Press, 1980.
118. Williamson JW, Hudson JI, Nevins MM. Principles of Quality Assurance and Cost Containment in Health Care: A Guide for Medical Students, Residents, and other Health Professionals. San Francisco: Jossey Bass, 1982.
119. Williamson JW, Barr DM, Fee E, et al. Teaching Quality Assurance and Cost Containment in Health Care: A Faculty Guide. San Francisco: Jossey Bass, 1982.
120. Boyd DR. Comprehensive regional trauma and emergency medical service delivery systems: a goal of the 1980s. Crit Care Q 1982;5:1-21.

31

Health Policy Research: A Surgical Perspective

H.B. Devlin

Professor Francis Moore has divided surgical research into three classical phases: the *discovery* of a new bioscience fact or process of some importance for surgical care; the development of this fundamental scientific fact (the applied biotechnical improvement so familiar to academic surgeons); and finally, the *delivery component* of this advance by all clinical surgeons, which often necessitates changes in the modes of surgical care offered to individual patients and the population in general. Elsewhere in this book research methods relevant to the discovery and development phases of surgery are reviewed. In this chapter we concern ourselves with the delivery of surgical care, how it can and should be monitored, and how the quality of surgical and anaesthetic care can be assured. No matter what our perspective is, we must accept the societal implications of surgery; economists, politicians, sociologists, jurists, and the man in the street all have cogent views of our surgical activities. These extra dimensions are approached hesitantly by many surgeons. The once almighty surgical decision maker is today relegated to a role subsidiary to the health care planner or the funding organization; but unless we reassert our role and research health care delivery for ourselves, others, nonsurgeons and nonsympathetic to our ideals, will invade our demesne and determine the future of surgery for us.

Contrary to the impression conveyed in textbooks and the perception of the public, surgical care is clouded by uncertainty. Surgery has developed, as has all science, by trial and error, by inductive and deductive reasoning, and sometimes by chance or serendipity. These uncertainties are reflected in the many aspects of the surgeon's work: Which patients should be referred for bladder neck surgery? How should this wound be closed? Which prophylactic antibiotic should be given? What range of movement should the patient expect after this arthroplasty? And so on. All these questions are reflected by disagreements among surgeons about their answers. While we surgeons rationalize these disagreements and regard them as part of the kaleidoscope of our professional life, to the administrator they represent resource shifts or problems of unmet need, danger zones for the politicians and economists who determine our activities.

The components of health care delivery can be divided into the *access* to care (structure)—who gets to the clinic, who gets treatment, and who gets the *operation*; the *process* of care, to include all the pre-, peri- and post-operative management by surgeon and anesthetist, and the *outcome*, which is the final and most difficult component to measure. When the alternative to surgery was death, "no death" was an excellent outcome and easy to measure; today, in the Western world, the crude death rate for elective surgery is less than 1%, so death from surgery is very rare. Indeed, in some surgical specialties—dental surgery and cosmetic surgery, for instance—postoperative deaths are unknown. Measuring death as a sole outcome is clearly no longer appropriate to modern surgery.

While surgeons go for an accurate diagnosis, a neat operation and no post-operative complications again the manager or politician has a different perspective. They equate process with efficiency and currently apply cost containment to promote this.

Having rehearsed the scenario within which Health Policy Research operates we can eyeball some key contributions and identify horizons which need urgent research attention and redefinition if we are to push back the frontiers of surgical practice.

Access

Throughout the developed world rates of surgical operations vary enormously. Even within the United Kingdom, with the universal provision of the National Health Service and where the population is demographically homogenous, rates of surgical intervention vary in different locations.

Studies of the international variation in rates of surgical operations have attracted much epidemiological interest, sadly this academic interest has not caught on with surgeons. Tonsillectomy and adenoidectomy are performed twice as often in the United States than in the United Kingdom; cholecystectomy is three times as common in Canada than in the United Kingdom with the United States in an intermediate position. Hysterectomy shows the widest international variation, the rate for the United States being 700 per 100,000 population at risk while the rate for Norway is 100 per 100,000. The United Kingdom occupies the middle ground at 250 per 100,000. It is unlikely that these variations in operation rates reflect a difference incidence of disease; it is much more likely that they reflect different perceptions of the indications for operation and clearly, if each surgical operation has to be justified for conferring some benefit on the patient, there is clearly a large measure of confusion about the definition of "benefit" employed by surgeons here. It has been suggested that high rates of operation (e.g., for cholecystectomy) may confer a negative benefit on the patients and population by generating unnecessary perioperative deaths and morbidity and by consuming resources that could more usefully be employed elsewhere.

Various factors have been suggested to explain these variations: different population morbidity is an obvious explanation. On the other hand, the supply side of medicine, the availability of surgeons, is said to contribute to higher operation rates. Financial incentives to surgery are most frequently suggested, with the evidence of higher rates of surgery in the United States, where there is item-for-service payment compared with the United Kingdom; but this explanation cannot be entirely true, for there are wide variations in operation rates—for example, hysterectomy within Massachussetts and elsewhere in North America. Clearly these differences in operation rates ("small-area variations") reflect different indications for surgery by surgeons in different localities, hence a different case mix of patients have surgery. Surgeons are used to comparing their results with those of colleagues, but differences of case mix of these magnitudes may well invalidate critical comparison of techniques and outcomes. There is much space for surgical research into these problems.

Apart from the operation rates, studying of access to surgical care throws up other issues: the location of surgical facilities, logistics, and economics of entitlement to an operating table space are among these. The opportunity costs of doing one operation rather than another are a major issue in today's economic climate.

These are questions of great relevance to the provision of surgical care and are legitimate areas of surgical inquiry.

Process

Process includes all the clinical and administrative stages through which the patient must progress to receive surgical care and a satisfactory relief from disease or injury. We include here consideration of the adequacy of initial assessment, clinical resuscitation, operative technique, postoperative care, and rehabilitation. Surgical technical expertise in the operating room, the prevention of sepsis and pulmonary embolism, and postoperative managing of comorbidities are just a few features that must be considered under the process heading. Surprisingly these clinical features of surgical practice reveal the greatest uncertainties, one though will remind every visceral surgeon that 30% of appendixes removed surgically are normal, this figure rises to 45% when the patient group considered is young women. The leak rate for colon anastomoses varies from 0.5% to 30% in a survey of the best British surgical practice, but this statement requires expanding: when the leak rate is 0.5%, the duration of inpatient stay was 25.4 days and the perioperative death rate 7.1%; surgeons reporting a leak rate exceeding >30% reported a mean duration of stay of 45.7 days and a perioperative death rate of 22.0%. These "surgeon-related variables" have dramatic consequences for the patient and the provider of health care and are now a legitimate area of political interest. They should interest surgeons, too.

The behaviorial aspects of surgical care, communication with the patient and his family, and advice regarding future life style and employment are measurable indices of patient care. The "good bedside manner" of yesteryear has been replaced by the "patient satisfaction index." Although cultural norms vary from country to country, civility in clinical practice is a universal jewel in our medical ethic. Patient satisfaction is the ultimate validator of a clinical intervention. Despite serious interest in patient satisfaction, there are considerable methodological difficulties to be overcome, and in neither the American nor the British literature has any standardization yet been settled. Marketing surveys are frequently used in the commercial world, and this approach undoubtedly has relevance for medicine.

Outcome

Traditionally, outcome has been most easily measured estimate of surgical endeavor. The worst outcome in surgery has always been death. Measurements of mortality rates have been a traditional benchmark for surgeons marketing a new operation. However, mortality rates are no longer relevant in most surgical practice. In the United Kingdom, the overall perioperative mortality rate for all surgery (emergency and elective), all specialties included, was 1.5% for 1985. No deaths are ever recorded in association with elective dental surgery and elective cosmetic surgery. Other specialties, other than acute neurosurgery, neonatal cardiac surgery, and vascular surgery, have death rates so low that a postoperative mortality is a very rare event. Although death is rare and can probably be discarded as a surgical indicator when large samples of surgical processes are sought, then aggregated and analyzed, high death rates, long durations of stay, high sepsis, and complication rates seem to cluster geographically—around one surgeon? One team? One hospital? We don't know which. We do however know, or the data strongly suggest, that outcome after surgery is related to surgeon training, to the volume of the operation the surgeon undertakes regularly, and to the management structure of the hospital. What is beyond dispute is that the well-trained surgeon who keeps himself up-to-date and participates in continuing education—who undertakes the operation regularly and works in an institution where the clinicians have a significant role in the hospital management—will achieve significantly better outcomes than one who does not.

Outcome measurement, now that we can no longer use death as an indicator, is a very vexed topic. "Quality of life" is an obvious concept, but there are many uncertainties in its measurement. These are discussed elsewhere in this book. It is suggested that multiplying indices of quality of life by years survived after therapy, a Quality-Adjusted Life Years (QALYS) index offers a way forward. Surgeons criticize the use of psychological or social parameters to measure outcomes after operation, but many of our own technical ways of comparing surgical outcomes involve intangible value-ridden concepts; the classical Visick scale for post-gastric surgery is an example. So we must not lightly dismiss the attempts of behaviorial scientists to assist in this process of refinement of outcome measures.

The development of universally applicable outcome measured after surgical intervention, indeed after any medical intervention, is a matter of urgency, and we would hope that research workers in many disciplines will address this problem urgently.

Changing the ground slightly, we are faced in surgical science with some major philosophical problems if we are to optimize our contribution to human well-being. No longer are surgeons at the cutting edge of medical science, no longer are we the lonely leaders in medicine. Today, no longer are we all Billroths or Halsteds. Medicine has changed. Science is now led by molecular biologists or biochemists; but surgeons have an important role in alleviating human distress. In today's world distress is unacceptable, health is perceived as a human right, and all physicians and politicians are inevitably involved in the delivery of health. Health is a universal commodity.

As the structure of society changes, we must question how we surgeons should provide our skills; should they be sold to patients, or distributed according to patients' ability to pay? Or is there a societal obligation to provide care for all? How much surgery? And for whom? Features on the agenda. Where does our professional ethic place us within this philosophical debate?

Clearly, we must optimize our use of finite resources, but how should this optimization be achieved? And how do we measure it?

Within the United Kingdom we have traveled some way down each of these roads. Since the 1930's we have had the Confidential Enquiry into Maternal Mortality. This inquiry has reviewed all maternal deaths throughout this period and published triennial reports that have signposted new directions for obstetric care. The Confidential Enquiry is nationally based and has led to an improvement in obstetric management and obstetric anesthesia. Its approach is elitist: peers review the management of each dead patient; they identify any clinical and administrative shortcomings, and then set guidelines designed to bring the best medical care to benefit all mothers. We have also developed similar Confidential Enquiries into Perinatal Mortality, which are regionally based and use a similar form of peer review to judge standards of care of the newborn; again, these studies draw conclusions and publish recommendations that are virtually mandatory standards.

Anesthetic morbidity and mortality have been reviewed with staggering improvements in anesthetic mortality over the years. Credit for the study of anesthetic mortality rightly rests with the American Henry Beecher. Beecher and Todd[1] in 1954 reported an anesthetic mortality of 1:1560 anesthetics; subsequent anesthetic studies have documented how this has improved – 1:10,000 mortality reported by Lunn and Mushin[2] in 1982. Most recently the Confidential Enquiry into Perioperative Deaths[3] has investigated deaths associated with surgery and anesthesia in three regions of England and found the incidence of avoidable deaths associated with anesthesia to be 1:185,000.

The Confidential Enquiry into Perioperative Deaths (CEPOD, now the National CEPOD) is a significant advance in the search for quality assurance in surgical and anesthetic practice. The first prerequisite for this exercise was the development of foolproof, litigation-resistant rules of confidentiality so that even the most sensitive areas of clinical practice could be investigated without the risk of malpractice litigation against the individual surgeon or anesthetist. Such legal protection had to be obtained at the highest level of government within the United Kingdom.

CEPOD investigated deaths occurring within 30 days of a surgical intervention in three National Health Service regions; 4034 deaths were reported (there were 485,580 operations performed), and 83% of these deaths were fully investigated by a peer group of surgical and anesthetic "assessors." The overall crude death rate was 0.7%. Most deaths occurred in elderly patients, 70% of deaths occurring in patients aged >70 years old; 30% of all deaths were due to the progress of the initially presenting surgical disease (e.g., cancer or atherosclerosis), but 30% of deaths were related to suboptimal surgical performance and 2% to suboptimal anesthetic performance. Surgical failure was the sole cause of one death for every 2860 operations performed; anesthetic failure accounted for one death in 185,056 anesthetics.

The Confidential Enquiry into Perioperative Deaths has now been extended to include England, Wales, Northern Ireland, the UK defense services and the private sector in the United Kingdom. National CEPOD has devised a more rigid mode of peer review by using paired controls and randomly selected samples from practices in all surgical specialties. NCEPOD published its first report in June 1990 and reviewed the care of children by surgeons.[4] Only 0.2% of consultants have failed to participate in this exercise. Again the problems associated with low volume surgical operators have been identified and recommendations to improve the surgical and anesthetic care of children made.

Studies of clinical practice or audits require the participants to record routine data about their practice. These data are then compared with similar data from other institutions and the results subjected to independent peer review. The results of this peer review are relayed back to the participating clinicians. The completion of this individual "feedback" leads to alteration and improvement in practice. Apart from this specific feedback, the regular collection and appreciation of clinical data beneficially alters practice – the Hawthorne effect. National studies allow large samples to be recruited; this allows small differences to be identified with confidence, an important issue when complications are infrequent.

Audit of clinical practice requires tact and sensitivity. Clearly protection of the individual patient, alive or dead, and particularly protection of the relatives and interests of the dead, should be a prime objective. A close second in importance is protection of the anonymity and good standing of the clinicians being audited. Down the line the hospital and the community it serves must be protected from unwarranted condemnation, though how far the protection must be extended to protect the frankly bad performer is an issue as yet unaddressed. Is there a public right to know? Should the audit process include some professional duty to protect the public interest? By disbarring abberant individuals from practice?

For audit to be successful, there must be commitment by all the participants – by the clinicians to supply the data and by the scrutinizers to review it dispassionately and fairly. National studies depersonalize data collection and thereby assist compliance and confidentiality. Most important, the feedback mechanism must be able to address the clinical problems that are identified.

The funders and providers of health care also have a legitimate interest in the quality of surgeons' activities. The use of administrative and clinical data aggregated by computer have highlighted the many ambiguities and confusions in surgeon behavior and operation outcomes. Administrators and politicians have a legitimate interest in these, though how far surgical policy should be driven by each of these factors and by the funders of the system is a question of importance to all surgeons.

Quality, quality assurance, and the inevitable sting in the tail, recertification, are issues that confront surgeons. The response must come from us. Major research into requirements for efficient surgery and into outcomes after surgery are needed. We now have the technical tools to resolve many of these problems – modern computers will handle almost infinite amounts of data. Audit and peer review are today a necessity. Every surgeon must seek to optimize his results. At the unit and hospital surgeons should cooperate to achieve improved outcomes. Multiparticipant exercises and national audits need designing and pursuing if some of the pressing problems are to be solved. But we surgeons are inhibited by our history of individuality and the surgeon-related variables that still haunt our profession. Nonetheless, we must embrace research into the socioeconomics of practice and undertake clinical audit; if we do not, others will do these tasks for us.

References

1. Beecher HK, Todd DP. A study of the deaths associated with anesthesia and surgery based on a study of 599,548 anesthesias in 10 institutions 1948–1952, inclusive. Annals of Surgery 1954;140:2–35.
2. Lunn JN, Mushin WW. Mortality associated with anesthesia. London: Nuffield Provincial Hospitals Trust, 1982.
3. Buck N, Devlin HB, Lunn JN. The Report of a Confidential Enquiry into Perioperative Deaths. London: Nuffield Provincial Hospitals Trust and the King's Fund, 1987.
4. Campling EA, Devlin HB, Lunn JN. Report of the National Confidential Enquiry into Perioperative Deaths. London: Royal College of Surgeons, 1990.

Additional Reading

Devlin HB, Professional audit: quality control: keeping up to date. Balliere's Clin anaesthesiol 1988;2:299–324. A comprehensive literature review that includes all the instances cited in this chapter.

Hann C, ed. Health Care Variations. London: the King's Fund, 1988.

The Report of a Confidential Enquiry into Perioperative Deaths. N Buck, HB Devlin, JN Lunn, The Nuffield Provincial Hospitals Trust and the King's Fund, London 1987.

Jolly D. L'hôpital de XXIe siècle. Paris: Economica, 1988.

Rutkow IM, ed. The Socioeconomics of Surgery. St. Louis: Mosby, 1989.

Audit and the quality of clinical care. College and Faculty Bulletin: Supplement to the Annals. pp 3–14. Ann Roy Coll Surg Engl 1990;i:72.

32

Technology Assessment

J.S. Barkun, A.N. Barkun, D.S. Mulder, and R.N. Battista

"...It is difficult enough when one's therapeutic management is based on nothing more than the memories of personal experiences because it is important to realize how fallacious some of these memories can be... because what a cautious person calls "sometimes" is "often" or even "always" to the overly enthusiastic, and "seldom" or "never" to the overly sceptic."

Theodor Billroth, 1898

The twentieth century has witnessed tremendous changes in all aspects of medicine. The industrial revolution and the postwar boom have reinforced the technical aspects of medicine. The practice of surgery is increasingly modulated by the appearance of new technologies. Indeed, different imaging modalities have emerged in the past decade, including computerized tomographic and magnetic resonance imaging, as well as the several diagnostic tools provided by nuclear medicine. In addition, ultrasound is increasingly used, not only for diagnostic purposes, but also as a therapeutic tool in draining abdominal abscesses, and even in breaking up gallbladder and common bile duct stones. The multiple applications of laser technology have also expanded in a great variety of surgical disciplines.

These new developments will continue to influence the delivery of health care at all levels, and consequently to alter the distribution of medical manpower and the burden of primary clinical responsibilities. Although these emerging technologies will not obviate the need for many surgical procedures, some operations may disappear as less invasive and possibly more effective techniques become available. Surgeons increasingly are turning to adjuvant techniques such as endoscopy, laparoscopic surgery, and lasers, anticipating that these may complement or even replace more traditional approaches to the treatment of surgical conditions. Likewise, radiologists have successfully applied the skills they initially developed in diagnostic ultrasound and computed tomography to treat both medical and surgical patients. Certain specialties will develop a particular expertise in emerging technologies, and this will help to shape the face of medicine in the next century.

In parallel to these exciting new developments, policy makers and politicians worry about the rising costs of medical care. As a consequence, we hear an increasing number of pleas for a careful evaluation of the efficacy, effectiveness, and efficiency of these new techniques.[1-4] This trend toward a more formal assessment of new technologies in health care gives rise to a more delicate task of reevaluating already existing technologies. National and regional governing bodies, as well as academic organizations devoted to technology assessment, have emerged and are helping to establish and consolidate vital links between clinicians and policy makers. Although we all welcome the new developments in technology, developers as well as the potential users, the health care professionals must become much more critical before accepting new tools in medicine's expanding black bag.

Health professionals, after several decades of resistance to the idea of rationalization, are now becoming its prime movers. We all want to put novel approaches into practice if we can clearly establish that they will replace more cumbersome, less effective, and less efficient alternatives. The combination of innovations and the need to justify their introduction as replacements for traditional approaches will have a determining impact on the shaping of modern medicine. Thus, beyond the establishment of the efficacy, effectiveness, and efficiency of a given technology, we see a mounting need for a clear definition of criteria for utilization, which could then determine its use in the practice of surgery.

Technology assessment can be viewed as an integrative exercise aimed at establishing state of the art knowledge of a specific technology with a view to shaping policy recommendations concerning its adoption and utilization in practice. Hence, technology assessment is the necessary link between health science and health policy.

Technology assessment draws on information generated by research studies, pursues the ultimate synthesis and critical appraisal of this information, and culminates in a policy recommendation concerning the diffusion of a given technology. Given the comprehensive nature of this exercise, technology assessment in surgery will integrate several of the concepts and approaches discussed in greater depth in other chapters of this book. We shall describe the several steps involved in this all-encompassing activity that bridges the gap between surgical science and surgical practice. Several examples will illustrate our discussion, and the case of cholelithotripsy in particular will be presented in more detail.

Generating Science

The far-reaching process of technology assessment starts with the necessary generation of scientific information on different aspects of a technology, including efficacy (Does the technology work in ideal circumstances?), effectiveness (Does the technology work under real-life conditions?), efficiency (If the technology works, what is the relationship between the benefits and the costs of this technology?), safety, acceptability, availability, and ethical considerations.

Efficacy and Effectiveness

The assessment of the efficacy and effectiveness of surgical procedures is certainly the first step in any overall assessment. Indeed, we would not consider introducing a surgical procedure if it did not work, or if it did not produce more good than harm. As discussed elsewhere in the book, different designs are available to conduct these efficacy and effectiveness studies.

The randomized controlled trial is our most powerful research tool to answer the fundamental question of whether any intervention is beneficial. Important features of randomized clinical trials are discussed in Section II, Chapter 14. One of the best-known surgical examples of a randomized controlled trial, the National Surgical Adjuvant Breast Project trial, compared modified radical mastectomy to segmental resection and radiotherapy in the treatment of localized breast cancer and its recurrence.[5] This study led to a new and less aggressive therapeutic approach to the condition (see Chapter 26).

Randomization may not always seem feasible for different ethical and logistical reasons. When randomization is not desired, if the investigators can control the allocation of the surgical procedure to different groups of individuals, they can perform a clinical trial without randomization. For example, consider a study in which the question relates to the incidence of recurrent hernias following two different herniorrhaphy techniques. At institution A, all patients included in the study would be treated with the Bassini method, and all patients at institution B would be treated using the Shouldice Clinic method. The patients could be matched for age, sex, and body size. In this example, although the interventions would be overseen and controlled by the investigators, patient accrual into each group would not, as it would depend on the hospital in which the patient is operated on, and there would be no randomization. In this case, the equalization of the groups with respect to possible confounding factors will be more difficult to achieve and will necessitate an important conceptual effort from the investigators. (Of course, even if later readers of such a trial's published reports were to accept that the treatment groups were initially similar, they may not be willing to ascribe outcome differences to differences between the two types of herniorraphy. Perhaps the surgeons or the anesthetists were more skillful in institution A?)

When neither randomization nor allocation of the intervention under investigation is possible, other designs can still be used to give information about the efficacy and effectiveness of a procedure (non-experimental designs) (see Section II, Chapter 13). Using the same clinical example as above, a cohort study to assess the better herniorrhaphy technique would investigate patients divided into two groups determined by the type of hernia repair to be performed. After surgery, all patients would be followed over time and recurrence rates in each group compared. Perhaps a case-control study might look at patients with recurrent hernias following any repair and retrospectively assess which patient had been treated by which surgical technique. Clearly, as we move farther away from the randomized clinical trial, the internal validity of a study is more difficult to ensure as control of biases and confounding factors will be harder to achieve. (Later, readers of published reports may be even more skeptical of study's findings.)

In each of the aforementioned study designs, there is a comparison group. This is not so for cross-sectional studies, case series, and case studies. Although the absence of a comparison group severely limits their usefulness, in rare cases, especially if the benefit is obvious and of a large magnitude, these designs can provide useful information.

A recent example of such a case study was the publication of the first insertion of the "artificial heart." A single treated patient was enough to illustrate the limitations of this technology from effectiveness, ethical, and social perspectives.[6]

One example of the use of a case series, and there are many, was the introduction of the Ramstedt-Fredet pyloromyotomy in infants with hypertrophic pyloric stenosis. Although it has never been formally tested against conservative treatment alone, the drastic improvement in prognosis of these infants following the introduction of the procedure has been accepted by most observers as sufficient evidence of its efficacy and effectiveness.[7]

The case series remains a commonly used design in surgery. At a surgical congress in 1990, the Society of American Gastroenterological Endoscopic Surgeons meeting in Atlanta, more than 90% of all abstracts presented were based on data from series of cases. After a review of structured reports published in the *New England Journal of Medicine* and *The Lancet* over a recent 6-month period, Feinstein found that up to 15% of all articles fell into this category.[8] The popularity of the use of case series is attributable to a number of factors: the false belief that historical control groups are often adequate; the ethical dilemma stemming from a prejudice that the new, unproven technology is "best"; the fact that absence of a true control group allows for a greater number of subjects to receive the "wonderful" new intervention; and the desire to publish quickly as a result of peer pressure. Because of their inherent limitations, case studies and case series are most useful for the generation of hypotheses rather than the assessment of efficacy and effectiveness.

Up to this point, we have described a number of design methods; their strengths and weaknesses were covered in previous chapters. However, a number of limitations in the selection of these methods to generate data on efficacy relate to their application to surgery rather than to any intrinsic methodological characteristic. We will now address certain of these aspects as they specifically pertain to surgical studies. A number of points relate to the nature of the procedures themselves: surgical procedures are often irreversible (e.g. in the case of organ ablation) and, unlike most medical randomized controlled trials, once an operation has been performed, there often cannot be patient crossover from one group to another. A paired study using a surgical patient as his own control can, therefore, never be undertaken. Note that this, in a sense, seems to be an infringement on patients' rights as defined in the Declaration of Helsinki.[9]

Furthermore, differences in the levels of technical skill of the operator (performance bias[10]), or patient morphology, may significantly alter outcome or be a source of selection bias. For example, racial differences in patient morphology may limit the external validity of a study, as hypothesized from Oriental series on gastric cancer operations. Technical considerations of such a lean population can differ from a North American series, which would include many more obese patients.

For many new surgical techniques to achieve optimal performance, investigators must learn the new procedures. Investigators and study designs must address this learning curve issue to allow for a more precise and fairer assessment of efficacy and effectiveness.

We cannot blind investigators or patients to the presence of a scar, since sham operations are usually not ethically acceptable.

Some study limitations in modern surgery pertain to outcome measures: unlike many drug trials, long-term follow-up is often required and difficult to document. Moreover, in the light of improved surgical and anesthetic techniques, the occurrence of traditional outcomes such as morbidity and mortality is often so low that the detection of significant rate differences between study groups becomes difficult (insufficient power of the study). Outcome scale or scores may be used.[11] Other, more sensitive endpoints such as aesthetic results and measures of quality of life are introduced.[12]

There may be difficulties that pertain to specific ethical, philosophical, and legal aspects involving the practice of surgery. Treatment bias (the tendency in medicine to opt for intervention in the natural course of disease) is very prominent in surgery because of the nature of surgical thinking.

In addition, surgical teaching in many countries is carried out by apprenticeship, which makes the application of randomized controlled trials more difficult. Surgeons may fear that patients will view true informed consent as evidence of indecisiveness on the part of an unsure operator. Some surgeons fear this will hinder the surgeon-patient relationship.[13,14]

Last, in contradistinction to drug trials, surgeons fear a tendency to attribute all side effects of a surgical intervention to the surgeon, thus making the operator more prone to liability.[13]

Efficiency

Once we have documented the efficacy and effectiveness of an intervention, the notion of resources invested to achieve a level of effectiveness becomes important. Different techniques can assess the efficiency of procedures; they depend on the availability of outcome information, and the units in which the investigators wish the comparisons to be made.[15-17] In comparing two procedures, if their effectiveness is similar, we can perform a "cost minimization" analysis, to ask a single question, Which procedure carries the least cost? One example could be the comparison of hospital-use-generated costs for inpatient and ambulatory surgery herniorrhaphy.

If the effectiveness between two procedures is different or thought to be possibly different, we then select a "cost-effectiveness" analysis. We compare interventions in terms of their respective costs per unit of common effectiveness. Imagine a comparison of laparoscopic and conventional cholecystectomy, where the unit of effectiveness would relate to the length of postoperative disability before the patient can return to active employment. Typically the amount of postoperative disability saved by the use of a laparoscopic, instead of a muscle splitting approach, would be compared on the basis of "cost (of the procedure) per day of occupational disability."

Cost-benefit comparisons examine the costs and benefits in monetary terms. We often restrict this type of analysis to comparing technologies with outcomes or units of effectiveness that are different—for example, the institution of a preoperative antibiotic side effect prevention program versus the purchase of an intraoperative hepatic ultrasonographic unit. We attempt to convert the amount of prevented morbidity from the prevention program into dollars and compare it to the dollar value attributed to the number of days of prolonged life due to the increase in early metastatic tumor liver resections. Yet, how can one properly assign arbitrary monetary value to such disparate outcomes? Also, how will the analysis take into account secondary future benefits that will result from the acquisition of a still developing technology? One can easily see the multiple difficulties involved in the application of a cost-benefit analysis. The truth is, cost-benefit studies entail serious difficulties when policies with widely different benefits are compared, despite the theoretical possibility of reducing both costs and benefits to the same monetary unit.

We sometimes convert units of effectiveness into quality-adjusted life years (QALY), to assess the level of health status and its effect on the patient's life. For example, consider the development of an epileptogenic cerebral scar following craniotomy for benign disease in a desk clerk and in a commercial airline pilot. Whereas the former could well pursue his normal activities and thus give his potential disability a low score (say a 2 out of 10), the latter would be unable to resume his profession and thus would likely report a higher disability score (say a 7 out of 10). This is an example of the use of "utility" units of analysis. Transforming units of effectiveness into units of utility constitutes a "cost-utility" analysis.

Safety, Availability, Acceptability, and Ethical Considerations

In assessing a surgical technique, broad safety specifications pertaining to the use of this technology need to be documented. In effect, we must clearly establish the potential risks to all involved in using a given technology. Practical aspects of availability and accessibility of this technology should be considered. Finally, we need to establish ethical considerations pertaining to the use or nonuse of a given procedure.

We must generate clear and valid information on all these aspects of a surgical procedure in any technology assessment exercise.

Synthesizing Information and Formulating Recommendations

We try to use a number of studies and sources to develop information on the different aspects of a given technology. Synthesizing this information by combining the results from different studies is the next important step in any overall technology assessment effort. The well-known (simple) review of the literature is one approach that uses a qualitative assessment of available evidence.

Critical appraisal of the scientific literature increasingly involves the use of quantitative approaches to combine information: one example is "overview analysis" (often referred to as meta-analysis) (see Section II, Chapter 9).[18,19] "Decision-analytic" approaches combine information from research studies to determine the preferred courses of action in given situations. We use these to summarize information and determine the best alternatives.[20] An example would be a recent meta-analysis confirming the harm of portacaval shunting in the prophylactic treatment of esophageal varices in regards to bleeding.[21]

Specifically mandated task forces, consensus conferences, or technology assessment councils all represent formal attempts to synthesize the state of knowledge with respect to health-related technology. When critically appraising results from published studies, panels of experts meet to sift through a large amount of data to decide what is actually known about a given intervention. This process has become an intense area for research.[22,23] Such a group must agree on some rules of evidence that will enable them to examine existing information and reach a consensual decision on the appropriateness of introducing or keeping a given technology. A possible approach used by different task forces has been to grade the level of evidence according to the strength of the design used to assess efficacy and effectiveness.[24] In this classification, of course, the randomized clinical trial constitutes the highest level of evidence, followed by a nonrandomized clinical trial, a trial with so-called historical controls, cohort studies, case-control studies, and finally cross-sectional studies, case series, and case studies, as well as expert opinions. The consensus process enables the panel to further integrate all the pieces of information provided by the studies with additional factors that would be less quantifiable, such as ethical and logistical considerations. The panel finally formulates recommendations as to whether a given procedure is fit for diffusion (see Section IV, Chapter 53.)

Implementation of Practice: Recommendations and Diffusion of Surgical Technologies

The ultimate aim of technology assessment is to provide decision makers with the necessary information to enable them to take action and implement a given recommendation.[25] The decision makers can be individual clinicians, health administrators, politicians, or the public at large. All these actors could certainly use the results of technology assessment within their own spheres of activity. Clinicians could use this information in shaping their own clinical practice and deciding on specific criteria for utilization of a given procedure. Health administrators could use the information to decide on a global policy for diffusion of a given technology, determining, for example, the number of computerized tomographic (CT) scanners that should become available in a region or a country. In effect, coordinated actions by all interested participants will minimize tensions between groups pursuing different objectives.

Quality Assessment and Quality Assurance of Surgical Care

Once technology assessment recommendations have become policy decisions for diffusion and specific criteria for patterns of practice, we need to monitor quality of practice and to ensure compliance with practice guidelines.[26,27] We call this "process evaluation." It occurs at many levels, ranging from the government to clinicians themselves at mortality and morbidity rounds. The objective is to compare the practice in use with practice guidelines derived from the overall technology assessment exercise. The evaluative process may apply to patterns of practice, programs, or institutions. In any case, the different levels the evaluator(s) report to may include governing or licensing bodies, institutional boards of directors, department heads, or peer review groups. The evaluation goals should be clear and explicit from the outset; yet not infrequently they are implicit, hidden, and different from the presumed intent (so-called "pseudoevaluation").

The assessment of a technique, therefore, involves many different levels, which become important as the process matures in the scientific, clinical, and sociopolitical settings.

We now trace the different steps of such a technological assessment by taking the example of extracorporeal shock wave lithotripsy, or cholelithotripsy, a new technology for treatment of gallstones. Since the status of common bile duct stone lithotripsy is entirely different,[28] for the sake of brevity, we will discuss gallbladder stones only.

Gallbladder Stone Lithotripsy

Following Langenbuch's original report, cholecystectomy has been the treatment of choice for patients with gallbladder stones for more than 100 years.[29] With the advent of modern operative techniques, overall mortality in the elective setting is about 0.5% with morbidity approximating 4%.[30,31]

Disadvantages of elective cholecystectomy, one of the two most common surgical procedure in the United States today, include the need for a general anesthetic, a hospital stay that averages about 6 days, the resultant surgical scar, and a postcholecystectomy period of convalescence that translates into a decrease in patients' quality of life, as well as a loss of function and sociofinancial productivity. Many nonoperative alternatives to cholecystectomy have recently been developed in the hope of obviating the need for surgical intervention and its associated convalescence. Extracorporeal shock wave lithotripsy (ESWL) has been one of the most widely publicized of these, since it avoids a laparotomy, may be performed with minimal pain, often in the outpatient setting, and is safe.

We discuss the example of ESWL as therapy for elective cholelithiasis because it highlights the difficulties encountered today in assessing a promising new technology amidst social, financial, and industrial pressures.

Efficacy

In vitro studies have shown that about 90% of all gallstones can be broken with ESWL, but "satisfactory" fragmentation[32] is achieved in only 35% of cases.[33,34] Stone size and number are the most important determinants of fragmentation and have led to the concept of "total stone burden." Thus the first set of clinical inclusion criteria: patients would be offered ESWL only if they carried solitary stones measuring 30 mm in diameter or less, or up to three radiolucent stones with a similar total stone mass.[35] The chemical stone composition does not appear to affect fragmentation,[33,34] but certain CT morphological criteria may be helpful[34] determinants.

Animal studies, as well as pathological human data, have shown that the propagation of shock waves through tissues leads to few histological changes using most machines.[36-39] In animal studies, minor hemorrhages were noted in the gallbladder, liver, and kidneys, and a few cases of significant lung hemorrhage have been reported.[40] These may, in part, be attributable to anatomic differences in the canine model.[36,38] Minor short-lived hematologic and biochemical abnormalities have been noted with the first-generation machines, but conditions have reverted to normal within 4 weeks following lithotripsy.[38]

Effectiveness

The first published clinical case series have used the above mentioned inclusion criteria and selected only patients with visualized gallbladders on oral cholecystography.[28,35] These data confirmed a selective fragmentation efficacy in which the patients most likely to benefit from ESWL are those with small (diameter $\leq$ 20 mm) and few (solitary) calculi. After satisfactory fragmentation has been achieved, 90% of patients are stone-free a year after ESWL if given adjuvant oral bile acid.[32] This result, however, is achieved in only 10% to 15% of patients who would originally present to a surgeon[41] with symptomatic gallstone disease as defined by the presence of biliary colic.[42,43] In other words, about 85% of patients with symptomatic gallstones are not candidates for this treatment modality. In the hope of broadening indications for lithotripsy, investigators have treated patients with more numerous, larger, and calcified stones[32,35,44] with limited efficacy. Adjuvant oral bile acid therapy has proven to be necessary both to decrease recurrence rates and to achieve more rapid dissolution of remaining stone fragments.[45] Side effects following the lithotripsy session are minor[28] and self-limited, and many have disappeared with the advent of second-generation machines. The use of second-generation lithotripters has permitted outpatient treatment under intravenous analgesia, if any, but has led to diminished fragmentation efficacy and a more frequent need for repeat treatment sessions.[28]

During the dissolution period, biliary colic is experienced by 35% of patients,[28] in contrast to an expected 69% over 2 years, as reported in the control group of the National Cooperative Gallstone Study.[46] Fragment migration has occasionally led to pancreatitis and cystic duct obstruction (1-2%), and over the next 18 months, 1% to 6% of patients have required cholecystectomy because of recurrent symptoms or acute cholecystitis.[28] There has been no reported mortality attributable to gallstone lithotripsy with more than 10,000 patients treated worldwide. Note that this technique, at present, is used only in the elective setting to treat patients who, for the most part, are young and otherwise healthy and therefore would be expected to experience minimal morbidity and near-negligible mortality following cholecystectomy.

Although case series suggest a benefit for highly selected patients, no comparative controlled trial have so far been published. As a consequence, the effectiveness of cholelithotripsy remains unproven, especially in comparison to cholecystectomy.

From the data above, one cannot help noticing how sorely controlled trials are needed; yet it is difficult to initiate a randomized controlled trial at this time for many reasons. The need to maintain institutional prestige and practical aspects of patient recruitment creates pressure to acquire a machine rapidly. In areas where the technique is accepted and widespread (such as in Europe) it would be difficult to get both patients and physicians to agree to randomizing subjects to a surgical procedure within the context of a trial of cholelithotripsy. For example, this is the case in Lyons, France, where three biliary lithotripters are available for a population of 1.2 million. On the other hand, in areas where the technique has not yet been implanted, advocates want to cumulate as many patients as possible to get approval for use of the lithotripter; or alternatively, local authorities and funding agencies decline to invest resources until more data on its applicability to patients with gallstones appear. This difficult state of affairs explains why only one group in the world so far has undertaken an evaluative assessment comparing biliary ESWL to cholecystectomy.[45]

Safety, Availability, Acceptability, and Ethical Considerations

Early reports from the Münich group suggest that the stone recurrence rate quickly levels off at 11% within 2 to 3 years following stone disappearance.[47] The persistence of a diseased gallbladder and the resultant risk of stone recurrence are perhaps the most important issues needing to be addressed, especially when dealing with young patients. The unknown teratogenic potential of oral bile acids in humans requires that women of child-bearing age practice some type of contraception during the stone dissolution period.[48] Although data are scarce, there is no evidence of harm being caused by the discontinuation of the oral dissolution therapy (only a slower stone disappearance rate).

Overall, ESWL and bile acids appear to be safe over the short term, but we have not investigated long-term complications. Recent very weak epidemiological data suggest an 8% rate of systemic hypertension in patients treated for renal stones with ESWL.[49] Only careful long-term follow-up will provide more interpretable evidence. Finally, since ESWL and oral bile acids do not preclude cholecystectomy, acceptability of this therapeutic alternative has been a problem.

Synthesizing Information and Making Recommendations

Biliary ESWL is widely used in Europe, where it has been the opinion of regulating bodies that efficacy has been proved with no prohibitive safety or ethical concerns. Regional financial and political considerations may have also played a role in reaching these conclusions quickly. For the reasons mentioned above, however, one cannot yet draw conclusions on the true effectiveness of this technique.

At present more than 80 centers in the United States are evaluating nine different lithotripter systems (Baillie J, Affronti J, personal communication). Regulations of the Food and Drug Administration will require for each to be tested on at least 300 patients with a 6-month follow-up. At the time of writing, no lithotripter had yet been approved for biliary use in the United States, and two machines recently had their applications rejected because of poor clinical results.[50] At present, one can recommend the use of cholelithotripsy only within the context of ongoing clinical trials, which will help determine the effectiveness of the technique.

Diffusion, Implementation, and Quality Assessment of Cholelithotripsy

Very important questions remain unanswered: How does this new technique compare to cholecystectomy (The present gold standard)? Will gallbladder stone ESWL justify its initial cost? (the purchase cost of some systems approached $2 million in 1990.)

In addition to a comparative study of benefit as measured by the incidence of symptoms, complications, recurrences, and quality of life issues, governing bodies require cost analyses. Although the latter may vary according to the health care system, they need to include the costs of purchase, maintenance, technician support, any further equipment acquisition or upgrade; the adjuvant dissolution treatment, as well as the equivalent cost attributable to time lost from work, complications, and recurrences. In the next few years, only limited data will be available to address these issues.

There is no doubt that diffusion of the technique must await confirmation of effectiveness and must, therefore, remain limited at this time. Third-party payers, policy makers, and governments need to decide whether to acquire such machines, and how to integrate them into the overall planning of equipment expenses despite the lack of data to counsel such decisions. It is unfortunate that patient pressure in a competitive private market motivates the acquisition of this tool in many institutions.

It is likewise premature to discuss the issues of implementation and quality assessment of cholelithotripsy at this time. The establishment of specific utilization guidelines requires carefully conducted controlled trials, but there are already foreseeable problems in reaching such recommendations. The interpretation of an evaluative trial must consider issues that may alter efficacy; for example: ESWL machines have been significantly modified since initially coming onto the market. Moreover, optimal treatment schedules have not been determined with certainty for most machines. Adjuvant methods for improving fragmentation such as the administration of cholecystokinin remain unstudied, as does tailoring of associated dissolution methods (oral bile acid or methyl-*tert*-butyl ether) as a function of the extent of fragmentation. Finally, three (soon four) types of generator system are clinically available; thus comparative trials may need to be performed between all these, because retreatment rates and the feasibility of inpatient versus outpatient treatment settings vary among them. Since mortality and morbidity rates for untreated symptomatic cholelithiasis[51] are already low, significant differences in outcome measures of any comparative therapeutic trial will be difficult to detect and must rather focus on quality of life issues. The ongoing introduction of newer surgical techniques, such as laparoscopic cholecystectomy, which may well replace the previous "gold standard," only compounds the dilemma.[52]

The assessment of ESWL as a new technology requires consideration of medical and sociopolitical issues. So-called turf issues amid the physician communities may complicate the problem further.[53] The medical profession must ensure the adequate assessment of this technique before premature diffusion occurs, as has too often been the case in medicine.

Conclusion

Technology assessment in surgical care is prompted by the realization that we must make a greater effort to use resources provided for health care in a more rational fashion. As a complex and all-encompassing process that bridges science, practice, and policy making, technology assessment is a modern way of applying the fundamental principles of medicine enunciated by Hippocrates, Osler, and Billroth when they stated that clinical actions must always have justification.

References

1. Fineberg HV, Hiatt HH. Evaluation of medical practices—the case for technology assessment. N Engl J Med 1979;301:1086–91.
2. Banta HD, Behney CJ, Willens JS. Toward National Technology in Medicine. New York: Springer Verlag, 1981.
3. Jennett B. High Technology Medicine—Benefits and Burdens. Oxford: Oxford Medical Publications, 1986.
4. Committee for Evaluating Medical Technologies in Clinical Use—Institute of Medicine, Assessing Medical Technologies. Washington, DC: National Academy Press, 1985.
5. Fisher B, Bauer M, et al. Five year results of a randomized clinical trial comparing total mastectomy and segmental mastectomy with or without radiation in the treatment of breast cancer. N Engl J Med. 1985;312:655.
6. Office of Technology Assessment, US Congress. Abstracts of case studies. In: Health Technology Case Study series, Ota-P-225. Washington, DC: Government Printing Office, 1983.
7. Spicer RD. Infantile hypertrophic pyloric stenosis: a review. Br J Surg 1982;69:128.
8. Feinstein AR. Clinical biostatistics: XLIV. Clin Pharmacol Ther 1978;24:117–25.
9. Levine RJ. Ethics and Regulation of Clinical Research. Baltimore, Urban and Schwarzenberg, 1981.
10. Feinstein AR. Clinical Epidemiology: The Architecture of Clinical Research. Philadelphia: Saunders. 1985.
11. McPeek B, Gasko M, Mosteller F. Measuring outcome from anesthesia and operation. Theor Surg 1986;1:2–9.
12. Schipper H, Why measure quality of life? Can Med Assoc J 1983;128:1367–70.
13. Taylor KM, Margolese RG, Soskolne CL. Physicians' reasons for not entering eligible patients in a randomized clinical trial of surgery for breast cancer. N Engl J Med 1984;310:1363–67.
14. Rudicel S, Esdaile J. The randomized clinical; trial in orthopedics: obligation or option? J Bone Joint Surg 1985;67–a,8:1284–93.
15. Soloniuk L, McPeek B. Do the pluses outweigh the minuses? A quality checklist for cost analysis studies in anesthesia and surgery. Theor Surg 1988;2:209–14.
16. Department of Clinical Epidemiology and Biostatistics, McMaster University. How to read clinical journals: to understand an economic evaluation: Part A. Can Med Assoc J 1984;130:1428–33.
17. Department of Clinical Epidemiology and Biostatistics, McMaster University. How to read clinical journals: to understand an economic evaluation: Part B. Can Med Assoc J 1984;130:1542–49.
18. Louis TA, Fineberg HV, Mosteller F. Findings for public health from meta-analysis. Ann Rev Public Health 1985;6:1–20.
19. Sacks HS, Berrier J, Reitman D, et al. Meta-analysis of randomized clinical trials. N Engl J Med 1987; 316:450–55.
20. Pauker SG, Kassirer JP. Decision analysis. N Engl J Med 1987;316(5):250–58.
21. Pagliarao L, Burroughs AK, Sorensen TIA, et al. Therapeutic controversies and randomised controlled trials (RCTs): prevention of bleeding and rebleeding in cirrhosis. Gastroenterol Int. 1989;2:71–84.
22. Battista RN, Fletcher SW. Making recommendations on preventive practices: methodological issues. Am J Prev Med 1988;4(4)(Suppl):53–67.
23. Woolf SH, Battista RN, Anderson G, Wang E. Assessing the effectiveness of preventive maneuvers: analytic principles and systematic methods in reviewing evidence and developing clinical practice recommendation. J Clin Epidemiol (in press, 1990).
24. Canadian Task Force on the Periodic Health Examination. The periodic health examination. Can Med Assoc J 1979;121(Suppl):1–45.

25. Battista RN. Innovation and diffusion of health-related technologies – a conceptual framework. Int J Technol Assess Health Care 1989;5:227–48.
26. Greene R, ed. Assuring Quality in Medical Care. Cambridge: Ballinger, 1976:11–134.
27. Donabedian A. Aspects of Medical Care Administration: Specifying Requirements for Health Care. Cambridge, MA: Harvard University Press, 1973.
28. Barkun AN, Ponchon T. Extracorporeal biliary lithotripsy: review of experimental studies and a clinical update. Ann Intern Med 1990;112:126–37.
29. Langenbuch C. Ein Fall von Exstirpation der Gallenblase wegen chronischer Cholelithiasis. Berliner Klin Wochenschr 1882;18:725–77.
30. DenBesten L, Berci G. The current status of biliary tract surgery: an international study of 1072 consecutive patients. World J Surg 1986; 10:116–22.
31. Houghton PWJ, Jenkinson LR, Donaldson LA. Cholecystectomy in the elderly: a prospective study. Br J Surg 1985; 72:220–22.
32. Schachler R, Sauerbruch T, Wosiewitz U, et al. Fragmentation of gallstones using extracorporeal shock waves: an in vitro study. Hepatology 1988; 8:925–29.
33. Barkun AN, Ponchon T, Valette PJ, Cathignol D. Stone density distribution index: a CT scan index that predicts the in vitro success of biliary extracorporal lithotripsy. Gastroenterology 1989;96:A574.
34. Ponchon T, Barkun AN, Pujol B, Mestas JL, Lambert R. Gallstone disappearance following extracorporeal lithotripsy and oral bile acid dissolution. Gastroenterology 1989;97:457–63.
35. Sackmann M, Delius M, Sauerbruch T, et al. Shockwave lithotripsy of gallbladder stones. The first 175 patients. N Engl J Med 1988;318:393–403.
36. Brendel W, Enders G. Shock waves for gallstones: animal studies. Lancet 1983:1054.
37. Johnson AG, Ross B, Stephenston TJ. The short term effects of extracorporeal shock wave lithotripsy on the human gallbladder. In: Biliary Lithotripsy, Ferrucci JT, Delius M, Burhenne HJ, eds. Chicago: Year-Book Medical Publishers, 1989:59–62.
38. Ponchon T, Barkun AN, Berger F, Ayela P, Margonari J, Capron F. Extracorporeal biliary lithotripsy: tissue lesions in dogs. Surg Gynecol Obstet 1989; 169:435–41.
39. Eli CH, Kerzel W, Heyder N, et al. Tissue reactons under piezoelectric shockwave: application for the fragmentation of biliary calculi. Gut 1989;30:680–85.
40. Delius M, Enders G, Heine G, Start J, Remberger K, Brendel W. Biological effects of shock waves: lung hemorrhage by shock waves in dogs-pressure dependence. Ultrasound Med Biol 1987;13:61–67.
41. Heberer G, Paumgartner G, Sauerbruch T, et al. A retrospective analysis of 3 year's experience of an interdisciplinary approach to gallstone disease including shock-waves. Ann Surg 1988;208:274–78.
42. Gracie WA, Ransohoff DF. The natural history of silent gallstones: the innocent gallstone is not a myth. N Engl J Med 1982; 307:798–800.
43. McSherry CK, Ferstenberg H, Calhoun WF, Lahman E, Virshup M. The natural history of diagnosed gallstone disease in symptomatic and asymptomatic patients. Ann Surg 1985;302:59–63.
44. Darzi A, Monson JRT, O'Morain C, Tanner WA, Keane FBV. Extension of selection criteria for extracorporeal shockwave lithotripsy for gallstones. Br Med J 1989;299:302–3.
45. Johnson AG, Ross B, Frost E, et al. A randomized controlled trial of lithotripsy and cholecystectomy: Interim report. In: Biliary Lithotripsy, Vol. II, Burhenne HJ, Paumgartner G, Ferrucci JT, eds. Chicago: Year-Book Medical Publishers, 1990; pp 151–54.
46. Thistle JL, Cleary PA, Lachin JM, Tyor MP, Hersh T. The steering committees and the National Cooperative Gallstone Study Group. The natural history of cholelithiasis: the National Cooperative Gallstone Study. Ann Intern Med 1984;101:171–75.
47. Sackmann M, Ippisch E, Tilman S, et al. Early gallstone recurrence rate after successful shock wave therapy. Gastroenterology 1990;98:392–96.
48. Heywood R, Palmer AK, Foll CV, Lee MR. Pathological changes in fetal rhesus monkey induced by oral chenodeoxycholic acid. Lancet 1973;1021.
49. Williams CM, Kaude JV, Newman RC, Peterson JC, Thomas WC. Extracorporeal shock-wave lithotripsy: long term complications. Am J Radiol. 1988;150: 311–15.
50. Stern W, et al. (ACG Ad Hoc Committee on FDA-related matters). Summary of the FDA Gastroenterology-Urology Device Section advisory panel meeting on extracorporeal shock wave lithotripsy for gallbladder stones. Am J Gastroenterol 1990; 85:(in press).
51. Ransohoff DF, Gracie WA. Management of patients with symptomatic gallstones: a quantitative analysis. Am J Med 1990;88:154–60.
52. Dubois F, Icard P, Barthelot G, Levard H. Coelioscopic cholecystectomy. Preliminary reports of 36 cases. Ann Surg 1990; 211:60–62.
53. Ferrucci JT. Biliary lithotripsy: What will the issues be? Am J Roentgenol 1987;149:227–31.

Additional Reading

Special issue of the *International Journal of Technology Assessment in Health Care* on "Technology Assessment and Surgical Policy," edited by JP Bunker and M Baum. Int J Technol Assess Health Care 1989;5:1: 305–472. Cambridge University Press.

Committee for Evaluating Medical Technologies in Clinical Use (F Mosteller, Chairman). *Evaluating Medical Technology.* Washington, DC: National Academy Press, 1985.

33

From the Bedside to the Laboratory and Back

R.C.-J. Chiu and D.S. Mulder

A number of strategies for planning a research project and organizing a competent team of clinician–scientists to execute it are discussed in this book. The "horizontal interaction" approach, illustrated by the Marburg Experiment, joins a team of basic scientists with clinicians to attack a problem. "Vertical interaction," another effective approach, draws collaborators with differing areas of expertise into a study as it progresses.

The vertical approach may be more cost-effective for a complex project, because collaborators are recruited as and when the need for their particular areas of expertise arises. Success with this approach depends on the availability of a wide variety of experts and the establishment of an extensive communication network within the research community. An attempt to develop a new "biomechanically activated cardiac assist device," undertaken in our laboratory at McGill University, illustrates the vertical approach to a research project in the North American context.

The Clinical Problems To Be Addressed

The problem addressed by our study is chronic heart failure, which afflicts approximately 2.3 million patients in the United States alone; 400,000 new cases occur each year, and the 5-year survival rate is about 50%. The patients who fall into the New York Heart Association class IV functional category have a one-year survival rate of only 50%, and half their deaths are sudden. Long-term cardiac assist devices might benefit between 35,000 (NIH study) and 160,000 (Heart Failure study) patients per year. For many of these patients, cardiac transplantation is the most established and acceptable mode of therapy now available; but even the most optimistic estimate of cardiac donors is only about 2000 per year in the United States, for the foreseeable future.

Despite considerable relaxation in donor criteria in recent years, the waiting period for donor organs has increased eightfold in some cardiac transplantation centers in North America. The epidemiologic impact of this mode of therapy is obviously very limited, without even considering that cyclosporin has not solved all the allograft rejection problems, and that continued monitoring with endomyocardial biopsies is required for all the transplant recipients. The alternative is to use mechanical artificial hearts or cardiac assist devices; but existing long-term devices are plagued by thromboembolitic and external power source problems. The tethers connecting the patient to the external power source limit the patient's mobility and are a constant potential source of infection. Another approach to cardiac assist would be valuable, if feasible.

The Conceptualization of a Hypothesis

We postulated that powering a cardiac assist device from an intrinsic energy source, such as the patient's skeletal muscle, would offer many advantages. Accordingly, the research question of our project was "Can the energy generated by skeletal muscle be harvested and modified, if necessary, to activate a totally implantable cardiac assist device capable of producing significant hemodynamic improvement?"

The Rationale

Using the patient's skeletal muscle as the power source would eliminate the need for donors, immunosuppression, and external power sources; it also would restore patients' mobility and avoid the risk of infection by eradicating tethers. Careful selection of the assist mode could also exclude such thrombogenic components in existing cardiac assist devices as artificial valves. Obviously, an effective skeletal-muscle-powered device would be a useful addition to the spectrum of cardiac assist devices currently under development.

Review of the Literature and Identification of Specific Problems To Be Solved

An extensive literature review revealed that the idea of utilizing skeletal muscle to assist circulation was expressed several decades ago. Two types of approach were described. One uses a skeletal muscle flap to replace damaged myocardium, or to enlarge a hypoplastic right or left ventricle, and is called today "dynamic cardiomyoplasty." The second approach uses skeletal muscle to activate a pump device, in series or in parallel with the heart, to improve the circulation. Critical appraisal of previous experiments identified two major problems that must be addressed before either technique can become clinically applicable. The first problem is skeletal muscle fatigue; the second is that skeletal muscle's response to stimulation by a single electrical impulse is a contraction of much shorter duration and smaller amplitude than a cardiac muscle contraction. Nevertheless, we felt that recent advances in muscle physiology and electronics could make these problems resolvable.

Physiologists have discovered that electrical stimulation at 10 Hz for 4 to 6 weeks can transform type II, fast-twitch skeletal muscle fibers, into type I, slow, fatigue-resistant muscle fibers. This conferred fatigue resistance may solve the first problem; microchip and computer technology now make it feasible to construct miniaturized, implantable, programmable electronic stimulators to solve the second problem.

Our research plans were developed and pursued in the light shed by the work on transforming skeletal muscle to confer resistance performed by John Macoviak and Larry Stephenson and associates at the University of Pennsylvania, in collaboration with Stanley Salmons, a muscle biologist and pioneer in muscle transformation at the University of Birmingham. We learned the technique of muscle transformation from these investigators and adopted it for the purpose of cardiac assists, particularly the augmentation of left ventricular function.

Simultaneously, we pushed the idea that a new stimulator that sensed the R-wave of the heart, processed the signal with appropriate delay and added a burst of electrical "pulse train" stimuli that could produce summation of the skeletal muscle contraction and modulate it to match the duration and amplitude of a myocardial contraction. This would compensate for the fact that skeletal muscle, even after transformation, consists of individual muscle fibers and "motor units," whereas cardiac muscle is a syncitium in which all the myocytes are connected by the intercalated discs. To be hemodynamically effective, the pulse train stimuli would have to be injected precisely into the selected segment of the cardiac cycle.

Preliminary Studies and the Animal Model

To evaluate the feasibility of the foregoing ideas, we consulted an electrical engineer to work out the specifications for a pulse train stimulator capable of being synchronized with the R-waves of the electrocardiogram. We then connected an available generator, the bulky model 5837 of Medtronics, Inc., to an Interstate Electronics Corporation stimulator, purchased with a modest grant from the Quebec Heart Foundation, to obtain the desired capabilities.

A canine model was chosen, primarily on the grounds of size and availability. The new stimulator was tested, using a rectus muscle pouch; it produced the expected effects and was then used for a cardiomyoplasty approach to augmenting left ventricular function. The isometric left ventricular function was assessed by intraventricular balloon measurement during cardiopulmonary bypass, with the pulse train stimulator turned on, and turned off. This on–off "paired design" was advantageous, as discussed in Chapter 16, because it reduced the sample size required for the study.

A preliminary report on the concept of pulse train stimulation timed to the cardiac cycle was published in 1980.[1] The efficacy of synchronously stimulated skeletal muscle graft for myocardial repair was reported in 1984.[2] In 1985 the feasibility of transforming a skeletal muscle to make it fatigue-resistant for myocardial assist and for powering an accessory ventricle was described.[3]

To obtain maximum muscle stretch prior to contraction, and thereby derive a powerful contractile force (Frank Starling's law), we selected the extra-aortic balloon pump as the most feasible design for our skeletal-muscle-powered assist device. Hemodynamically significant diastolic augmentation was achieved with it, in a canine study reported in 1985,[4] and further improvements were made in subsequent years.[5,6]

Progress and Interaction with Other Disciplines

Throughout this project, we interacted with various experts in muscle physiology and electronic technology. In 1985 a symposium sponsored by the Neuroelectric Society brought together for the first time international groups of investigators in this field and facilitated their interaction.[7]

To continue the elucidation of the muscle transformation phenomenon, we collaborated with David Ianuzzo, an expert in muscle biochemistry at York University in Toronto, Canada, in an investigation of changes in phenotype expression of genes during transformation, species differences, and the effects of various stimulation parameters.[8] Our concept of "working transformation"–achieving muscle transformation while extracting a measure of hemodynamic work–has gained acceptance in both laboratory and clinical settings.

While all the foregoing was happening, we also interacted with electronic and device engineers at Medtronics, Inc., in Minneapolis and in Maastricht, Holland. The engineers of this leading pacemaker company improved and miniaturized our prototype stimulator; an implantable, synchronized burst stimulator (Medtronics model SP1005)–the first of its kind–is currently undergoing clinical trial[9]

To expand the capability of our stimulator to muscle-powered counterpulsation systems, we acted as consultants to Medtronics in their project to develop a new generation of pacemakers–"Prometheus" is currently being tested in our laboratory.[10] Thus, as the project progresses, it obtains necessary expertise from both academic and industrial sources.

From the Bedside to the Lab and Back Again

The clinical problem we chose for investigation was taken to the laboratory, where the feasibility of muscle-powered cardiac assist was demonstrated; we are now trying to bring the results back to the patient.

Clinically, we perform "dynamic cardiomyoplasty" by wrapping the latissimus dorsi muscle around the patient's failing heart and stimulating it to contract during systole. Bruce Williams, a plastic surgeon with experience in muscle flap procedure, and John Burgess, a senior cardiologist who coordinates case selection and pre- and postoperative studies, joined us for this phase of our continuing "vertical interaction" in this project.

Worldwide, more than 90 patients have now undergone dynamic cardiomyoplasty, and rigorous clinical evaluations are in progress to define its clinical efficacy. We anticipate its clinical application with further refinement of the muscle-powered assist device.[11]

In conclusion, a surgical research project can be initiated, guided, and coordinated by a principal investigator who freely consults needed experts and interacts with collaborators to achieve success for the project. It can be done by "horizontal interaction" within a research team composed of a variety of experts from the outset, or by "vertical interaction" with experts and collaborators who are consulted as the project progresses. Horizontal and vertical interaction may occur simultaneously in a large project. Given the increasing sophistication of science and technology, ability to communicate and willingness to collaborate are becoming important attributes in a surgical investigator.

References

1. Drinkwater DC, Chiu RC-J, Modry D, Wittnich C, Brown PR. Cardiac assist and myocardial repair with synchronously stimulated skeletal muscle. Surg Forum 1980;31:271–74.
2. Dewar ML, Drinkwater DC, Wittnich C, Chiu RC-J. Synchronously stimulated skeletal muscle graft for myocardial repair: an experimental study. J. Thorac Cardiovasc Surg 1984;87:325–31.
3. Brister S, Fradet G, Dewar M, Wittnich C, Lough J, Chiu RC-J. Transforming skeletal muscle for myocardial assist: a feasibility study. Can J Surg 1985;28:341–44.
4. Neilson IR, Brister SJ, Khalafalla AS, Chiu RC-J. Left ventricular assist using a skeletal muscle powered device for diastolic augmentation: a canine study. J. Heart Transplant 1985;4:343–47.
5. Chiu RC-J, Walsh GL, Dewar ML, De Simon JH, Khalafalla A, Ianuzzo D. Implantable extra-aortic balloon assist powered by transformed fatigue resistant skeletal muscle. J Thorac Cardiovasc Surg 1987;94:694–701.
6. Kochamba G, Desrosiers C, Dewar ML, Chiu RC-J. The muscle powered dual-chamber counter-pulsator: rheologically superior implantable cardiac assist device. Ann Thorac Surg 1988;45:620–25.
7. Chiu RC-J, ed. Biomechanical Cardiac Assist–Cardiomyoplasty and Muscle Powered Devices. Mount Kisco, NY: Futura, 1986.
8. Ianuzzo CD, Hamilton N, O'Brien PJ, Desrosiers C, Chiu R. Biochemical transformation of canine skeletal muscle for use in cardiac assist devices. J Appl Physiol 1990.
9. Hill A, Chiu RC-J. Dynamic cardiomyoplasty for treatment of heart failure. Clin Cardiol 1989;12: 681–88.
10. Li CM, Hill A, Desrosiers C, Grandjean P, Chiu

RC-J. A new implantable burst generator for skeletal muscle powered aortic counterpulsation. Proc Am Soc Artif Int Organs 1989;35:405–07.

11. Chiu RC-J, Bourgeois I, eds. Transformed Muscle for Cardiac Assist and Repair. Mount Kisco, NY: Futura, 1990.

34

Research in the Surgical Laboratory: A Brief Historical Appraisal

G.H. Brieger

The words science, technology, and research denote three highly complex concepts of human activity. All have become closely linked to late twentieth century medicine and surgery. Although all three activities were part of European medicine by the mid-1800s, their linkage with North American medicine did not become indissoluble until the early decades of the twentieth century. Surgical research, now a common activity in medical centers around the world, has a history that goes considerably farther back than the beginning of this century.

This section of the book focuses on the surgeon in the laboratory, but it is well to remember that however crucial the exploits of the research pioneers may have been to the development of clinical practice, merely retelling their stories gives a glimpse of only a part of the research story. It is more interesting, and more difficult, to explore the fascinating question of creativity. How is clinical knowledge created? What conditions cause some to do only what they are taught, while others are stimulated to push on to find new techniques, new understanding, or even new cures? Fame is elusive, but it is safe to say that surgical leaders, now and in the foreseeable future, must be good biologists as well as good surgeons; the care of the patient is an exercise in human biology.

We tend to view surgical research as a recent development – maybe 30 or 40 years old – but it was clearly evident in the work of John Hunter, in the late 1700s, and of Joseph Lister in the 1860s and 1870s.[1]

Some of Lister's contemporaries cited his work in their clearly voiced calls for research. In Vienna in the 1870s, Theodor Billroth, one of the greatest surgical teachers of his century, told his students that the duty of all physicians was "to find the causes of the morbid processes, to foretell their course correctly, to conduct them to a favorable issue or to check them. . . ."[2] The means at hand to find the solution for such problems, Billroth noted, were scientific research and refined empiricism.

John Shaw Billings, a leader of medicine in the United States and a contemporary of Billroth, said "Besides his duties to his patients, the physician is under certain obligation to contribute, by way of interest, his quota of the common stock of medical knowledge from which he has drawn so freely."[3] Billings wrote those words to open a review of American medical literature for the centennial of 1876. In the next few years, he was engaged in bringing out the monumental *Index Catalog of the Surgeon General's Library*; the first volume appeared in 1880. Here was a compilation of the world's medical books, monographs, and reprints in one of the world's best medical libraries. For access to the medical journal literature, Billings, in 1879, began the monthly compilation known as *Index Medicus*. These two magnificent reference guides provided the primary research tool for generations of medical investigators to gain access to the world's medical practices and research findings – a tool that was and is crucial to the pursuit of surgical research or medical work of any kind.

Since ancient man first made empirical observations about appropriate diets for the sick, or effective ways to splint broken bones, the aim of surgical research has been to increase our understanding of health and disease in order, ultimately, to relieve pain and illness.

The authors of the summary report of the Study on Surgical Services for the United States (1975) claimed they had difficulty in defining surgical research. Discoveries from many medical, scientific, and technical fields have certainly contributed to the care of surgical patients, but for the purpose of introducing this section, "surgical research" will be used as the shorthand expression for the process required to create surgical knowledge. The aim of most research is to create new knowledge, technology, and understanding. Since early in this century, the reigning ideology in medicine has been that new knowledge comes from teaching and research centers (i.e., from the clinics and laboratories).

Sometimes the facilities were very rudimentary, as they were in 1921 when a young Canadian surgeon became convinced that, if he tied the pancreatic duct, he might be able to isolate the hormone that controlled the metabolism of sugar when the pancreatic enzymes could no longer interfere. The discovery of insulin by Frederick Banting and his medical student assistant Charles Best, working with borrowed facilities and equipment, had one of the most profound effects on medical practice, research, and education since Lister's work 50 years earlier.[4] While the introduction of antiseptic surgery, based on the new science of microbiology, moved surgery from the kitchen table to the sanitized atmosphere of new hospitals, the advent of insulin confirmed the notion of medical scientists that the average physician had to know something about human physiology and biochemistry to practice medicine in the new and exciting era of therapeutics. This was a clear and early example of a shift in medical education prompted by a new relationship between knowledge to practice.

George Crile, the Cleveland surgeon, began to apply physiological methods to the study of shock in 1895,[5] and as the 1920s began, the results of this and other surgical research were becoming evident. When we review surgery in that presulfa, preantibiotic era—especially the work of those who were developing the new fields of intracranial and intrathoracic surgery—we usually think of it as a time when postsurgical infections played a decisive role in limiting the surgeon's field of action. In the thinking of surgeons, however, infection was no longer as threatening as it had been around the turn of the century.

In his Shattuck Lecture to the Massachusetts Medical Society in the summer of 1933, Elliott Cutler said,

> Today, however, physiological experimentation and bacteriological study, advances in surgical technique and competent methods of anesthesia have made it possible for the surgeon who knows of these things to enter the chest with as much relative safety to his patient as when he enters the abdomen. This is the last great field for the surgeon to explore, and now that he has methods which make it safe for him to enter this field, it is only right and proper that the information should be disseminated and patients with certain thoracic disorders should be given the hope which surgical therapy may promise them.[6]

Thus did Cutler proclaim not only a new era, but also his clear belief that his own work and the work of many others in the laboratory had advanced surgery sufficiently to make it much safer for patients. We are accustomed to thinking that safety arrived after the antimicrobial drugs became available, but those working in the vineyards of surgery felt otherwise. They were quite confident with what they knew and had achieved by the mid-1930s. Yet, others were not so satisfied.[7]

Creativity in science has been receiving more attention from historians and sociologists in recent years, but relatively little work of a comparable nature has been devoted to creativity in medicine. Except for Peter Medawar and Julius Comroe—medical scientists of wide accomplishments—very few historians have been interested in the subject. In a paper describing the research ideas and techniques used by cardiovascular surgeons early in this century and again just after the second world war to elucidate a more effective therapy for mitral stenosis, I described the surgical research carried on in laboratories in the United States and England.[8] The techniques of empirical clinical observation were illustrated in a second study on the introduction of early ambulation after surgery.[9]

Julius Comroe wrote about the use of his instrument, the retrospectroscope, not to establish who did what first, but as an exploration of science as a creative process.[10] He was not satisfied with telling what happened; he wanted to know why scientific investigators arrived at the questions they asked and urged his colleagues to "tell it like it was." Comroe urged that medical papers go beyond the IMRAD formula (i.e., introduction, methods, results, and discussion) to get at the unreported elements of why the investigator undertook the study, whether the initial idea was correct, and how the correct track was found.

The introduction of microvascular surgery in 1960 was one of Comroe's most telling illustrations of his point. In their very modest paper of barely 2 pages, Jacobson and Suarez described how much accuracy could be achieved, even in large-vessel surgery, with the aid of a microscope. The authors summarized their technique, concisely, but they neglected—Comroe pointed out—to tell their readers and colleagues why they took up the method in 1960. This was an astute historical comment, given that ears, nose, and throat surgeons had been operating with magnification for nearly 40 years. It took a letter from Comroe to Jacobson to elicit some pertinent facts about the process of creativity in surgical research. Jacobson had indeed seen ENT microscopes and had become comfortable and proficient with them during several summers of work at Woods Hole. When the complexity and detail of the blood vessel wall became much clearer to Jacobson later in his surgical career, it was perfectly natural for him to use a microscope when suturing during anastomosis.[11,12]

The literature on the psychological aspects of creativity in nonscientific fields is vast; for medicine and science it is growing slowly, but it is still rare to find much mention of the process of surgical discovery. Francis D. Moore, one of the few surgeons to write about it, spoke of creative science in surgery when he described the work of Dwight Harken on the mitral valve in his 1950 annual report as surgeon-in-chief of the Peter Bent Brigham Hospital.[13] Building on the earlier work of Cutler and Samuel Levine, Harken and Charles Bailey brought mitral valve repair into common surgical practice within 20 years of its use as a laboratory research technique. A remarkable 130-page report appeared in *Archives of Surgery*, November 1924, entitled "The Surgical Treatment of Mitral Stenosis: Experimental and Clinical Studies." In it, Cutler, Levine, and Beck described the history of surgical treatment of this common disorder; their rationale for attempting to alleviate it surgically; and their experiments, clinical cases, new instrument, and results in four cases. Their necessarily tentative conclusions were: "We feel that the proposal that certain cases of mitral stenosis may be relieved by surgery has not been contradicted by our experiences. . . ."—a clear attempt to "tell it like it was." Nevertheless, Comroe was right when he bemoaned the rarity of such writing, 50 years later.

Four years after their report, Cutler and his coworkers called for a moratorium because the results did not justify further use of their method of opening the stenotic mitral valve.

The surgical laboratory, a now common feature of medical centers around the world, probably had its origins in Renaissance anatomical theaters and mid-nineteenth-century physiological laboratories. The history of surgical research merits a book, but in the limited space available here I will cite only one example of a laboratory founded specifically to advance surgical knowledge and to teach students how to handle living tissues—the Hunterian Laboratory of the Johns Hopkins University School of Medicine. This facility has been an important model for teaching and investigation since its founding in 1905.

In 1895 William S. Halsted began a course on operative surgery—for the first clinical class at Hopkins—and Harvey Cushing took it over in 1901. Cushing persuaded the university to build a separate structure to combine teaching and experimental work in surgery. Part of Halsted's success as a surgical teacher is attributable to his firm belief in the German method of training, which included practical as well as scientific experiences for the young surgeons. In 1904 in his oft-cited Yale address, "The Training of the Surgeon," Halsted proclaimed:

"We need a system, and we shall surely have it, which will produce not only surgeons but surgeons of the highest type, men who will stimulate the first youths of our country to study surgery and to devote their energies and their lives to raising the standard of surgical science."[14]

The Hunterian Laboratory, a rectangular, well-lit, two-story building with its own paddock for animals was opened in 1905. The faculty rooms for research were used by members of the departments of medicine, surgery, and pathology. The prevailing philosophy of medicine taught early in this century at Hopkins and a few other places, was concisely stated by the professor of anatomy, Franklin P. Mall: "The object of the laboratory is to teach students, to train investigators, and to investigate." This philosophy was very evident in the building named for John Hunter, the experimental surgeon of the eighteenth century.[15]

Shortly after the opening of the Hunterian, where he carried out his first studies on the pituitary, Cushing wrote: "We have endeavored to combine this instruction in operative work with the necessary experimentation of the various laboratories . . ."[16]

Cushing firmly believed that the principles of surgery, including diagnosis, sterile technique, gentle handling of tissues during dissection, and careful control of bleeding, could be learned best on living animal bodies rather than on cadavers.

A student may read surgery, may hear and see surgery [Cushing wrote], and yet, without having himself practiced operations and those on the living body, he remains totally incapable of carrying out those measures which alone distinguish this branch of medicine. One would not expect to play the violin after a course of lectures on music and merely by watching a performer for a few semesters. Just so with the looking on at operations. . . ."[17]

Cushing believed that, in addition to teaching the principles of surgery, such a course made the future physician more appreciative of the surgical point of view and might awaken the interest of some in surgical research as a result of being brought into direct contact with surgery. He also knew that stressing laboratory teaching at Hopkins was equally important in awakening that interest, and he cited his own experience "of working for a few semesters in physiological laboratories abroad, during which time, it seems to me, I acquired more of real value for my surgical work than in my previous six years service as a hospital intern."[18]

Fifty years later, Lester Dragstedt and James Clarke wrote: "Perhaps the most important reason for the continued advance of surgery during the past fifty years has been the incorporation of physiological thinking and knowledge into surgical practice."[19]

A regular series of reports flowed from the Hunterian Laboratory of Experimental Medicine. Cushing, with several young assistants, carried out important experimental studies on the mitral valve.[20] In 1907 Stephen Watts published an important review of papers and some of his own experimental work on the suture of blood vessels and the transplantation of organs.[21] The Hunterian was neither the first nor the only laboratory engaged in surgical research, but it certainly set an important example.

This brief introduction to the history of surgical research in the laboratory is not even a cursory survey of the subject, but it may impart some historical perspective to the chapters on the experimental approach that follow.

References

1. (a) Kobler J. The Reluctant Surgeon, A biography of John Hunter. Garden City, NY: Doubleday, 1960. (b) Godlee RJ. Lord Lister. London: Macmillan, 1917.
2. Billroth T. Lectures on Surgical Pathology and Therapeutics, 2 vols. London: New Sydenham Society, 1877;1:3.
3. Billings JS. A century of American medicine: IV. Literature and institutions. Am J Med Sci 1876; 72:439.
4. Bliss M. The Discovery of Insulin. Chicago: University of Chicago Press, 1982.
5. English PC. Shock, Physiological Surgery and George Washington Crile. Westport, CT: Greenwood Press, 1980.
6. Cutler EC. The origins of thoracic surgery. N Engl J Med 1933;208:1235.
7. Walter CW. Finding a better way. JAMA 1990;263: 1675–78.
8. Brieger GH. Mitral stenosis: a case study in the history of surgery. In: De Novis Inventis. Kerkhoff AHM, Luyendijk-Elshout AM, Poulisseu, MJD, eds. Amsterdam: APA-Holland University Press, 1984:28–44.
9. Brieger GH. Early ambulation, a study in the history of surgery. Ann Surg 1983;197:443–49. See also Holmes FL. The fine structure of scientific creativity. Bull Hist Sci 1981;19:60–70; Patterns of scientific creativity. Bull Hist Med 1986;60:19–35.
10. Comroe JH, Jr. Retrospectroscope. Menlo Park, CA: Von Gehr Press, 1977.
11. Comroe JH Jr. Retrospectroscope, pp 94–5.
12. Jacobson IH, Suarez EL. Micro-surgery on anastomoses and small vessels. Surg Forum 1960; 11:243–245.
13. Thirty-Seventh Annual Report of the Peter Bent Brigham Hospital for the Year 1950. Boston, 1951:54.
14. Halsted WS. The training of the surgeon. Bull Johns Hopkins Hosp 1904;15:267–75.
15. Harvey AM, Brieger GH, Abrams SL, and McKusick VA. A Model of Its Kind, a centennial history of medicine at Johns Hopkins, 2 vols. Baltimore: Johns Hopkins University Press, 1989. See especially Vol. 2:61–7.
16. Cushing H. Comparative surgery. Bull. Johns Hopkins Hosp. 1905;16:180.
17. Cushing H. Instruction in operative medicine. Bull. Johns Hopkins Hosp. 1906;17:127.
18. Cushing H. Instruction in operative medicine, Bull Johns Hopkins Hosp 1906;17:134.
19. Dragstedt LR. and Clarke JS. The contributions of physiology to surgery, 1905–1955. In: Fifty Years of Surgical Progress, 1905–1955, Davis L, ed. Chicago: FH Martin Memorial Foundation, 1955:52.
20. Tilney NL, Cushing, Cutler, and the mitral valve. Surg Gyn Obs 1981;152:91–6.
21. Watts SH. The suture of blood vessels. Implantation and transplantation of vessels and organs. An historical and experimental study. Bull. Johns Hopkins Hosp. 1907;18:153–79.

Additional Reading

Comroe JH, Jr. Retrospectroscope. Menlo Park, CA: Von Gehr Press, 1977.

35

Animal Experimentation

W.H. Isselhard and J. Kusche

Animal experimentation and research with animals is an integral part of clinical research, including surgery. The goal is to solve problems encountered in clinical practice and develop new methods and approaches to the cure and alleviation of disease and disability. Animal experimentation is to be understood as research that will benefit both man and animals.

Scientific and biomedical research employing animals has a long, productive, and exciting history. To pass over this history in a single paragraph does an injustice to many researchers and their innumerable accomplishments. The long list of names may be represented by John Hunter (1728–1793), the surgeon, anatomist, and naturalist, and by Claude Bernard (1813–1878), the physiologist. Hunter introduced arterial ligation for treating aneurysms, after the study of collateral circulation in the deer. He also conducted transplantation experiments in fowl, in the hope of establishing a technique for transplanting the human tooth. At the end of the Age of Enlightenment, he anticipated the value of research in animals for medical activities in man. Bernard elucidated functions of liver and pancreas and advocated the still modern concept of the "milieu intérieur." At the threshold of modern natural sciences and medicine, he contributed to the development of medical sciences by insisting on the use of strict experimental methods in the study of biological problems. This history provides convincing proof that progress in clinical medicine is, in large part, linked to advances in other "basic" sciences and that animal experimentation often was, and still is, the absolutely necessary key. A large body of facts, and a remarkable knowledge of interactions in physiology, pathophysiology, biochemistry, microbiology, and normal and pathological morphology, stem from research in animals, the value of which cannot be overestimated. They provide the fundamental scientific basis for contemporary medicine and surgery.

The scientist working with animals as a scientific tool must be aware of, and prepared for, the fact that research with animals and animal experimentation give rise to scientific, ethical, legal, and technical problems and controversies. These problems and the controversy they generate have existed for a long time. They change with times. To a large extent, they present themselves differently in different cultures and social communities. In countries where animal research has grown to major dimensions, questions concerning animals and animal experimentation have attracted considerable public interest. Unfortunately, the discussion of totally opposite views on and interests in animals has become emotionalized. This is regrettable, because it makes mutual consent nearly impossible and hinders pragmatic solutions.

Every scientist working with animals should be familiar with the problems of animal experimentation and local legal and ethical requirements for animal care. Animal experimentation demands the highest level of scientific and humane responsibility.

While it is not possible to provide the reader with a complete list of books, protocols and statements on animal experimentation, references 1–18 provide coverage of relevant publications.

The Role of Animal Experimentation in Clinical Research

Animal experimentation has made it possible for surgery and most other disciplines of human and veterinary medicine to reach their present high standards. An enumeration of the achievements made in surgery, alone, with the help and sacrifice of animals, is beyond the scope of this chapter; a catalog of surgical developments accomplished without animal experimentation would be much shorter. Our relatively vast knowledge of facts and interactions in physiology, pathophysiology, biochemistry, and morphology is largely the result of research in animals and provides the roots of today's surgery. Careful and judicious research in animals of various species preceded the introduction, and accompanies the continuous amendment, of surgical procedures and other therapeutic measures.

Examples of the contributions such research has made include development of gastrointestinal surgery, including gastrectomy for the treatment of ulcers and malignancies; development of modern thoracic and pulmonary surgery; elaboration of essential components of our knowledge of peri- and postoperative pathophysiology and its consequences for prophylaxis and therapy; establishment of open heart and coronary artery surgery, including development of the heart–lung machine, hypothermia, induced cardiac arrest, and myocardial protection; advances in microsurgery; treatment of terminal renal insufficiency by dialysis or transplantation; transplantation of tissues and such life-supporting organs as the kidney, liver, heart, and pancreas; preservation of live tissues and organs; development of neurosurgery; analysis and therapy of the various forms of shock; pilot preparation of the Open Reduction and Internal Fixation (ORIF) techniques and other techniques of osteosynthesis; testing of artificial joints; and biological and synthetic replacement of bone defects.

Research involving animals will continue to be necessary in the future if we wish to enjoy the advantages of innovation, widening knowledge of biological processes, and the possibility of curing as-yet incurable diseases and disorders.

Research in animals is usually the first step in attempts to make established operative interventions less cumbersome and stressful for patients. The development of endoscopy from a technique for direct inspection and diagnosis to a method for curative surgical intervention is an example. Many affected regions of the body can now be reached via natural apertures or small incisions, in comparison with earlier approaches that involved substantial disturbances to, or even destruction of, normal tissues. Similarly, animal experimentation has played an essential role in the development of the kidney lithotripter and its routine application in patients with nephrolithiasis. A similar method for the destruction of stones in the biliary system is now being introduced.

Work with and in animals is also an important constituent of teaching and learning prior to practice involving humans. The acquisition of medical and surgical skills, the avoidance of mistakes and wrong reactions that may have unfortunate consequences, and the development of sensitivity based on personal experience with extremely complex biological systems can be achieved only by means of intensive study of living organisms. Books, films, models, and modern audiovisual teaching methods are undoubtedly helpful in the teaching and learning processes, but they cannot completely replace work with living matter. The mandate and ethics of medicine require that the restoration and improvement of health be sought with the least possible risk to human patients. Lofty as this goal is, it does not absolve the investigator from a deep and continuing moral obligation to handle other than human life with care, responsibility, consideration, and respect.

The Differentiation of Living Matter

To appraise the importance, usefulness and yield of experimentation in intact animals versus the use of alternative methods, it is worth devoting some discussion to the differentiation of living matter.

All living matter is subject to very similar, if not identical, biological laws; that is, all living matter functions according to very similar principles and mechanisms, even though the degree of differentiation is extremely wide.

The cell is the smallest entity of self-supporting life. It may exist as a separate unicellular organism comprising all the attributes required to maintain its own existence and the continuation and evolution of its species. Alternatively, the cell may be bound to the coexistence and cofunctioning of many different cells whose number may be uncountable and whose potentialities for differentiation and performing different specific functions may be neither known nor understood definitively. The latter statement can be easily illustrated by a little reflection.

What information and conclusions could a physician derive from a white blood cell count and a differential blood smear 30 years ago compared to the early hints the specialist now gets for discriminating an early episode of rejection from a viral or bacterial infection after organ transplantation? Only one generation ago, the endothelium was assigned hardly any roles other than separating the blood from tissues and participating physiologically in the blood clotting processes and pathophysiologically in some vascular diseases and disorders. Today, biomedical science has started to realize that the endothelium has many differentiated physiological attributes like an organ, and may initiate or contribute to numerous pathologic processes.

A multicellular living system originates from unicellular living matter. In its unicellular state, it comprises all the species-specific characteristics of all the cells in the eventual multicellular organism. Multicellular living systems are able to exist independently and to continue the propagation and evolution of their species only after they have reached a sufficiently differentiated multicellular state of ontogenesis, as determined by phylogenesis.

An increase in the differentiation of cells usually means an enhancement of abilities and specialized functions that accompanies the evolution of the special cells, tissues, organs, and organ systems that, with their multiple interdependencies, constitute the body of the organism. For most of the specialized cells and organs, differentiation implies the loss of certain properties; for example, many differentiated cells totally lack potential for regeneration. As a rule, more differentiated living systems are considered to be higher forms of animal life than less differentiated forms. This view does not negate the fact that lower animal life has given rise to remarkable differentiations and capabilities. Human life can be rightfully regarded as the most differentiated living system.

Surgery is the art of palliative, curative, or restorative intervention in highly differentiated organisms. It cannot be learned or taught, nor can it progress, without access to adequately differentiated living systems.

Alternatives to Animal Experimentation?

So-called alternative methods, as originally defined, are alternatives to animal experimentation. A definition that classifies such methods and approaches as substitutes that will reduce animal experimentation is more realistic.[10,13,16,17] An animal experiment is defined as an intervention in, or treatment of, a living animal under strict scientific conditions. In the past few decades, the so-called alternative methods have been persistently propagated, often in an irrelevant way on the basis of an overvaluation of their efficiency. The apparent aim is to represent animal experimentation as being useless and needless. The excessive zeal of antivivisectionists sometimes causes occupational and personal defamation, and discrimination against the experimental investigator.[18]

For more than a century, biomedical research has taken advantage of experiments with living matter other than animals. It continuously improves these methods and designs new approaches. The scientific community distinguishes between in vivo studies in living animals and in vitro experiments with tissues or organs from sacrificed animals. The culturing of cells and the controlled growth of fetal organs, in whole or in part, are now established laboratory procedures, and studies in these preparations must be classified as in vitro experiments.

The important distinction between "schmerzfähiger und nicht schmerzfähiger Materie" (matter capable of suffering and not capable of suffering), is fully accepted by expert investigators[10] although it did not originate in the scientific community.[15] An in vivo experiment with animals is an experiment with living matter capable of suffering, whereas an in vitro experiment makes use of living matter that is no longer capable of suffering.

Current biomedical and surgical research employs the following approaches, when they are appropriate:

1. Experiments with surviving cells, tissues, organs, parts of organs, and organ systems.
2. Experiments with cultured cells, tissues, and organs.
3. Experiments with lower organisms.
4. Work with nonbiological materials.
5. Calculations in immaterial models.
6. Experiments involving a large variety of chemical, biochemical, molecular biological, microbiological, physical, and immunological methods of in vitro analysis.

It must be recognized, nevertheless, that cells, tissues, and organs for in vitro studies have their origin in living animals. It should also be realized that numerous animal experiments are still needed for development, testing, quality control, and comparative studies.

The prohibition of all animal experimentation and the exclusive use of alternative methods are not feasible, given the present state of scientific knowledge. This is particularly true for surgical research and experimental surgery. Problems like the care of the polytraumatized organism; the elaboration of more effective therapeutic approaches to different kinds of shock; management of multiorgan failure; the effect of rejection of organs, in whole or in part; tissue or organ substitution by biological or nonbiological matter; the improvement of existing and the development of new devices like the heart–lung machine or the artificial heart; and the trial of new concepts of surgical interventions can only be studied in whole animals.

Results obtained in an in vitro study cannot always be transferred directly to the in vivo situation; for example, an early cardioplegic agent[19] proved to be rather toxic in in vitro studies with isolated cells,[20] but under in vivo conditions it was found to be only slightly inferior to more modern therapeutic agents.[21,22] The scientific value of in vitro research must not, however, be underestimated. In vitro studies can reveal biological facts that may remain unrecognized in whole-animal experiments due to their complexity. Even in surgical research, in vitro experiments may be of help in the solution of special problems—for example for the screening of cardioplegic and organ-protecting solutions and principles, and the determination of tolerances to various forms of deprivation (ischemia, anoxia, hypoxia, hypoperfusion, etc.). Work with isolated or cultured cells, such as the preservation and transplantation of Langerhans' islets or the preoperative "endothelialization" of vascular prostheses is part of surgical research. The researcher has to be aware of the advantages, the disadvantages, and the limits of this scientific tool.

In 1959 *Russell* and *Burch*[20] enunciated the 3 R's for research in animals: replacement, reduction, and refinement. Replacement, as originally defined, refers:

> to a wide range of techniques in which animals were not required at all in the actual experiment or in which they were exposed to no distress. For example, a terminal experiment in which the animal is always under anesthesia until it is humanely killed would fall into the category of replacement. The use of tissue cultures and computer modeling represent the former category. The concept of reduction focused on reducing the number of animals required by better experimental planning, statistical design, and statistical analysis . . . The trial and error approach is less desirable than the hypothetico-deductive approach in which the researcher formulates a testable hypothesis . . . Refinement dealt exclusively with experimentation in which the animal was subjected to some degree of stress during the investigation. The 3 R's principle thus centers mainly on the question of stress research.

Within the concept of the 3 R's "it is permissible to use an animal in research provided that the animal suffers no pain whatsoever."[16] *Rowan*[16] finds this concept to have changed its meaning "with the advent of the term 'alternatives' to laboratory animals." Now,

> the main thrust is aimed at the total numbers of animals used, rather than at the question of stressful research. AS a result, replacement and reduction refer solely to the number of animals used while refinement refers to the overall question of reducing the stress suffered by the laboratory animal . . . An "alternative" includes any system or method that covers one or more of the following:
>
> 1. Replacing the use of laboratory animals altogether.
> 2. Reducing the number of animals required.
> 3. Refining an existing procedure or technique so as to minimize the level of stress or pain endured by the animal.

But, there is also the statement that "any 'alternative' must provide information or results which allow the investigator to draw the same conclusions with at least the same degree of confidence."[16,23] *Smyth*[13] has argued similarly.

It is important to know that not only the in vitro methods but also the commitment to humane in vivo experimentation with animals originated in the scientific community. Renowned scientific societies and science promotion societies have supported animals protection laws in various countries.

Animal Models

For clinical and surgical research, Wessler's definition of an animal model of human disease may be useful. An animal model is "a living organism with an inherited, naturally acquired or induced pathological process that in one or more respects closely resembles the same phenomenon in man."[24]

A more general definition covering all aspects of biomedical research was adapted from this definition by the Institute of Laboratory Animal Resources (ILAR).[25] An animal model might vary from a one-cell protozoan, the study of which can lead to a better understanding of cellular function, to the chimpanzee, one of the species phylogenetically closest to humans which may be the only species other than humans susceptible to a particular infectious agent.[26] Animal models, according to Gill[27] are used mainly for three reasons:

1. To elucidate host defense mechanisms.
2. To point the way for subsequent studies in humans.
3. To screen substances for effectiveness or toxicity.

There is no doubt that animal models have great merit in relation to points 1 and 2. An early example is the work of Edward Jenner (1749–1823), who observed that milk maids affected by cowpox did not contract the malignant smallpox then epidemic in England. Another important example is the finding of Robert Koch that guinea pigs are highly susceptible to tuberculosis. He used it to establish the causal relationship between the tubercle bacillus and tuberculosis. Koch's postulates concerning infectious diseases cannot be fulfilled without a susceptible animal model. For further important historical animal models, see the paper by Jones.[28]

Point 3, above, is the subject of much debate, because it is doubtful whether animal experiments can accurately predict the toxicity of substances in humans, whether the current extent of animal experiments is necessary, and whether alternatives can replace animal experiments.

If animal models are used, they should be appropriate for the situation that is to be studied. For instance, a model of prostatic cancer that depends on a tumor growth that is insensitive to hormonal influence is not relevant to the clinical situation, nor is an animal model of duodenal ulcer production that occurs without elevated acid output in the stomach.

There is probably no ideal model for any disease. The disease itself may be variable and may have many facets so that more than one animal model may be required. Although the ideal model may not exist, we should seek "its more modest cousin"[26] (i.e., the most appropriate model available).

During a workshop on needs for new animal models, Leader and Padgett[29] listed nine criteria for a good animal model:

1. It should accurately reproduce the disease or lesions under study.
2. It should be available to multiple investigations. Sharing of animals and data among institutions has been an important factor in many research successes. It allows monitoring of the scientific validity of observations and stimulates further investigation.
3. It should be exportable.
4. If the disease under study is genetic, the species should be polytocous—producing multiple young at each birth.
5. The animal should be large enough for multiple biopsy samples.
6. It should fit into the available animal facilities of most laboratories. The accelerating costs of any changes in animal housing and care standards make this criterion particularly relevant.
7. The animal should be easily handled by most investigators. However, convenience should not be the determinating factor in the selection of the model.
8. It should be available in multiple species.
9. The animals used in the model should survive long enough to be usable.

To ensure maximum comparability of results, another point should be added to the list of criteria. The animals for induced or spontaneous models of human disease should be genetically defined.

Although several populations of animals can be distinguished and their use has special advantages and disadvantages,[27] it is difficult to say which is the most appropriate for mimicking a particular disease or effect of therapy in a human population.

1. Randomly mating animal populations:

There are two types, those that are colony-bred and those found in the wild. The major use of the first type is testing the effects of drugs; the second type may be useful for developing studies relevant to human disease, because it generates mutants and mimics a disease process.[27]

2. Outbred populations:

These animals are systematically bred to maintain maximal genetic heterogeneity and are useful for drug screening.

3. Inbred strains:

An inbred strain is defined as being the product of 20 generations of brother–sister matings. Inbreeding implies a genetic drift. When an inbred strain has been separated from its primary source for eight or more generations, it should be identified as a subline by giving it a laboratory designation that follows the strain name. For the mouse, a standardized nomenclature exists,[30] but not for other species, such as the rat. The same rules for listing inbred strains should be used for species other than the mouse.[31] The major use of inbred strains is the study of specific questions, such as drug effects on a tumor, in a genetically defined population.

4. F_1 hybrids:

Two progenitor inbred strains are mated to form F_1 hybrids, which are more resistant to environmental influences than the parent inbred strains. The F_1 hybrid provides a well-defined population with limited genetic diversity.

5. Coisogenic and congenic strains:

Two isogenic (i.e., genetically identical) strains that differ only at a single locus, the differential locus, are known as "coisogenic" strains. Such strains arise as a result of mutation within an inbred strain. Strains that approximate the coisogenic status can be developed by backcrossing a gene from a donor strain into an inbred strain (the background strain of the inbred partner). The resulting partially coisogenic strains that differ at the differential locus and an associated segment of chromosome, are known as "congenic" strains.[30] The major use of

TABLE 35.1.

Animal Models of Human Disease	Handbook published by the Registry of Comparative Pathology, U.S. Armed Forces Institute of Pathology, continuing series of fascioles.
Experimental Cardiovascular Diseases	Salye H, New York: Springer-Verlag, 1970.
Naturally Occurring Animal Models of Human Disease	Appendix to the paper: "Animal Models" by Bustad UK, Hegreberg GA, Padgett GA. In: The Future of Animals, Cells, Models and Symptoms in Research, Development, Education and Testing. Washington, DC: National Academy Press, 1975.
Animal Models for Biomedical Research VI-Metabolic Disease	Fed Proc 1976; 35: 1992–1236.
Animal Models of Thrombosis and Haemorrhagic Diseases	National Institute of Health, Bethesda, Md., 1976.
Experimental Models of Chronic Inflammatory Diseases	Glynn LE, Schlumberger HD, eds. Heidelberg, New York: Springer-Verlag, 1977
Spontaneous Models of Human Diseases	Andrews EJ, Ward EJ, Altman NH, eds. New York: Academic Press, 1979.
Animal Quality and Models in Biomedical Research	Spiegel A, Ericks S, Vollevald HA, eds. New York: 8 Fischer Verlag, 1980.
Animal Models for Diabetes Mellitus: A Bibliography	ILAR News, 1981; 24: 5–22.
Animal Models for Research on Aging	Washington, DC: National Academy Press, 1981.
Animal Models and Hypoxia	Stefanovich V, ed. New York: Pergamon Press, 1981.
Bibliography of Naturally Occurring Animal Models of Human Diseases	Hegreberg GA, Leathers C, eds. Pullman, WA: Human Student Books, 1982
Bibliography of Induced Animal Models of Human Disease	Hegreberg GA, Leathers C, eds. Pullman, WA: Human Student Books, 1982
Animal Models for Tumor Progression	Leibovici J, Wolman M, Anticancer Res., 1984; 4: 165–168.
Recent Advances in Molecular Pathology. Animal Models in Athereosclerosis Research	Jokinen MP, Clarkson TB, Prichard RW, Exp Mol Path, 1985; 42: 1–28.
Animal Models of Gastrointestinal Diseases	Pfeiffer JC, Boca Raton: CRC Press, 1985.
Animal Models of Human Diseases	Cohen D, Boca Raton: CRC Press, 1985.
Experimental Models of Exocrine Pancreatic Tumors	Longnecker DS, In: Go VWL et al., eds. Pancreas: Biology, Pathobiology and Diseases. New York: Raven Press, 1986.
Animal Models: Assessing the Scope of their Use in Biomedical Research	Kawamata J, Melby EC, eds. New York: Alan R. Liss Inc., 1987.
Use of Animal Models for Research in Human Nutrition	Bayan AC, West CE, eds. Basel: S. Karger AG, 1988.
Animal Models in Chronic Renal Failure	Gretz N, Strauch M, eds. Basel: S. Karger AG, 1988.
Animal Models for Human Nutrition Physiology	Kirchgessner M, ed. Berlin-Hamburg: Verlag Paul Parey, 1990

these animals is to study the effects of one specific gene.

This chapter is not the place to describe the characteristics of the various animal models described in the literature. Bustad and coworkers[32] embarked on this task when they wrote a chapter in *The Future of Animals, Cells, Models and Systems in Research, Development, Education and Testing.* When they exceeded 6000 references for animal models, they decided to publish their list as an appendix. We have limited ourselves to preparing Table 35.1 to give you some help in finding the animal model you need in a special situation. If you intend to study duodenal ulcer disease, for example, you can look for spontaneous animal models[33] or for an experimentally induced model that was presented as a chemically induced duodenal ulcer by Szabo.[34,35] Even if your search does not produce the ideal animal model of this human disease, there are some models that come close to the human situation (e.g., the "Executive Monkey"[36]), or resemble human duodenal ulcer disease in many ways (e.g., the cysteamine ulcer[37]; see Table 35.2).

Remember, when a human disease is to be studied, you should reflect on the criteria for the appropriateness of an animal model, study the information that is available, and not leave animal models as a "neglected medical resource."[38]

Quality Control

Quality of Experiments

In several studies, the quality of publications has been evaluated by reporting the frequency and accuracy of the statistical data and criteria published in them.[3,40] In a similar exercise that focused on experimentation in animals, Juhr[41] investigated some volumes of *Laboratory Animal Science*. The result of his study (Table 35.3) provides a useful

TABLE 35.2. Comparison of chemically induced duodenal ulcer with human duodenal ulcer.

Condition	Experimental duodenal ulcer	Human duodenal ulcer
Localization of the ulcer	Anterior and posterior wall	Anterior and posterior wall
Tendency to perforate	Yes	Yes
Penetration into the liver and/or pancreas	Yes	Yes
Occurrence of "giant ulcer forms" and massive bleedings	Yes	Yes
Presence of chronic healed and/or active ulcers	Yes	Yes
Occurrence of pyloric ulcers with deformities of the pylorus	Yes	Yes
Accompanying adrenocortical necrosis	Frequent	Rare(?)
Presence of functional and/or organic brain disorders	±	+
Increased gastric acid output	±	±
Elevated basal serum gastrin levels	+	±
Supersensitivity of serum gastrin to food intake	Yes	Yes
Response to:		
Antacids	+	±
Antisecretory agents	+	+
H_2 receptor antagonists	+	+
Vagotomy	+	+
Availability to study preulcerogenic and very early ulcerogenic functional and morphologic changes	Yes	No

Reprinted with permission from Szabo S[40] (1980).

checklist of criteria that should be adhered to in a well-designed animal experiment. Control groups were described in only 14% of papers. Aspects of breeding, sex, and age of the animals are frequently reported, but the conditions of animal care are rarely given. The environment and the handling of animals can have an important input on study parameters of interest. If these factors are not recognized and controlled, the validity of the research results may be questioned. For example, transportation of test animals affects such factors as total leukocyte counts and ACTH levels.[42]

The principles of experimental design are discussed in Section II, but Table 35.3 shows that the calculation of sample sizes, or the choice of statistical tests, is not very different from those for clinical trials. Many people mistakenly assume that random allocation of animals is not necessary, because the animals represent a random sample taken from a well-defined population. Immich[43] has demonstrated that this technique is as necessary in animal experiments as it is in clinical trials.

Besides skillful design and presentation of the results, the optimum utilization of animal experiments includes attention to the possibility of reducing the number of animals necessary for each experiment. In every laboratory where several groups are performing animal experiments, information about planned studies should be exchanged to enable more than one research group to participate in a project. Sacrificing one rat today to obtain a colon sample, and another tomorrow to get a piece of muscle is wasting animals. Every effort should be made to reduce the number of animals needed by such measures as using a two-step experimental design or a sequential trial, or the replacement of a time- and animal-consuming dose–response curve by the up and down method of Dixon,[44] when the determination of an LD_{50} is required.

Last, but certainly not least, the quality of animal experiments depends on the correct handling and care of animals, and the proper use of anesthetics, analgesics, and tranquilizers. If a procedure must be conducted without the use of an anesthetic, analgesic, or tranquilizer, because such an agent would defeat the purpose of the experiment, the responsible investigator must personally supervise the procedure to ensure that it is carried out in accordance with institutional policies and local, state, or federal regulations. Muscle relaxants or paralytic drugs (e.g., succinylcholine or other curariform drugs) are not anesthetics, and they should not be used, alone, for surgical restraint.

Appropriate facilities and equipment should be available for surgical procedures. A facility intended for aseptic surgery should be maintained and used for that purpose only, and its cleanliness should be assured. Surgery on animals should only be performed by persons who are properly qualified by training and experience, and should be conducted in the same formal and respectful manner that characterizes the operating theater during surgery on humans.

Postsurgical care should include observation of the animal until it has recovered from anesthesia, administration of supportive fluids and drugs, care of surgical incisions, and regular monitoring to ensure the animal's physical comfort and optimal recovery. Appropriate medical records should be maintained.

Euthanasia should be performed by trained persons in accordance with institutional policies and

TABLE 35.3. Frequency of items reported in papers involving animal experiments.

Item	%
General Declarations	
Strain	91
Genetics	70
Origin	67
Sex	61
Age	80
Class of age	80
Experimental Design	
Total number	94
Number of	61
Body weight	31
Bacteriological state	43
Selection	22
Randomization	14
Environment and Care	
Adaptation to environment	27
to humans	14
to the experiment	27
Light/dark change	14
Temperature	20
Animal laboratory	20
Humidity	16
Air change	8
Noise	0
Feed	49
Drinking	22
Animals per cage	16
Cage material	29
Size of cages	18
Litter	10
Change of litter	18
Course of the Experiment	
Duration	71
Mortality	12
Diagnosis	12
Analysis of the Experiment	
Number of groups	71
Animals/groups	59
Controls	14
Animals/control groups	18
Statistical tests	34
Statistical significance	39

Modified with permission from Juhr[44] (1980).

applicable laws. The choice of method depends on the species of animal and the project in which the animal was used (e.g., it should not interfere with postmortem examinations). Procedures for euthanasia should follow approved guidelines, such as those already established by the American Veterinary Medical Association Panel on Euthanasia. Animals of most species can be killed quickly and humanely by the intravenous or intraperitoneal injection of a concentrated solution of barbiturate. Mice, rats, and hamsters can be killed by cervical dislocation, or by exposure to gaseous nitrogen or carbon dioxide in an uncrowded chamber. Ether and chloroform are effective, but their use is hazardous to personnel; ether is flammable and explosive, chloroform is toxic and possibly carcinogenic. If animals are killed by ether, special facilities and procedures are required for storage and disposal of carcasses. Serious explosions can result from storage in refrigeration equipment that is not explosion-proof, and disposal by incineration.

The environment and dietary regimen should be suitable for each species. The components of the diet should be known and standardized, and should be adapted to the age of the animals when necessary. Young animals usually need a diet that is richer in protein than that given to adults. Information about normal values for the species used in an experiment can be very helpful in arriving at a first estimation of the reliability of your own measurements.

Quality of Animals

A quality assurance program to define and characterize research animals, adequately, is important. Various commonly occurring microorganisms cause subclinical infections in animals that may flare to produce high morbidity or mortality when the animals are stressed by an experiment. Such incidents frequently complicate the research results, invalidate the scientific data collected or their interpretation, and cause loss of money, time, and other research resources.[41] Rodents, for example, should be free from sendai virus, mouse hepatitis virus, Reo 3 virus, lactic dehydrogenase elevating virus, lymphatic choriomeningitis virus, ectromelia, *Salmonella, Hexamita, Pneumocystis, Haemobartonella, Eperythrozoon, Syphacia, Aspiculuris*, ectoparasites, and the microorganisms listed in Table 35.4. When these pathogens infect and proliferate in animals, they cause subtle, long-term or short-term changes in organ and cell function, metabolism, and physiology, even though the animals appear to be clinically healthy. A sampling plan for the microbiological or pathological monitoring of animals to detect the presence of diseased animals, within adequate confidence limits, has been published by Hsu,[45] along with a list of the pathogens and parasites that may be encountered.

All laboratory animals should be observed daily for clinical signs of illness, injury, or abnormal behavior by a person trained to recognize such signs. All deviations from normal, and all deaths from unknown causes, should be reported promptly to the person responsible for animal disease control.

The most important link in a quality assurance program is probably the producer of the animals. Producers must ensure proper breeding systems for both the inbred strains and outbred stocks to maintain their genetic integrity and characteristics. They should periodically perform health characterization and genetic monitoring of their animal colonies, and make their findings available at regular intervals or on request by those who purchase their animals. The methods used in genetic monitoring are listed in Table 35.5. Research animals should always be obtained from a reliable vendor who consistently supplies high-quality, genetically defined animals. Vendors should be periodically evaluated according to the management, economic, and other criteria listed in Table 35.6.

The aim of all these measures it to lower costs, reduce the number of animals necessary for an experiment, and improve the reliability of the results. The experimenter will feel better about a well-designed experiment when he has taken care to avoid any unnecessary injury to, and sacrifice of, whatever creatures have been involved.

Some Personal Comments

Learning to use animals in clinical and surgical research, recognizing the possibilities and limits of animal experimentation, and accepting the attendant responsibilities should be seen as privileges. Competence in animal experimentation has to be learned like any other skill. The fact that living matter is involved, whatever its place in the classification of living organisms, imposes a particular obligation on you, as the investigator.

The researcher and all coworkers—those involved directly in the experiment and those taking care of the animals in the animal quarters—ought to be aware that animals have their joys and feel discomfort, are sensitive, are capable of suf-

TABLE 35.4. Bacteria for which routine monitoring is recommended.

Mice	Rats	Guinea pigs	Hamsters
Salmonella	*Salmonella*	*Salmonella*	*Salmonella*
Pseudomonas	*Pasteurella*	*Streptococcus*	*Pasteurella*
Corynebacterium	*Diplococcus*	*Zooepidemicus*	*Bordetella*
Pasteurella	*Klebsiella*	*Bordtella*	
Klebsiella	*Pseudomonas*	*Klebsiella*	
Bordetella bronchiseptica	*Corynebacterium*	*Diplococcus*	
Diplococcus pneumoniae	*Bordetella*		
Mycoplasma	*Mycoplasm*		

Modified with permission from Hsu CK, New AE, Mayo JG[48] (1980).

TABLE 35.5. Methods for genetic monitoring.

A. Breeding methods
B. *In vivo* histocompatibility testing
1. Skin grafting
2. Lymphoid tissue transplantation
3. Tumor transplantation
C. *In vitro* histocompatibility testing
1. Mixed lymphocyte reaction (MLR)
2. Cell-mediated lympholysis (CML)
3. Serology
D. Biochemical marker analysis
E. Embryo cryopreservation
F. Chromosomal banding
G. Mandible analysis

Modified with permission from Hsu CK, New AE, Mayo JG[48] (1980).

TABLE 35.6. Vendor evaluation.

1. Type of practice (producer or dealer)
2. Type of facility (barrier or conventional)
3. Management and operation (accredited or not)
4. Professional and technical staff
5. Availability of animal quality data
6. Genetic uniformity and compatibility
7. Methods of transportation
8. Number, strain, and species that can be supplied
9. Reliability in meeting ordering specification
10. Cost
11. Quality of animals

Modified with permission from Hsu CK, New AE, Mayo JG[48] (1980).

fering and enduring pain, can be afraid, and have memory. Members of the team who lack and cannot be taught respect, responsibility, and correct treatment of the animal as a fellow living being should not be allowed to use or handle animals.

You should go beyond the legal regulations in meticulously scrutinizing the scientific necessity, value, and mode of implementing each experiment.[11] You bear ultimate moral responsibility for your actions and choices related to animal experimentation.[46] There must always be a reasonable expectation that your study will contribute significantly to clinical knowledge and progress.

Experiments in animals should always be carefully thought out. A study of the literature relevant to the topic should precede the planning, and especially the implementation of any series of experiments. Helpful information can almost always be gained about the selection of relevant parameters, adequate methods of analysis, and appropriate animal model species. An animal species should not be used just because it is the one that is most readily available and most familiar to you. You should not find it repugnant to ask for advice and help. The animal is to be the surrogate of man!

The conception, planning, preparation, and performance of animal experiments is a major scientific responsibility. It requires time. It can rarely be discharged properly by adding it onto the end of a long day's work.

In vivo experiments and the sacrificing of animals without pain or fright at the end of experiments, or to obtain tissues or organs for in vitro experiments, must be performed by, or under the immediate and continuous supervision of, an appropriately qualified scientist. Experiments in animals should be performed with the assistance of a sufficient number of properly trained personnel; individual research has given way to the team approach. Work on a do-it-yourself basis using self-taught techniques in a distant corner of a laboratory is contrary to the principles of experimentation in animals. Surgical research in animals should be confined to specialized and adequately equipped institutes, departments, or units.

The 3 R's—replacement, reduction, refinement[17]—are important guides for research in animals. Animals should be used only after careful consideration has convinced you that no method other than an animal experiment can solve a problem, or provide the information that is needed. The scientific question should be formulated in such a way that a clear and valid answer can be reached with a minimum number of experiments. As many data as possible should be collected in each experiment, provided overinstrumentation does not invalidate the model.

> The care and use of animals for experimental purposes should be based on the principle that pain and discomfort must be avoided. To this end, anesthetics and analgesic agents should be employed in an appropriate manner, unless specifically withheld as a requirement of the experiment. Pain-relieving drugs should be continued as long as necessary. Experiments in which pain and discomfort are an unavoidable consequence should be undertaken only when, on the basis of expert opinion, there are reasonable expectations that such studies will contribute to the ultimate enhancement of our knowledge of life. The degree of pain should never exceed that determined by the humanitarian importance of the problem to be solved by the experimental study.[47]

Surgical research and postoperative care, particularly in higher animals, should be conducted according to the same standards as surgery in humans.

The decision on the fate of an animal depends on the purpose of an experiment. Either the animal must be sacrificed when the experiment is completed, or its subsequent life must be free from pain, grief, and discomfort.

References

1. American Association of Pathologists: A workshop on needs for new animal models of human disease. Am J Pathol December 1980 (Suppl); 101(35).
2. Tierexperimentelle Forschung und Tierschutz/Dt. Forschungsgemeinschaft, Mitteilung III, Boldt Verlag, Boppard, 1981.
3. Gartner K, Hackbarth H, Stolte H. eds. Symposium on research animals and concepts of applicability to clinical medicine. Hannover FRG, 1981, Exp Biol Med Vol. 7. Basel: Karger, 1982.
4. Hoel DG. Animal experimentation and its relevance to man. Environ Health Perspect 1980;32:25–30.
5. Hoff, C. Immoral and moral uses of animals. N Engl J Med 1980;302:115–18.
6. IABS 16th Congress for Biological Standardization, San Antonio, 1979: The standardization of animals to improve biomedical research. Basel: Production and Control S. Karger, 1980.
7. ILAR Symposium. The Future of Animals, Cells, Models and Systems in Research, Development, Education, and Testing. Washington, DC: National Academy of Sciences, 1977.
8. Kubler K, ed. Der Tierversuch in der Arzneimittelforschung (interdisziplinäres Fachgesprach im Bundesgesundheitsant) bga-Berichte 1980;1:1–111. Dietrich Reimer Verlag, Berlin.
9. McDaniel CG. Animal rights or human health? Med J Aust 1984;141:855–57.
10. Merkenschlager M, Wilk W. Gutachten über tierschutzgerechte Haltung von Versuchstieren. Gutachten über Tierversuche, Möglichkeiten ihrer Einschraenkung und Ersetzbarkeit. Recommendations for the keeping of laboratory animals in accordance with animal protection principles. Verlag Paul, Parey, Berlin-Hamburg: 1979.
11. Riecker G. Aerztliche Ethik und Tierversuche Arzt und Krankenhaus 1984;11:306–12.
12. Sechzer JA, ed. The role of animals in biomedical research. Ann NY Acad Sci 1983;406.
13. Smyth HD. Alternatives to Animal Experimentation. London: Scolar Press, 1978.
14. Sontag KH. Der Tierversuch nach dem Stand der wissenschaftlichen Kenntnis, Pharm Ind 1982; 44:4.
15. Weihe WH. Das Problem der Alternativen zum wissenschaftlichen Tierversuch. Fortschr Med 1982; 100:2162–66.
16. Ullrich KJ, Creutzfeldt OD (Ed). Gesundheit und Tierschutz. Wissenschaftler melden sich zu Wort ECON Verlag, Düsseldorf-Wien (1985).
17. Sedlacek H. Tierschutz: Güterabwägung oder Gleichheitsprinzip Klinikarzt 1986;15:508–10.
18. The Ethics of Animal Experimentation: Proceedings of the Second CFN Symposium Acta Physiol Scand 1986; 128 (Suppl. 554):4–250.
19. Rowan AN. The concept of the three R's, and introduction. 16th IABS Congress: the standardization of animals to improve biomedical research, production and control, San Antonio, 1979. In: Develop Biol Standard. Vol. 45, Basel: Karger, S, 1980;45:175–180.
20. Russell, WMS, Burch RL. The Principle of Humane Experimental Technique. London: Methuen, 1959.
21. Stiller H, Stiller M. Tierversuch und Tierexperimentator. F. Hirthammer Verlag, München. 1977.
22. Kirsch U. Untersuchungen zum Eintritt der Totenstarre an ischamischen Meerschweinchenherzen in Normothermie. Arzneim Forsch 1970;20:1071–74.
23. Carrentier S, Murawsky M, Carpentier A. Cytotoxicity of cardioplegic solutions: evaluation by tissue culture. Circulation 1981;64 (Suppl. II),II:90–II-95.
24. Isselhard W, Schorn B, Huegel W, Uekermann U. Comparison of three methods of myocardial protection. Thorac Cardiovasc Surgeon 1980;28:329–126.
25. Hügel W, Lübbing H, Isselhard W, et al. Hemodynamics and metabolic status of the human heart after application of different forms of cardioplegic solutions. In: Myocardial Protection for Cardiovascular Surgery, Isselhard W, ed. München Pharmazeutische Verlagsgesellschaft, 1981.
26. Rowan AN. Laboratory animals and alternatives in the 80s. Int J Study Anim Probl 1980;1:162–69.
27. Wessler S. Introduction: what is a model? In: Animal Models of Thrombosis and Hemorrhagic Diseases. Bethesda, MD: National Institutes of Health, 1976:XI–XVI.
28. ILAR National Research Council Committee on Animal Models for Research on Aging. Mammalian Models for Research on Aging. Washington, DC: National Academy Press, 1981.
29. Held JR. Appropriate animal models. In: The Role of Animals in Biomedical Research, Sechzer, JA, ed. Ann NY Acad Sci 1983;406:13–19.
30. Gill THJ. The use of randomly bred and genetically defined animals in biomedical research. Am J Pathol 1981;100:21–32.
31. Jones TC. The value of animal models. Am J Pathol 1981;101:3–9.
32. Leader RW, Padgett GA: The genesis and validation of animal models. Am J Pathol 1981;101:11–17.
33. Festing FW. Inbred Strains in Biochemical Research. London and Basingstoke: Macmillan, 1979.
34. Jay GE. Genetic strains and stocks. In: Durdette WJ, ed. Methodology in mammalian genetics. Holden-Day, San Francisco, 1963:83–126.
35. Bustad LK, Hegreberg GA, Padgett GA. Animal models. In: The future of animals, cells, models and systems in research development, education and testing. Nat Acad of Sci, 1977.
36. Andrews EJ, Ward BC, Altman NH, eds. Spontaneous models of human diseases. Academic Press, 1979.
37. Szabo S. Animal model of human disease: duodenal ulcer disease. Animal model: cysteamine–induced acute and chronic duodenal ulcer in the rat. Amer J Pathol. 1978;93:273–76.
38. Szabo S, Haith LR Jr, Reynolds ES. Pathogenesis of duodenal ulceration produced by cysteamine or

proprionitrile: influence of vagotomy, sympathectomy, histamine depletion. H_2 – receptor antagonists and hormones. Am J Dig Dis 1979;24:471–74.
39. Brady JV. Ulcers in "Executive" Monkeys. Sci Am 1958;199:99–100.
40. Szabo S. Discussion. Am J Pathol 1980;100:78–82.
41. Cornelius CE. Animal models: a neglected medical resource. N Engl J Med 1969;281:933–944.
42. McPeek B. Darstellung von Elementen des Designs und derer Analyse in klinischen Studien. In: Rohde H, Troidl H, eds. Das Margenkarzinom, Thieme Verlag, Stuttgart, 1984;35–9.
43. Pollock AV. Design and interpretation of clinical trials Br Med J 1985;290:243.
44. Juhr NC. Die Optimierung des Tierversuchs – Aufgabe einer Tierversuchskunde. In: Kübler K ed. Der Tierversuch in der Arzneimittelforschung bga-Berichte. Dietrich Reimer-Verlag, Berlin, 1980; 1:57–62.
45. Held JR. Mühlbock memorial lecture: consideration in the provision and characterization of animal models. In: Spiegel A, Erichsen S, Solleveld HA, eds. Animal quality and models in biomedical research. Stuttgart, New York: G. Fischer Verlag, 1980;9–16.
46. Immich H. Medizinische Statistik. Stuttgart, New York: Schattauer Verlag, 1974.
47. Dixon WJ. The up-and-down method for small samples Am. Statis. Assoc., 1965;60:967–978.
48. Hsu CK, New AE, Mayo JG. Quality assurance of rodent models. 7th ICLAS Symp., Utrecht 1979 G. Fischer, Stuttgart, New York: 1980;17–28.
49. Bonnod J. Principles of ethics in animal experimentation. 16th IABS Congress: the standardization of animals to improve biomedical research, production and control. San Antonio 1979, Developments in Biological Standardization. S. Karger, Basel. 1980;45:185–187.
50. Rowsell HC. The ethics of biomedical experimentation. In: the future of animals, cells, models and systems in research, development, education, and testing. Washington, D.C.: Nat Acad of Sci, 1977.

36

Recombinant DNA Technology

J.A. Drebin, S.W. Hartzell, and J.E. Niederhuber

It has become clear in recent years that man is now a truly accessible genetic system for study. The tremendous advances in the development of new techniques in molecular genetics have made it possible to propose mapping and sequencing the entire human genome. To most of us, the rate at which these technologies have been producing new knowledge in such clinically relevant areas as the inherited diseases, cancer-related oncogenes, growth factors, and cellular receptors has been staggering; and the emergence of molecular genetics as a powerful research tool has touched every area of biomedical research. As a result, the surgeon scientist has a growing opportunity to use recombinant DNA techniques to identify, isolate, and characterize the molecular elements involved in the pathophysiology of surgical disorders. In this chapter, the terms and techniques most common to the molecular genetic laboratory will be introduced as a stimulus to further reading and, it is hoped, to facilitate the application of these techniques in the surgeon's laboratory.

One Gene, One Protein

The process of cell function (e.g., the production of functional proteins) has its beginning in each cell at the level of the chromosomal DNA. The sequence of amino acids in the protein and, therefore, its tertiary structure and function, are determined by the precise order of purine and pyrimidine nucleotides in the DNA sequence.[1] For each cellular protein, a specific DNA sequence or code exists, and it determines the order of the 20 different amino acids that can be used to form the protein.[2,3] The DNA molecules exist as long, linear polymers built from four different nucleotides connected together by phosphodiester linkages.[3-5] Two of the four nucleotides contain purine bases, adenine [A] and guanine [G], while the other two are pyrimidine bases (thymine [T] and cytosine [C]). The polynucleotide chains of a DNA molecule are paired in a double helix held together by hydrogen bonds between base pairs (Figure 36.1). The paired polynucleotide chains are not identical but are complementary, with adenine always paired to thymine and guanine always matched to cytosine. Thus, if the sequence of one chain is determined, the second is automatically known. Note that each strand of DNA has polarity that is indicated by a 5′ to 3′ labeling.

For the synthesis of proteins, the sequence of DNA base pairs serves as a template to generate another form of nucleic acid, RNA.[4,5] The RNA copies, found primarily in the cytoplasm, provide the final templates for protein synthesis. RNA, like DNA, is composed of four different nucleotide building blocks. Two are purines, adenine and guanine; two are pyrimidines, uracil [U] (which replaces the thymine used in DNA) and cytosine.

The process of generating an RNA copy of one strand of DNA is termed *transcription*, is accomplished by a specific enzyme, *RNA polymerase*. The resultant messenger RNA (mRNA) molecules move across the intracellular ribosomes that are the factories of protein synthesis. Within the ribosomes, specific enzymes, *aminoacyl synthetases*, attach a given amino acid to specific transfer RNA (tRNA) molecules that comprise three RNA nucleotides defined as an *anticodon*. The tRNA anticodon uses base pairing to find the appropriate codon of three base pairs on the mRNA, and successive codons are positioned on the ribosome for synthesis of polypeptide chains, a process termed *translation*. Of the 64 (4 × 4 × 4) potential triplets (codons), 61 determine specific amino acids and three provide chain termination signals.

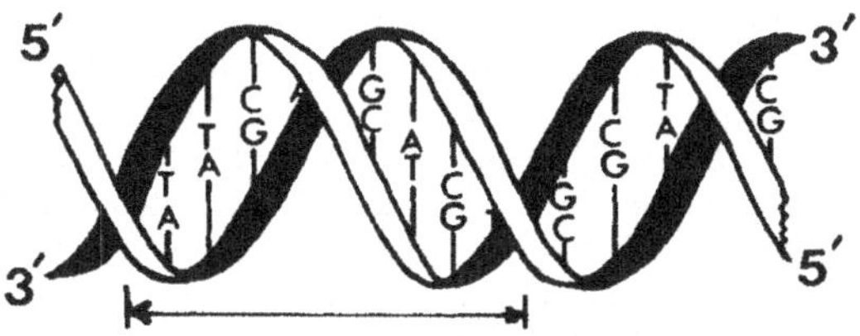

FIGURE 36.1. The DNA double helix. Complementary strands are held together by hydrogen bonds between purine and pyrimidine base pairs. Each DNA strand in the helix has polarity indicated by the 5′ to 3′ labeling.

TABLE 36.1. Examples of recognition sequences of restriction enzymes.

Enzyme	Enzyme recognition sequence and site of cleavage
Eco RI	5′ G|AA TTC 3′
	3′ CTT AA|G 5′
Hind III	5′ A|AG CTT 3′
	3′ TTC GA|A 5′
*Bam*H I	5′ G|GA TCC 3′
	3′ CCT AG|G 5′
Hpa II	5′ C|C GG 3′
	3′ GG C|C 5′
Hae III	5′ GG| CC 3′
	3′ CC| GG 5′
Hpa I	5′ GTT|AAC 3′
	3′ CAA|TTG 5′

Utilization of DNA Properties Involved in Nucleic Acid Hybridization

The chemical bonds holding complementary nucleotide strands together are relatively weak and, in the laboratory, helical duplex DNA can be denatured (separated into single strands) by heating in a water bath to a temperature of 70 to 80°C or by extremes of alkaline pH. Similarly, the separated strands will reanneal at low temperatures and at neutral pH. This ability to denature and anneal DNA sequences, in the laboratory, is involved in almost all phases of genetic engineering and nucleic acid analysis.

Hybridization between DNA strands can occur when as few as 75% of the bases are complementary (A–T and C–G). Thus, a gene isolated in an animal model can form a DNA–DNA hybrid with its human counterpart if there is at least 75% sequence homology. Under the electron microscope, this hybridization would appear as regions of double-stranded DNA where sequence homology occurred, interspersed with regions of single-stranded DNA representing non-homologous sequences. Labeling of one DNA sequence, usually with [α^{32}P](deoxycylosine triphosphate), (to be discussed), can be used to confirm hybridization and to isolate desired DNA sequences using gel electrophoresis and autoradiography.

Restriction Enzymes

The functions of DNA include self-replication and transcription of mRNA leading to protein synthesis—processes that involve specific DNA binding enzymes. In addition, bacteria have evolved the means to protect their DNA from damage by externally introduced DNA or from defects in replication. One such protection system is a series of enzymes termed *restriction enzymes,* which cut DNA at specific nucleotide sequences.[6-8] Restriction enzymes with more than 100 different nucleotide sequence specificities have been isolated from various bacteria. For each bacterial restriction enzyme, a corresponding DNA methylase enzyme protects the restriction enzyme target sequence of the native bacterial DNA. These DNA methylases add methyl groups only to adenine or cytosine bases within the target sequence of the native DNA to protect it from cutting.

Highly purified bacterial restriction enzymes provide a very powerful laboratory tool for cutting double-stranded DNA at known recognition sequences. An array of different restriction enzymes that recognize sequences of four, five, or six base pairs is now commercially available. The DNA fragments generated by cutting with one or more restriction enzymes can be easily separated by size, using electrophoresis on agarose gels, and visualized by staining with ethidium bromide and fluorescing with long wave UV light.[9]

DNA fragments separated by gel electrophoresis can be recovered from the gel as intact DNA for further analysis or use in cloning. The various sites of cutting along a chromosome or chromosome segment are used to generate a series of "restriction fragments," the determined order of which is called a *restriction map* of the DNA segment. Restriction enzymes with rarely occurring cutting sequence sites tend to be the most useful. The maps generated by different enzymes or combinations of enzymes will be different, and these differences can be used to order the restriction fragments.

Restriction enzymes used in the laboratory cleave double-stranded DNA in a staggered fashion leaving a four-base 5″ overhang on each strand. There are other restriction enzymes that create only blunt ends—no overhang (Table 36.1). The presence of the overhang facilitates the ligation (joining) of identically cut DNA fragments derived from different DNA molecules to produce *recombinant DNA*. The ligation process is accomplished in the laboratory using the enzyme DNA-ligase and a mixture of the cut DNA fragments to be joined.[9] The most common use of ligation is the insertion of a DNA sequence under study into an autonomously replicating DNA cloning vector—a topic addressed in more detail later in the chapter.

Southern and Northern Transfer Analysis

Detection of particular sequences of cloned DNA, or digests of total eukaryotic DNA, is most often accompanied by a transfer technique originally described by Southern.[10] In this method, fragments generated by cutting with various restriction endonucleases are separated according to their size (number of base pairs) using one-dimensional agarose gel electrophoresis. The gel is denatured and the DNA is transferred directly to a cellulose membrane where it is immobilized. A ^{32}P-labeled DNA or RNA probe of known sequence is hybridized to the membrane-bound DNA, and the membrane is exposed to x-ray film. Only the DNA fragments complementary to the DNA sequence of the probe used will bind (hybridize) to the radioactive probe, detected as a dark band on autoradiography (Figure 36.2).

When this technique is used with RNA, it is known as a Northern blot; when used to transfer proteins, a Western blot. A Northern blot is generated by separating total RNA or poly-A^+ selected mRNA in a denaturing agarose gel. The RNA species are transferred to a cellulose membrane and hybridized to specific radiolabeled DNA probes.[11]

A variation on this technique is the use of dot or slot blotting. For example, to detect the presence of a particular mRNA species in a variety of cell types, total RNA harvests from each of the cell lines are spotted adjacent to each other on a cellulose filter. The filter is hybridized to a 32P-labeled DNA probe of interest. If the RNA sequence is present in a given cell line, the dot or slot representing that RNA will be detected by autoradiography. The intensity of the signal is a reasonable measure of the degree to which the mRNA is represented in the cell.

Gene Cloning

The ability to isolate genetic sequences of particular interest—*gene cloning*—is the cornerstone of molecular biology (for technical details, see reference 9). By introducing mammalian DNA into self-replicating genetic agents (vectors), it is possible to rapidly duplicate any DNA segment to milligram quantities within a bacterial host, most commonly *E. coli*. The origins of gene cloning came from researchers studying bacterial genetics. These investigators identified and specifically engineered genetic vectors capable of autonomous replication in bacterial hosts. These vectors include viruses, called *bacteriophage* or *phage*, and miniature chromosomes, called *plasmids*. Such structures function in nature to parasitize bacteria by replicating independently within the bacterial cell.

Molecular biologists have adapted phage and plasmids as a way to isolate and replicate specific genes. Essentially, all cloning schemes depend on the ligation of novel DNA segments, such as those derived from mammalian cells, into a phage or plasmid vector in a manner that allows the vector to replicate itself and the introduced DNA segment.

Bacteriophage undergo a process of replication leading to lysis of the host bacterium within a time as short as an hour (lytic growth cycle), or they may integrate into the bacterial chromosome and be replicated with subsequent bacterial division (lysogenic growth cycle). As lytic bacteriophage is most commonly employed in cloning strategies, it will be discussed here. Infection by lytic phage of a single bacterium on a lawn of susceptible bacteria in a petri dish will lead to rapid replication of phage within the infected bacterium. This is followed by lysis of the bacterial host, and the release of large numbers of new bacteriophage that may sequentially infect and lyse adjacent bacteria. In this fashion, a single phage may destroy all bacteria on an area of a petri plate, while replicating itself to a high density, visible to the investigator as a clear area on an otherwise cloudy bacteria-coated plate. Such an area of clearing is called a *plaque*.

Exogenous DNA sequences can be introduced into bacteriophage without altering the phage's ability to undergo the lytic growth cycle in bacteria. Such exogenous DNA is referred to as an *insert*. Phage containing an insert (recombinant phage) will reproduce the insert along with its own genomes, with a resultant rapid amplification of inserted sequences.

Unlike lytic phage, plasmids replicate in parallel with their bacterial hosts and generally do not produce bacterial lysis. The presence of plasmids may actually confer advantages on the parasitized bacterial host. The presence within many plasmids of the antibiotic resistance gene, penicillinase, is an example. The presence of such a gene within a plasmid confers a selective advantage on bacteria

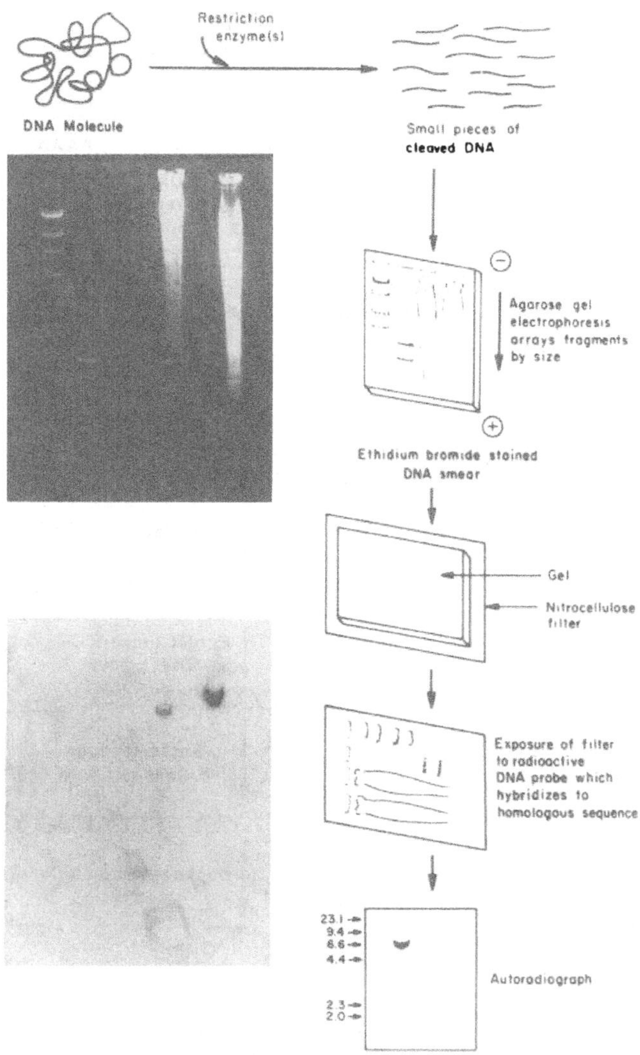

FIGURE 36.2. Genomic DNA was cu with either *Sac* I or *Bam*H I restrictioı enzymes. The cleaved DNA was sepa rated by size of a 0.7% agarose gel. Th upper photo insert represents the ethid ium-stained gel. The two left-hand lane: are size markers. The first DNA lane ha: been cut with *Sac* I. The second lane i: DNA cut with *Bam*H I. The DNA is the transferred from the gel to a nitrocellu lose filter and the filter is immobilized DNA is hybridized with a ^{32}P-labele DNA sequence representing the huma *blk* gene. The lower photo insert show: the autoradiograph of the probed filte showing a single band of 5Kb and 7Kb ir the respective lanes.

infected by it when they are in an environment containing penicillin. The presence of such selectable genetic markers within plasmid vectors has also been of great use to molecular biologists attempting to clone genes. Placing a novel DNA insert into a plasmid containing an antibiotic resistance gene and introducing the plasmid into susceptible bacteria in the presence of the appropriate antibiotic permits large scale growth of bacteria containing the plasmid (and its insert), while selecting against bacteria lacking the plasmid.

An enormous array of bacteriophage and plasmid vectors has been developed for use in gene cloning. Many of these vectors have particular advantages for certain types of cloning problem, but their complexity precludes their discussion within the limits of this chapter. You are encouraged to consult Sanbrook et al.[9] for further technical information about cloning vectors.

Most cloning strategies involve the isolation of a vector containing a sequence of interest from a pool of vectors containing random DNA segments. Such pools of vectors, each containing a distinct genetic insert, are called *libraries*. DNA for construction of libraries may be derived from chromosomal (genomic) DNA cut to a certain size range with specific restriction endonucleases. Alternatively, complementary DNA (cDNA) synthesized from an mRNA template by the enzyme reverse transcriptase may be used (Figure 36.3). There are advantages and disadvantages to each method.

An example of this dichotomy is genomic cloning, in which both protein coding and noncoding sequences are likely to be included in any cloned

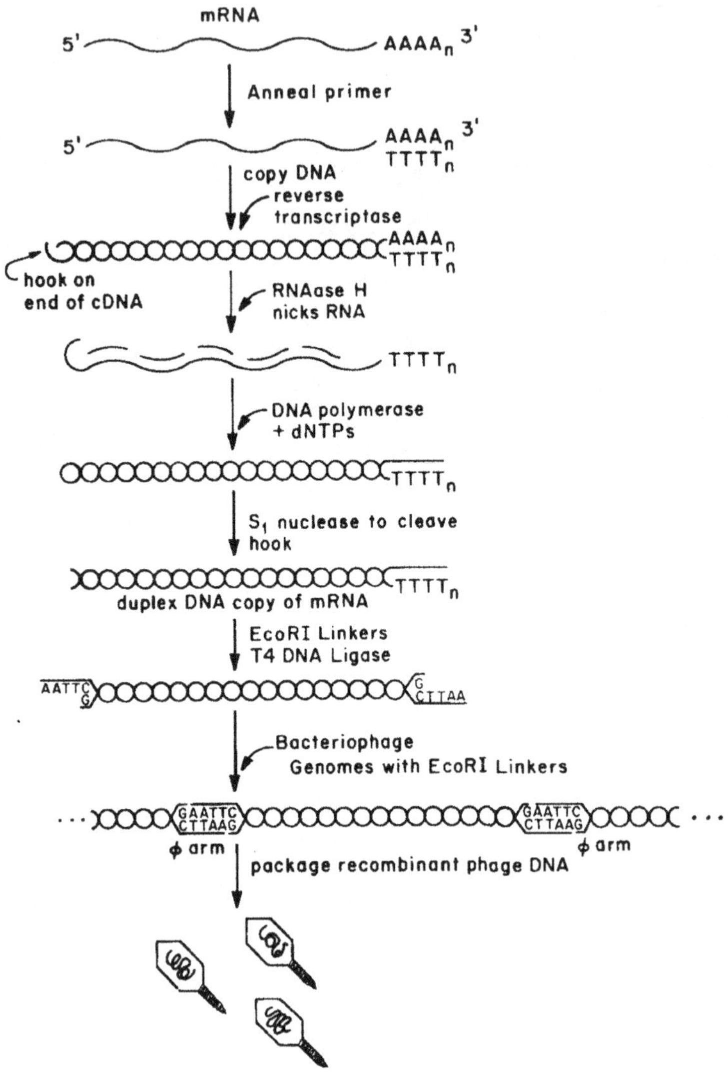

FIGURE 36.3. Schematic representation of the reactions to convert messenger RNA into complementary DNA for the purpose of generating a cDNA library. In this procedure, total cellular RNA is first passed through a column of oligo deoxythymidine, which hybridizes with all of the poly-A tails of the pool of mRNAs. The poly-A$^+$ enriched mRNA is then eluted from the column. An oligo dT primer is annealed to the poly A stretch of the mRNA and added to a reaction mix that includes a pool of the four different nucleotide bases (dNTPs) and the enzyme reverse transcriptase. The enzyme acts to copy the mRNA, creating a first strand of cDNA. The RNA is then enzymatically degraded from the DNA:RNA complex by RNase H, and the second strand of DNA is synthesized by adding a pool of the four nucleotide bases and the enzyme DNA polymerase.

The naturally occurring "hook" on the end of the first strand serves as the primer for extension of second-strand synthesis. This loop is subsequently cut by the enzyme S_1 nuclease. In this experiment, *Eco* RI linkers are attached to each end of the duplex DNA using T_4 DNA ligase and the DNA inserted into λ gt_{10} bacteriophage constructed with appropriate *Eco* RI linkers to receive the inserts. The recombinant phage are packaged into phage heads to make them infective to host bacteria.

DNA segment of reasonable size. This is an advantage if studies of chromosomal structure are contemplated, but it may complicate DNA sequencing or use of cloned segments as probes of gene expression in Northern blots. Furthermore, any particular sequence in a library composed of random genomic segments is likely to be represented in the library at a relatively low frequency. (Since the human genome contains about 3×10^9 nucleotide bases of DNA, a 10^4 base segment would represent less than 0.001% of the library.) It may, therefore, be necessary to screen 10^5 to 10^6 random recombinant phage to find a specific sequence of interest.

Libraries composed of cDNA offer solutions to some of these problems. Since cDNA reflects mRNA organization rather than chromosomal DNA organization, it is composed of protein coding sequences. In addition, because certain mRNA species are expressed at high levels in specific tissues or cell lines (e.g., immunoglobulin mRNA is abundantly expressed in B lymphocytes), cDNA libraries constructed from mRNA derived from these tissues is likely to be selectively enriched for certain sequences. If the investigator designs a library appropriately, it may be possible to obtain a higher percentage of the specific clones of interest than would be possible using a genomic library. The major disadvantage of cDNA libraries is related to the fragility of mRNA. Unlike DNA, which is remarkably stable, RNA is rapidly broken down by RNAase enzymes found, among other places, in sweat, saliva, and respiratory secretions, and almost ubiquitously in laboratories; cDNA libraries constructed from degraded mRNA are unlikely to be of much use. The synthesis of cDNA is also dependent on the fidelity with which reverse transcriptase converts mRNA to DNA; the enzyme may produce only partial copies of a particular mRNA. This problem can be overcome by isolating multiple overlapping cDNA clones, but it can become quite a laborious process. In summary, the choice of whether to use a genomic or a cDNA library depends very much on the overall goal of the project.

Screening libraries for clones of interest involves growing independent vectors on petri dishes and transferring small amounts of each vector to nitrocellulose paper, which will covalently bond both protein and nucleic acids (Fig. 36.4). By carefully applying the nitrocellulose to an agar plate and applying orientation marks to the plate and the paper, vectors can be bound to the paper in a precise mirror-image fashion. Because independent vectors can be grown at high density in petri dishes—more than $10^4/mm^2$—it is possible to screen 10^5 to 10^6 independent vectors of a particular library for sequences of interest in a single experiment using a reasonably small number of plates.

Screening of nitrocellulose filters can be based on the presence of particular sequences, as determined by nucleic acid hybridization. If nitrocellulose filters are incubated with a ^{32}P-labeled DNA sequence (probe) under appropriate conditions, the probe will hybridize with related sequences, but not with unrelated sequences. Figure 36.5 demonstrates an autoradiograph showing the presence of phage-containing DNA that hybridized with a sequence specific probe; a segment of the murine *blk* oncogene[12] was used as probe and hybridized to the homologous human gene in a phage vector.[13] This plate actually contained about 5×10^3 phage plaques, but only one phage contained sufficient homologous sequence to react in this assay. The part of the nitrocellulose filter containing the vector of interest can be determined after identification of the homologous sequence on the autoradiograph. Since the filter is a mirror image of the original agar plate, the area on the plate containing the plaque of interest can be identified and the phage isolated as a pure clone containing the sequence of interest inserted within its genome. Although our example shows screening of a phage library, it is also possible to screen plasmid libraries by quite similar methods.

The example above used a mouse gene to identify and clone the homologous human gene. However, it is possible to clone genes for which no related gene clones are available. Synthetic DNA probes can be generated inexpensively by an automated oligonucleotide synthesizer. Thus, if a small amount of protein amino acid sequence is known for any protein of interest, it is possible to synthesize a probe corresponding to the homologous nucleotide sequence and to isolate the specific gene encoding the protein by screening an appropriate library with the synthetic oligonucleotide probe. Another screening strategy uses immunoselection. Certain libraries have been designed to express the protein product of inserted genes in *E. coli*. Following mirror-image transfer of libraries to nitrocellulose, it may be possible to identify a portion of the filter containing a particular protein using a monoclonal or polyclonal antiserum reactive with the protein.[14] The corresponding phage containing the genetic insert responsible for expressing this protein can then be isolated.

DNA Sequencing

The Nobel Prize awarded to Sanger, Gilbert and Berg in 1980 recognized the significant contributions to science of their DNA sequencing tech-

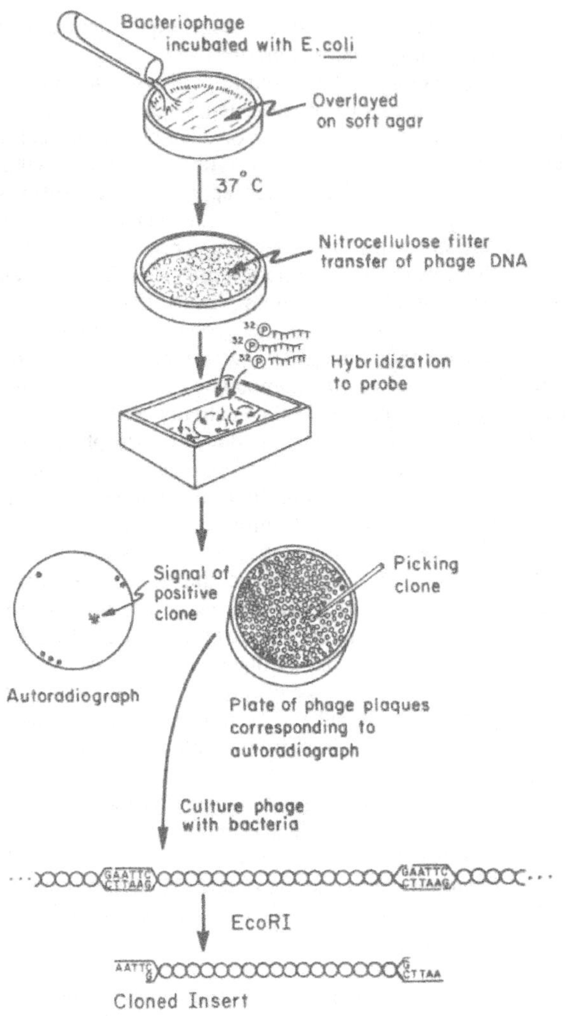

FIGURE 36.4. Continuation of the cloning demonstrated schematically in Figure 36.3. The recombinant phage are incubated with *E. coli* and overlayered on a plate of soft agar. *E. coli* infected with the phage are lysed, forming a lytic plaque of concentrated phage DNA on the *E. coli* bacterial lawn. A nitrocellulose filter is placed carefully on the plate for 2 minutes to absorb the spots of DNA. The filter is then probed in this experiment with ^{32}P-labeled murine *blk* DNA (the 5′-most portion of the *blk* sequence). An autoradiograph of the filter showed a single positive colony. The filter was aligned with the original plate so that the appropriate positive colony could be picked from the plate. The cone is reexposed to *E. coli* until the lytic phase is reached. The recombinant phage DNA is harvested and purified so that the desired insert can be removed using digestion with *Eco* RI.

niques. Sequencing DNA reveals information about the nucleotide order composing a given gene. Because the nucleotide code determines the order in which amino acids are arranged for a given protein, it also reveals important information about amino acid sequence and structure.

The two basic methods of DNA sequencing are those of Maxam and Gilbert and of Sanger[15]; although their technical aspects differ, they share a common overall strategy. The simpler and more widely used method of Sanger is described below.

DNA sequencing takes advantage of the ability of purified DNA polymerase—actually the Klenow fragment of *E. coli* DNA polymerase—to faithfully synthesize the complementary strand of any particular single-stranded piece of DNA from the 5′ toward the 3′ direction. In the absence of a single-stranded template from which to work, the DNA polymerase is enzymatically inactive. Furthermore, the polymerase enzyme requires a small region of double-stranded DNA at the 5′ end to act as a primer and free nucleotides of all four types (A, C, G, T). It will then extend the primer in a 3′ direction, adding only the complementary nucleotides (A for T, G for C, etc.). In practice, a common start site for DNA polymerase can be obtained by adding a primer complementary to the 5′ region of the vector where the gene to be sequenced is cloned. Polymerase will always initiate DNA synthesis from this common 5′ site.

Sanger observed that, whereas normal nucleotides are able to be sequentially added to growing complementary strands by DNA polymerase, chemically modified nucleotides lacking free hydroxyl

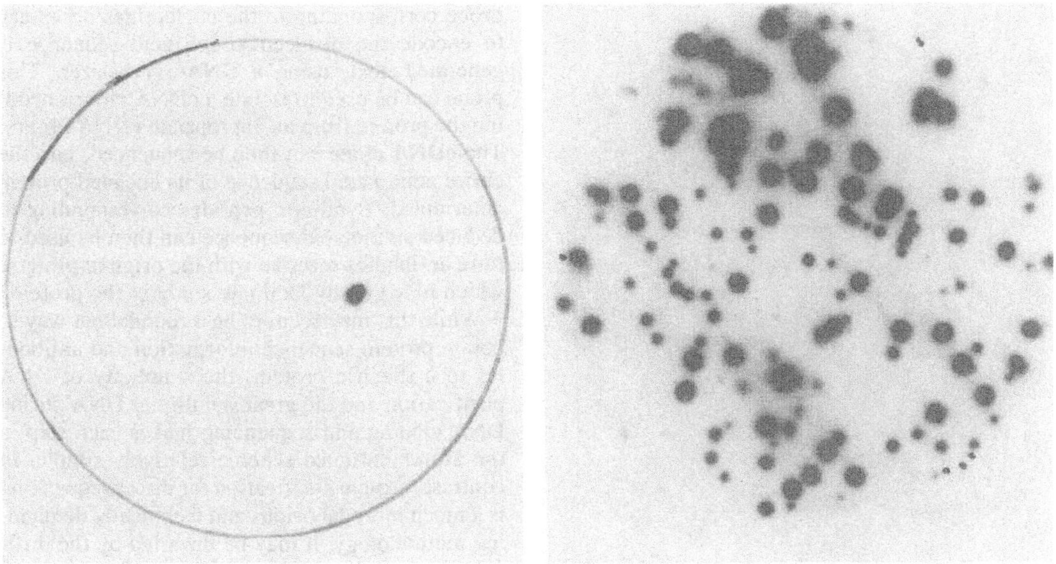

FIGURE 36.5. Autoradiographs of primary screen that identified a single positive phage clone. The panel on the right is an autoradiograph of the same clone after tertiary screening.

groups (dideoxynucleotides) cause termination of chain extension when added to growing strands. Thus, a DNA polymerase molecule that adds a dideoxycytosine opposite a guanine is unable to continue creating a complementary strand beyond this point.

In the Sanger sequencing method, four samples of DNA are prepared simultaneously, each containing the same gene of interest in its appropriate vector, as well as DNA polymerase, an appropriate primer, and all four types of free nucleotide, one or more of which are radioactive to facilitate subsequent identification of newly synthesized strands. In addition, a different dideoxy nucleotide is added to each of the four samples. The dideoxy nucleotide concentration is adjusted so that chain termination will occur infrequently at any particular nucleotide.

Following the action of DNA polymerase on the mixture described above, the sample containing dideoxyadenine would contain a mixture of newly synthesized radioactive DNA strands of varying lengths—each starting exactly at the primer site and ending at one of the adenine sites at which termination was effected by the dideoxyadenine. Similarly, in the sample containing dideoxyguanine, there will be a mixture of newly synthesized strands, each ending where a dideoxyguanine was added to the growing chain. The parallel reaction mixtures using dideoxycytosine and dideoxythymidine will, likewise, contain mixtures terminated at the corresponding nucleotide.

All four reaction mixtures are then loaded in parallel wells on a high-resolution polyacrylamide gel and subjected to electrophoresis. In such gels, it is possible to distinguish even a single nucleotide difference in chain length. Since all chains are initiated at an identical 5′ primer site, chain length will be determined by the termination site of the chain extension at a dideoxynucleotide. For a hypothetical nucleic acid sequence 12 bases long—ATTCGAAACCTG—subjected to the sequencing described above, the dideoxyadenine lane would contain chains 1, 6, 7, and 8 nucleotides long; the dideoxythymidine lane would contain chains 2, 3, and 11 nucleotides long; the dideoxycytosine lane would contain chains 4, 9, and 10 nucleotides long; and the dideoxyguanine lane would contain chains 5 and 12 nucleotides long. Since smaller chains run faster (closer to the bottom) on polyacrylamide gel electrophoresis, the lane containing the bottom band represents the first nucleotide in a given sequence—in our example, adenine. Similarly, the lane containing the next lowest band (in our example, thymidine), represents the second nucleotide, and so on.

This methodology can be utilized over large numbers of nucleotides; with a large gel apparatus,

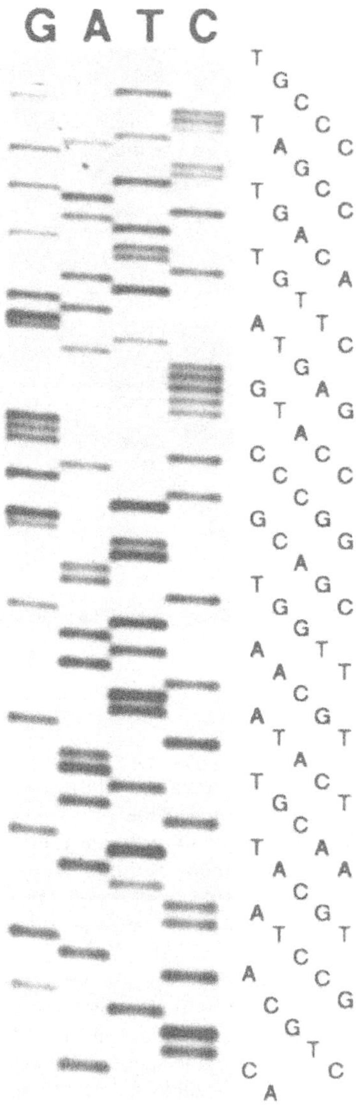

FIGURE 36.6. Example of an autoradiograph of an actual DNA sequence deduced from a sequencing gel. The dideoxyl chain termination method was used.

500 bases can be sequenced in a single experiment. Figure 36.6 shows an actual DNA sequence deduced from a sequencing gel.

Because DNA sequencing is much simpler from a technical point of view than protein sequencing, some investigators have obtained complete protein sequences from rare and difficult to purify proteins by first sequencing a small number of amino acids from one end of the protein. A synthetic DNA probe corresponding to the nucleotides necessary to encode the deduced amino acid sequence is generated next, using a DNA synthesizer. This probe can be used to isolate a cDNA clone encoding the protein from an appropriate cDNA library. The cDNA clone can then be sequenced, and the entire amino acid sequence of its encoded protein determined. Synthetic peptides corresponding to deduced amino acid sequence can then be used to raise antibodies reactive with the original protein, which may greatly facilitate study of the protein.

While this may seem to be a roundabout way to obtain protein sequence information and antibodies to a specific protein, the simplicity of DNA purification and the great stability of DNA during DNA cloning and sequencing makes each step in the aforementioned scheme relatively simple. In contrast, protein purification for direct sequencing is a much more laborious and technically demanding methodology. It may be thwarted by the difficulty of obtaining the large amounts of a given protein necessary for complete amino acid sequencing and by the labile nature of most purified proteins. Thus, DNA sequencing methodology, in addition to providing direct information about the organization of specific genes, gives the investigator the ability to understand and manipulate their protein products.

Polymerase Chain Reaction

The analysis of DNA sequences is increasingly important to an understanding of many genetic and infectious diseases. Many of the conventional analytical methods of molecular biology are difficult to use without relatively large quantities of DNA, which may be difficult to obtain from clinical samples. Recently, a powerful new technique, called the *polymerase chain reaction* (PCR), has been developed.[16] This technique can be used to amplify any segment of DNA lying between two areas of known sequence. Using PCR, a millionfold amplification of a given sequence of DNA is possible in 2 hours.

PCR amplification is accomplished by using DNA polymerase and two synthetic oligonucleotide primers that are complementary to the flanking regions of the DNA sequence to be amplified (Fig. 36.7). The primers hybridize to opposite strands of the DNA and are oriented with their 3′ ends facing each other. In this orientation, DNA polymerase can extend the primers, and synthesis proceeds across the original DNA template. Both the newly synthesized strands of DNA will contain sites that are complementary to one of the primers;

consequently, both the new strands can participate as a template in subsequent rounds of primer extension and amplification. Provided there is a large excess of primer, this cycle can be repeated many times with a doubling of the newly synthesized DNA, each time around.

A denaturation step is required between each round of synthesis to separate the double-stranded DNA into single strands, which are then available for annealing a primer. This step requires heating to 92 to 93°C—a temperature that inactivates *E. coli* DNA polymerase I; if the latter is used, a fresh amount must be added at each cycle, but the problem has been solved by purifying DNA polymerase from the thermophilic bacterium *Thermus aquaticus*. This enzyme, called *Taq DNA polymerase*, survives incubation at 95°C and is not inactivated by the heat denaturation step. The ability of Taq DNA polymerase to work at high temperatures provides the additional benefit of allowing the annealing step to occur at temperatures up to 55°C. Annealing at high temperature increases the specificity of base pairing between the primer and the target DNA. This lowers the amount of nonspecific binding and increases the amount of specific product yield.

One drawback to using the Taq DNA polymerase is the small rate of misincorporation of nucleotide by the polymerase that will not be corrected, because Taq DNA polymerase has no "proofreading" activity. This is not a significant problem and can be minimized experimentally by varying the concentration of nucleotides in the reaction. Because of the possibility of an error in any given extension product, it is important to attain a consensus sequence from two or three different clones when the PCR products are analyzed.

In addition to the purification of the Taq DNA polymerase, several other new technological developments make PCR an attractive technique. For example, the production of synthetic oligonucleotides for use as primers has become relatively easy and inexpensive with automated DNA synthesizers. In addition, the PCR cycle contains annealing, extension, and denaturation steps that require different temperatures; a machine—called a DNA thermal cycler—has been developed to control the temperature of heating blocks using a microprocessor, and it automatically runs polymerase chain reactions of programmed duration and cycle number.

The polymerase chain reaction technique has been applied to a number of clinical and basic research problems. For example, PCR can be used to prepare cDNA libraries from the mRNA derived from fewer than 10 cells and to clone unknown members of gene families. In clinical research, PCR can be used to detect polymorphisms, mutations of single bases, deletions and insertions, and even the presence of specific pathogens. This new methodology promises great enhancement of scientists' ability to address important clinical questions.

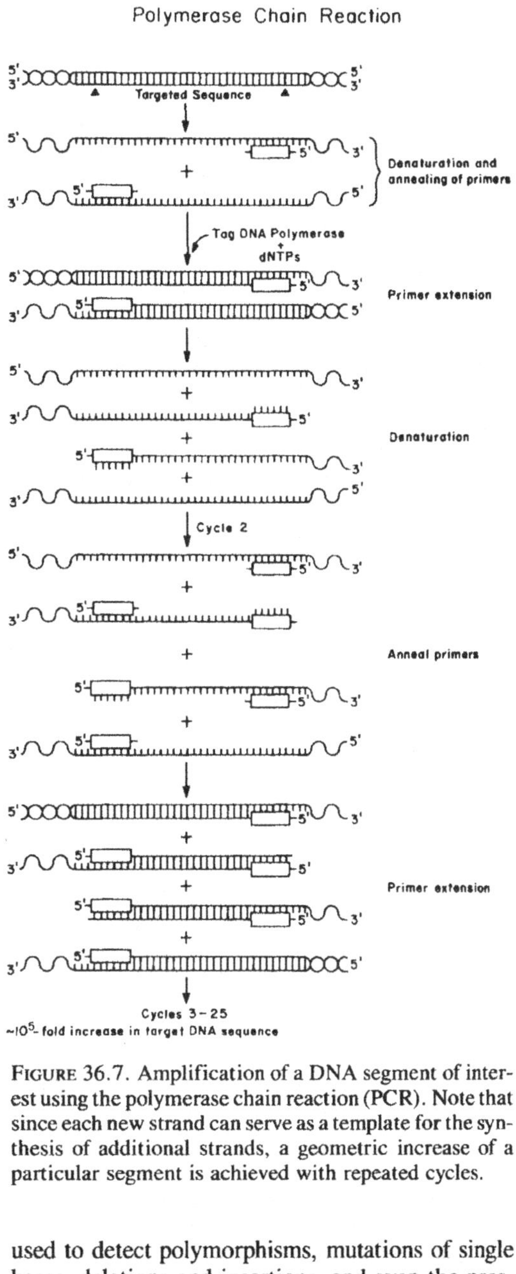

FIGURE 36.7. Amplification of a DNA segment of interest using the polymerase chain reaction (PCR). Note that since each new strand can serve as a template for the synthesis of additional strands, a geometric increase of a particular segment is achieved with repeated cycles.

Gene Transfer

The ability of bacteria to take up and express exogenously added DNA has been known since the classic experiments of Avery and colleagues in the

1940s, but only in the 1970s did it become apparent that mammalian cells could also take up and express foreign DNA.[14] Initial studies with calcium-phosphate DNA coprecipitates demonstrated that a variety of genes could be introduced into mammalian cells in a way that maintained the function of their encoded proteins. Such gene transfer is called *transfection*. For example, a purified gene for the enzyme thymidine kinase can be suspended in phosphate buffer. When calcium chloride is added to this mixture, a fine precipitate of calcium phosphate will form in the solution. DNA trapped in this precipitate can be added directly to cell cultures, where it is taken up and integrated into the chromosomes of recipient cells in a stable configuration allowing expression of the gene. (The frequency of stable integration following transfection for a purified gene is usually of the order of 1 in 10^4 to 1 in 10^5 cells). When the purified gene for thymidine kinase is transfected into cells rendered drug-sensitive by deletion of their own thymidine kinase gene, the introduced gene can cause some of the cells to revert to a drug-resistant state. The use of transfection techniques has been crucial to the identification and characterization of genes involved in the etiology of cancer (oncogenes).

Although transfection using the calcium phosphate technique is the most widely used method of introducing exogenous DNA into mammalian cells, a number of other existing methods may permit more efficient transfection or allow larger amounts of DNA to be introduced into particular recipient cells. Such methods (described in detail in reference 14) include transfection of whole chromosomes, incorporation of DNA into liposomes, and *electroporation* – the use of electrical charge to drive DNA into cells. These methods may be especially useful for gene transfer experiments of certain types, but they are not yet in widespread use.

Retroviral vectors are used in the method of gene transfer currently holding the greatest clinical promise. We can now generate recombinant retroviruses containing a gene of interest adjacent to a viral promoter to drive expression of the inserted gene. By deleting viral genes necessary for viral replication from such recombinants, it is possible to produce a retrovirus vector that will infect cells at high efficiency and lead to expression of the inserted gene. Such a virus will not undergo viral replication or infect additional cells, so that it targets a specific gene only to the cells initially infected.

This methodology was used by Rosenberg and colleagues in a widely publicized National Cancer Institute study in which tumor-infiltrating lymphocytes were infected with a noninfectious recombinant retrovirus encoding a drug resistance gene.[17] This is the first successful use of this technique in human trials, but other applications will undoubtedly follow.

Gene transfer experiments are also possible in vivo. If fertilized eggs are microinjected with cloned genes and implanted into a uterus, some of the progeny will express the introduced genes in their own tissues.[18] Such organisms are referred to as transgenic. Because the microinjected gene is incorporated into germ cells, transgenic mice will generally pass the gene to their progeny by normal mating. Although these techniques require considerable expertise, they are already being carried out in a number of labs and are revealing important information about cancer genes and transplantation immunology.

Applications

Our goal has been to review some of the basic molecular biological techniques that researchers may employ to address a variety of questions. The power of these techniques to reveal fundamental aspects of biology may be quite relevant to research on diseases commonly considered "surgical"; the best example may be cancer (reviewed in reference 19). The original experiments of Bishop and Varmus, using nucleic acid hybridization techniques, demonstrated that all higher organisms contain genes (cellular oncogenes) that are very similar to genes found in some cancer viruses. Using DNA transfection techniques, Weinberg's laboratory demonstrated that tumor tissues, but not normal tissues, contain activated oncogenes that can neoplastically transform nonmalignant cells in tissue culture. Cloning and sequencing these genes established that small changes, even single nucleotide mutations, could be sufficient to activate the malignant potential of certain oncogenes. The use of Southern and Northern blotting techniques with cloned oncogene probes established that other genetic abnormalities involving oncogenes are seen in certain tumors, including gene amplification, chromosomal rearrangement, and aberrant expression. The applications of PCR technology to this process have logarithmically increased the efficiency with which such information is generated. Finally, researchers are now using transgenic mice to further characterize the role of specific oncogenes in tumorigenesis in vivo; one such line of transgenic mice carrying a recombinant oncogene is already available commercially.

While the prognostic and therapeutic possibilities of oncogene research are just beginning to be developed, its enormous potential is already apparent. The use of molecular biological techniques in other research areas as diverse as transplant immunology, shock, metabolism, circulatory physiology, and hormone-receptor interactions underscores the importance of an understanding of these techniques for the surgical investigator.

Training the Surgeon in Molecular Biology

While the technologies reviewed here are widely applicable to research questions posed in surgical laboratories, it should be obvious that such endeavors require significant training and a serious long-term commitment to running a sophisticated laboratory. To be competitive in the biomedical research environment of the future will require, for many surgeons, a period of research training comparable in length and effort to that devoted to attaining their clinical skills. Indeed, it is more apparent than ever that a 2-year research training experience is not enough to ensure competence and competitiveness. In the future, research training for the surgeon-investigator will often include obtaining a Ph.D. degree. While this may seem to be an impossible task, the rewards of such efforts to develop a balanced training experience for academic surgeons will pay great dividends—both personal and departmental—during the years of faculty appointment.

In today's environment, the surgeon scientist must not only be willing to make a substantial commitment to research training; once he or she is appointed to the faculty, the laboratory must occupy an appropriate and perhaps equal share of daily effort. If such is not the case, funding and scientific credibility will prove elusive.

Additional Reading

Berger SB, Kimmel AR. Guide to Molecular Cloning Techniques. San Diego: Academic Press, 1987.

Lewin B. Genes III. New York: Wiley 1987.

Sambrook J, Fritsch EF, Maniatis T. Molecular Cloning. Cold Spring Harbor, NY: Cold Spring Harbor Laboratory Press, (1989).

Watson JD, Hopkins DH, Roberts JW, Steitz JA, Weiner AM. Molecular Biology of the Gene. Benjamin/Cummings, CA: (1987).

References

1. Crick FHC. The recent excitement in the coding problem. Prog Nucleic Acid Res 1963;1:164–217.
2. Sarabhai AS, Stretton AOW, Brenner S, Bolte A. Collinearity of the gene with the polypeptide chain. Nature 1964;201:13–17.
3. Yanofsky C, Carlton BC, Guest JR, Helinski DR, Henning U. On the collinearity of gene structure and protein structure. Proc Natl Acad Sci 1964;51:266–72.
4. Hoagland MB, Stephenson ML, Scott JF, Hecht LI, Samecnik PC. A soluble ribonucleic acid intermediate in protein synthesis. J Biol Chem 1958;231: 241–57.
5. Jacob F, Monod V. Genetic regulatory mechanisms in the synthesis of proteins. J Mol Biol 1961;3:318–56.
6. Smith HO, Wilcox KW. A restriction enzyme from *Hemophilus influenzae*: I. Purification and general properties. J Mol Biol 1970;51:379–92.
7. Dana K, Nathans D. Sequence specific cleavage of Simian Virus 40 DNA by restriction endonucleases of *Hemophilus influenzae*. Proc Natl Acad Sci 1971; 68:2913–17.
8. Smith HO, Nucleotide sequence specificity of restriction endonucleases. Science 1979;205:455–62.
9. Sanbrook J, Fritsch ER, Maniatis T. Molecular Cloning. Cold Spring Harbor, ME: Cold Spring Harbor Laboratory Press, 1989:5–10.
10. Southern EM. Detection of specific sequences among DNA fragments separated by gel electrophoresis. J Mol Biol 1975;98:503.
11. Thomas PS. Hybridization of denatured RNA and small DNA fragments transferred to nitrocellulose. Proc Natl Acad Sci 1900;77:5201.
12. Dymecki SM, Niederhuber JE, Desiderio SV. Specific expression of a novel tyrosine kinase gene, *blk*, in B lymphoid cells. Science 1990;247–332.
13. Drebin JA, Hartzell SW, Niederhuber JE. Molecular cloning of the human *blk* oncogene. Manuscript in preparation.
14. Sanbrook J, Fritsch EF, Maniatis T. Molecular Cloning. Cold Spring Harbor, NY: Cold Spring Harbor Laboratory Press, 1989; Chapter 16.
15. Sanbrook J, Fritsch ER, Maniatis T. Molecular Cloning. Cold Spring Harbor, NY: Cold Spring Harbor Press, 1989;Chapter 17.
16. Sanbrook J, Fritsch ER, Maniatis T. Molecular Cloning. Cold Spring Harbor, NY: Cold Spring Harbor Press, 1989;Chapter 14.
17. Varmus H. Retroviruses. Science 1988;240:1427.
18. Hanahan D. Transgenic mice as probes into complex systems. Science 1989;246:1265.
19. Bishop MJ. The molecular genetics of cancer. Science 1987;235:305.

37

The Isolated Organ in Research

T. Yeh, Jr. and A.S. Wechsler

Technological advances in artificial perfusion allow effective isolated perfusion of a wide variety of organs and tissues including, but not limited to, brain, heart, lung, heart–lung, liver, kidney, spleen, pancreas, thymus, gastrointestinal tract, urinary tract, reproductive tract, skeletal muscle, nerves, and blood vessels. The option of extended pharmacological or surgical treatment of animals before organ isolation makes this an extremely powerful technique.

Tissue similarities make possible in virtually any organ system the evaluation of certain phenomena: metabolic or biochemical processes and their related enzyme systems, oxygen consumption, organ weight, water content, electrolyte content, tissue compartment size, and measurement and analysis of organ blood or lymph flow. It was pointed out by Doring and Dehner[1] in their classic treatise *The Isolated Perfused Warm-Blooded Heart* (pp. 89–90) that perfusion with disaggregating solutions dissociates cells for molecular biological analysis, cell culture, cellular separation, and subcellular fractionation. Direct perfusion of tissue with fixatives or histochemical stains, such as vital dyes, provides excellent material for light or electron microscopy. Modification of perfusate composition or administration conditions permits the study of drugs, toxins, hypoxia, ischemia, hypotension, or hypertension on organ function.

Organ-specific investigations depend on the presence of specialized organ function such as exocrine secretion by the liver or pancreas, or endocrine secretion (hormone production) in the pancreas, thymus, or adrenal. Kidney or liver preparations permit evaluation of organ clearance capacity for drugs, metabolites, or toxins. With beating hearts, peristalsing gastrointestinal tract, or isolated tissue (muscles, nerves, or vessels), we can study mechanical or electrical function (i.e., depolarization, automaticity, or rhythmicity). The possibilities are myriad.

Advantages and Disadvantages of Isolated Perfusion

Isolating an organ for study confers several experimental advantages. Surgical access to the organ is simplified. Arteries are easily cannulated for perfusion and precise drug administration. Lymph, venous blood, or exocrine secretions are obtained simply by cannulating the appropriate system. The entire organ can be continuously weighed, biopsied, or monitored for mechanical or electrical function.

Precise control of experimental variables is a second advantage. Perfusion parameters—that is, perfusate composition, oxygenation (and therefore hypoxia), pressure, flow, and temperature—are rigorously controlled. In evaluating contractility of cardiac, skeletal, or smooth muscle, loading conditions can be uniformly standardized. Cellular depolarization can be electronically stimulated for in vitro analysis of electrical activity or mechanical contraction. Because isolated preparations are free of hemodynamic instability and untoward neural or hormonal influences, organ response is unaffected by confounding systemic factors.

A third advantage is economy. The preparation of isolated organs is generally faster and less expensive than preparing intact animals. A single preparation of the apparatus often permits multiple studies, conserving investigator resources and time. An isolated preparation is ideal for screening new hypotheses before initiating more extensive experiments. Finally, because organs are rapidly excised and the donor animal immediately sacrificed, isolated preparations may be a more humane form of animal experimentation.

The major disadvantages of isolated perfusion result from the unphysiologic facets of the technique. Perfusates are either nonblood or modified blood preparations and are administered with artificial pumps and conduits without benefit of normal systemic homeostasis (although the parabiotic system discussed below may be an exception). These unavoidable limitations inevitably cause deterioration in organ function, making extended or chronic isolated perfusion impractical. Finally, experimental results obtained from isolated organs may not be entirely applicable to in vivo organ response; this caveat was expressed in 1973 by Ritchie and Hardcastle[2] in their seminal work *Isolated Organ Perfusion* (p. 9).

System Design, Implementation, and Maintenance

As typified by clinical surgery, the implementation of isolated organs is best learned by doing. Isolated organs are widely employed in university environments, and an academic colleague who employs a similar model will often teach or collaborate with a novice. Even if the precise model differs, many of the techniques can be generalized.

Choice of Animal Species

Conservation of resources requires careful planning in the early stages of any experiment. The need for well-attended, healthy animals in obtaining meaningful data is self-evident.[3] Although smaller animals may be more cost-effective in evaluating biochemical or cellular phenomena, the chosen species must allow adequate assessment of the parameter of interest. Tissue, metabolites, exocrine secretions, or endocrine products must be available or produced in sufficient quantities for subsequent analysis. Organ size must permit cannulation of small vessels, ducts, lymphatics, or organ chambers of interest. Biochemical and physiologic response may vary between species, and the investigator must determine whether a given species is appropriate for investigating a particular hypothesis.

Anesthesia

To avoid hypoxia or respiratory arrest, consider the use of ventilatory support. Choose anesthetic agents rationally, avoiding those with detrimental effects on the organ of interest, such as irreversible myocardial depression when halogenated hydrocarbons are used in studies of cardiac physiology.[4] Precision in dosage is required. Underdosage is not only inhumane, but concomitant pain-associated catecholamine release may have profound and undesirable effects on organ vasculature.[5] If muscle relaxants are used, their interference with assessment of anesthetic adequacy may have the same ultimate outcome as underdosage.[6] After induction, overdosage may prematurely kill the donor or unnecessarily depress the organ of interest.

Route of administration is generally a matter of convenience. Intraperitoneal administration is often simplest in smaller animals. Intravenous administration is usually possible in larger animals, although intramuscular injection may enhance investigator safety with ferocious carnivores. Inhalational methods require calibrated vaporizers and close monitoring but are also an option.[7]

In protracted organ harvests, even closer monitoring of ventilatory hemodynamic, hydration, thermal, and metabolic status is indicated. The same holds true for parabiotic systems in which a support animal supplies oxygenated blood perfusate to an isolated organ for the duration of experiment.

Surgery

Although surgical preparation of isolated organs varies between specific organs, animal species, and experimental protocols, minimizing organ hypoxia with rapid, consistent harvest and expeditious reperfusion is absolutely essential for reproducible results.[8] Fortunately, protocols to expedite harvest and minimize ischemia exist for most organs; for example, liver harvests can be performed without any period of total ischemia. Mechanical organ trauma also should be minimized by avoiding unnecessary tissue handling.

Perfusion System Design

Choice of Perfusate

Design a perfusion system that meets experimental requirements but simplifies daily use and maintenance. Basic requirements in choosing one of the many available formulations oxygenation of tissue, provision of nutrients, and removal of metabolic wastes.

Perfusates are generally classified as nonblood perfusates or blood-based perfusates. In studies of cardiac physiology, Langendorff in 1895 first demonstrated that sufficient quantities of oxygen

TABLE 37.1. Modified Krebs–Henseleit solution.

Component	Amount (mmol/l)
NaCl	118.0
KCl	4.70
$CaCl_2$	2.53
$MgSO_4$	1.64
$NaHCO_3$	24.88
KH_2PO_4	1.18
Glucose	5.55

could be dissolved in crystalloid solution to support isolated rat hearts.[9] Such nonblood perfusates are generally more economical and convenient than blood-based perfusates but are, not surprisingly, less physiologic. First, the oxygen-carrying capacity of pure crystalloid is limited.[10] Second, aqueous solutions are less viscous and yield higher flow rates than blood-based perfusates.[11] Finally, crystalloid is without the normal complement of cells and proteins found in blood. Nevertheless many important, well-accepted studies have been executed with nonblood perfusates. The composition of a commonly employed formulation, modified Krebs–Henseleit buffer, is given in Table 37.1, but many solutions have been formulated for specific uses.[12]

Meticulous preparation of nonblood perfusates is imperative. All components must be accurately measured and, once in, adequately filtered. In Figure 37.1, a filter used for nonblood perfusate demonstrates that even analytical-grade chemicals have impurities that can form microemboli in organ capillaries and compromise performance.[13,14] Filters of silk, wool, or membrane[15-17] are recommended; paper filters are unacceptable because they release cellulose fibers. Finally, advance preparation of sufficient quantities of perfusate is strongly advised. Nothing is more disheartening than a smoothly running preparation that suddenly runs out of perfusate for a period of unwanted ischemia whose duration is limited solely by the investigator's land speed.

The second class of perfusates, blood-based perfusates, are generally more costly and troublesome, but they are more physiologic. Use of any blood-based perfusate necessitates anticoagulation. Heparin is most commonly employed, but other anticoagulants are available if heparin is contraindicated.[18] Be cognizant of alterations in blood components that occur in any extracorporeal system and degrade tissue perfusion.[19] These include protein denaturation,[20] fat embolism,[21] erythrocyte and platelet aggregation,[22] viscosity changes,[23] and cellular disruption of erythrocytes, leukocytes, and platelets.[24]

Regardless of perfusate class, the concentration of perfusate components (e.g., sodium, potassium,

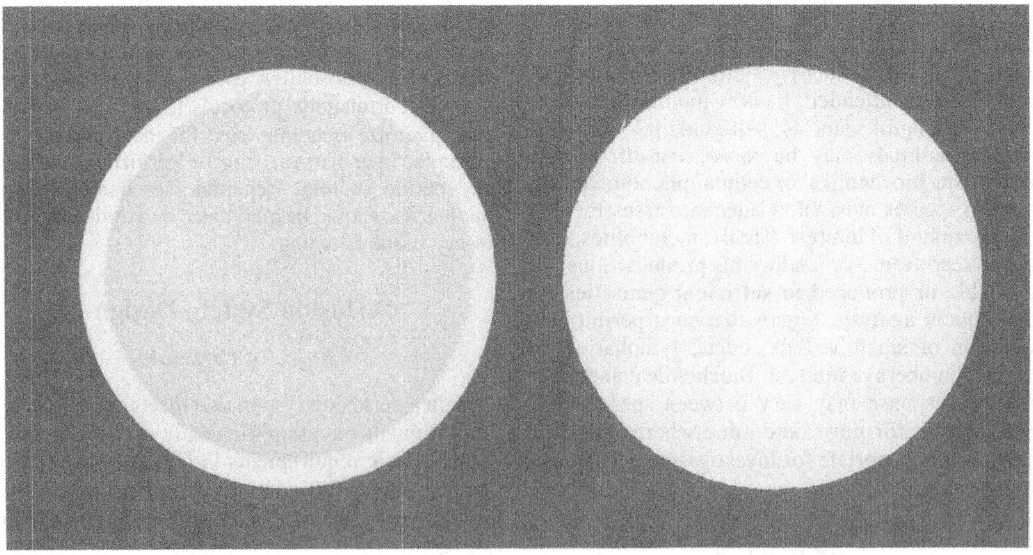

FIGURE 37.1. Used filter: a 5 μm membrane filter (left) used to filter crystalloid perfusates prepared with analytical-grade chemicals versus unused filter (right). Even though prepared perfusate was clear to visual inspection, the necessity for filtration is apparent.

chloride, calcium, magnesium, glucose, as well as experimental additives) should be periodically analyzed. Blood-based perfusates are prone to hemolysis, which lowers hematocrit and raises potassium and plasma-free hemoglobin, all of which should be assessed when using blood-primed systems.[25-29] Remember that free hemoglobin is damaging and is cleared by liver preparations. Blood-based perfusate are also more prone to hyperkalemia (from hemolysis), and fluctuations in calcium levels with changes in pH.

If blood from a second animal is used, blood-tissue incompatibility may result. To avoid this phenomenon, autologous blood is preferable—some claim essential—for success.[30] The use of autologous blood presents the logistical difficulty of increasing organ ischemia, since organ and perfusate must be simultaneously obtained from the same subject.[31]

Constant Pressure or Constant Flow Perfusion

An important advantage of isolated perfusion is that either pressure or flow can be strictly controlled. As illustrated in Figure 37.2, a constant pressure system is implemented by the action of gravity on a column of perfusate that is maintained at constant height above the perfused organ with a mechanical pump. In this method, perfusion pressure remains constant, but flow varies with the vascular resistance of organ. Proponents of constant pressure perfusion argue that mean perfusion pressure is constant in intact circulations and is therefore physiologically more relevant in isolated systems.[32]

As illustrated in Figure 37.3, a constant flow system is implemented by pumping perfusate directly to an isolated organ. Flow remains constant, but perfusion pressure varies with the vascular resistance of the organ. Perfusion pressures are generally lower than in vivo arterial pressure, probably a result of autonomic denervation, the absence of circulating catecholamines,[33] and decreased perfusate viscosity (in crystalloid or diluted blood-based perfusates). Proponents of constant flow perfusion argue that loss of normal neural and endocrine medication of vascular tone,[34] as well as altered vascular reactivity, lead to abnormal vascular resistances and that only constant flow perfusion assures flow rates in the physiologic range.[35]

Overperfusion should be carefully avoided, otherwise irreversible damage, in the form of edema, increased vascular resistance, petechial hemorrhage, or frank hematoma, may result. Exocrine secretions may become tinged with blood. Underperfusion is generally less serious, and many organs will tolerate brief periods of moderately reduced flow.[36]

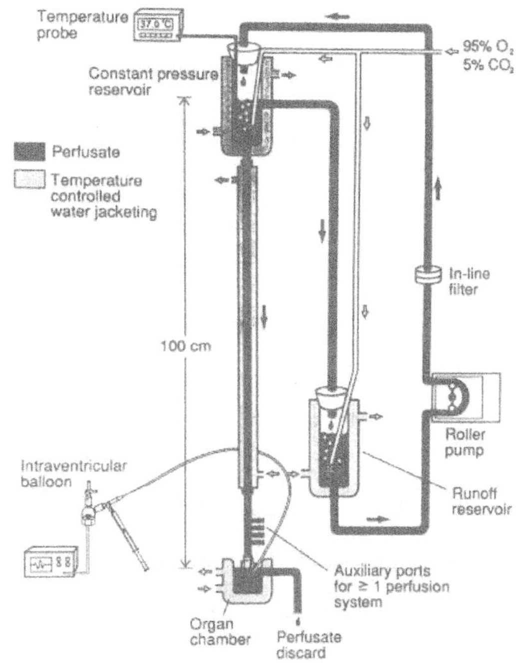

FIGURE 37.2. Simple constant pressure preparation (crystalloid perfusate, nonrecirculating). Constant pressure is effected by maintaining a column of perfusate at constant height above the organ. Perfusate is continuously pumped from the runoff reservoir to the constant pressure reservoir. After the desired level is achieved (e.g., 100 cm above the heart), perfusate overflows to the runoff reservoir through the overflow conduit. In this system, perfusate is discarded after one pass through the organ and is replenished by adding warmed, oxygenated perfusate to the runoff reservoir. Perfusate temperature is monitored and controlled by water jacketing of perfusate conduits. System oxygenation and pH are maintained by bubbling both reservoirs with a mixture of 95% O_2 and 5% CO_2. The organ chamber maintains constant temperature (with water jacketing) and hydration (by bathing the organ in its effluent). Continuous in-line filtration (e.g., 5 μm) removes residual particulate matter from the perfusate before it reaches the constant pressure reservoir. Auxiliary inputs of the organ cannula allow other columns to be added in parallel for rapid or repetitive switching of perfusates, drugs, etc. An intraventricular balloon attached to a pressure transducer is used to monitor ventricular function.

Whether constant flow or constant pressure is utilized, pumps must be of adequate capacity. Perfusate flow and pressure should be monitored during experimentation. Pulsatile flow, an option in constant flow preparation, mimics the function of the intact cardiovascular system with pumps that simulate arterial pressure waveforms. Several

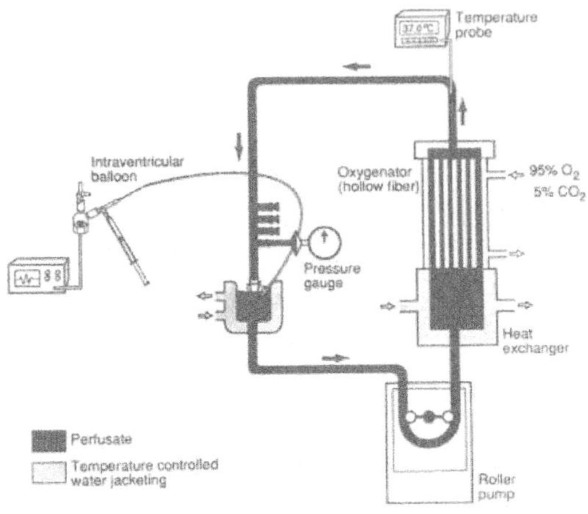

FIGURE 37.3. Simple constant flow preparation (blood-based perfusate, recirculating). Many features of this preparation (temperature control, oxygenation, and pH control) are similar to the constant pressure preparation. Remarkable differences are that a commercially available hollow-fiber oxygenator oxygenates blood. An occlusive roller pump supplies constant flow to perfuse the organ (rather than constant pressure), and perfusate pressure is monitored with a pressure gauge (or pressure transducer). Because of expense and limited availability, blood is usually recirculated rather than discarded. Note that Figures 37.2 and 37.3 represent only two of many examples, depending on one's experimental needs.

studies have shown its benefit in isolated organs,[37-40] as well as in cardiopulmonary bypass surgery.[41-43] The use of pulsatile flow may be more important in vascular system studies.[44] Pulse pressure must be monitored closely; otherwise, the poor compliance of artificial tubing may transmit undampened system pressures and damage the organ. A side arm in the circuit filled with a column of air or incorporation of excess aorta into the perfusion circuit functions as an effective compliance chamber. The advantages of pulsatile perfusion must be weighed against its cost and complexity, and the additional blood trauma introduced.[45]

Recirculation Versus Nonrecirculation of Perfusate

If perfusate is recirculated, waste products accumulate and nutrients or substrates are depleted, not only with time, but also in proportion to the size and metabolic rate of the organ being studied. Although nonrecirculating systems eliminate these problems, recirculation may be required to study minute changes in perfusate composition, or if expensive admixtures or blood-based perfusates are used.[13,46-48] The sheer volume of perfusate required by organs from larger animals may prohibit a one-pass system. Regardless of the method chosen, the supply of perfusate in a nonrecirculating system, or losses from recirculating preparations, must be monitored and repleted as necessary.

Choice of Oxygenator

For reproducible results, accurate standardization of perfusate gas tensions between studies is essential and requires that an oxygenator be of sufficient size to handle maximum anticipated flow while maintaining adequate gas exchange. Oxygenators have evolved into two commonly employed designs: bubble oxygenators and membrane oxygenators. The less expensive bubble devices are ideally suited for pure crystalloid perfusates; however they are more destructive to the blood cells and proteins present in blood-based perfusates.[49] For pure crystalloid perfusates, a bubble oxygenator is easily implemented with commercially available aquarium aerators (generically known as "airstones") that deliver fine gas bubbles into any chamber.[50] Membrane oxygenators are more costly but minimize blood element damage[51] and require smaller priming volumes.

A parabiotic system, first described in 1904[52] and depicted in Figure 37.4, directly perfuses an isolated organ with arterial blood from a support animal. Several variations on this method exist,[53-55]

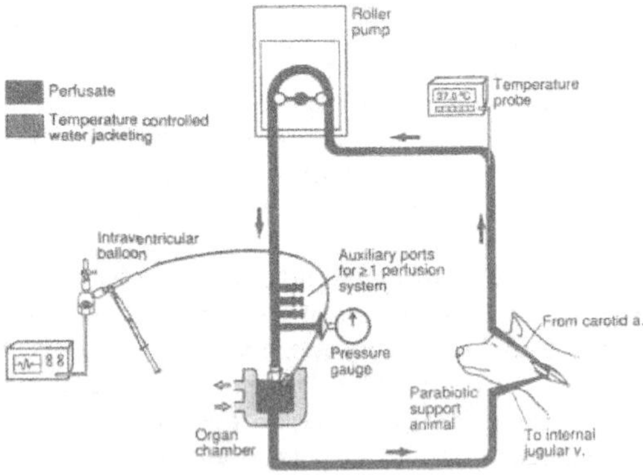

FIGURE 37.4. Parabiotic isolated heart (constant flow, blood-based perfusate, recirculating). This ingenious variation employs a parabiotic support animal to supply arterial blood (with a pump) to an isolated organ. After perfusion, venous blood is recaptured and returned to the support animal, in which it is oxygenated and homeostatically regulated. Constant pressure or constant flow can be implemented. If desired, the support animal's arterial pressure can directly supply the isolated organ.

but in general, venous blood is captured and returned via the jugular vein to the support animal, which not only functions as a living "oxygenator" but also maintains perfusate homeostasis. One disadvantage is the risk of an incompatibility reaction between blood and isolated organ tissue.[56]

The gas typically employed for oxygenation and buffering of nonblood perfusates is a 95% oxygen/5% carbon dioxide mixture,[57] although carbon dioxide is generally not required in blood-based systems. Gas supplies must be verified prior to experimentation for the same reason adequate quantities of perfusate were prepared in advance. Continued gas flow is imperative for oxygenation and is assessed visually in bubble oxygenators or tactually at the exhaust port of membrane oxygenators. Periodically monitor perfusate gas tensions and pH during experimentation, adjusting gas flows as necessary. Extracorporeal gassing allows precise control of oxygenation. Hypoxia is induced by bubbling perfusate with nitrogen.

Conduits, Cannulas, and Reservoirs

Choose tubing of sufficient caliber to handle anticipated flow rates without undue turbulence; but within that limit, minimize caliber and length to reduce priming volume. Silicone rubber and polyvinyl chloride (PVC) tubing are commonly employed. Silicone rubber has the advantages of being inert and is more compliant than PVC tubing; however, it is expensive and, because of its permeability to gases, is more prone to bubble formation if flow ceases for moderate periods of time. PVC tubing is cheaper and impermeable, but it is relatively rigid and can harbor detrimental contaminants from the manufacturing process.[58,59] Its use may be more deleterious with whole blood than with crystalloid solutions.[59,60]

Choose tubing connectors that minimize turbulence and are air- and watertight, particularly on the arterial side of the circuit, to prevent leakage of perfusate or aspiration of air into the system (Venturi effect). Banding of connections may alleviate these problems.[61]

Cannula tips should have a lip or groove so that cannulated structures can be secured with ties. If a metal cannula is used, a groove can be ground on a lathe. If a plastic or glass cannula is used, flaming the tip and touching it to a cool surface will form a satisfactory lip. Cannulas should be carefully positioned to avoid obstruction of smaller supply arteries (e.g., the coronary ostia when cannulating the ascending aorta of the heart).[62] Consider, also, that a metal cannula may serve as a grounding electrode for electrical stimulation or for monitoring electrical depolarization.

If the venous circulation is cannulated, particularly in recirculating systems, larger tubing is generally required than for arterial cannulation to achieve adequate venous drainage.[63] The venous reservoir should accommodate necessary volumes and flow without increasing venous hydrostatic pressure, be of adjustable height, allow exclusion of air, and minimize stagnation of blood.[64] Some investigators believe that preservation of normal venous pressure is important in successful long-term perfusion, and monitoring venous pressure (e.g., portal venous pressure in liver perfusions), therefore, becomes important.[65]

Avoidance of Emboli

Microscopic or macroscopic emboli can be troublesome in artificial perfusion. Microemboli can be avoided with appropriate filtration of perfusate. For crystalloid systems, filtration can be performed in line with a 5μm filter. During extended perfusions, filter clogging occurs and manifests itself, at best, as decreased forward flow, or less ideally, as sudden tubing decompression that showers everyone within range. In-line filters occasionally rupture and seed an organ with microemboli; the only manifestation may be a precipitous deterioration in organ function. Regular replacement and careful seating of the filter in its holder may prevent such incidents.

Macroscopic emboli are usually air bubbles that can be avoided by carefully priming the system, using air traps where appropriate, securing tubing connections, and inspecting conduits after periods of perfusate stasis. Foaming and protein denaturation[19] can be problematic in colloid or blood-primed systems and may require the use of such antifoaming agents[66] as Silicone MS Anti-foam A (Hopkins and Williams Ltd, Chadwell Heath, Essex).

Temperature Control

An organ chamber is required to control organ temperature and prevent tissue desiccation.[67] Two varieties of chamber are commonly used: a temperature-controlled, humidified gas chamber and a physiologic fluid bath into which the organ is immersed for temperature and humidity control. The fluid bath may confer hydrostatic advantages and limit the edema formation inherent in isolated preparations by increasing tissue pressure (see below).[68] Organ chamber and perfusate temperature are generally controlled with supplemental water baths and some combination of water jacketing, heat exchangers, or warming blankets (in parabiotic systems).

On System Stability

In an isolated system, physiologic homeostasis and organ stimulation become the responsibility of the investigator. During experimentation, all system parameters [arterial pressure and flow, venous pressure (if applicable), perfusate levels, gas flows, temperature, oxygenation, acid–base status, perfusate chemistry, electrical stimulators and recorders], as well as functional stability of the organ, must be continuously monitored.

A period of stabilization is mandatory as an isolated organ adjusts to its new environment. Depending on the organ, 15 to 60 minutes are required, but experimental parameter(s) of interest (e.g., ventricular mechanical function, hepatic bile production) should be assessed to confirm that stabilization has occurred. Documentation of stability with extended trial perfusions is essential before bona fide experimentation begins, so that results are not merely a reflection of system instability. Many investigators perfuse control organs at regular intervals to ensure quality control. At any point during actual experimentation, deteriorating organ function may indicate a problem in the system. Once this relatively late alarm has sounded, the further experimental validity of that preparation is suspect. Remember that organ function inevitably deteriorates and that experimentation should be performed within an organ's window of stability.

Some organs have idiosyncratic reactions to isolated perfusion. Livers develop hepatic venous spasm. Kidneys tend toward arterial spasm. Lung is prone to edema formation. These problems can generally be circumvented, if their existence is known.[69]

System Maintenance

The importance of appropriately maintaining and cleaning the system cannot be overstated. In blood-primed or protein-containing systems, disassemble the apparatus, discard disposable items, scrub reusable apparatus to remove blood residues, and soak overnight in hydrogen peroxide. The next day copiously rinse the apparatus with hot running tap water and recirculate with distilled water, followed by saline, and finally by physiologic crystalloid.[70]

When using crystalloid primes, the regimen can be simplified. Before and after use, copiously rinse the apparatus with hot tap water, then with filtered, deionized water. Some advocate boiling water for removal of the residual glucose used in most perfusates. Change all filters before priming with crystalloid perfusate. On a periodic basis (depending on usage or for unexplained system instability), soak all glassware and nondisposable items in chromic sulfuric acid for 24 hours, then in reagent grade water for 24 to 48 hours.[71] After copious rinsing, reassemble the system, preferably with new tubing.

Although sterility is unnecessary for most short term studies, bacterial contamination of the apparatus may occur, especially in nutrient-rich, blood-primed systems. Consider sterilization for persistent unexplained instability.

Physiology of Isolated Organs

Isolated organs have a time-dependent tendency to acquire weight. With protein-free crystalloid solutions, water gradually escapes from the vascular bed and interstitial edema develops. This phenomenon can be limited in two ways.

1. Increase the colloidal osmotic pressure of the perfusate with albumin,[72] other colloids, or osmotic agents.[73,74]
2. Increase tissue pressure, as is commonly done in isolated hearts, by immersion (1–2 cm) into a bath filled with perfusate.

Immersion is believed to increase hydrostatic pressure, thereby reducing transcapillary fluid escape and minimizing tissue edema. Without immersion, the dry weight (weight of dried tissue/weight of wet tissue) of guinea pig hearts after perfusion with saline solution decreases from 20% to 21% (in situ) to 16.5% after 30 minutes.[75] Rat hearts perfused with Krebs–Henseleit solution increase their extracellular volume by 2% after 15 minutes, 5% after 30 minutes, and 17% after 60 minutes.[76] After 4 hours of perfusion combined with immersion, the dry weight of the left ventricular myocardial tissue is limited to $17.2 \pm 0.2\%$[77] and viability is extended.[78]

Eventually, the function of all isolated organs deteriorates, presumably because normal homeostasis is absent and the perfusates and apparatus of isolated perfusion are unphysiologic. In blood-primed systems, the gradual destruction of cellular elements and proteins contributes to this deterioration. Distinguishing unphysiologic deterioration from physiologic response to experimental manipulation is critical.

Examples

Two examples are presented. For comprehensive details of implementation see the references; these details are much more easily read than "rediscovered."

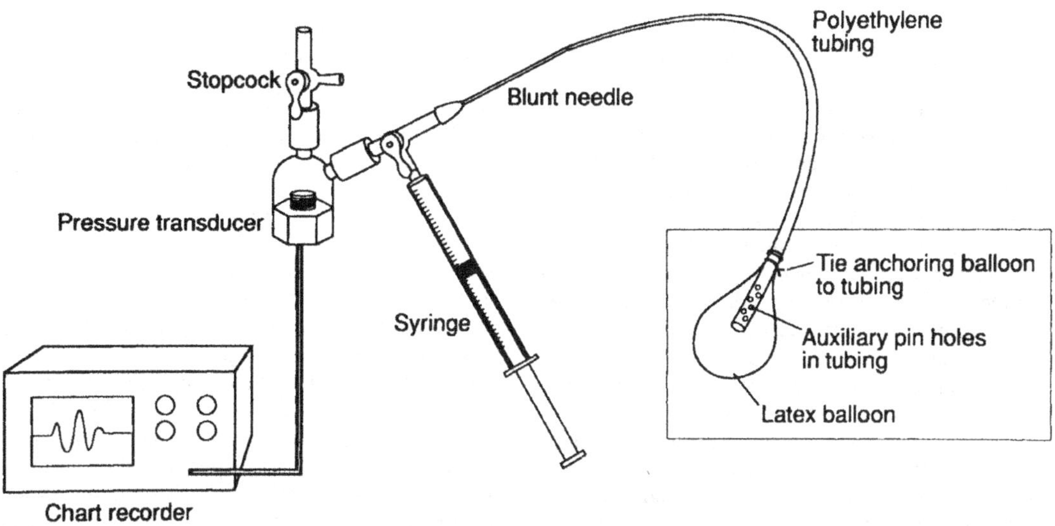

FIGURE 37.5. Construction and use of intraventricular balloon. A blunt needle is used to attach polyethylene (PE) tubing to the stopcock. Additional pinholes are made in the end of the tubing that is to be within the balloon so that fluid flow (from the syringe) and transmission of pressure waves to the transducer is unimpeded by the latex itself. Latex balloons may be purchased commercially or constructed from condom rubber. They should be slightly larger than the ventricle of interest so that no pressure is generated by the balloon itself at maximal volume. A silk tie firmly secures the balloon to the PE tubing. Intraventricular pressure is transmitted from the balloon to a standard electromagnetic pressure transducer. An appropriately sized syringe is used to precisely vary balloon volume and is subsequently isolated from the system (with the stopcock) when measurements are made.

Heart

Oscar Langendorff was the first to devise a method for investigating the isolated mammalian heart. He demonstrated that retrograde perfusion of the ascending aorta in the presence of a competent aortic valve, both closed the valve and perfused the coronary arteries. Except for coronary venous drainage, the cardiac cavities remained empty. An excellent technical reference to Langendorff's original technique and modern modifications is: H.J. Doring and H. Dehnert's *The Isolated Perfused Warm-Blooded Heart According to Langendorff*, referenced frequently in this chapter. A wide variety of parameters are assessed in isolated hearts. Coronary flow and autoregulation in response to endogenous or exogenous vasoactive substances may be assessed with or without the modulation of endothelium.[79] Myocardial rate, rhythm and rhythm disturbances, electrical potentials and depolarization, and refractory period can be studied in response to cardioactive drugs, hypoxia, ischemia, or electrical stimuli. Biochemical, metabolic, and histologic investigations discussed in the introductory material are all possible. Pharmaceutical pretreatment, experimentally induced myocardial infarction, chronic cardiac overload, and transplantation are all fertile areas for investigation.

Historically, cardiac contractility was difficult to evaluate because fluctuations in heart rate, perfusion pressure, afterload, and preload often confounded the evaluation of true changes in contractility. The isolated heart allows precise standardization of such variables so that ventricular function can be accurately assessed, typically with one of two basic models: the nonworking heart or the working heart.

In both models, crushing or excising the sinus node and the use of external pacing produce a constant heart rate. Right atrial pacing, either with two atrial microelectrodes or a metal aortic cannula and a single atrial microelectrode, is preferable for normal ventricular conduction and contraction. Stimulus amplitude should not exceed 4 volts, or norepinephrine release from cardiac sympathetic nerve fibers may exert a positive inotropic effect.[80]

The nonworking heart standardizes preload and afterload with a left ventricular balloon that is also used to assess ventricular function.[81] As illustrated in Figure 37.5, construct the balloon[82] by tying an appropriately sized piece of latex (latex condom) onto a semirigid (polyethylene) catheter attached to a stopcock. Prime the balloon with fluid to eliminate air bubbles, withdraw the fluid, and connect the apparatus to a mechanoelectrical pressure transducer. Confirm air- and watertightness of the balloon by adding volume (thus applying a test pressure), and observe for a pressure drift indicative of a leak. Potential leakage sites are a hole in the balloon (condom rubber ages and eventually leaks), the ligature holding the balloon on the catheter, the catheter, the stopcock, the transducer dome, the transducer itself, or connections between any parts of the apparatus. Insert the balloon via a left atriotomy through the mitral valve into the left ventricle for accurate assessment of ventricular pressure and performance assessments. Make certain that, after placement, the catheter tip does not press on the apex of the heart and impede pressure recording.[83]

Incremental increases in balloon volume effectively increase left ventricular preload and allow independent assessment of diastolic and systolic ventricular function. Analyze diastolic function by (a) plotting compliance curves of end diastolic pressure versus balloon volumes, or (b) comparing end diastolic pressure at the baseline volume that generates a predetermined end diastolic pressure (e.g., 5 or 10 mm Hg) and remeasuring end diastolic pressure at that same volume after an intervention. Similarly, assess systolic performance by comparing (a) peak systolic pressures or developed pressures (maximal systolic pressure minus end diastolic pressure) at the same volumes described above or (a) maximal developed pressure over a range of balloon volumes.[84] Electronically differentiating the pressure signal yields the rate of ventricular contraction (a measure of systolic function) and relaxation (a measure of diastolic function). Normal functional parameters are known for many species.[85] Of particular interest is that the isovolumic left ventricular balloon does not cause recognizable myocardial lesions and that at even relatively high preloads ($\leq$ 60 mm Hg) coronary flow is unimpeded.[86]

The second basic model for assessing ventricular function is the working heart. As illustrated in Figure 37.6, the working heart is implemented by inserting a second cannula into the left atrium and allowing perfusate to flow under constant pressure (i.e., constant preload) through the mitral valve into the left ventricle. During systole, perfusate is ejected against constant afterload (i.e., a column of perfusate in the aortic cannula), and work is performed. System design allows easy switching between nonworking and working modes. Working hearts require a compliance chamber to avoid injury from pumping against noncompliant tubing.[87,88] They may be more physiologic because the heart actually pumps perfusate and is forced, by system design, to supply its own perfusion pressure. However, consider also that constant pressure atrial filling does not standardize ventricular volumes in the presence of changing ventricular compliance. Ventricular function is assessed by simply measuring cardiac output, or with more sophisticated dimensional analyses of cardiac function, such as sonomicrometric crystals and pressure transducers or impedance catheters.[89]

Liver

The isolated liver permits the study of standard biochemical processes, blood flow, lymph flow, oxygen consumption, tissue composition, or histology; however, other unique opportunities also exist to study hepatic bile flow and composition (bilirubin, bile salts, alkaline phosphatase, pH, and electrolytes), liver regulation of perfusate composition, hepatocyte function (glycogen metabolism), and metabolism and clearance of drugs or toxins, as well as subsequent excretion of metabolites into the bile. Animal pretreatment with drugs or surgery to alter liver parenchyma or the biliary tree adds tremendous potential to the technique.[90]

The isolated perfused liver went through its own technical evolution largely because of its predisposition to develop a phenomenon known as hepatic venous outflow block. The problem was first reported in 1915, in response to histamine or peptone in constant pressure, crystalloid perfused canine

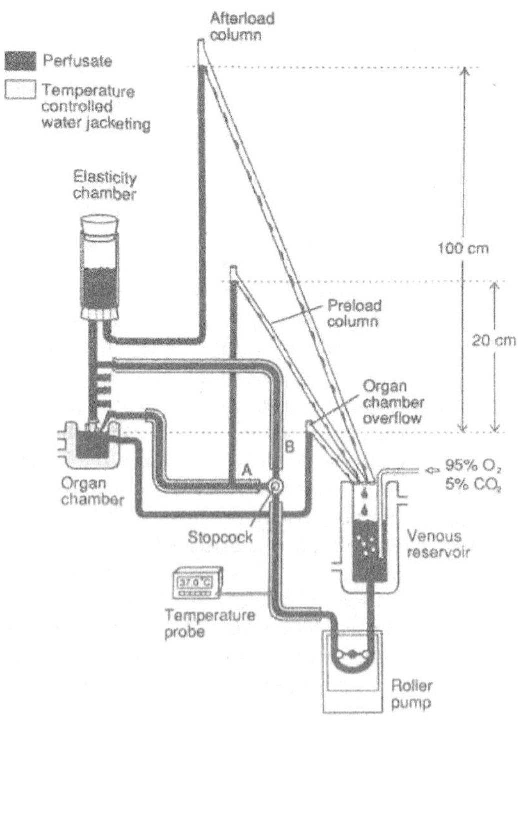

livers.[91] In 1928 blood-based, constant pressure perfusion improved organ survival,[92] but constant pressure perfusion was eventually criticized because progressively increasing organ resistance diminished portal venous flow. As a result, constant flow perfusion was attempted.[93] In 1951 a description of constant flow, sanguineous perfusion was published[94] and subsequently modified in 1953, with autologous blood, adjustable pumps, and avoidance of any total ischemia, in a preparation that became firmly established as a model for physiological studies.[95] H.D. Ritchie and J.D. Hardcastle's *Isolated Organ Perfusion*, cited throughout, provides an excellent review of the specifics of isolated liver perfusion.

Hepatic venous outflow block is variably evident after initiation of perfusion by edema, cyanosis, and mottling of the organ. Serous fluid streams from the liver surface as portal pressure rises and bile flow diminishes in a virtually irreversible process. In early preparations, venous outflow block occurred within 30 minutes of initiating perfusion.[93] Current techniques afford several hours of stability before the onset of serious deterioration. Many factors, including histamine, endotoxin, pharmacologic agents,[96] and a rise in hepatic venous pressure are thought to precipitate this phenomenon. Its physiologic basis may be spasm of smooth muscle in the walls of small hepatic venous radicles.[97]

Minimize hepatic venous outflow block by observing several salient points. Surgically, avoid unnecessary organ manipulation and any period of total ischemia with staggered cannulation of portal vein and hepatic artery.[98] Some consider the use of autologous blood to be essential. The addition of uncrossmatched homologous blood to a porcine liver preparation causes a marked fall in total hepatic blood flow.[99] Even with crossmatching, early outflow block occurs when homologous blood is used.[5] Fully oxygenated, diluted blood is also preferred, since a lower hematocrit facilitates perfusion and lessens hemolysis. A mixture of autologous blood and modified Krebs solution is usually employed to obtain a hematocrit of 35% for isolated greyhound livers.[100] Maintaining pH above 7.30 may also aid in maintaining stable vascular resistance. Constant flow perfusion has proved to be more successful than constant pressure. Steady portal venous pressure is useful in confirming stability. With initiation of artificial perfusion, portal venous pressure is high but gradually settles to less than 10 cm H_2O. Pressures that steadily rise or exceed 15 cm H_2O indicate a deteriorating preparation and impending outflow block.[101] Meticulous maintenance of the perfusion apparatus is essential to avoid contamination by substances or foreign proteins that precipitate hepatic venous outflow block. The excessive blood trauma and protein denaturation of bubble oxygenators may contribute to hepatic venous outflow block.[19] Silastic tubing is preferred over PVC tubing because vasoconstrictor substances can be leached out of the latter by the perfusate.[60]

Livers generally require one hour of stabilization. Stability is achieved after portal venous pressure falls and plateaus, bile flow rises and plateaus, and bile composition stabilizes. Plasma potassium and glucose concentrations usually rise from parenchymal cell loss and then stabilize. Studies should not be undertaken before stability is achieved.[102]

Summary

The isolated organ is a model rich in possibilities. Its limitations are few and, for the most part, reflect deficient knowledge of the physiologic requisites necessary for extended survival in isolated

◄

FIGURE 37.6. Working heart preparation (constant pressure, recirculating). The intraventricular balloon has been criticized for the unphysiologic (isovolumic) load it places on the heart. The working heart preparation forces the heart to supply its own perfusion pressure and pump blood, thereby performing work that can be measured. With the stopcock open to the left atrium (A), oxygenated perfusate enters the left atrium under a constant pressure controlled by the height of the preload column, traverses the mitral valve, and is pumped by the left ventricle into the aortic cannula. Ejection occurs against an afterload determined by the height of the afterload column. The same column also supplies a constant pressure head, which in retrograde fashion perfuses the heart with oxygenated perfusate.

Closing the stopcock to the left atrium (A) and opening the stopcock to the aortic cannula (B) converts the system to a nonworking preparation. Perfusate is delivered to the coronaries in the usual retrograde fashion.

Note that the design of this apparatus requires that perfusate be pumped faster than coronary flow (in the nonworking mode) or faster than cardiac output (in the working mode) so that perfusate continuously overflows the constant pressure columns. This minimizes perfusate oxygen desaturation or temperature loss by avoiding stagnation. Also note that construction of the preload column prevents aspiration of air into the left atrium in the nonworking mode, even after the preload column pressure has dropped to zero. Clamping the preload column instantaneously eliminates preload from the heart. Finally, note that overflow columns (afterload, preload) have air inlets that promote free runoff and avoid lowered column pressures from siphoning effects.

systems. Consequently, markedly extended perfusion is currently not practical. Furthermore, caution is required in generalizing results obtained in isolated systems to in situ organ response. Nevertheless, for the meticulous investigator, isolated perfusion is an extremely powerful tool, economically conferring a host of experimental advantages in a model whose potential is limited primarily by the imagination.

References

1. Doring HJ, Dehnert H. The isolated perfused warm-blooded heart according to Langendorff. Methods in experimental physiology and pharmacology. Biological measurement techniques. Germany: Biomesstechnik-Verlag, March 1987;5:89–90.
2. Ritchie HD, Hardcastle JD. Isolated Organ Perfusion. Baltimore: University Park Press, 1973;9.
3. Ritchie HD. 16–21.
4. Doring HJ. Reversible and irreversible forms of contractile failure caused by disturbances of general anesthetics in myocardial ATP utilization. In: Fleckenstein A, Dhalla NS eds. Recent advances in studies on cardiac structure and metabolism. Basic functions of cations in myocardial activity. Baltimore: University Park Press, 1975;5:395–403.
5. Andrews WHH, Hecker R, Maegraith BG, Ritchie HD. The action of adrenaline, 1-noradrenaline, acetyl choline and other substances on the blood vessels of the perfused canine liver. J Physiol (Lond) 1955;128:413–34.
6. Ritchie HD. 24.
7. Ritchie HD. 21–23.
8. Ritchie HD. 10.
9. Langendorff O. Untersuchungen am überlebenden säugetierherzen. Arch f d ges Physiol 1895;61: 291–332.
10. Kammermeier H, Rudroff W. Funktion und energiestoffwechsel des isolierten herzens bei variation von pH, pCO_2 und HCO_3. Pflugers Arch 1972;334: 439–49.
11. Doring HJ. 4.
12. Doring HJ. 93.
13. Bleehen NM, Fisher RB. The action of insulin in the isolated rat heart. J Physiol (Lond) 1954;123: 260–76.
14. Doring HJ. 28.
15. Doring HJ. 28.
16. Fallen EL, Elliott WC, Gorlin R. Apparatus for study of ventricular function and metabolism in the isolated perfused rat heart. J Appl Physiol 1967; 22:836–9.
17. Taylor IM, Huffines WD, Young DT. Tissue water and electrolytes in an isolated perfused rat's heart preparation. J Appl Physiol 1961;16:95–102.
18. Cole CW, Bormanis J. Ancrod: a practical alternative to heparin. J Vasc Surg 1988;8:59–63.
19. Miller JH, McDonald RK. The effect of hemoglobin on renal function in the human. J Clin Invest 1951;30:1033–40.
20. Lee Jr WH, Krumhaar D, Fonkalsrud EW, Schjeide OA, Maloney Jr JV. Denaturation of plasma proteins as a cause of morbidity and death after intracardiac operations. Surgery 1961;50:29–39.
21. Miller JA, Fonkalsrud EW, Latta HL, Maloney Jr JV. Fat embolism associated with extracorporeal circulation and blood transfusion. Surgery 1962; 51:448–51.
22. Long Jr DM, Folkman MJ, McClenathan JE. The use of low molecular weight dextran in extracorporeal circulation, hypothermia, and hypercapnia. J Cardiovasc Surg 1963;4:617–41.
23. Rand PW, Lacombe E, Barker N, Derman U. Effects of open-heart surgery on blood viscosity. J Thorac Cardiovasc Surg 1966;51:616–25.
24. Ritchie HD. 13.
25. Cahill JJ, Kolff WJ. Hemolysis caused by pumps in extracorporeal circulation (in vitro evaluation of pumps). J Appl Physiol 1959;14:1039–44.
26. Ferbers EW, Kirklin JW. Studies of hemolysis with a plastic-sheet bubble oxygenator. J Thorac Surg 1958;36:23–32.
27. Indeglia RA, Shea MA, Varco RL, Bernstein EF. Mechanical and biologic considerations in erythrocyte damage. Surgery 1967;62:47–55.
28. Paton BC, Grover FL, Herson MW, Bess H, Moore AR. The use of a nonionic detergent added to organ perfusates. In: Norman JC, Folkman J, Hardison WG, Rudolf LE, Veith FJ, eds. Organ perfusion and preservation. New York: Appleton-Century-Crofts, 1968;105–20.
29. Ritchie HD. 13.
30. Ritchie HD. 53.
31. Ritchie HD. 12.
32. Doring HJ. 4.
33. Ritchie HD. 57.
34. Ritchie HD. 57.
35. Doring HJ. 4.
36. Ritchie HD. 57–58.
37. Brodie TG. The perfusion of surviving organs. J Physiol (Lond) 1903;39:266–75.
38. Hooker DR. A study of the isolated kidney—the influence of pulse pressure upon renal function. Am J Physiol 1910;27:24–45.
39. McMaster PD, Parsons RJ. The effect of the pulse on the spread of substances through tissues. J Exp Med 1938;68:377–99.
40. Giron F, Birtwell WC, Soroff HS, Deterling RA. Hemodynamic effects of pulsatile and non-pulsatile flow. Arch Surg 1966;93:802–10.
41. Trinkle JK, Helton NE, Bryant LR, Word RC. Metabolic comparison of pulsatile and mean flow for cardipulmonary bypass. Circulation 1968:38 (Suppl VI):VI-196.
42. Trinkle JK, Helton NE, Bryant LR, Griffen WO. Pulsatile cardiopulmonary bypass: clinical evaluation. Surgery 1971;68:1074–8.
43. Shepard RB, Kirklin JW. Relation of pulsatile flow to oxygen consumption and other variables during cardiopulmonary bypass. J Thorac Cardiovasc Surg 1969;58:694–702.
44. Ritchie HD. 38–39.

45. Ritchie HD. 38–9.
46. Doring HJ. 77.
47. Bacaner, MB, Lioy F, Visscher MB. Induced change in heart metabolism as a primary determinant of heart performance. Am J Physiol 1965; 209:519–31.
48. Brink AJ, Lochner A. Work performance of the isolated perfused beating heart in the hereditary myocardiopathy of the Syrian hamster. Circ Res 1967;21:391–401.
49. Ritchie HD. 40.
50. Rebeyka IM. Personal communication.
51. Lee JR WH, Krumhaar D, Derry G, Sachs D, Lawrence SH, Clowes Jr GHA, Maloney Jr JV. Comparison of the effects of membrane and nonmembrane oxygenators on the biochemical and biophysical characteristics of blood. Surgical Forum 1961;12:200–2:
52. Heymans JR, Kochmann M. Une nouvelle méthode de circulation artificielle à travers le coeur isolé de mammifère. Arch Internat Pharmacodyn et Therapie 1904;XIII:27–36.
53. Osher WJ. Pressure-flow relationship of the coronary system. Am J Physiol 1953;172:403–16.
54. Mendler N, Hagl S, Sebening F, Theobald KP. Metabolite des energiestoffwechsels im parabiotisch perfundierten rattenherzen während und nach kardioplegie durch ischämie, kaliumchlorid und kalium-magnesium-aspartat. Arzneimittelforschgung 1972;22:909–12.
55. Weiss M, Zehl U, Förster W. Koronare autoregulation des isolierten kaninchenherzens. Acta Biol Med Germ 1978;37:291–9.
56. Doring HJ. 77.
57. Ritchie HD. 42.
58. Little K, Parkhouse J. Tissue reactions to polymers. Lancet 1962;2:857–61.
59. Guess WL, Stetson JB. Tissue reactions to organotin-stabilized polyvinyl chloride catheters. JAMA 1968;204:580–4.
60. Duke HN, Vane JR. An adverse effect of polyvinylchloride tubing used in extracorporeal circulation. Lancet 1968;ii:21–3.
61. Ritchie HD. 48.
62. Doring HJ. ii.
63. Ritchie HD. 43.
64. Ritchie HD. 48.
65. Fisk RL, Brownlee RT, Brown DR, McFarlane DF, Budney D, Dritsas KG, Kowalewski K, Couves CM. Perfusion of isolated organs for prolonged functional preservation. Norman JC, Folkman J, Hardison WG, Rudolf LE, Veith FJ, eds. Organ perfusion and preservation. New York: Appleton-Century-Crofts, 1968;217–27.
66. Ritchie HD. 42.
67. Doring HJ. 17.
68. Doring HJ. 30.
69. Ritchie HD. 3.
70. Ritchie HD. 50.
71. Personal Communication. David Hearse.
72. Ritchie HD. 54–5.
73. Ferrans VJ, Buja LM, Levitsky S, Roberts WC. Effects of hyperosmotic perfusate on ultrastructure and function of the isolated canine heart. Lab Invest 1971;24:265–72.
74. Weisfeldt ML, Shock NW. Effect of perfusion pressure on coronary flow and oxygen usage of nonworking heart. Am J Physiol 1970;218:95–101.
75. Doring HJ. 20.
76. Fisher RB, Williamson JR. The oxygen uptake of the perfused rat heart. J Physiol (Lond) 1961;158: 86–101.
77. Doring HJ. 29–30.
78. Doring HJ. 79.
79. Furchgott RF, Zawadzki JV. The obligatory role of endothelial cells in the relaxation of arterial smooth muscle by acetylcholine. Nature 1980;288 373–6.
80. Doring HJ. 58.
81. Doring HJ. 51.
82. Gottlieb R, Magnus R. Digitalis und herzarbeit. Nach versuchen am überlebenden warmblüterherzen. Arch f exper Path u Pharmakol 1904;51:30–63.
83. Doring HJ. 43–7.
84. Coulson RL, Rusy BF. A system for assessing mechanical performance, heat production, and oxygen utilization of isolated perfused whole hearts. Cardiovascular Res 1973;7:859–69.
85. Doring HJ. 67–8.
86. Doring HJ. 51.
87. Ritchie HD. 39.
88. Ritchie HD. 34.
89. Sagawa K, Maughan L, Suga H, Sunagawa K. Cardiac contraction and the pressure-volume relationship. New York: Oxford University Press, 1988; 428–44.
90. Ritchie HD. 87–96.
91. Mautner H, Pick EP. (1915) Ueber die durch schockgifte erzeugten zirkulations-störungen. Münchener Medizinische Wochenschrift 1915;62:1141–3.
92. Bauer W, Dale HH, Poulsson LT, Richards DW. The control of circulation through the liver. J Physiol (Lond) 1932;74:343–75.
93. Trowell OA. Urea formation in the isolated perfused liver of the rat. J Physiol (Lond) 1942;100:432–58.
94. Brauer RW, Pessotti RL, Pizzolato P. Isolated rat liver preparation. Bile production and other basic properties. Proc Soc Exp Biol Med. 1951;78:174–81.
95. Andrews WHH. A technique for perfusion of the canine liver. Ann Trop Med 1953;47:146–55.
96. Greenway CV, Stark RD. The hepatic vascular bed. Physiol Rev 1971;51:23–65.
97. Arey LB. Throttling veins in the livers of certain mammals. Anat Rec 1941;81:21–33.
98. Ritchie HD. 76–81.
99. Eiseman B, Knipe P, Koh Y, Normell L, Spencer FC. Factors affecting hepatic vascular resistance in the perfused liver. Ann Surg 1963;157:532–47.
100. Ritchie HD. 75.
101. Ritchie HD. 82.
102. Ritchie HD. 73.

38

Using Computer Models

H.L. Galiana

Introduction

Experimental and theoretical methods can be two complementary arms in clinical research. Mathematical or geometrical models implemented on computers provide the means of testing new medical procedures, or evaluating the effects of surgery and drugs on patient recovery and functional limits. When sufficiently accurate physiological or structural models are available, it is preferable to perform 'bloodless' experiments on the computer models before attempting actual treatment. In clinical applications, predictions from model simulations can be used to explore new protocols for the evaluation of patients; if the models relate well with known anatomy and physiology, they can even be used to evaluate the function of selected central nervous system pathways, noninvasively. Examples of the potential role of computer models in medical research and practice are presented below, followed by an application in the study of the human vestibulo-ocular system.

Geometric and Dynamic System Models

The three-dimensional (3-D) reconstruction of anatomical parts is one of the most dramatic applications of computer modeling. Most physicians are familiar with the impressive images that can be acquired with tomographic scanners or nuclear magnetic resonance (NMR) imaging. These instruments are supported by sophisticated computer algorithms to permit high resolution 3-D visualization of selected body sections.[1] Fewer clinicians are aware of the availability of highly sophisticated tools for the geometrical reconstruction of biological interfaces, which can be very useful in the analysis of biological processes and the design of prostheses. (See also Chapter 21.)

Several software programs from industrial sources are based on finite-element meshes that permit the 3-D computer image reconstruction of tissues—from the ossicles of the inner ear to the skeletal knee or hip joint, complete with muscle insertions. The data base for such geometric models can be defined theoretically—algebraic surface definitions—or experimentally from sequential serial sections. This means that, in principle, joint prostheses could be designed to replace the form and function of a diseased joint, exactly (i.e., tailored for each patient). Once a structure, including the physical properties of its tissues, has been well defined geometrically, it is quite feasible to study its biomechanical properties with real-time graphics interfaces. The distribution of stress and strain in a real joint can be studied under various load conditions, and prosthetic designs evaluated to improve their matching to the existing interface.[2] In the case of hearing, the transmission of vibrations through the middle ear, including the ossicles and such interconnecting tissues as ligaments and muscle, can be simulated. Recently, favorable comparison of vibrations in a finite-element model of the eardrum[3] with experimental data[4] has improved our understanding of sound transmission at this level. Accurate biomechanical models are not only graphically impressive they illustrate dynamic action on a computer screen; they also permit the identification in each system of critical geometric or material parameters that must be embedded in any prosthesis and those that can be modified harmlessly to simplify construction and design (i.e., form vs. function).

Computer models can also represent such dynamic central nervous system processes as motor control, reflexes, or vision. Whole textbooks have been dedicated to the study of nonlinear mathematical models for the transmission of signals between neurons,[5,6] or other bioelectrical phenomena. Much of this work explored the electrical properties of neural tissue, but research is now expanding to include theoretical models of the chemical and hormonal factors affecting signal transmission. Models of neural processes are being interfaced with sensors (e.g., touch or pain receptors, vestibular system) and effectors (muscles and skeleton). Such work on central neural systems has contributed to development of the new field of neural networks, which is finding applications in natural and artificial intelligence,[7] and in new theories on learning and development.[8,9] These can, in turn, lead to the design of new computer chips. Neural network theories are also being combined with nonlinear dynamics (chaos) in studies ranging from epidemiology to blood chemistry, from retinal models to cardiology.[10]

Another aspect of mathematical modeling borrows engineering from methods in signal processing and system theory to deduce the control strategies used by the CNS in various sensory-motor systems.[11-13] As noted below, such studies are relevant not only to neuroscience, but also to the clinical environment and the design of new robotic control strategies.

Signal processing in medicine can take many forms. When an electrocardiogram (ECG) is scanned to detect the QRS complex and possible abnormalities, matched filtering techniques are often applied: a filter is designed using the shape of the ideal waveform (i.e., a "model" of the waveform), and its interaction with the ECG can flag heartbeat occurrences by producing large peaks. Similarly, a good model for a process can be implemented as a filter: a comparison of on-line observations with those predicted by the filter can be used to detect deviations from normal. Such model-based filtering could be useful in monitoring the metabolism of drugs, or respiration or motor functions as varied as the spinal and oculomotor reflexes.

Systems approaches are generally applied to the understanding of more complex dynamic processes. The idea is to formulate a general mathematical representation, called a transfer function or impulse response, that can predict the system response (output) to any potential stimuli (inputs). A dynamic process is one in which responses depend on past history, not only on the current stimulus levels; in a static process, only the instantaneous level of a stimulus is relevant. The difference is clear if one considers a response to a simple change in stimulus level—called a step input. In a static model, the new constant response level is sufficient to describe the sensitivity (or gain) of the process; theoretically, the response should reach its new level immediately. In a dynamic model, the new response level may be reached only gradually, or may reach a peak only temporarily, and subsequently decay back to zero. With dynamic models, the time of the measurement becomes important; ideally, to define the process properly, the whole response profile should be recorded.

Most data base analyses in medical research rely on a static assumption, when a search for linear correlations between observations is being implemented. Static processes are very rare in nature, but the resulting linear models—straight-line fits—are certainly useful when the variables of a dynamic problem are being selected (see below), and in certain clinical studies, they can be sufficient.

The Evolution of a Model

There are several steps in the definition of models for a biomedical problem.

Selecting Relevant Variables

All modeling studies must be based on an evaluation of the variables that fully define the problem. This is true whether you are evaluating new drugs in the treatment of disease, or epidemiologic factors, blood circulation, cardiac mechanics, or gas exchange in the lungs. At the outset, we normally select one or several variables as the subject of study; but it is not always clear which are independent, or which directly affect others. In these circumstances, one can resort to classical medical data base analysis, or to more complicated engineering analyses. The goal is to eliminate irrelevant information and concentrate careful measurement and analysis on the key variables; a decision to divide the candidates into stimuli (input) and response (output) sets must be made. Normally, this is done by labeling as stimuli only those variables over which one has full control.

Defining the Parameters of the Problem

Any known parameters in the system under study must be defined, because they will directly influence how data are collected or analyzed. Parameters and variables are distinguishable by their roles in potential model descriptions: variables can be related qualitatively by an equation; the parameters in the equation will define the quantitative results. For example, the general form of an equation expresses force in a spring as a function of its

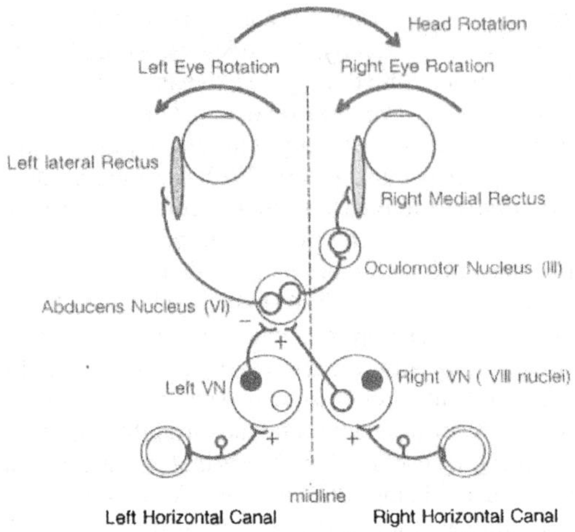

FIGURE 38.1. Schematic of direct excitatory connections in the vestibulo-ocular reflex. Horizontal head rotation to the right increases activity in the right canal and decreases activity in the left canal. Open cells are excitatory; solid cells (soma) are inhibitory. Adapted with permission from Galiana H. A nystagmus strategy to linearize the vestibulo-ocular reflex. Engineering. To be published in 1991. © 1989 IEEE.

length: the exact force in a given spring requires a definition of its spring constant. The variables in this example are force (output) and length (input); the parameter is the spring constant.

In geometric models, both variables and parameters will depend on spatial coordinates. The physical properties of tissue (viscosity, fiber directions, etc.), membrane properties in gas exchange, and blood viscosity and vessel diameter in rheology are examples of parameters. Some estimate of parameter values should be available before attempting the final modeling process, because these values will affect the complexity of the final model form.

Proposing and Testing a Model

When reasonable estimates of both variables and parameters are available, you can proceed to a mathematical description of the problem on the computer, that is, building the model. This is normally done in collaboration with a biomedical engineer, or someone with a background in physics and mathematics. It is best to start such a collaboration as early as possible, since the insights of the engineer may help you formulate the spatial and temporal aspects of the problem and reduce the necessary experimental load. The engineer's role is normally to select the appropriate modeling form using basic physics and systems principles (e.g., fluid dynamics principles, mechanics, electrical network equations). The engineer can indicate efficient experimental procedures to probe for potential nonlinearities and reduce the experimental overhead. Often, simulations from a preliminary attempt will provide new insight and lead to alternative experimental questions. As a result, new observations may be required before you achieve the desired result.

Modeling the Vestibulo-Ocular Reflex

We can now explore a particular study in more detail to illustrate the advantages of drawing on theoretical models to complement surgical and clinical research. The sensory-motor system under study is the horizontal vestibulo-ocular reflex (VOR), which controls eye movements in response to head movements in space. This reflex stabilizes visual scenes on the retina during active or passive (unexpected) head movement. As a result, the line of sight, or gaze (gaze = eye − re-head + head − re-space), can be maintained on a target despite environmental interference.

Gaze stabilization relies heavily on both visual and vestibular cues, but it operates effectively even in the dark. In the absence of vision, the VOR relies on sensory signals from the vestibular apparatus, which provides information on the linear and angular components of head motion with respect to a head coordinate system. If we now restrict head motion to rotation in a horizontal (coronal) plane, the relevant sensors are the horizontal semicircular canals—one in each inner ear. Observation of the firing rates on the primary vestibular nerve shows that the information relayed by the canals is most directly related to angular head velocity, during normal, rapid head turns. This information is degraded during slow movements and decays to zero if rotation is maintained in one direction for more than about 10 seconds. Because such low-frequency stimuli are not encountered in daily life, the function of the canals should be considered to be the monitoring of angular head velocity during normal activities. This brief review indicates that the variables of interest in a study of the VOR system in the dark would be angular head velocity as the input and eye position or eye velocity in the orbit as the output.

The next step is the selection of an appropriate form, or structure, for a potential model that would provide dynamic relations between head and eye profiles. Figure 38.1, a simplified sketch of the most direct excitatory pathways in the VOR, omits complementary inhibitory pathways and parallel connections to both eyes during conjugate eye movements.

Two properties are immediately obvious; the system is bilateral, despite previous tendencies to

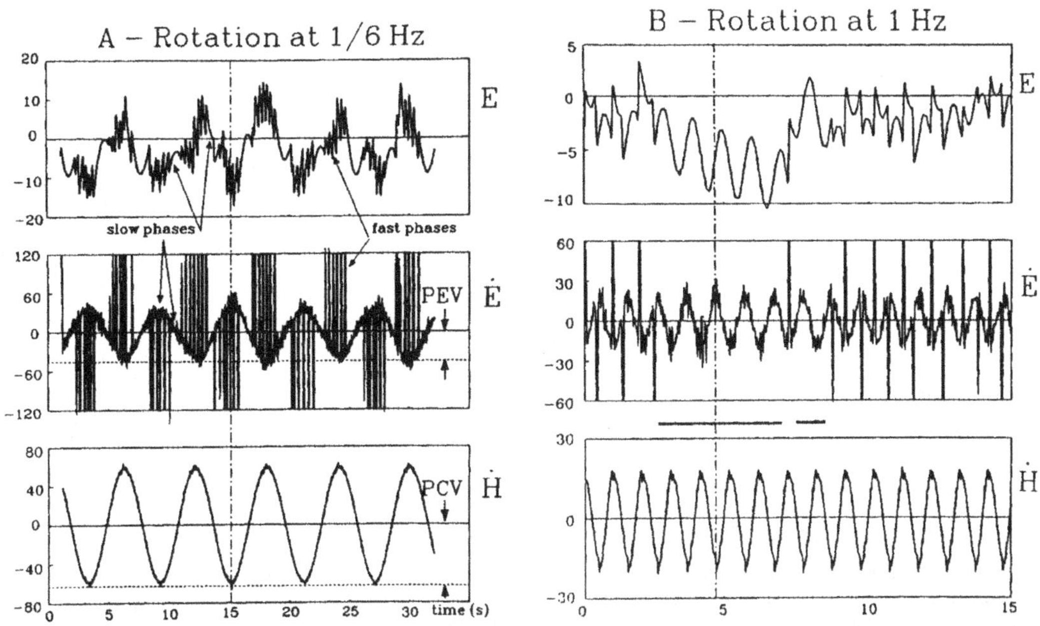

FIGURE 38.2. Examples of VOR responses in a normal subject, using bitemporal surface electrodes (EOG). PCV is peak head velocity in the sinusoidal profile, PEV is resulting peak slow-phase eye velocity; vertical dashed line indicates near zero phase between the two peaks (no time lag) at these rotation frequencies; E, angular eye position in degrees; $\dot{E}$, angular eye velocity in degrees per second; $\dot{H}$, angular head velocity in degrees per second. Heavy horizontal bars in Band B denote periods devoid of quick phases, often observed during rotation at high frequencies. Rotations to the right (clockwise seen from above) are termed positive with upward deflection in the graphs. Reprinted with permission from Galiana H. A nystagmus strategy to linearize the vestibulo-ocular reflex. IEEE-Transactions on Biomedical Engineering. To be published in 1991. © 1989 IEEE.

model it in block forms lumping both sides of the brain; and sophisticated processing is required to transform head velocity estimates from the semicircular canals into appropriate oculomotor drives during nystagmus. Figure 38.2 provides sample nystagmus records obtained in a normal human subject during sinusoidal, passive head rotation in the dark. Note that ocular responses have a sawtoothlike pattern (called nystagmus), where slow phase segments stabilize gaze in space (eye velocity = head velocity), while quick phases redirect the eye to a new position in space. In other words, the function of gaze stabilization cannot be sustained by the VOR because of limitations involving both the central premotor system and the ocular muscle. Consequently, the slow-phase segments must be interrupted regularly to redirect gaze.

In clinical environments, the VOR is normally characterized by measurements on the slow phase. The properties of quick phases are ignored, unless visual saccades are being evaluated. For example, the VOR can be defined by two parameters in response to sinusoidal head rotation (see head trace in Fig. 38.2): first the "gain" at the selected rotation frequency (1/period of oscillation; 1/6s = 1/6 Hz in Fig. 38.2) is calculated from the ratio of peak observed slow-phase eye velocity to peak imposed head velocity (PEV/PCV in Fig. 38.2); second, the time T between opposite and adjacent eye velocity and head velocity peaks is measured (vertical dashed line in Fig. 38.2) to determine the "phase" of the slow-phase response, as $360 \times T$/period in degrees. An ideal VOR should have a gain of one and a phase of 0°, so that any head movement is matched by the same but opposite eye movement. In Figure 38.2, the subject has an apparent gain of approximately 0.7, and a phase of 0°. Patients normally have lower gains, and phase leads of as much as 45°—that is, peak eye velocity occurs before the peak head velocity.

From systems theory, one must repeat this measurement at all frequencies in the range of interest to define a dynamic model properly. Testing at one frequency is never sufficient, unless we are dealing with a linear static model, such as a pure gain. Alternatives to sinusoidal testing are step inputs, or

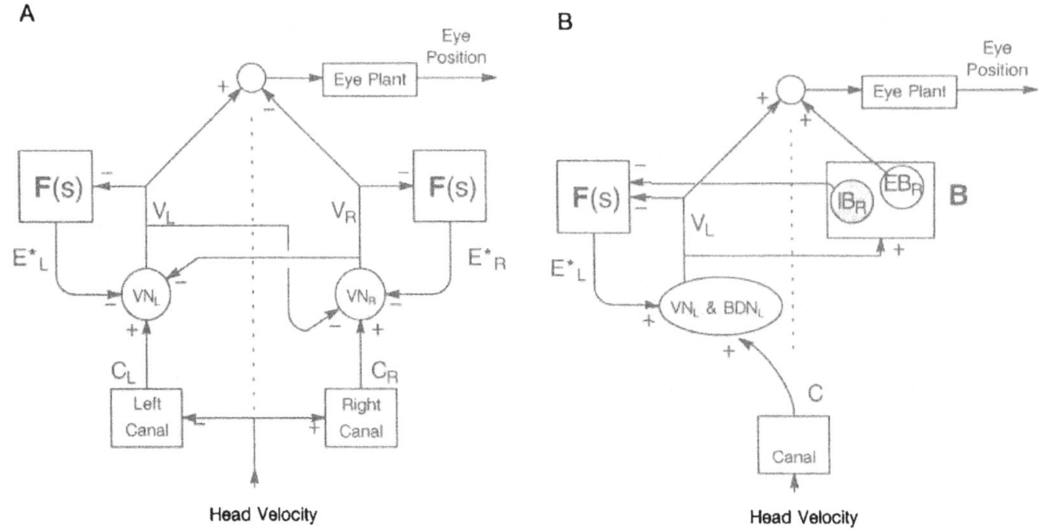

FIGURE 38.3. Bilateral model for the vestibulo-ocular reflex. (A) System is bilateral and symmetric during compensatory slow phases of nystagmus. (B) Asymmetric structure, shown here for quick phases directed toward the right side of the head, combines signals from the left vestibular nuclei (VN) from left burster driving neurons (BDN_6) in propositus hypoglossi,[15] and from reticular bursters (IB and EB) on the right side of the brainstem. Filtering processes (F) on each side act as internal models of the eye plant and provide efference copies of each eye's position to pre-motor control circuits $E^*_{R,L}$. Adapted with permission from Galiana H. A nystagmus strategy to linearize the vestibulo-ocular reflex. IEEE-Transactions on Biomedical Engineering. To be published in 1991. © 1989 IEEE.

random (noise) inputs, which can be used to define the dynamics of a system fully if the whole response profile is recorded.

Given recent behavioral and neurophysiological data, a bilateral model of the VOR has been proposed and discussed in detail elsewhere.[12,14] It incorporates the bilateral nature of the oculomotor system and the known burst cells in the paramedian pontine reticular formation, which are selectively activated during visual saccades or vestibular quick phases (see Figure 38.3). This model can successfully simulate both the slow and fast phases of vestibular nystagmus under various head velocity profiles (see Figure 38.4). It also implies a novel automatic strategy for the timing and characteristics of rapid eye movements that could linearize the premotor system, despite sensory and central neural nonlinearities.[15] This has led to the development of an alternate view for the coordination of eye and head movements during natural gaze shifts[16,17] that emphasizes strong coupling of the two motor systems in gaze control. These strategies are finding applications in the control of mobile robotic vision systems.

Simulations of the bilateral VOR model lead to theoretical predictions that could have implications in the clinical evaluation of vestibular patients. Only the slow phase of nystagmus is normally used to make clinical measures of the VOR, but our model indicates that nystagmus can increase the linear range of the reflex. What is more surprising is that the nystagmus pattern itself (beat frequency and endpoints) can also affect the shape of the slow-phase velocity envelopes and modify the measured VOR parameters; that is, both slow- and fast-phase segments contain valuable indices of VOR function and integrity, which should be considered in the clinic. An example follows.

The VOR model presented in Figure 38.3 attempts to duplicate the behavioral (ocular) responses to vestibular stimuli and the many known central firing rates at the levels of the vestibular nuclei (VN), reticular burst cells (IB and EB), and motor nuclei. Since the model is related to anatomy and physiology, it can be used to test the effects of lesions and to probe potential parametric changes that could subserve compensation or adaptation during recovery. Figure 38.5 illustrates the effects on the VOR model of removing one of the vestibular sensors, as would occur after vestibular neurectomy. Background resting rates in central cells are assumed to have recovered their symmetry on the two sides, so that no spontaneous nystagmus is present in the absence of rotation.

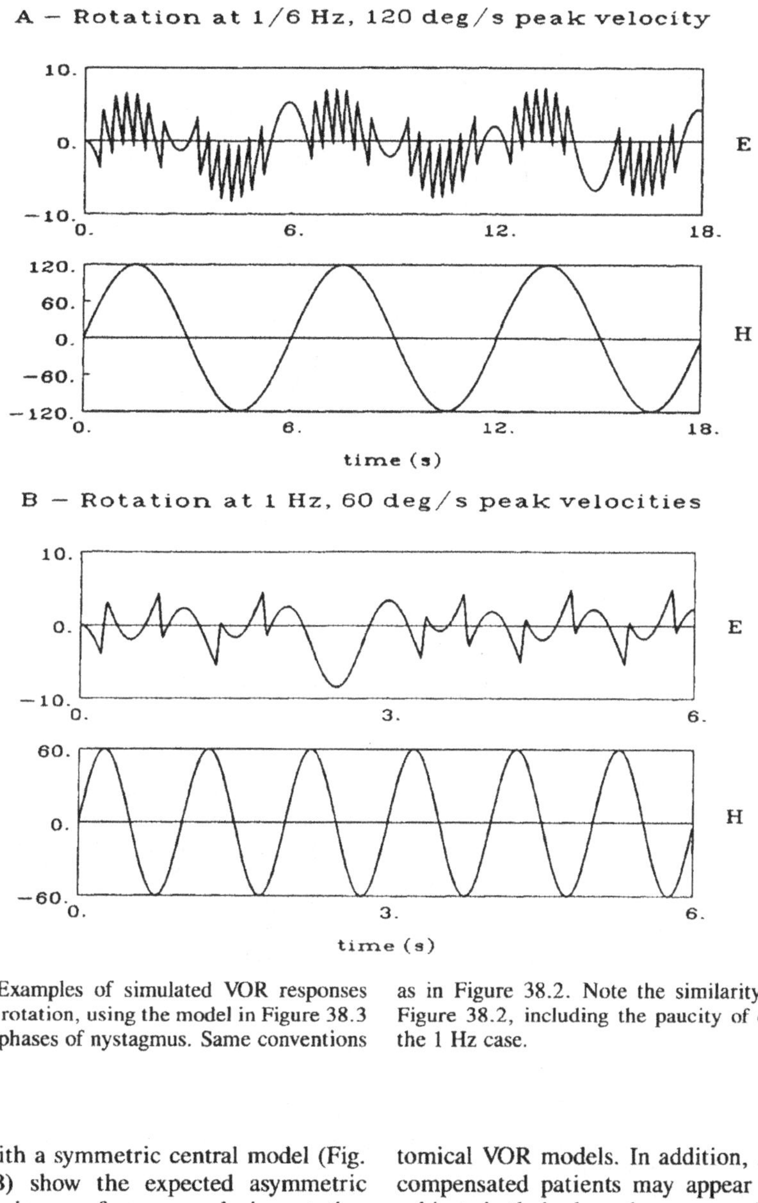

FIGURE 38.4. Examples of simulated VOR responses to passive head rotation, using the model in Figure 38.3 to generate all phases of nystagmus. Same conventions as in Figure 38.2. Note the similarity to the data in Figure 38.2, including the paucity of quick phases in the 1 Hz case.

The results with a symmetric central model (Fig. 38.5A and B) show the expected asymmetric responses (dominance of responses during rotation to the healthy left side) in the slow-phase gain, and even the appearance of saturations and d.c. biases at high head velocities. If asymmetric fast phase thresholds are now used, the predicted interactions between slow-and fast-phase dynamics permit the appearance of symmetric responses at low head velocities (Fig. 38.5C), and an improvement in the nonlinear properties at high velocities (Fig. 38.5D). The modification of fast-phase strategies to linearize the VOR is a testable hypothesis now being explored in vestibular patients. It is an unexpected mechanism for vestibular compensation that could not have evolved from previous nonanatomical VOR models. In addition, it implies that compensated patients may appear to be normal subjects in their slow-phase properties, but still be distinguishable as peripherally lesioned upon examination of the fast phases. New clinical measures may evolve.

Conclusions

The applications of geometric and dynamic 3-D computer models are still in the research or development phase but, as computer power and software tools evolve, they will become a standard tool for surgeons and clinicians. They have already become indispensable in the biomedical engineer-

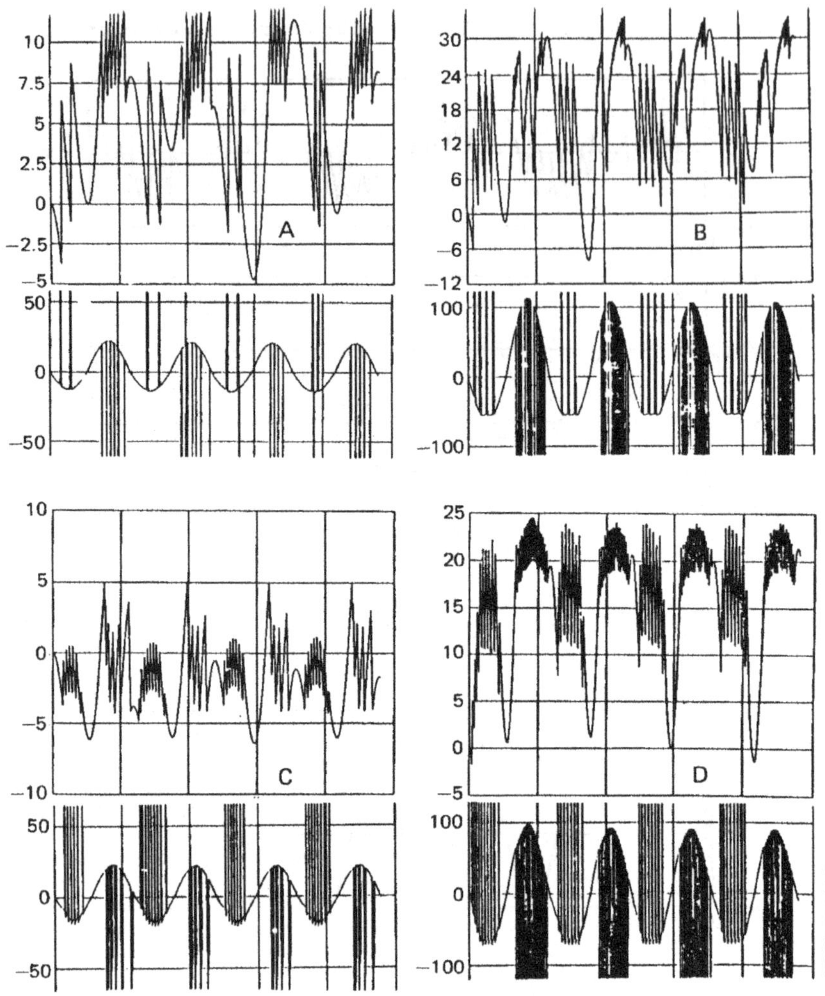

FIGURE 38.5. Examples of simulated eye position (top curves, deg) and eye velocity (bottom curves, deg/s) in the case of unilateral sensory signals from the left canal, and no spontaneous nystagmus using model in Figure 38.3. The two top panels (A,B) show asymmetric slow-phase velocities, when the central model parameters are the same on both sides. Appropriate asymmetries in the quick-phase strategies, on the other hand, are predicted to lead to an improvement in the slow-phase eye velocities: for example, near-normal symmetric responses at low head velocities (C, 60 deg/s), and improvement in the nonlinear asymmetry for higher velocities (D, 300 deg/s). (Left/right gain ratio = 1.5 in A, 1.0 in C; dc bias in B is reduced in D.) Note that mean eye position with the asymmetric strategy is then shifted toward the healthy side.

ing area, where they are being applied to the study of inhomogeneous, nonlinear muscle tissue, the evaluation of speech mechanics by ultrasound imaging, the design of implants to scanner tolerances,[2,18] the on-line guidance of brain surgery,[1] and the modeling and simulation of physiological systems as diverse as joint reflexes,[11] metabolic processes, and molecular biology.

References

1. Henri CJ, Pike GB, Collins DL, Peters T. Three-dimensional display of cortical anatomy and vasculature; MR angiography vs multi-modality integration. In: Medical Imaging IV: Proceedings of the SPIE, Newport Beach, CA, 1990. in press.
2. Doré S, Kearney RE, De Guise J. Experimental determination of CT point spread function. In:

Images of the Twenty-First Century, Proc IEEE Eng Med Biol Soc 1989;11:620–21.

3. Funnell WRJ, Decraemer WF, Khanna SM. On the damped frequency response of a finite-element model of the cat eardrum, J Acoust Soc Am 1987; 81(6):1851–59.
4. Decraemer WF, Khanna SM, Funnell WRJ. Interferometric measurement of the amplitude and phase of tympanic membrane vibrations in cat. Hear Res 1989;38(1):1–18.
5. Cronin J. Mathematical Aspects of Hodgkin-Huxley Neural Theory. Cambridge: Cambridge University Press, 1987.
6. MacGregor RJ. Neural and Brain Modeling. New York: Academic Press, 1987.
7. Szentágothai J, Arbib MA, Conceptual Models of Neural Organization. Cambridge, MA: MIT Press, 1974.
8. Grossberg S, Kuperstein M. Neural Dynamics of Adaptive Sensory-Motor Control. In: Advances in Psychology, no 30, Amsterdam: North-Holland, 1986.
9. Grossberg S. Studies of Mind and Brain: Neural Principles of Learning, Perception, Development, Cognition and Motor Control. Boston: Reidel, 1982.
10. Koslow SH, Mandell AJ, Shlesinger MF, eds. Perspectives in biological dynamics and theoretical medicine. Ann N Y Acad Sci. 1987;504.
11. Kearney RE, Hunter IW. System Identification of Human Joint Dynamics. Boca Raton, FL: CRC Press, 1990.
12. Galiana HL. Oculomotor control. In: An Introduction to Cognitive Science, Vol 2, Visual Cognition and Action, DN Osherson, SM Kosslyn, JM Hollerbach, eds. Cambridge, MA: MIT Press, 1990: 243–83.
13. Marmarelis PZ, Marmarelis VZ. Analysis of Physiological Systems–The White Noise Approach. New York: Plenum Press, 1978.
14. Galiana HL, Outerbridge JS. A bilateral model for central neural pathways in the vestibulo-ocular reflex, J Neurophysiol. 1984;51:210–41.
15. Galiana HL. A nystagmus strategy to linearize the vestibulo-ocular reflex–a strategy for ocular nystagmus. IEEE Trans. Biomed. Eng., in press 1990.
16. Galiana HL, Guitton D, Munoz D. Modeling head-free gaze control in cat. In: The Head-Neck Sensory Motor System, A Berthoz, PP Vidal, W Graf, eds. New York, Oxford Univ. Press, 1990.
17. Guitton D, Munoz DP, Galiana HL. Gaze control in the cat: studies and modeling of the coupling between orienting eye and head movements in different behavioral tasks. J Neurophysiol., in press, 1990.
18. Doré S, Kearney RE, De Guise J. Quantitative assessment of CT PSF isotropicity and isoplanicity In: Proc. 16th CMBEC. 1990, in press.

Section IV

Reporting Your Work

When you have completed the analysis of a research project, you should consider your work only half-completed. Communicating your research effectively, through a variety of oral presentations, abstracts, and scientific articles, is just as important as conducting the research itself. Even when your research has been well designed, responsibly conducted, and judiciously analyzed, it is all a sterile exercise if the results fail to reach your target audience. Many scientists who are brilliant in the conception of ideas or the execution of research never receive the recognition they deserve because of problems in communication. Communicating is a vital component of research, and its principles must be learned and practiced at a high level of sophistication.

The chapters in this section have been written to provide helpful suggestions about writing abstracts, presenting short reports, writing and submitting articles to peer-reviewed scientific journals, preparing audiovisual aids, giving lectures, chairing panels, and acquiring the other communication skills that are such essential components of success in any research endeavor. Reading about them is not enough; you can develop skill in communicating only by communicating.

39

Your First Abstract

A.V. Pollock and M.E. Evans

There are two kinds of abstract: one you send to a learned society to be considered for presentation at a meeting; the other you write to summarize a paper for a journal. The first kind must interest the selection committee and make it want to accept your work for presentation; the second must interest the reader and make him want to read the rest of your paper. (See also Chapters 40, 41, 42, and 44.)

Abstracts are usually written in the passive voice: "Plasma was incubated with endotoxin . . . ," not "We [or worse still, "the authors"] incubated plasma with endotoxin . . ." The main reason for this requirement is that abstracts are often published unaltered in abstracting journals, and the presence of an occasional abstract written in the active voice introduces a discordant note.

Abstracts for Presentation at Meetings

Your first job is to read, and reread, the instructions enclosed with notices of meetings. They may stipulate that the abstract shall (a) contain no more than 200 words, (b) be typed with double line spacing, (c) have no more than two references and (d) be submitted in 10 or 12 copies. Most surgical societies send abstract forms in box format for "camera-ready copy." The box usually measures 200 × 150 mm and is contained on a sheet of A4 (297 × 210 mm) paper. In the box you must type in single line spacing using 10 or 12 pitch letter spacing (10 or 12 characters to the inch). If the abstract is accepted, it will be reduced and printed by photolithography straight into the book of abstracts. This means that you must start by photocopying the blank form to make sure your abstract will fit in the box. It also means that dot matrix printing is unacceptable, unless it is of letter quality.

Abbreviations and Acronyms

The box format is undoubtedly a cost-effective way of producing a book of abstracts, but it tempts authors into a proliferation of abbreviations and acronyms. An abstract should be easy to read and abbreviations make it more difficult. We have chosen this example at random: "LYM play a significant role in potentiating LTB4 production in CTL PMN." We accept that certain abbreviations have no equivalent, or are so hallowed by usage that they have become part of everyday medical writing and speaking. These include commercial descriptions of strains of experimental animals (e.g., C_3H/HeJ mice) and of new chemicals (e.g., calcium ionophore A23187); they also include DNA, RNA, AIDS, TNM classification of cancers, T and B lymphocytes, and PO_2 and PCO_2.

We analyzed all 122 abstracts in the program book of the meeting of the Association of Surgeons of Great Britain and Ireland held in Edinburgh in 1989, and all 50 in that of the Surgical Infection Society held in Denver in 1989. Table 39.1 shows that the use of abbreviations in abstracts was more widespread in the American program book than in the European. Even when abbreviations were explained earlier in the abstract—in more than a quarter of the cases they were not—the reader had to look back through the text to find their meaning.

The Content of an Abstract for Presentation at a Meeting

Your abstract must have a title and, on the whole, the shorter and more arresting it is, the better. It should contain no abbreviations and usually should not make a statement about the results. Here are two contrasting titles from the program book of the Surgical Infection Society, 1989: "Wound

TABLE 39.1. Number (%) of abbreviations in abstracts at scientific meetings.

No. abbreviations per abstract	Association of Surgeons (U.K.)	Surgical Infection Society (U.S.A.)
0	53 (43)	1 (2)
1	40 (33)	3 (6)
2	18 (15)	9 (18)
3	4 (3)	8 (16)
4	3 (2)	7 (14)
5	3 (2)	5 (10)
6 or more	1 (1)	17 (34)
Total abstracts	122	50

$\chi^2 = 87.8$; df = 6: $p < .001$

cytokines in the sponge matrix model" and "Development of a bacterial-independent experimental model which faithfully simulates the pathophysiology and histopathology (HPa) of the multiple organ failure syndrome (MOF)."

An abstract must reflect the whole paper: it must start with a statement—in one sentence—of why you did the research. It must continue with an easily understood description of your patients or materials, and methods; and it must show your main results, giving whole numbers, not just percentages. If you are comparing two groups treated in different ways, it is not enough to give a p value—a confidence interval is more revealing, but in any case the statistical test must be mentioned. Results may be better expressed in a concise, eye-catching table. The abstract must end with a brief discussion of the relevance of your work to previous knowledge, and a concluding sentence.

An abstract must include statements about the objective of the research, the methods, the results, and the conclusion. It should contain no abbreviations, and unusual words should be avoided or explained. Here are examples of a good abstract and a poor one. First, the good one:

The aim of the study was to determine the fate of cultured skin allografts in patients with burns. In situ DNA hybridization with a Y probe (pHY 2.1) was used to detect cells carrying the Y chromosome (the probe being visualized by the alkaline phosphatase-antialkaline phosphatase method) in biopsy specimens taken from cultured allografts derived from donors of the opposite sex to the recipients (20 patients with burns). Specimens were taken within a week, between 1 and 3 weeks, between 4 and 6 weeks, and more than 6 weeks after grafting. Only 2 of the 27 biopsy specimens contained cells that were the same sex as the donor; both were taken within a week after grafting. In the 25 other specimens the epithelial cells were the same sex as the recipient.

Cultured skin allografts showed no evidence of survival in patients with burns, which suggests that they are probably not suitable for long-term management of burns but may be useful as short-term biological dressings.[1]

This one is poor and uninformative:

The details of inquests concerning 104 deaths due to trauma were studied in the Sheffield and Barnsley Coroner's district for the year 1986. Fifty-four of these patients did not reach hospital alive. In those patients where some form of resuscitation was attempted, the hospital notes were reviewed and the deaths occurring unexpectedly were identified using TRISS methodology. This method uses the Trauma Score, the Injury Severity Score and the patient's age to predict the probability of survival in an injured patient. It showed that some of the deaths were unexpected and the implications of these findings are discussed.[2]

Structured Abstracts

An international working group set up by R.B. Haynes of McMaster University Center, Hamilton, Ontario, published a proposal for more informative abstracts in clinical research papers.[3] This group suggested that the abstract—which need not have fully formed sentences—should contain the following information:

1. Objective: the exact question(s) addressed by the article.
2. Design: the basic design of the study.
3. Setting: the location and level of clinical care.
4. Patients or participants: the manner of selection and number of patients or participants who entered and completed the study.
5. Interventions: the exact treatment or intervention, if any.
6. Measurements and results: the methods of assessing patients and key results.
7. Conclusions: key conclusions including direct clinical applications.

The following example of a structured abstract is taken from the *British Medical Journal*[4]:

Objective—To evaluate the outcome of pregnancy in Finnish women after the accident at the Chernobyl nuclear power plant on 26 April 1986.
Design—Geographic and temporal cohort study.
Setting—Finland divided into three zones according to amount of radioactive fallout.
Subjects—All children who were exposed to radiation during their fetal development. Children born before any effects of the accident could be postulated—that is, between 1 January 1984 and 30 June 1986—served as controls.

Interventions—Children were divided into three temporal groups: controls, children who were expected to be born in August to December 1986, and children who were expected to be born in February to December 1987. They were also divided, separately, into three groups according to the three geographic zones.

Endpoint—Incidence of congenital malformations, preterm births, and perinatal deaths.

Measurements and main results—There were no significant differences in the incidence of malformations or perinatal deaths among the three temporal and three geographic groups. A significant increase in preterm births occurred among children who were exposed to radiation during the first trimester whose mothers lived in zones 2 and 3, where the external dose rate and estimated surface activity of cesium-137 were highest.

Conclusions—The results suggest that the amount of radioactive fallout that Finnish people were exposed to after the accident at Chernobyl was not high enough to cause fetal damage in children born at term. The higher incidence of premature births among malformed children in the most heavily polluted areas, however, remains unexplained.[4]

You may feel, when you have finished writing and editing a research paper, that your job is done. It is not finished until you have put the message of that paper into a short, accurate, and interesting form. You will have wasted a lot of time and money on your research if the finished product does not attract listeners and readers.

References

1. Burt AM, Pallett CD, Sloane JP, et al. Survival of cultured allografts in patients with burns assessed with probe specific for Y chromosome. Br Med J 1989; 298:915–17.
2. Wardrope J. Traumatic deaths in the Sheffield and Barnsley areas. J R Coll Surg Edinb 1989;34:69–73.
3. Ad Hoc Working Group for Critical Appraisal of the Medical Literature. A proposal for more informative abstracts of clinical articles. Ann Intern Med 1987; 106:598–604.
4. Harjulehto T, Aro T, Rita H, Rytomaa T, Saxen L. The accident at Chernobyl and outcome of pregnancy in Finland. Br Med J 1989;298:995–97.

40

Writing an Effective Abstract

B.A. Pruitt, Jr. and A.D. Mason, Jr.

An abstract should be a concise distillate or synopsis of the work being reported and must emphasize what was done, how it was done, the results obtained, and how the author interprets them. In most instances, the organization or publication to which the abstract is submitted defines its length (usually one standard size double-spaced typewritten page, i.e., approximately 200 to 250 words), and that limit is inviolable. This required brevity precludes all extraneous material.

Mechanical and technical factors, as well as presentation and content, determine the strength and attractiveness of an abstract. If the source of the abstract is to be "blinded" to the reviewer, the originating institution should not be surreptitiously identified in the body of the abstract. A dot matrix printer should not be used to prepare an abstract since most reviewers find a typed abstract easier to read. A grammatically correct abstract, free of typographic errors, jargon, and colloquialisms will be viewed with favor but requires meticulous proofreading of each successive draft—capricious word processors have been known to drop out words, phrases, and even entire sentences. Acronyms should be used sparingly (never in the title) and only if widely accepted. Each acronym must be presented in parentheses after its first citation in the abstract. Data tables should be easily read, with entries kept to the essential minimum, units of measurement defined, the number of entries or observations stated, and levels of statistical significance defined and indicated by conventional symbols.

Format

The format of an abstract is usually that of a scientific report or presentation (i.e., title, introduction, materials and methods, results, discussion, and conclusions). An interesting or even clever *title* can enhance attractiveness, but cuteness is to be avoided at all costs. It is sometimes appropriate for the title to be presented as the question addressed by the reported research, thus reducing or even eliminating the need for an introduction. In general, the *introduction* should be limited to a sentence or, at the most, two sentences, which establish the importance of the problem addressed and the rationale for the study.

The abstract should emphasize results and materials and methods, in that order of importance. *Materials and methods* should be described in generic or categorical terms, with specific details of data processing, experimental procedure, and fine points of technology or technique left for the presentation or publication. Control or comparison groups or proposed models should also be described in general terms, but with sufficient detail to verify relevance and appropriateness. All the information contained in these two sections must be covered in the presentation and the final publication. The abstract itself must focus on the *results* of greatest importance and widest applicability and provide the basis for any conclusions drawn. The materials, and methods and results sections of an abstract are customarily written in the past tense, but in the other sections the present tense can be used, as appropriate.[1]

The *discussion* should focus on the present study and explain in concise fashion the applicability of the results to the problem addressed, omitting needless reference to the work of others or even the author's previous work in that field. The word "significant" should be applied only when a difference has been statistically verified.

The *conclusions* section should consist of one or, at the most, two sentences and should be confined to the work being reported. In the conclusions, hypotheses should be clearly separated from facts,[2] and one should not make unwarranted extrapolations of the findings beyond the point supported by the data presented. In the case of a clinical study, the conclusions should make clear how the results influence patient management or outcome. In the case of a laboratory study, the conclusions should explain the importance of the findings to understanding of biologic processes and disease mechanisms or, if relevant, clinical application.

Study Design

It is obvious that the potential quality of an abstract is directly related to the quality of the study being reported. Any clinical or laboratory study should be conducted according to an experimental design that will permit appropriate statistical assay and answer the question being asked. A priori statistical comparisons reported in the abstract must be comparisons that were planned before the study began; *a posteriori* comparisons should be clearly identified. Serial comparisons of multiple nonindependent test groups by means of *t*-tests without appropriate adjustment is considered to be a fatal flaw by many reviewers. The attribution of a trend to data that approach but do not reach a level of statistical significance is apt to be regarded by reviewers as wading by the "no swimming" sign. In the preparation of an abstract reporting a chronologically lengthy series of cases, one should keep in mind improvements in general care and changes in treatment modalities that have occurred across time and stratify patients within appropriate time segments.

Topic Relevance

The acceptability of an abstract will be enhanced if the abstract topic is related to the subject of the meeting, conforms to the interests of the membership of the sponsoring organization, and deals with a subject that has not been featured at recent meetings of the organization to which it is being submitted. Topics of clinical relevance and significance will be most favorably considered for programs in which clinical medicine is emphasized. Similarly, laboratory studies will be most favorably reviewed for programs in which research and the understanding of disease processes are emphasized. An abstract addressing a nonexistent, archaic, or even a recently well-covered problem or one that could be perceived as a reinvention of the wheel will elicit little enthusiasm on the part of reviewers. Single case reports are similarly lightly regarded unless the information presented illustrates a general principle or reports a spectacular result of importance to an entire class of patients. Negative studies will, in general, receive little consideration unless they refute established dogma, break icons, gore oxen, or dispel myths.

Things to Avoid

There are certain features of an abstract that are likely to dampen the enthusiasm of all but the most inexperienced of reviewers.[3] Although brevity is essential, an abstract should not read like a telegram. The abstract should not represent merely a review of the work of others or address a self-created straw man. In the introduction, one should avoid sentences that begin with "The following experiment was performed to . . . ," since it should be obvious from the introduction and body of the abstract why the experiment was performed. In the discussion section, space should not be devoted to things "not done" or "not found," and one should consider only the data that were generated in the study being reported. There should be no surprise endings, with conclusions unrelated to the information provided in the abstract or not supported by the data presented. The conclusions can usually be stated without a preamble, such as "The results of this study showed . . ."

The abstract should not intermix materials and methods with results or conclusions; the integrity of each section should be maintained. The abstract should not promise any answer that is not provided, and the authors should not request carte blanche for "work in progress" or "to be done." Vague generalizations regarding data to be presented, results to be discussed, experience to be reviewed, or techniques to be described should be avoided. References to a nondescript "extensive experience" or self-denigrating comments regarding a "limited" or "modest" experience will not excite the enthusiasm of reviewers. It goes without saying that the abstract should contain only information at hand, since subsequently generated data may significantly alter the results and interpretation of the research and necessitate an embarrassing withdrawal of an accepted paper. Important research results are not so perishable that one cannot delay submission until the research is completed.

Reviewing and Editing

It is much more difficult to describe the key aspects of a study, in an abstract, than to write the paper for publication. A first draft is never submittable, and

TABLE 40.1. Abstract "detractors."

1.	Typographic, grammatic, and spelling errors
2.	Use of jargon and colloquialisms
3.	Failure to define acronyms
4.	Failure to define units of measurement or identify numbers of cases, experimental subjects, or observations
5.	Extensive review of the work of others
6.	Excessive experimental detail
7.	Needless reference to earlier work of author or other investigators
8.	Inclusion of what was "not done" or "not found" in the discussion
9.	Intermingling of hypothesis and facts
10.	Unwarranted extrapolation of findings
11.	A surprise ending
12.	Promises of work "to be done"

even the final draft should be reviewed by each coauthor as well as selected peers. Even in these antipaternalistic times, it is a courtesy to offer the department chairman the opportunity to review the abstract, particularly if he will have to answer to his colleagues for the results and conclusions. Good abstracts are made better by rewriting, and the need for this "aging" process speaks against writing the abstract the night before the submission deadline. Though robust results often speak for themselves, even the best are enhanced by an outstanding presentation; the fate of a report of more fragile results frequently hinges on the quality of the abstract.

The Rejected Abstract

Because more abstracts are submitted to program committees than can be accepted for presentation at professional meetings, almost every author will receive a rejection notice, sooner or later. When you have recovered from the emotional impact of being rejected, you must decide whether to attempt resuscitation of the failed abstract.

An understanding of the sorting and selection process followed by a program committee is helpful when you are performing such a triage. The committee will unanimously approve 10% to 15% of every batch of abstracts and reject 20% or so, with equal enthusiasm. Abstracts prepared hurriedly at the last minute, and those reporting marginal modifications of previously published material, usually fall into this ill-fated 20% and are best left to die unmourned. The reasons for the rejection of the remaining 65% to 70% vary, and some of this material will deserve rescue.

Postpone revision of your potentially viable abstract for a few weeks; you may be asked to serve as an invited discussant of similar papers accepted for presentation. If, by the time of the meeting, your series is larger than the one to be reported in an accepted paper, or if you can present a different and well-supported conclusion, you may be able to savor the pleasure of being one-up.

Diagnosing and Correcting the Problem

Rejection may reflect a surfeit of recent papers on your topic, at meetings of the society you chose or in the literature. As an author, you will usually be aware of such focused increases in publication density; but if you are in doubt, a search of the literature, by title, over the past 5 years, will usually clarify the situation. If your subject is faddish or a commonly encountered surgical problem, undertake a revision of your abstract only if your results illuminate significant pathogenetic factors, validate a new treatment, or significantly enhance understanding of the area you have studied. Even if you think this is true, you should honestly try to identify why these sterling qualities were not perceived by the program committee.

Some abstracts fail because they are messy. Organization, neatness, grammar, and spelling really do count; careful revision and reorganization will sometimes reveal the prince within the toad. Every sentence should be reviewed for clarity and economy of wording.[4] Invite uninvolved colleagues to review your abstract and correct any deficiencies they find. Shear away the "detractors," listed in Table 40.1, and incorporate as many of the "enhancers" in Table 40.2 as possible.[5] Presenting your data in a table will often rid your abstract of a jumble of abbreviations and wordy descriptions. A graphic display, easily produced by desktop publishing and computer enhancement techniques, is even better; a picture worth a thousand words can be put in the space required for sixty. The same techniques allow you to employ stylish arrange-

TABLE 40.2. Abstract "enhancers."

1.	A clever, specific, and concise title
2.	Conformity to interests of program committee and sponsoring organization
3.	Emphasis on new or unique findings and observations
4.	Grammatically correct, error free typescript
5.	Easily read, minimal entry data tables
6.	Properly defined and appropriately applied statistical assessment
7.	Definition of all measurements units
8.	Identification of number of cases, experimental subjects, and observations
9.	Use of graphic display to emphasize important relationships
10.	Use of "typeset" format

ment, font selection, and laser printing to enhance the appearance of your abstract. Significantly higher acceptance rates are reported for such "typeset" abstracts.[6] While the necessity for such embellishments may be inversely related to the importance of the content on your first submission, they are almost certainly desirable in your revised abstract.

If there were few observations in your original abstract, make every effort to buttress your new one with more data, even if gathering them entails some delay. The new material should include supplemental observations that confirm an initially tenuous hypothesis or logically extend your original data. Next, review your conclusions to ensure that they are appropriately supported by the data you have presented and that they relate your results to a topic that interests the organization to which you are submitting your abstract.

Accepting a Second Rejection

If your diagnosis of the cause of your abstract's rejection is correct, these prescriptions may save it. If, however, a second rejection ensues, consider your abstract moribund and move on to more fruitful endeavors. At such a time, you may find it comforting to remember that almost every successful scientist has, tucked away somewhere, a copy of an abstract that only he or she still cherishes and believes to be important.

References

1. Warren R. The abstract. Arch Surg 1976;111:635–36.
2. Baue AE. Writing a good abstract is not abstract writing. Arch Surg 1979;114:11–12.
3. Pruitt BA Jr. Improve your next abstract. Presented at the Seventh Annual Meeting of the American Burn Association, Denver, March 20–22, 1975.
4. American Association for Laboratory Animal Science. How to prepare an abstract. Cordova, TN: AALAS, January 1990.
5. Pruitt, BA Jr. Tips on how to write abstracts for newer members of the American Burn Association. Presented at the 21st Annual Meeting of the American Burn Association, New Orleans, March 30, 1989.
6. Koren G. Letter to the editor—a simple way to improve the chances for acceptance of your scientific paper. N Engl J Med 1986;315:1298.

41

The Ten-Minute Talk

A.V. Pollock and M.E. Evans

Most learned societies require presentations to be in the form of talks of no more than 10 minutes' duration, followed by 5 minutes for discussion. Surgical investigators should attend such meetings and should contribute to them. Young investigators are seldom included among the invited speakers; they are usually required to submit abstracts for consideration by the society's selection committee for presentations to be given in the free paper sessions.

Preparation of an Abstract

A meticulously structured abstract describing original work has a good chance of being accepted. A selection committee faced with choosing 20 out of 100 candidate abstracts will automatically reject those that are badly thought out or noncompliant with the society's requirements. An abstract must be clear and concise. It must stand on its own and state precisely the objective, the methods, the results, and the conclusions of the research. It should normally be written in the passive voice: "Four hundred patients were enrolled in a trial . . .," not "We enrolled 400 patients in a trial . . ." It is preferable to avoid abbreviations altogether: an abstract prepared with acronyms and abbreviations is almost impossible to understand and may well lead to rejection of an otherwise sound piece of work. The piece must be edited several times; as much time and care are needed to produce a good abstract as to produce a good paper (see Chapter 40).

Designing the Talk

The acceptance letter for your abstract has arrived; waste no time in preparing your talk. The paramount consideration is scientific reliability. When you have to describe your objectives, methods, results, and conclusions in a 10-minute talk, you have to take some short cuts. The first thing to remember is that there is a big difference between what is essential in writing and what is acceptable in speaking, though absolute honesty is fundamental to both. You have to condense and clarify your data when you give a short talk: graphs are preferable to tables in spoken presentations, tables to graphs in written reports. When people read a journal, they have time to study tables or figures; when they hear a speech, you, the speaker, must convey the essentials as clearly and concisely as possible.

You must be prepared to spend hours and hours preparing, editing, and reediting your work. Constructing an after dinner speech is admittedly outside the scope of this chapter, but the remarks of a polished after-dinner speaker (Sir Hugh Casson) also apply to the 10-minute talk. He said that he spent an hour preparing for every minute he was going to speak. You do not grudge the time you spent gathering your data, so you must not grudge the time it takes to put the results and conclusions into an intelligible form.

The first thing you must do is make a table of the results and decide on the important outcome events. You have used the methods so often that the preparation of this section might seem to be easy, but try out the draft on a colleague who was not part of the research team – he or she will probably help you to clarify it. When you have surmounted the difficulties of these two sections, the introduction and conclusion should follow logically. It is impossible to lay down strict rules for the amount of time you should spend on each section. The best guide is that nothing you say should be obscure, nothing boring, and nothing unjustified by the results you present. These requirements mean that your talk must nearly always be accompanied by slides.

Designing Slides

Slides provide background, evidence, and illustration.[1] They must not be merely prompts for the speaker. They must be appropriate, accurate, legible, comprehensible, and well-executed. If possible, they should also be interesting and memorable. The audience should be able to absorb the information on one slide in 4 seconds. The standard slide measures 35 × 22 mm, in a frame 50 mm square; the artwork should be drawn in the proportions of 35:22. This can be achieved on A4 paper or card by drawing a line with a pencil 30 mm from each edge and using the whole of the remaining space. If you are using A4 paper, you must use a type size not less than 24 point (capital letters 6 mm high and lowercase 5 mm); this is most conveniently and neatly done on a Kroy printer.

If you have to use a typewriter, you must make the artwork fit into a space 95 × 60 mm: the type size will usually be 10 or 12 pitch (lowercase letters 2 mm high), and you must remember to clean the keys and use a carbon ribbon. Only by obeying these rules can you be certain that you will not overcrowd your slides and that they will be visible to the whole audience. Computer graphics are great fun to play with but, they can make poor slides unless the outline of the letters is perfectly clear. Often, you are tempted to put too much on the slide.

There are three common ways of producing transparencies from lettered artwork: the Diazo process gives white letters on a translucent, usually blue, background; positive transparencies give black letters on a white background: and the negative (Kodalith) process produces white letters—which can be colored on the transparency using felt-tipped pens—on an opaque black background. All these methods are relatively cheap, but some people find Diazo slides boring, and the blue background tends to fade, producing an effect known as "aged professorial." Slides with black lettering on a white background show dirty marks easily.

There is a fourth way of making transparencies that can either please by judicious use of colors or offend by garish display: this is the Color-Key process. It is used to good effect by the illustration department of the Mayo Clinic, for example, but it requires a professional laboratory and is considerably more expensive and time-consuming than any of the other three methods.

A few other rules about lettered slides are sometimes flouted with disagreeable results. Most slides, unlike printed words, look better if the typeface is sans serif; suitable typefaces are Helvetica and Universe. Ruled lines should be used sparingly, and punctuation marks, except question marks, should be avoided. Each item in a list should be preceded by a dot, known as a bullet, of the same diameter as the size of the typeface, not by a number—numbers should be used only when they signify either increasing or decreasing order of importance, or ordered steps in a method. Finally, capital and lowercase letters must be used logically, not at random. Slides with scattered upper- and lowercase letters are unattractive. Lettered slides should always be wider than they are tall—"landscape" style. The proportion of 35:22, forced upon us by the standard 50 mm slide, is close to that of the "Golden Rectangle" of aesthetics.[2] The Golden Rectangle has a proportion of 1.62:1, whereas a slide has a proportion of 1.59:1.

So much for the lettering on slides. On many occasions it is necessary to use line drawings, photographs, or graphs. Line drawings are often used to depict apparatus, and photographs are essential in showing radiographs and microscopic sections. Graphs are indispensable particularly to show results; they must, however, be constructed with considerable care and kept as simple as possible.

Designing Graphs

Tufte[2] gave this advice: "What is to be sought in designs for the display of information is the clear portrayal of complexity." Among the essentials demanded by Tufte for the graphic display of data are the following: graphs must not lie; the data must be shown; the "data/ink ratio" must be maximized, and all "nondata/ink" and "redundant data/ink" must be erased. The data/ink ratio is the ratio of the parts of the graph that disclose the data to the total amount of ink used to make the graph. Overcrowded slides are always irritating, and the lettering on graphs and other diagrams must be horizontal, not vertical.

A large number of data can be shown most effectively by a scattergram, which should include a mean and standard deviation if the data are normally distributed, or a median and quartiles if they are not. For the graphic display of proportions, bar diagrams and pie charts are more suitable. Line graphs on x and y-axes are essential to illustrate the progress of one variable against another (e.g., the concentration of an antibiotic in serum against time); they are always shown as curved lines. Such lines should not be used for such discontinuous data as life tables; they should be drawn in steps.

It is allowable in slides, unlike written papers, to use percentages without whole numbers, and probability values without their parent test statistic. Somerset Maugham wrote that simplicity and naturalness are the truest marks of distinction, and you must aim for them in designing your slides. "Graphic elegance is often found in simplicity of design and complexity of data."[2]

Line drawings, photographs, and graphs, like lettered slides, should be in landscape form, if possible. It is sometimes impossible to avoid the alternative "portrait" style, but the number of such slides should be kept to a minimum; surprisingly few lecture theaters have screens that are as tall as they are wide.

All slides must be mounted with plastic or glass and have a mark on the left-hand bottom corner of the mount to ensure they are put into the projector magazine correctly. It is sensible to put your slides into the magazine yourself, and then check that all is well in the room set aside for previewing slides. (See also Chapter 48.)

Technique of Presentation

The usual form of words implies that a 10-minute talk is read from a manuscript–Dr. Jones read a paper at a meeting of the Society of Omphalologists. There is, however, considerable variation from country to country. The Surgical Research Society in Britain positively discourages speakers from taking manuscripts up to the lectern, unless English is not their native language. In contrast, many of the papers presented at the Society of University Surgeons and other research societies in the United States are read from manuscripts.

There are pros and cons of both techniques. British surgeons claim that the omission of a manuscript results in a more interesting presentation: an enthusiastic research worker can talk rather than lecture to his peers, and tell them about, and illustrate, the hypothesis, methods, results, and conclusions. Obviously he or she has rehearsed many times to be confident of not drying up or exceeding the allotted 10 minutes. The American view is that the words that are spoken should be the words on the manuscript. This has the merit that every word is accurate–or, at least, as accurate as the written work–and that the pace of reading can be judged to allow the presentation to last exactly 10-minutes. Critics of this method believe that it encourages a stilted, unconversational, monotonous recitation that may embarrass both speaker and audience. It is doubtful if consensus can be reached on whether 10 minute talks should be spoken or read, but whichever method you choose, the result will be pleasing only if sufficient preparation has gone into your talk.

Dual projection of slides is becoming increasingly common. The technique does have a place, but it is a limited one. A courtesy to an audience whose first language is not English is to project at least the most important slides in the language of your host country at the same time as the slides in English. To synchronize the showing of two slides, side by side, it is often necessary to use blanks so that both projectors can be advanced simultaneously. Dual projection should never be used merely to fit twice the number of slides into your talk.

Personal Appearance and Manners

You should dress formally and not flamboyantly; you must keep still; and you must beware of irritating mannerisms either in speech or in actions. If you have a friend with a video camera, get him or her to record your talk during a rehearsal; you will be surprised how many mannerisms you have that need to be corrected. One of the common faults of an inexperienced speaker is using a light pointer to draw attention to part of a slide, forgetting to turn it off, and waving it about so that the roving spot distracts the audience's attention–the "mad moth" syndrome.

There is no place for jokes in a 10-minute talk. A witty aphorism or a juxtaposition of the serious and the ridiculous can relieve the tedium of what might otherwise be a dull talk, but it must not be contrived. Rudeness about previous speakers or previous workers in the field of your research is indefensible. Yet during question time, somebody in the audience may make disparaging remarks about your work. However vexed you feel and however unjustified the criticism, avoid the temptation to reply in kind; thanking the person for his or her observations is far more effective.

Burkhart wrote the following description of an inept lecturer: ". . . verbosity overtakes conciseness; disorganized presentation overtakes clear thinking and careful preparation; mumbles overtake articulateness: and, worst of all, you can't read the slides beyond the third row."[3]

The ideal speaker does not wander about the platform, as if searching for a way out; does not wave his or her arms, or the pointer, for emphasis; rather, the speaker establishes rapport with the audience by being enthusiastic about the subject and by referring to a previous speaker's comments. In the ideal case, the slides can be read easily by people sitting in the back row, and the talk will have a beginning, a middle, and an end.

Although speakers who follow all these rules make it look easy, you can be sure they have taken a lot of trouble to get their manuscripts and slides correct; they have rehearsed, with their slides, in front of a critical audience of colleagues; they have changed the order of their slides several times; they have not memorized their speech like an actor—and they will always have room for spontaneous remarks.

It is just as important to present your work in a polished form as it is to conduct your research carefully. Making a presentation is an integral part of any research project, and it can be a stimulating exercise.

References

1. Evans M. Use slides. In: How To Do It, 2nd ed, Lock S, ed. London: British Medical Association, 1985: 152.
2. Tufte ER. The Visual Display of Quantitative Information. Cheshire, CT: Graphics Press, 1983.
3. Burkhart S. Do as I say, not as I do? Br Med J 1983; 287:893.

42

Commenting on a Ten-Minute Talk

A.S. Wechsler

Scientific societies usually afford authors the opportunity to present their work in the format of a 10-minute talk. A program committee has invariably reviewed the work on the basis of submitted abstracts, and has chosen it because it will inform the audience or provoke discussion. Members of the audience are encouraged to ask the speaker questions at the conclusion of the talk, and those who are knowledgeable about the work, or the field, have an obligation to make constructive comments and pose appropriate questions.

Asking Questions

Critical discussion is a source of important new knowledge. The program director frequently encourages younger members of the audience to comment on work that touches on their own investigations. Commenting, in this context, increases the knowledge of other members of the audience and directs attention to the speaker. Depending on how a comment is made, it may be favorable, constructive or detrimental. We offer some fundamental philosophy, in the form of a list of "do's and don't's."

Do

1. Do be sure you understand the data before you comment.
2. Do formulate a question that clarifies or contrasts the data, or puts them into perspective.
3. Do write your question out in advance.
4. Do initiate discussion that is likely to be of general interest.
5. Do feel a responsibility to participate if the field is within your area of expertise or close to your own work.
6. Do remember that criticism can be politely raised in the form of a question.
7. Do put yourself in the speaker's position.
8. Do, if you wish, bring a simple highly pertinent slide, but prearrange for its projection to avoid creating a delay in the flow of the program.
9. Do know and follow the rules of the meeting.
10. Do let the chair know, in advance whenever possible, that you wish to discuss the paper.
11. Do feel comfortable about referring to a specific slide used by the speaker.
12. Do realize the importance of the discussion to the science, the speaker, and yourself.
13. Do prepare yourself in advance by carefully reviewing the abstract(s) prior to the meeting.

Don't

1. Do not take more than your fair share of the session time.
2. Do not personalize your comments; deal with the scientific data only.
3. Do not use your comments for self-glorification.
4. Do not waste time with excessive compliments.
5. Do not ask incriminating questions.
6. Do not set up a series of questions to make your point.
7. Do not bring a handful of slides.
8. Do not give another paper.
9. *Do not even consider using a public forum to ventilate personal animosity or attempt to embarrass another scientist.*
10. Do not entertain your colleagues with tutorative comments as an alternative to standing up and contributing to the quality of the session.

Responding to Questions

The program moderator will usually organize this facet of a presentation and should protect speakers from excessively long, abusive, or inappropriate forms of commentary. You, as a speaker, will have to do some thinking on your feet, but thoughtful preparation will pay off. We offer some helpful advice.

Do

1. Do jot down critical aspects of questions, as they are asked.
2. Do try to anticipate questions by talking with your peers and others prior to the meeting.
3. Do remember that the knowledge gradient is in your favor for your focus paper and do not be disconcerted by the sudden appearance of an "expert" in the audience.
4. Do recognize each questioner visually, or by name.
5. Do give the shortest answer possible.
6. Do answer the question specifically, and do not use it as an opportunity to speak about marginally related topics.
7. Do prepare a couple of slides you think you may need, but keep them simple.

Don't

1. Do not waste time thanking questioners excessively.
2. Do not belittle the question, or the questioner, no matter how off-the-mark the question may be.
3. Do not be afraid to admit a lack of knowledge or data.
4. Do not promise to do the suggested experiment next year.
5. Do not be afraid to ask for clarification of a confusing question.
6. Do not use the question period as an opportunity to show how much you know.

43

Facing the Blank Page

J.A. Bennett and M.F. McKneally

Reading maketh a full man, conference a ready man, and writing an exact man.

Of Studies, Francis Bacon (1561–1626)

Writer's Block Is a Good Thing

We try to be exact when we write, because writing carries the onus of permanently associating the author with a final product that will be read by an audience of potentially unlimited size and critical powers. This imaginary readership intimidates the writing process in a salutary way, because it reduces the presentation of totally spontaneous, ill-considered rubbish. In this sense, the writer's block that prevents easy generation of the written word is probably beneficial to society. The trait is certainly conserved in the evolution of surgical scholars, as 77% of our authors described blocking symptoms in response to a questionnaire about writing their chapter for this book (Fig. 43.1).

The contributors who experienced writer's block during preparation of this book are all widely published in their fields of concentration. It seems that blocks are the rule rather than the exception, and effective ways have been found to help the writer overcome them. This chapter discusses the problem as experienced by our authors, and provides some suggestions that have been helpful to others who were faced with the task of communicating their ideas in writing. The subject is well presented in the very helpful book entitled *Overcoming Writing Blocks*.[1]

Pathogenesis

The pathogenesis of writer's block has been described as intimidation by the internal critic. Since the skill of writing is developed by trial and error, with a heavy emphasis on correction by the teacher, students of writing develop an internal critic that censors words being selected to express an idea before the words reach the page. This censorship, especially in people who tend toward perfectionism, can severely restrict the ability to formulate ideas in written words, even when the ideas are well developed. This power of the internal critic is actually helpful to the writer if it can be saved for the editing stage of writing and inactivated during the drafting stage.

Getting Started

Starting the flow of words generally requires a very considerable amount of preliminary reading and thought, and a locus that separates the writer from interruptions and distractions. The distractions of daily practice and life are extremely tempting, because they are immediate, concrete, circumscribed, and familiar. A ritualized reorganization of the environment seems to be quite helpful and necessary for many writers. This pencil-sharpening, desk-clearing preparation can become very significantly elongated into procrastination, usually a symptom of inadequate mental preparation for the writing task. Mary Evans, one of the authors of Chapter 44, recommends that we not take our blocks too seriously, but leave the writing task alone for a few more days, reading or thinking about the assignment more extensively before readdressing the blank page.

The intellectual process of assembling the background information is carried out in many ways by different authors. Popular techniques included developing a large legal folder or loose-leaf notebook into which are entered references, useful phrases, "single pages with single ideas," any subsequent notes on such ideas, and blackboard brain-

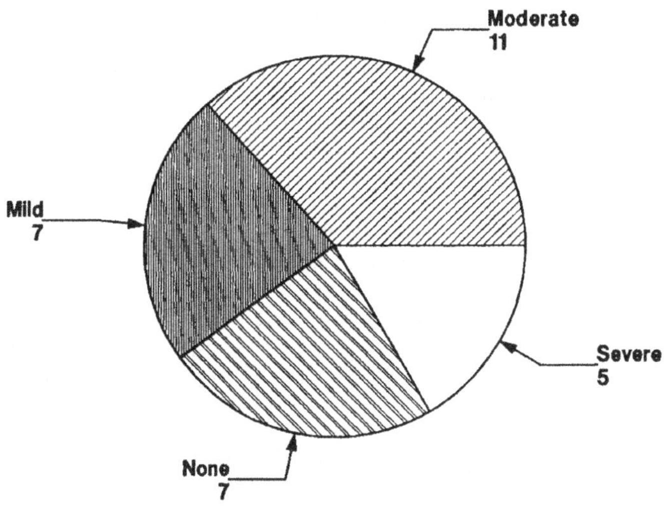

FIGURE 43.1. Responses of contributors to this book to the question: "Did you have blocking symptoms preparing your chapter?"

storming sessions with coauthors or students; dinner with a friend to discuss the writing project—particularly useful when the friend is a coauthor; or giving a 10-minute lecture to an imaginary audience followed by writing down an outline of the lecture.

The Outline

Following this prewriting phase, some authors found it most effective to develop an outline, either conventional (Table 43.1) or spoke-wheel (Figure 43.2).

Many of our authors found writing the outline as difficult as writing the first draft. When the outline is finished, blocking symptoms diminish and writing proceeds more smoothly for many authors. Dr. Neugebauer: "When my (conventional) outline is complete, my symptoms disappear and I am happy!" Scattered pages of notes, a separate page for each individual topic, can serve as a surrogate or prelude to the outline. This technique has been developed into computer software called, "Tornado Notes" [Tornado: Micro Logic Corp., Hackensack, NJ 07602], which allows the author to summon up notes on various subtopics within the writing assignment by a keystroke, and to work on them individually, as some of us work on randomly scattered pages. A miscellaneous but progressively more structured set of lists replaces the outline for Dr. Mosteller.

Drafting

Once the prewriting phase of gathering and organizing the information for the written assignment has been completed, the drafting of the first version is begun. As one begins drafting, it is crucial to get the words out, past the critic, regardless of how they sound, averting the review or editing process as much as possible. Some writers find it necessary to get started by writing a letter that describes the writing assignment to an imaginary, unconditionally accepting friend. Many speak into a tape recorder, because the critic has far less influence over the spoken word compared to the written word in most people's experience. Our editors prefer to consider this the "zero draft," whose principal function is to violate the blank page and to provide material for editing and reworking. Since the zero draft is not permanent, you can proceed without interruptions, never seeking the perfect word or spelling or reference until the manuscript is complete. Some of us put parentheses around incompletely developed thoughts or poorly chosen words, deferring critical review until the whole draft or outline is in hand to make corrections. Most authors found editing far easier than drafting or outlining. The symptoms of anxiety associated with writer's block seemed to diminish progressively as the manuscript moved from the prewriting phase through first draft, outline, and progressively edited rewrites. This is illustrated in Figure 43.3.

The traditional outline forces an ordered prioritization of ideas, which is very helpful for some writing assignments and quite difficult for others. For example, the rigid format of an original article on a scientific subject provides a basic outline generic to all such articles. The order in which these main headings are drafted (introduction, methods, results, discussion, abstract) varies with the preference of the author. Many recommend that the author, like Alice in Wonderland, "begin at the beginning and continue until the end, then stop!" A larger number preferred beginning with

TABLE 43.1. Facing the blank page.

Introduction: Writer's block is a good thing.
Writing is permanent.
Audience intimidates.
Blocking is good.
Most of us have it.
Pathogenesis? The internal critic.
Internal critic like our teachers.
Defer criticism.
Write a letter, or dictate.
Getting Started
Preliminary reading and thought
Procrastination and pencil-sharpening
Collecting information; examples
Brainstorming
The Outline
Conventional
Spoke-wheel
Pages of notes
Lists
Drafting
"Zero draft"
Order
Key phrases
Distracting thoughts
Capturing the right words
Signposts
Editing
Reread, rewrite.
Get critique from others.
Save "diamond chips."
Avoid telegraphic writing.
Environment for Writing
Right time; schedule
Divide assignment
Set deadlines
The right place
How we do it
David Mulder's list
Quotes from authors
End with Francis Moore

some very concrete and simple segment, such as the methods or the tables and figures, which "trick us to overcome procrastination." Writing about the most exciting and interesting points first energizes the writing process. In this phase, key phrases and words that communicate your ideas effectively should be captured on paper, even in incomplete or awkward sentences if they seem to fit the ideas well, regardless of the flow. As you write, let your thoughts evolve, and accept the fact that the language to communicate the thoughts is also evolving. Remind yourself: "It is not a finished product," and you need not expect the perfect sentence to communicate the drift of your ideas. As you are developing your draft, you will have many thoughts that do not fit the outline or the segment you are working on. It is useful to have a second tablet for text memoranda so that well-expressed thoughts can be recorded or reintroduced later. A third tablet for recording important distractions is useful to keep you from leaving the writing task simply because you remembered another obligation.

Writing assignments travel with us, and the right words or the best fit of ideas often come at unexpected moments, while driving home, walking the corridors, in the operating room, or sleeping at night. Have a note pad or recorder available to capture these words and thoughts as they appear. Frequent rereading aloud of what you have already written on the topic helps to keep your conscious and subconscious mind focused as you develop the draft. If the process is interrupted, leave signposts in the margin that briefly advertise the upcoming sequence of thoughts. These can be one-word descriptors, short phrases, drawings, or the names of authors of references containing the ideas you wish to discuss. Signposts facilitate reentry into the drafting process at your next sitting.

Editing

In the editing stage, reread the work several times yourself, rewriting where necessary, and then give the draft to others who are experienced in writing. To be sure that you are not misunderstood, you can tell them what you want the written work to communicate and ask if it succeeds. Alternatively, you can ask them to read it and communicate the main points of the work back to you. At this stage it is important to loosen your ownership over the piece and welcome criticism. Remember that the ultimate objective is to communicate your ideas to the readers. If different words or different arrangements of them accomplish this better than your

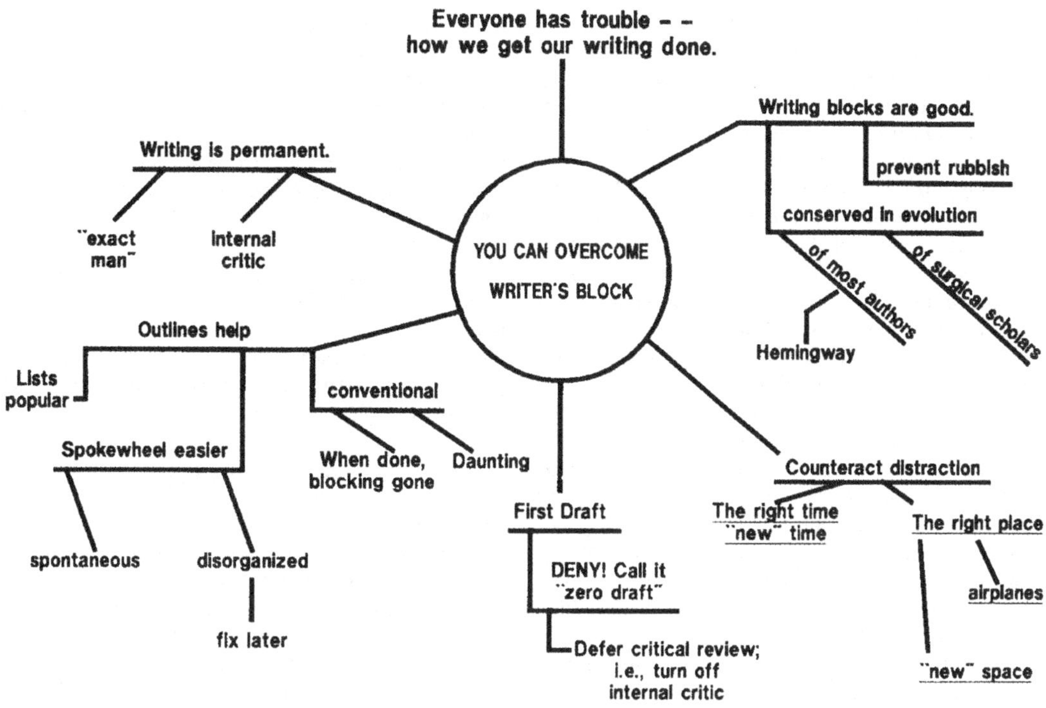

FIGURE 43.2. Spoke-wheel outline.

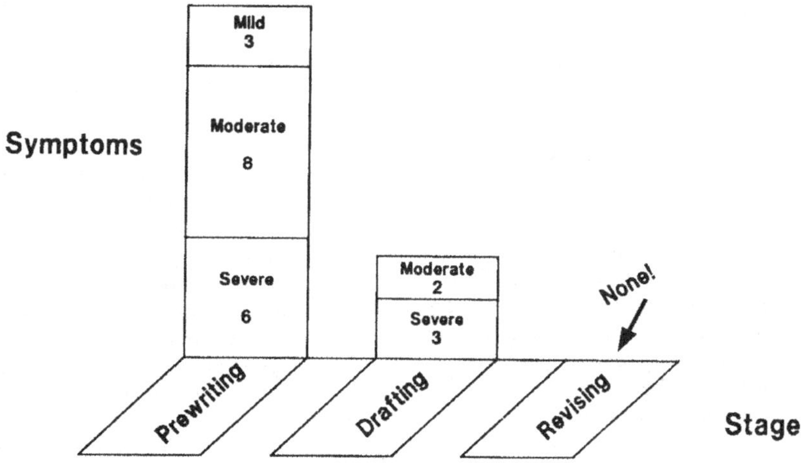

FIGURE 43.3. When the "zero draft" is done, blocking symptoms disappear.

original attempt, accept the new formulation. It is important that the writing be as reader-friendly as possible. The work is already friendly to you as author, since it is a part of you, but often the objective input of others is needed to season the work to the tastes of your readership.

When phrases, sentences, graphs, tables, and ideas dear to your heart are eliminated in the editing process, think of them as diamond chips that can be saved for use in future masterpieces. This will make the editing process easier to handle, and your treasury of unpublished material may provide the impetus or text for further development of your ideas in a subsequent publication.

Most writers are extremely well informed by the time they overcome their writer's block and move into the writing phase. As you consolidate your background material, be sure your familiarity with the subject does not cause you to omit the logical, transitional steps you made in your own thinking. John Bailar advises, "Focus on the message received, not the message sent by the writer. Take pains to be sure that you are not misunderstood." Don't presume that the logic of your readership is the same as your own. You may well have a patterned thought process that is not necessarily communicated in the words you selected to describe your thinking, although it is intuitively obvious to you. Align the readers with your thinking and logic by using connectors like, "Based on these findings we concluded that . . . ," or, "It seems reasonable to conclude that . . . ," "These data support the view . . ." It is easy to be telegraphic when you are well informed about a subject.

The Environment for Writing

Most readers of this chapter do not write for a living and their environment is not ideally suited to the writing process. One author stated, "Since I am paid to administer and teach, I have many interruptions." Making your environment safe for consecutive thinking is a very challenging project. This is particularly true when critically ill surgical patients are part of the environment.

The Right Time

Time has to be created for writing. Ideally, this time should be sufficient to allow you to establish momentum of thought and written word. Writing time should be placed in a fresh, creative phase of your biological cycle. Most of our authors preferred writing early in the morning, but some found it useful to write late at night. "Creating a new time" is very desirable. Ideally, this is done by completing a previous assignment and devoting the newfound time to your next writing assignment. It is important to realize, when you are accepting a large writing assignment, that some other part of your schedule will have to be eliminated. Without this conscious acceptance and reorganization of time, you will find yourself stealing time to write and resenting the writing assignment. Generally, writing time can be used more efficiently if the assignment is broken down into smaller, more manageable parts. Placement of deadlines for completion of each part helps to sustain motivation, prevent procrastination, verify productivity, and provide a feeling of accomplishment.

The Right Place

The locus for writing is a powerful factor in success. Some authors found that working outdoors or in a new setting, such as a library office or a colleague's conference room, out of the routine venue of daily practice, helped to stimulate the writing process and prevent distraction. Airplane trips provide a very satisfactory form of isolated, protected time for writing with minimal interruption.

The ideal writing space should be large enough to allow notes, pads, outlines, and books to be spread out. A dictionary, thesaurus, and appropriate reference books should be within easy arm's reach. If you work more efficiently with a word processor or typewriter, this equipment should be immediately available. The dictating machine and ready access to transcription should be provided in an effective writing center. Immediate feedback of preliminary drafts keeps the process moving.

Some writers find it helpful to have inspirational pictures in the environment, such as highly respected and productive mentors, leaders in the specialty, notable writers, thinkers, or family members. It is useful to have space in which to walk, to pace the floor while dictating or thinking about the next iteration of a draft. For many authors, this kind of physical activity is an outlet for the creative tension of writing. Some respondents mentioned the dining room table at home as a practical place for writing. This broad expanse, free of the clutter of the daily routine in the office or laboratory, provides a comfortable and reassuring setting for writing.

Taking control of your writing environment puts confidence and efficiency into the writing process. Periodically changing position, short walks, timed small rewards such as—a walk around the block, a cup of coffee, or a 10-minute break to talk to friends or family—will sustain your energy and keep your writing fresh and energized for a longer period of time.

How We Do It

David Mulder's recommendation to surgical residents is as follows.

1. Gather all the reprints about the subject, highlight or underline, choose additional references from the bibliography, read and reread them.
2. Then list the points in a very rough outline.
3. Based on this background and outline, dictate a long form of the zero draft, triple-spaced. (Mary Evans makes the point that written language is different from spoken language and that "much bad writing comes from a failure to make this distinction!" Be sure you dictate in written language.)
4. Revise by cutting, pasting, and deleting from the long zero draft.
5. Stop writing and let the project mature in your subconscious mind for the next several days or weeks, depending on the time pressure.
6. Proceed with the definitive revisions of the manuscript.

Writing in longhand is popular, particularly for writing the introduction. When the introduction is written and a rough or complete outline is available, many authors prefer to switch to dictation to accelerate the process. Walter Spitzer says, "Sit down, let it flow, then stand up, pace the floor and dictate. Consider the first typed draft as zero time. Then go." Ray Chiu advises, "Read extensively. Concentrate on organization and message, and then leave your subconscious to work it over. When you are ready, complete the whole essay rapidly." Mary Evans suggests, "Fill five pages before you stop . . . Edit five times." In our brainstorming sessions, idea circles on the blackboard or on large, conspicuous pieces of paper seemed to facilitate the creative process.

Many of our authors identified critical sessions with their mentors who were "liberal with red ink and time" as the most important training for scientific writing. Many felt that their medical school training "militated against good writing" or provided no useful background for writing. Writing essays in undergraduate school or in graduate school for Ph.D. degrees was very helpful. Interestingly, some felt that Latin and mathematical training provided pattern recognition and discipline that was very useful in writing. Reading Fowler's *Modern English Usage*[2] and Pope's "Essay on Criticism"[3] were specifically cited.

Some authors felt that having multiple writing assignments under way simultaneously allowed them to keep the creative process going when progress was slowed on one of the projects. Most authors, however, seemed to feel that juggling more than one writing assignment is detrimental.

Clearly there are many ways to overcome writer's block, and successful authors develop an approach which works most reliably to unlock their creative energies. The inspiration for this chapter was Francis Moore's description of playing the piano wildly to help himself get started writing when he was producing his landmark textbook *The Metabolic Care of the Surgical Patient*.[4] Thirty years later, his response to our questionnaire illustrates the consummate conquest of writer's block, and provides a fitting conclusion for this essay. Dr. Moore writes: "Most of my friends feel that I have written too much in my lifetime, and they would be convulsed with laughter if they thought I were answering a questionnaire on writing block."

References

1. Mack K, Skjei E. Overcoming Writing Blocks. Los Angeles: Tarcher, 1979.
2. Fowler HW. A Dictionary of Modern English Usage, 2nd ed, rev Gowers E. New York: Oxford University Press, paperback with corrections, 1983.
3. Pope A. An essay on criticism. In: Pope: Poems and Prose, Grant D, ed. New York: Penguin USA, 1985:14–35.
4. Moore FD. Metabolic Care of the Surgical Patient. Philadelphia: Saunders, 1959.

44

Writing Your First Scientific Paper

A.V. Pollock, M.E. Evans, N.J.B. Wiggin, and C.M. Balch

Science begins only when the worker has recorded his results and conclusions in terms intelligible to at least one other person qualified to dispute them.

Cooper BM, quoted by Dudley HAF[1]

Writing a research paper is an integral part of research, not just a tiresome appendage to swell your curriculum vitae. You must guarantee that your research was ethical, that your data are accurate, that you have concealed no relevant information, that you have not submitted the same data in another form to another journal, and that all the authors named have taken part in the research and in the preparation of your paper.

Research papers reporting either clinical or laboratory data usually follow the sequence introduction, methods, results, and discussion, or in the words of Bradford Hill, "Why did you start, what did you do, what answer did you get, and what does it mean anyway?"[2]

The International Committee of Medical Journal Editors has published uniform requirements for manuscripts submitted to biomedical journals.[3] These requirements have been adopted by more than 300 journals.

Preparing to Write a Paper

First, decide what your hypothesis is. It defines the purpose and scope of your subject—the "message" you wish to convey to your prospective readers. Next, familiarize yourself with relevant published work to ensure that your paper is original and that you present your data in a proper perspective, as different approaches may be appropriate for different papers. Next, assemble all the necessary information and data, including appropriate statistical analyses, and plan your paper. Finally, before you begin to write your first draft:

1. Organize your results, including tables and figures. Be sure the evidence you are providing is complete enough to permit your reader to draw an independent conclusion.
2. Prepare a sentence to define the limits and focus your paper.
3. Prepare an outline to guide your writing and ensure the logical coherent development of your message. Restrain the impulse to begin writing prematurely; fragmented, disorganized writing is a waste of time.
4. Prepare a strong, decisive conclusion.
5. Determine what recommendation(s) should be made.
6. Decide what audience you are trying to reach, and choose a journal that will reach it.
7. Consult the "Instructions to Authors" in the journal you have selected.

Writing Your First Draft

Sit down in front of a blank sheet of paper, or the blank screen of a word processor, and you will probably find that your mind is just as blank. You must start, and once you have started you must go on. Do not stop to polish your phrases—just get as much on paper as quickly as you can. Correct any obvious errors, but leave any editing until after the first draft is done.

There are at least three ways of starting to write.

1. Take a pen and a pad of lined paper and write. This is probably the most common approach. Always write on alternate lines to allow room for corrections.
2. Outline your thoughts in an organized fashion and use a tape recorder. Beware, however; spoken language is so different from written language that the typed manuscript will take

TABLE 44.1. Guidelines on authorship of medical papers.

Principle 1.	Each author should have participated sufficiently in the work represented by the article to take public responsibility for the content.
Principle 2.	Participation must include three steps: a. Conception or design of the work represented by the article, or analysis and interpretation of the data, or both. b. Drafting the article or revising it for critically important content. c. Final approval of the version to be published.
Principle 3.	Participation solely in the collection of data (or other evidence) does not justify authorship.
Principle 4.	Each part of the content of an article critical to its main conclusions and each step in the work that led to its publication (steps a, b, and c in Principle 2) must be attributable to at least one author.
Principle 5.	Persons who have contributed intellectually to the article but whose contributions do not justify authorship may be named and their contribution described—for example, "advice," "critical review of study proposal," "data collection," "participation in clinical trial." Such persons must have given their permission to be named. Technical help must be acknowledged in a separate paragraph.

Reprinted with permission from Huth EJ[4] (1986).

longer to edit than if it had been written or typed in the first place.

3. Type your ideas on paper or onto the screen of a word processor. Many writers are as confident at a keyboard as others are with pen and paper. Some find that seeing the printed word in front of them and having the ability to rearrange words, phrases, and paragraphs with ease, stimulates the flow of their thoughts. As an immediate benefit of using a word processor, software is available that enables you to insert references in their correct alphabetical or numerical order as soon as you mention them, and renumber them if you add a new one.

There is no standard order of writing and you may find it difficult to write in the order: abstract, introduction, materials and methods, etc. To make it easy to assemble your material, we recommend that you use the following order:

1. Authorship and acknowledgments.
2. Title.
3. Figures and tables.
4. Materials (or subjects) and methods.
5. Results.
6. Discussion/Conclusion.
7. Introduction.
8. References.
9. Abstract.
10. Keywords.
11. Covering letter.

If you try this order and find it just won't work for you, develop one that does and stick to it. If you are writing your first draft by hand, put each of the topics at the top of a separate sheet of paper.

Authorship

Determine who the authors are when—preferably before—you start to write a paper, because each author has responsibility for the accuracy of the data and the content of the manuscript. Individuals with only a casual involvement in the research or in the writing of the manuscript should be listed in the acknowledgments rather than as authors. Acknowledgments might include such contributions as supplying reagents, entering a limited number of patients in a protocol, performing a standard statistical analysis, or editing the manuscript.

Gift authorship is fraud. Specific criteria for determining authorship have been published,[4] and the extracted guiding principles are listed in Table 44.1.

The first author should be sure that all the authors have received the final manuscript and agree with its content before it is submitted to a journal.

Title

Draft a title that will attract readers' attention and permit the proper indexing of your paper in the literature. It should be accurate, brief, and clear. Avoid superfluous words, overgeneralizations, question marks, and exclamation points.

Figures and Tables

Construct tables and graphs, with statistical analyses, early in the preparation in your manuscript. Compare different methods of presenting your data to determine which one conveys the message in the quickest and easiest way. Avoid extensive, complicated tables. Use concise titles and legends that convey enough information to make reference to your text unnecessary.

If you find a particular table cumbersome, try a graph; it may be preferable. When the x-axis refers to time (or before and after an intervention) and the y-axis to the numerical results of a test, lines drawn between two or more points refer, like scattergrams, to a number of patients. Such lines are convincing if they all go up or down, but if some go up and others go down, it implies that some patients have responded differently from others and suggests a possible new avenue of research. This is illustrated by a graph (Figure 44.1).[5] Why

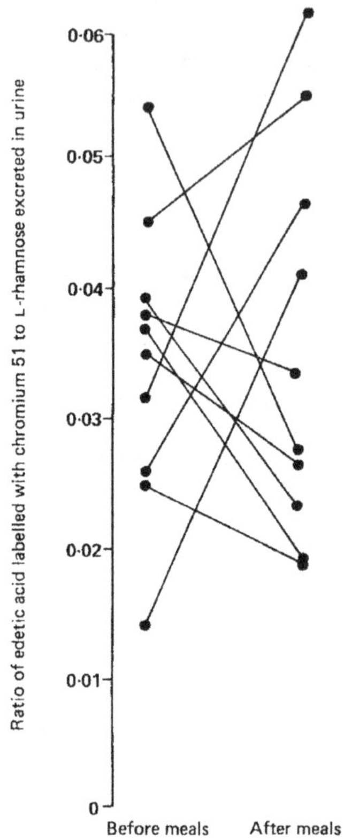

FIGURE 44.1. Pollock & Evans. Reprinted with permission from Bjarnson I, Levi S, Smethhurst P, Menzies IS, Levi AJ[5] (1988).

did the ratio rise in 4 subjects and fall in 6? Table 44.2 and Figure 44.2 convey the same information. The graph is, however, not as accurate as the table, and the reader has to guess at the figures by ruling horizontal lines from each point to the *y*-axis. The table is not cumbersome, in this case, because there are few data.

Life Table Charts

Survival data can be expressed in tables, but the impact of a chart is greater. The chart, however, is never as accurate. A life table chart should be drawn with interrupted horizontal lines, not as a smooth curve. The reason for doing this becomes obvious if you think about it: the number of survivors on the vertical or *y*-axis remains constant until the next time interval on the horizontal or *x*-axis. Table 44.3 and Figure 44.3 show the same information.[7] The accuracy of the figures cannot be guaranteed because we have had to guess them by ruling lines to the *y*-axis.

TABLE 44.2. Natural killer cell activity against K562 before and after operation; values are expressed as mean (SEM).

	Activity			
	Control group (n = 15)	Interferon α group (n = 15)	"t" value	p value
Before operation	38 (6)	41 (6)	.35	>.50
Postoperative				
day 1	15 (4)	33 (5)	2.81	>.01
day 3	16 (5)	36 (5)	2.83	>.01
day 5	16 (5)	30 (5)	1.98	>.05
day 10	22 (4)	22 (5)	0	1.0

Scattergrams

A table or tables, presenting as many data as are contained in the scattergram of Figure 44.4,[8] would be unmanageable. A scattergram on *x* and *y* axes shows whether the data are normally distributed. The illustration can be completed by a horizontal line, indicating a mean (or median), and lines to indicate standard deviation (or upper and lower quartiles). It is the only truly indispensable graphic. A graphic display of correlations is another kind of scattergram, which should normally be accompanied by a line, the slope of which is calculated from a stated correlation coefficient.

Tables

There are four absolute rules about tables:

1. They must not repeat results that you have detailed in the text.
2. Each table must stand on its own and not require reference to the text to explain it; that is, it must have a title, without abbreviations.
3. Each table should disclose whole numbers, with or without percentages.

TABLE 44.3. Percent graft survival after first cadaveric renal transplantation.

	Age	
Months postoperatively	< 55 years (n = 444)	> 55 years (n = 63)
1	90	90
3	77	80
6	70	77
18	65	70
24	65	65
36	60	65
55	55	60

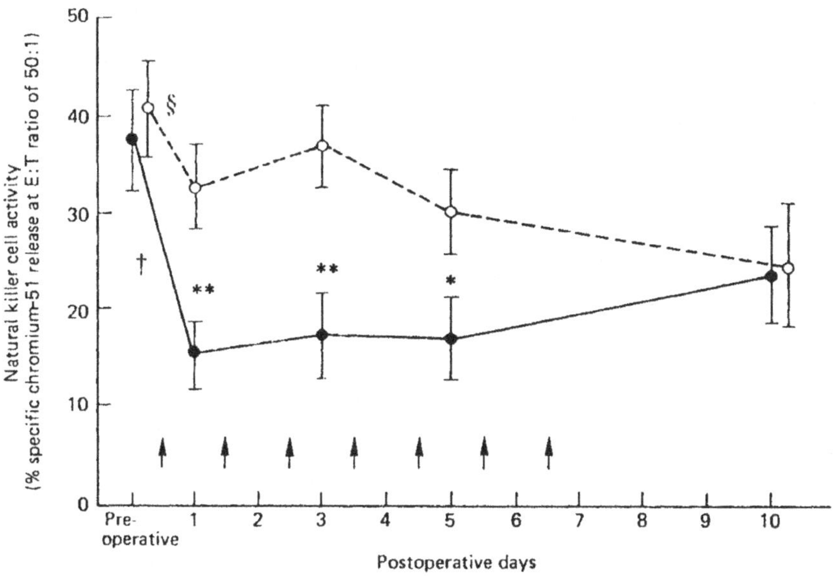

FIGURE 44.2. Natural killer cell activity against K562 levels before and after surgery. ●——● control group: ○——○ r-HuIFNα (2 megaunits/day) ($n = 15$ for both groups). r-HuIFNα versus controls. *$P < 0.05$. **$P < 0.01$. §Preoperative versus postoperative: ●, $P < 0.01$; ○, n.s. E:T, effector:target ratio. Reprinted with permission of Butterworth & Co., publishers, from Sedman PC, Ramsden CW, Brennan TG, Giles GR, Guillou PJ[6] (1988).

4. Tables, like everything else in a manuscript, must be double-spaced and must not have vertical lines.

The content of your tables is at your discretion, but you must pay close attention to the style of your selected journal. If you compare the results of an intervention in a randomly selected experimental group with those in a control group, you must publish a table of comparability to show that the composition of the two groups did not differ significantly. This table can incorporate the incidence of the main outcome event in each group for each variable (men and women, age groups, etc.). Tables of results that show significant differences between groups should be accompanied by confidence intervals, test statistics, and probability values. The vague abbreviation NS, meaning not significant, should never be used: always give the test statistic and the probability.

Materials (or Patients or Subjects) and Methods

This section should give sufficient detail to enable a competent worker to repeat your experiments. You can cite standard techniques, but explain the features or components of your methods that are new or modified. Describe the number and kind of subjects you used, your selection criteria, how you recorded the data, and the statistical tests you applied. Specific suggestions for reporting statistical or numerical issues can be found in Bailar and Mosteller.

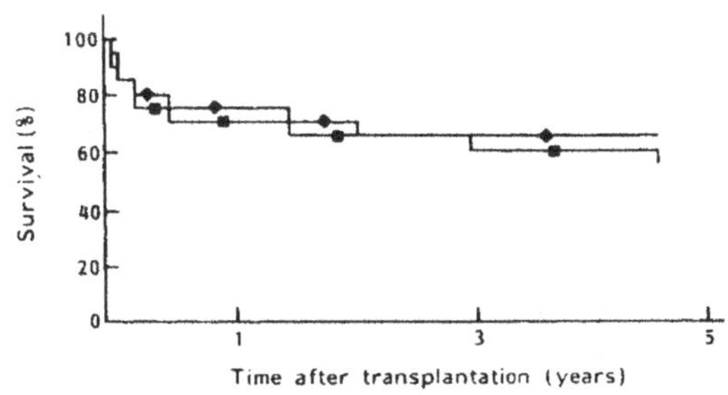

FIGURE 44.3. Actuarial graft survival for 5 years in 444 under-55-year-old (■) and 63 over-55-year-old (◆) first cadaver renal transplant recipients. Reprinted with permission of Butterworth & Co., publisher, from Lauffer G, Murie JA, Gray D, Ting A, Morris PJ[7] (1988).

Results

This section covers pertinent observations and data and involves the development of a complex interrelation between text and figures.

After you have assembled all your information, analyze it in different ways so that you will not omit any important correlations. Arrange the data to disclose significant information in an orderly fashion. You do not have to describe your results in the chronological order in which you performed your experiments. You may refer to material in the tables, graphs, and photographs, but do not repeat that material in the text. Do not put any interpretation, explanation, or discussion of your results in this section.

The headings of your main table will be your experimental group, with "main event" and "no main event" subheadings, and your control group, subheaded in the same way. The variable will be all the data you have amassed. You can then construct a table of comparability of the groups and a table of results. You will need to ask the computer about secondary events and complications in each group. The experimental arm of your research may show important differences from the control arm in the incidence, not only of the main event but also of other and perhaps less desirable outcomes. A trial, for example, of recombinant human tissue type plasminogen activator in the treatment of recent myocardial infarction showed a significant benefit in terms of myocardial function and short-term survival, but an increased incidence of cerebral hemorrhage.[10]

Presentation of Numerical Data

When you give a lecture, your goal is to have your audience grasp your message in a few seconds. A written paper is different. It should achieve precision combined with comprehensibility. Dudley quoted a referee's comment on a paper from his own department: "The methods and statistical analysis were most elegant, but no one could get within a mile of the raw data."[1] "Precision" is a relative term. You should make summary state-

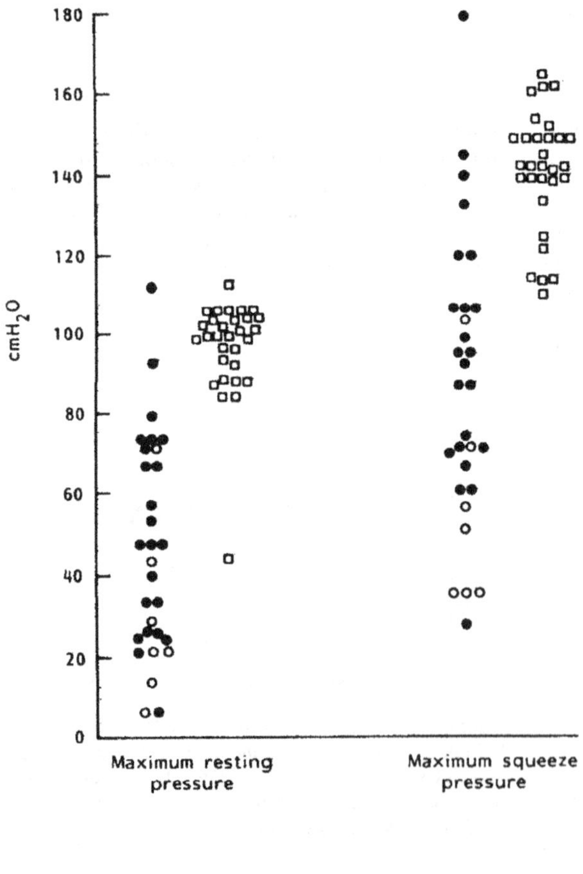

FIGURE 44.4. Maximum resting ($P < 0.005$) and maximum squeeze ($P < 0.01$) anal pressure (cm H_2O) after restorative proctocolectomy compared with controls. ●, Patients with good function; ○, patients with poor function; □, controls. Reprinted with permission of Butterworth & Co., publisher, from Keighley MRB, Yoshioka K, Kmiot W, Heyen F[8] (1988).

ments that allow the reader to understand what you did and what results you got. If your measurements are normally distributed, they can be expressed as means and standard deviations (i.e., measures of the scatter around the mean from which standard errors of means can be easily calculated). If, like most biological measurements, they are not normally distributed, they should be expressed as medians and ranges or medians and interquartiles. The expression $\pm$ must never be used: write mean (SD) or median (interquartile).

The requirements for precision and comprehensibility forbid such errors as dividing age groups into 20–25 and 25–30; groups must be mutually exclusive (20–24, 25–29, etc.). Nearly all journals require the use of Système Internationale (SI) units, except for blood pressure (mm Hg) and ventilator pressures (cm H_2O).

Discussion/Conclusion

The discussion should accomplish seven things.

1. Provide a brief summary of current knowledge and explain your results.
2. Discuss your interpretation of the importance of your results.
3. Outline any alternative explanation(s) to the one(s) you have chosen.
4. Discuss the relation between your data and all pertinent results reported by others.
5. Point out the strengths and weaknesses of your results.
6. Suggest possible refinements in methods for future studies.
7. Conclude with a statement or recommendation that relates your work to current surgical practice.

Do not allow your enthusiasm to override your common sense: never draw conclusions that are not justified by your results, or suggest that your experimental results have a wider application than you have shown.

Introduction

The introduction should be short, should arouse the reader's interest, and should define the purpose and scope of the work you are reporting; it should not be a review of the literature. One or two paragraphs will suffice to put the work into context and to outline any controversy you are trying to resolve or illuminate. Remember that controversy inspires most conjectures and hypotheses. If you can delineate the controversy, it will stimulate interest in what you have to say; but avoid pleas and exaggerated claims.

References

References are an essential ingredient of an original paper. Be sure they are correct. If you refer to a journal that is catalogued in *Index Medicus*, you must abbreviate its title to conform with the *Index*; if it is not, the journal's title must be given in full. Never copy a reference from another paper. Find the original and make sure you repeat every detail correctly. It is a mark of laziness, bordering on dishonesty, to quote a paper you have not read, and a mark of carelessness to refer to it inaccurately. When your manuscript has reached the "final draft" stage, put each reference on a separate index card and assemble a typed reference list in the format required by the journal you have chosen.

Abstract

Writing the abstract is your last task before editing the text and selecting keywords. As many readers will only read your abstract, make sure it contains all the important information in your paper—that is, hypothesis, methods, main results (including important numerical data), and the discussion/conclusion. Your abstract should not be more than two paragraphs long; most journals specify a maximum number of words, usually 150 to 200.

Keywords

Most journals require authors to supply keywords. They should be chosen in compliance with the Medical Subject Headings (MeSH) published each year by *Index Medicus*. Keywords are not merely words that epitomize the message of your paper. They are an important means of making your report retrievable by other investigators who are interested in your field of endeavor. Care taken in the selection of keywords will not only aid the people who index your chosen journal and the compilers of *Index Medicus*, but will help to ensure the optimal indexing and maximal accessibility of your paper.

Covering Letter to Editor of the Journal

When your manuscript is ready, write a covering letter to the editor of the journal you hope it will appear in. Describe the importance of your paper briefly, and tell the editor why you have chosen his journal. Be sure all figures are labeled on the back, and submit a separate set for each copy of the manuscript.

Some General Observations

There are two rules you must never violate: your manuscript must be typed in double spacing, with wide right and left margins; and it must conform to the style of the journal you have chosen.

Make your paper *interesting*. Write simply, directly, and clearly. If you or your coworkers have to read a sentence twice to grasp its meanings, reword it.

Slang words and colloquialisms are not appropriate in a scientific paper. Your paper will probably be read in parts of the world where such expressions will not be understood.

Reference Books

We recommend four instructive, interesting, and amusing books as a matter of personal choice. They are Strunk and White's *The Elements of Style*,[11] O'Connor and Woodford's *Writing Scientific Papers in English*,[12] Thorne's *Better Medical Writing*,[13] and Roberts's *Plain English: A User's Guide*.[14] Other useful specialist dictionaries are Partridge's *Usage and Abusage*,[15] the *Penguin Dictionary of Troublesome Words*,[16] and the *Oxford Dictionary for Writers and Editors*.[17]

Strunk and White's book contains only 85 pages, but they are packed with common sense and good advice. If you choose only one such aid, make it this one.

O'Connor and Woodford's book is a close second. All of its 98 pages are well worth reading, but the last six—"Expressions to Avoid"—should be in front of you whenever you write a paper. Some examples are "as already stated," "as follows," "it may be borne in mind that," "the statement may be made that," "it has long been known that," "it is of interest to note that," and the qualifying adjectives or adverbs "relatively," "fairly," "hopefully," "much," "quite," "rather," and "very."

Charles Thorne's *Better Medical Writing* was first published in 1970 and has been edited, more recently, by Stephen Lock, editor of the *British Medical Journal*. Its 89 pages are amusingly written and contain a wealth of good advice, particularly about how to keep original articles short and clear.

The chief merit of Roberts's book is its 103-page vocabulary of correct words juxtaposed with the "almost correct" ones (e.g., "try to" not "try and").

TABLE 44.4. Checklist for determining when manuscript is completed.

1. Be sure that the introduction is consistent with the content and conclusions.
2. Be sure that each paragraph is logically developed.
3. Be sure that the transitions between sentences, paragraphs, and sections are smooth.
4. Read the paper for clarity, coherence, unity, and consistency.
5. Check the adequacy and consistency of headings and subheadings.
6. Eliminate awkward expressions and faulty or monotonous sentence structures.
7. Check for grammatical, syntactic, and typographic errors.
8. Be sure that references to tables and illustrations and any illustrative material have been inserted in the proper position(s).
9. Verify all arithmetic in the text, tables, and graphs.
10. Verify all quotations.
11. Verify all references.
12. Have the references typed according to the "Instructions to Authors" in the journal you have chosen.

Editing

"Probably, indeed, the larger part of the labour of an author in composing his work is critical labour; the labour of sifting, combining, constructing, expunging, correcting, testing: this frightful toil is as much critical as creative."[18]

You have the first draft of your paper; now you must revise it. Cut out redundant words and phrases, look for sentences that may be misunderstood and, above all, simplify the text. Have the corrected version typed or printed by word processor, make copies, and give them to all your coauthors, interested colleagues, and a technical editor, if one is available. These people will suggest additional corrections and simplifications. Do not feel hurt if they cover your manuscript with red ink. Take it as a compliment: it means they think your work merits their devoting time and thought to helping you improve it.

Work all the useful suggestions into your paper and put it away for a week. When you pick it up again, you will find more to correct. Do not be satisfied with it until you have revised it five or six times and, even then, be prepared to find a few more defects. Table 44.4 offers a checklist for this stage of the work.

Conclusion

Sir Peter Medawar has written "The most heinous offense a scientist, as a scientist, can commit is to declare to be true that which is not so; if a scientist cannot interpret the phenomenon he is studying, it is a binding obligation upon him to make it possible for another to do so."[19]

Writing is hard work, but so is research. The writing of a good paper is as much a part of the research as the performance of the experiment and the accurate recording of data. We have drawn your attention to some aspects of writing scientific papers, but you will learn to write good papers only by writing and editing them.

References

1. Dudley HAF. The Presentation of Original Work in Medicine and Biology. Edinburgh: Churchill Livingstone, 1977.
2. Hill AB. The reasons for writing. Br Med J 1965;iv: 870–71.
3. International Committee of Medical Journal Editors. Uniform requirements for manuscripts submitted to biomedical journals. Ann Intern Med. 1982; 96:766–71.
4. Huth EJ. Guidelines on authorship of medical papers. Ann Intern Med. 1986;104:269–74.
5. Bjarnason I, Levi S, Smethurst P, Menzies IS, Levi AJ. Vindaloo and you. Br Med J 1988;297:1629–31.
6. Sedman PC, Ramsden CW, Brennan TG, Giles GR, Guillou PJ. Effects of low dose perioperative interferon on the surgically induced suppression of antitumour immune responses. Br J Surg 1988;75:976–81.
7. Lauffer G, Murie JA, Gray D, Ting A, Morris PJ. Renal transplantation in patients over 55 years old. Br J Surg 1988;75:984–87.
8. Keighley MRB, Yoshioka K, Kmiot W, Heyen F. Physiological parameters influencing function in restorative proctocolectomy and ileo-pouch-anal anastomosis. Br J Surg 1988;75:997–1002.
9. Bailar JC, Mosteller F. Guidelines for statistical reporting in articles for medical journals. Ann Intern Med. 1988;108:266–73.
10. Van de Werf F, Arnold AER. Intravenous tissue plasminogen activator and size of infarct, left ventricular function, and survival in acute myocardial infarction. Br Med J 1988;297:1374–79.
11. Strunk W, White EB. The Elements of Style, 3rd ed. New York: Macmillan, 1979.
12. O'Connor M, Woodford FP. Writing Scientific Papers in English. Tunbridge Wells, England: Pitman, 1978.
13. Thorne C. Better Medical Writing. London: Pitman, 1970.
14. Roberts PD. Plain English: A User's Guide. Harmondsworth: Penguin, 1987.
15. Partridge E. Usage and Abusage. Harmondsworth: Penguin, 1969.
16. Bryson B. The Penguin Dictionary of Troublesome Words. Harmondsworth: Penguin, 1984.
17. The Oxford Dictionary for Writers and Editors. Oxford: Clarendon, 1981.
18. Eliot TS. The functions of criticism. In: Selected Essays 1917–1932. New York: Harcourt-Brace, 1932:18.
19. Medawar P. The Limits of Science. Oxford: Oxford University Press, 1984:6.

Additional Reading

Eger EI II. A template for writing a scientific paper. Anesth Analg 1990;70:91–96.

45

Writing for Publication

N.J.B. Wiggin, J.C. Bailar III, B. McPeek, C.B. Mueller, and W.O. Spitzer

The final part of research is the publication of results, and good research deserves good writing. Methods, results, conclusions, ideas, and thoughts must be published if they are to last; unless they are put into the literature they can be committed only to a small circle of colleagues or students and will lie beyond recall once verbal communication ceases. The great body of recorded surgical knowledge is in the permanent collection of books and journals prepared by individuals so that others may read, reread, contemplate, refute, or accept their findings. Writing and publishing is more than an obligation of every sophisticated scholar or clinician; it is an essential part of any definition of a productive investigation.

It is helpful to discuss scientific writing in terms of *substance, content*, and *form*. All three are critical to communication, hence to good writing. By substance we mean the subject matter of the writing, considered at several different levels: the subject of a book, a paper, a paragraph, a sentence or phrase. By content we mean what is said about that subject: that the author had discovered a cure for hypochondria; that Figure 1 presents thus-and-so; that two patients were lost to follow-up. Accuracy and precision are critical aspects of content. By form we mean how the content is presented: organization, clarity, economy of language, adherence to the rules of good grammar, and style.

Effective written communication requires one more thing: concern for and empathy with the reader. Too many writers believe that it is enough to send a message; the message, however, must also be received and properly understood. Busy readers tend to be overwhelmed with material they find on their desks; they are not likely to work very hard at understanding a poorly written offering, whatever its relevance and importance. Some potential readers will also be lazy, or tired, or distracted by other matters, and some—perhaps a majority—will not be experts in the subject matter of the writing. None will know as much about the material they are reading as the author. If we have one point to add to the burden already borne by those who seek to write well, it is this: pay constant attention that your message be correctly received at the other end of the communication link; the words you write have no other purpose. This puts great stress on such matters as clarity and brevity. When an interested and qualified reader misunderstands or does not attend to some point of a paper, it is the author who has failed.

Characteristics of Good Writing

The works of great and near-great clinicians nearly always meet high standards in each aspect of writing. There is a reason; we believe that many other clinicians may be just as great in most ways, but they have not learned to write as well. In short, good writing helps the world to recognize good work more than good work elicits good writing. Careful attention to substance, content, and form—down to the last nuances of style—will not be sufficient, in itself, but it can be an invaluable professional asset. It is also an asset to readers and to the discipline as a whole, and that may be one reason why good writing is rewarded so well.

Good technical writing is not an accident, nor is ability in such writing a gift bestowed on a fortunate few. Thoughtful, conscientious, constant attention to what is—and what is not—put on paper can help. So can courses in writing given by qualified instructors. So can careful attention to the writing successes of others. So, we dare to hope, can reading a book or chapter on the subject—but only if the new knowledge is put to use. There is no substitute for practice, objective self-criticism, and as many rounds of revision as needed to do the job well.

Scientific writing must be lucid and carry a message that leaves the reader in no doubt about the concept or idea being stated. It requires a writing style much different from that used by great writers to stimulate image formation in the minds of their readers. Style is as important in scientific work as it is in literature, but the style is different. The scientist should generally try to write so that the style is unobtrusive, even transparent. We read with distress of some who think that a proper "scientific" style requires passive voice, complex sentences, and words of Latin origin. Would you rather read "Specimens were individually developed by exposure to the atmosphere at ambient temperatures" or "I dried each sample in room air." Which do you think is most likely to be found in a research report? Hemingway, in *Snows of Kilimanjaro* or *The Old Man and the Sea*, deliberately sought to evoke many images that would be unique to the individual reader. The intent of scientific writing is the direct antithesis; that is, to transmit a message with such clarity that all readers will receive the same information and arrive at the same conclusion. It demands that the writer be so precise that no one will be confused and no reader will be permitted to develop his or her own concept about what the writer wished to say.

Many books are available to instruct the novice or the expert author in "how to write"; a few are listed in the references.[1-10] Some deal with organization and logic; some cover style and the use of biologic words and abbreviations; some tell you how to use words and phrases to clarify, amplify, and communicate a clear message, and to bring power to your writing. For more than 30 years, the ultimate reference work has been Strunk and White.[8] Every author who writes in English should obtain a copy of this little book and read it carefully – many times.

It is always advisable to develop the overall scope of your message by thinking in terms of paragraphs of 5 to 20 sentences, with each paragraph containing a coherent concept that is developed sequentially. Some writers paste their paragraphs on the wall as they write. They can thus see the whole as they put technical procedures, data, ideas, or results into the appropriate paragraphs, and they can easily rearrange the paragraphs in a sequence that allows the reader's thoughts to flow from research question, to study design, to data, to analysis, to conclusions.

Good scientific writing requires that your words say exactly what you mean and that you construct sentences that are direct and pungent. The subject of every sentence must be easily identified and the verb readily visible. Each sentence must have a noun or pronoun as its subject, and each transitive verb must have a clearly stated object. Sentences often are most powerful when they begin with nouns accompanied by few adjectives and have action verbs with few qualifiers. Avoid the passive voice. Sentences that begin with clauses or dangling phrases referring to elements within the sentence are confusing and generally fail to convey a clear message. Eschew verbosity. Keep sentences short; half a dozen typewritten lines is usually too long. Write in good English, rather than jargon, and your ideas will stand out clearly. Multiple drafts before submission are always more rewarding than multiple drafts after a rejection.

Each communication must convey a significant message, such as a report of an original research study, a critical analysis and review of the work of others, or a brief appraisal of something that has been observed or written. The content and format of a written article depend on your purpose in writing it. Some of the common formats, arranged in an order that is didactically useful rather than a reflection of their relative importance, are:

Monographs.
Research papers.
Review Articles.
Editorials.
Letters to the editor.

Formats of Written Scientific Communication

Monograph

Senior clinicians in various academic posts often serve as leaders or members of research groups or task forces formed to study scientific problems of particular concern to some institution or to the public. The terms of reference of such research assignments, whether they are supported by a conventional research grant or undertaken in response to government or agency contract requests, often require that a lengthy monograph be written. The final product may comprise several hundred pages of double-spaced typed material, with numerous tables, figures, conclusions, recommendations, and references. One can easily see why the commissioning agency may require such a document. It not only constitutes an archival record of the deliberative process, research methods, results, and conclusions, but also serves as a basis for policy making.

Unfortunately, much valuable research or scholarly work is lost to the scientific community because it is buried in monographs that are replicated in very limited numbers and not subsequently published in peer-reviewed, indexed journals. Readers will find it difficult, or even impossible, to discover the existence of publications with such limited circulation. The net result, too often, is the creation of an obstruction to the normal widespread diffusion of good research. If you have a choice between writing a monograph or writing a series of research papers for publication in journals, choose the latter. An indexed journal is cited in the national and international biomedical indexing systems available in most academic libraries. The cross-referencing of key words and ideas in such research resources makes it relatively easy for your colleagues and other investigators throughout the world to discover your work.

Sometimes, you may find that the potential value of a monograph for you, the sponsoring agency, or the public is great enough to justify a substantial investment of your time and effort. If you have accepted a contractual or professional obligation to write a monograph, you can still have advantage of having a principal volume of reports that can be referred to by your research team as they prepare other articles for publication in journals. If you must write monographs, write only those that will be published in archival systems that provide ready access to them.

Scientists sometimes fear that the stringently limited space available for many journal articles will prevent adequate reporting of a large data set or the extensive deliberations of an expert task force. Yet monographs, journal articles, and book chapters are not mutually exclusive; monographs can be created, if necessary, as supplements to brief and focused shorter articles. The shorter articles in journals can reveal the source of supplementary data banks in footnotes and references. The availability of the longer documents can be enhanced by using microfiche and commercial microfilm firms to duplicate the information for those who need it, at nominal cost.

The traditional sequence, which you may alter if there is reason to do so, is to discuss your research findings with your peers, prepare a draft of your paper, revise your draft to take account of the constructive criticisms you have received, submit your paper for publication in a peer-reviewed journal, follow up with book chapters when your findings have been validated and accepted, and make reference to the foregoing in any monographs or journal articles you write on the same subject. A major research project or expert inquiry can easily generate several original, related, yet distinctive publications. As a final world on monographs, avoid contracts and grants that emphasize a requirement for a confidential report that will be given only limited circulation. If you are an autonomous academic or professional investigator, it is wise to refuse an assignment if there is no guarantee that your finished work will be released for open publication within a period of 6 months at most.

Research Papers

The most valuable advice anyone can give you, as a prospective author of a research paper, is to devote adequate time, thought, and expert collaboration to the refinement of your research question, the design of your study (including appropriate outcome measures), its careful performance, and the correct analysis and interpretation of the data. If you have fulfilled these requirements, you can easily get help in writing your paper, if you need it. If your study was poorly conceived and executed, no one can help you. No amount of analytical or writing skill can convert poor data into a good paper.

Getting started is a major hurdle for most of us. Although your paper will eventually end up in the standard format of introduction, methods, results, discussion, and abstract, you are not required to write it in that sequence. Start with whatever you find it easiest to write about (e.g., your methods or results). Another approach is to write and rewrite the first sentence, then the first two, and finally the first three sentences however many times it takes to get them into a form that you feel is exactly right. You may then discover, to your surprise and delight, that you can draft the rest of the paper without difficulty. As you write, your effort will often gather a momentum of its own that will carry you through the parts you considered most intimidating at the outset.

Remember that your intended reader is not only intelligent but also hard-pressed for reading time. You need state something only once, as clearly and directly as possible. Circling around what you want to say or saying it two or three times is more likely to drive your reader away than to drive your point home. Don't coin new words or define new meanings until you have assured yourself that the word and meaning you want do not exist already. A dictionary, Fowler's *Modern English Usage*,[11] and a thesaurus are useful aids. Be careful not to employ elegant variation where it might confuse your reader.

The *introduction* should be a straightforward account of why you embarked on your study, what you hoped to learn or achieve by doing it, and what others who have studied the same or a closely related problem have reported. Your review of other research reports need not be as exhaustive as it would be for a review article. A few significant and directly relevant articles may be enough. Review articles are often cited in introductions, and should be cited more often, because they can facilitate writing, reduce length, and still give interested readers a guided entry to the relevant literature.

When you are giving your reasons for carrying out the study, it is important to confine yourself to the questions or the hypothesis you had in mind when you started. Additional questions prompted by your results should be left for the discussion section.

The *methods* portion of your paper is very important to every sophisticated reader who wishes to be satisfied about the appropriateness of what you did and the validity or reliability of the results your methods produced. An adequate and precise description of the population you studied, your approach to randomization, the experimental intervention, your choice of outcome measures, etc., will enable readers to compare your results with those obtained by other investigators. Adequate description of methods is also needed if others are to contrast or combine your results with their own to gain new insights. This matter is discussed under meta-analysis in Chapter 9.

If your research project has involved a clinical trial, you will need to describe eligibility criteria, admission of patients to your study before allocation, random allocation to different treatment or control groups, the mechanisms you used to generate your random assignments, patients' blindness as to which treatment they received, blindness of the person assessing the outcome as to which treatment each patient received, the methods of statistical analysis included in your design, and how you determined your sample size or the size of detectable differences.[12]

All the foregoing are discussed later in this chapter or elsewhere in this book. They are listed here to remind you that you will need to deal with them in your paper.

The appropriate level of detail regarding statistical matters varies from one paper to another and even within one paper. Fully detailed descriptions of statistical design and methods are seldom required because few readers will wish to replicate your study exactly. It is usually sufficient to cite standard works on statistical design for important details and to provide technical references whenever the design is unusual or particularly complex. Your report should emphasize such features of your design as "partially balanced incomplete blocks," "treatments assigned by using a random number table, with numbers supplied in sealed opaque envelopes," or "status before and after treatment, as assessed and recorded by a person blind to the assigned treatment." You must, however, supply enough detail to allow readers to assess the most important potential sources of bias in your results. The omission of such basic information is a frequent and serious deficiency in published reports.[13]

Although much technical detail should be omitted, your paper must still be self-contained with respect to general aspects of your study's design, even if you repeat information provided in earlier reports on other aspects of your investigation. If the specific details are essential and require considerable space to present them, consider reporting them once as a separate paper in a methodology journal, or make them available on request from your laboratory, hospital, or university.

A good example of how to report the statistical design of your study is:

> Three hundred female patients were assigned to a control or a treatment group on the basis of the last digit of their hospital admission numbers. If the last digit was even, the patient was assigned to the control group; if odd, to the treatment group. Treatment patients were given two 250-mg tablets every 6 hours; control patients were given two lactose tablets, identical in appearance and taste to the drug tablets, also every 6 hours.

While this description is good, the method it describes is not. Someone who knows the allocation method can know the treatment group to which a specific patient will be allocated. Whether and when a patient is admitted to the study may then be influenced by a referring physician. The result can be a biased, nonrandom allocation of patients among treatment groups of the study.

Detailed statistical consideration of the data collection phase of a study, including quality control, is rarely needed in journals whose primary purpose is to report results. If your paper is accepted by and published in a respected, peer-reviewed scientific journal, its readers should have just enough information to know that your study was competently performed, that your data are accurate to the degree of precision you have specified, and that careful independent repetition of your work would produce essentially the same data within the limits of random variation.

In the *results* section of your paper, the appropriate level of statistical detail, including means, variances or standard errors, P values, and regression coefficients, depends on the nature of your subject and the purposes of your paper. Whatever statistical measures you use, they should be clearly labeled. A mean of precisely which set of observations? A variance of what statistic? A P value for what statistical method, testing what specific null hypothesis against what alternative(s), under what assumptions? A regression coefficient in what units of observations? An example of appropriate detail is:

> Pulse rate was measured for all 36 subjects immediately before and 10 minutes after the 3-minute infusion of the drug. The mean increase was 19.6 pulses per minute, with a standard error of the mean of 4.3. Although earlier studies suggested that pulse rate does not change, we found a consistent increase, with a two-sided P value of .023 on the basis of a matched-pairs t-test analysis that assumes the differences are approximately normally distributed.

Sufficient detail should be given regarding your methods of statistical analysis to enable a knowledgeable reader to reproduce your result if supplied with your raw data. This level of detail is particularly needed if your method of analysis is likely to be unfamiliar to most readers. Clinical journals will not often ask you to provide statistical computations that are familiar to most of their readers and they will rarely wish to publish computational formulas. When references are required or appropriate, standard works (e.g., refs. 14, 15) are preferable to original sources because the former are usually more readily available and easier to understand. Although it may be essential that you analyze your data in several ways, you should present only the most easily understood analysis that is technically correct. You may then state that, although other kinds of analyses were performed, the results obtained were in accord with those presented. If, however, different analyses lead to substantially different conclusions, the differences must be described and an attempt to reconcile them must be presented.

In most papers, the descriptions of statistical methods are best assigned to the appropriate parts of the results and discussion sections. Mosteller[16] has covered many additional aspects of reporting statistical studies, including construction of tables; presenting numeric values; overlap among text, tables, and figures; and standard statistical notation. Communication about statistical matters is often so important, and problems can be so frequent and subtle, that you should cultivate a close tie with an experienced professional statistician. A statistical review of your paper by such an individual, before you submit it, will often lead to suggestions that will improve it significantly.

Other matters must also be addressed in the results section of your paper. Demographic and clinical data on the patients in different treatment groups must be provided to demonstrate that they were in fact similar. You must also supply data on the complications experienced by your patients after treatment, the numbers of patients who were lost to follow-up, and the reasons why they were lost.

Carefully constructed tables offer you a way to present a large amount of data clearly and concisely. To avoid overly complex tables, divide your data into sets that convey information related to one or two specific points. Resist the temptation to present all the same data again in your written text. Once is enough!

In the *discussion* section, you will want to discuss potential sources of error and bias in your study, the conclusions that can be validly drawn from your data, the applicability of your findings to other patient groups, and any specific directions for future research suggested by your work. Do not overdo these matters, though. Few readers will need to know everything you have learned or speculated about. Discussion sections often offer more scope for creativity than introduction, methods, or results, but they should be kept short and pungent.

Now that your paper is written, writing the *abstract* is in order, regardless of whether it will appear at the beginning or the end of your paper. You must be brief, and you must not put anything in it that is not in your paper. In as few words as possible, tell the reader what your study is about, the essential features of its design, and the main results. Short abstracts are more likely to be read than long ones, and the abstract for a paper should be just long enough for a reader to decide whether to go on to the full text. ("Abstracts" for publication in the proceedings of a meeting are discussed in Chapters 39 and 40.)

Finally, go through your paper and pick out four to eight *key words* or phrases that will enable others who are interested in your findings to discover your paper by searching indexes to the literature using the words you have chosen from those listed as topic headings in the *Cumulated Index Medicus*.

Review Articles

Review articles are written to give perspective to previously published work. They are not original publications, although they may contain new findings from old data if they are based on meta-analysis rather than the traditional approach, as described in Chapter 9. Writing a review may appear to be dull work, but if it is well done you will gain an extensive knowledge and a comprehensive view of the subject. A good review paper is usually 10 to 50 manuscript pages in length. The subject may vary in breadth according to the extent of current knowledge: the more voluminous the related literature, the more narrowly focused your review should be. The accompanying bibliography should be comprehensive, and sometimes exhaustive. A good review offers critical evaluation of the literature and considered conclusions about the state of affairs in a special area. It is usually expected to include comments about every item in the bibliography. Reviews generally go beyond a historical account of a field to an exposition of the current state of knowledge and understanding in the subject area. As a consequence, attention to recent literature is usually more important than a retracing of historical development.

It is wise to contact the editor of the journal in which you wish to publish your review before you begin work on it. You will need to know whether the topic is suitable and acceptable, whether the proposed scope is appropriate, and whether you, the author, have the required credentials. Some journals stress bibliographic completeness, others stress critical evaluation; you should know exactly what is expected.

Organization of your review paper is important. Once you have assembled the bibliography, the preparation of an outline is essential. Although there is no prescribed order for traditional reviews, and the format of reviews employing meta-analysis varies, an appropriate outline is mandatory before you start writing. The outline imposes substantial structure on the intellectual content of the review, and it is not rare for the outline itself to be the main contribution to a confused and confusing field. If your outline is carefully thought out, the scope of your review will be defined, the logic of your sequence will be apparent, and the content of its sections can be easily deduced. This outline, which is so important to you as the author, is also important to the reader. It may be included as a quasi-index at the beginning of your review or be incorporated within the text, as topic and subtopic headings.

The anticipated readership of your review must be considered. Research papers are read by peers (i.e., individuals who are expert in the topic area); review papers are read by a wider readership from various backgrounds. You will have to take special care to avoid jargon and abbreviations and to use a writing style that is expansive and clear rather than telegraphic.

Because many review readers pick and choose rather than read the entire article, a special introductory paragraph is required for each section. This paragraph must cater to the readers, skimmers, and skippers by providing a comprehensive statement that leads logically into the material contained in the section.

A critical review always requires conclusions, while an annotated bibliography often does not. A *conclusion* section is a truly comprehensive summary that is succinctly stated and obviously drawn from the material under review. An authoritative conclusion is unique to you, the author, and it may be the most rewarding part of the review process, not only because your readers and their patients gain from it but also because your obligation to write it means that you will have to develop a consummate understanding of the topic.

Editorials

An editorial is usually a signed expression of personal opinion composed at the request of a journal editor or as a free-standing, unsolicited set of comments. As opinion, it carries an implicit weight of authority and need not concur with the general position of the journal, the authors of papers it discusses, or any one else. It frequently accompanies or follows a paper that has already been published; if so, it must relate closely to the same subject. A few sentences of historical background can set the topic in perspective, restate the content or conclusion of the work being discussed, and lead into your own comments. In general, editorial comments should amplify, expand, or give a sense of perspective to the major topic. You should rarely, or never, attack the manuscript under discussion, although you may express reservations about the conclusions that can be drawn from it.

An invited editorial usually carries weight because of the established credibility of its author, whose name should be well known to the expected readership. If you are not well known, you may establish your credibility by referring briefly to some special experience or expertise that gives you license to express your ideas with a minimum of referenced support. The supporting bibliography is always short, perhaps no more than half a dozen well-chosen citations. Editorials are usually supportive, broad in scope, and designed for a readership that may not be especially expert in the topic area. If your editorial is too long or wordy, you will lose your readers. If you devote thought to your subject and express your views clearly, you can make a significant contribution to current thinking on the chosen topic.

Letters to the Editor

The "letters" portion of a medical or surgical journal is usually one of its best read sections. As a result, letters have become important elements in communication. Letters must be brief and lively. They are often controversial, but never unfriendly. Occasionally, original studies appear first in the letters section. Brief case reports with a little interpretation, comments on previously published material, or statements of opinion may appear as letters. A good letter has one major constraint—it must deal with only one topic. To write a good letter, put the topic into perspective with two or three sentences that state or refer to the issue. Then, make observations or present ideas that may be new or may rebut material previously published. Close with a clear statement of your conclusions so that the readers will know what position you have taken.

Your letter may be accepted by the editor if it is appropriate for publication and suits the mission of the journal. If it refers to work that has been published, it is likely to be sent to the author of the original paper for his or her comments or rebuttal, which may be published with your letter. Be very careful to review the author's data and quote published observations correctly. Be prepared to have a challenge to your position—a position you are obliged to justify in a minimum of space.

References

1. CBE Style Manual Committee. CBE Style Manual: A Guide for Authors, Editors and Publishers in the Biologic Sciences, 5th ed. Bethesda, MD: Council of Biology Editors, 1983. Designed by the Council of Biology Editors, this book gives ideas about writing in acceptable format, tables, graphs, illustrations, abbreviations, and standard terminology. It discusses editors, the review process, and copyrights and contains all the required features to make it a reference work for everyone who writes in the biological field.
2. Day RA. How to Write and Publish a Scientific Paper. Philadelphia: ISI Press, 1983. Easily read, humorous, well-annotated, and full of helpful admonitions about the entire process of writing in the scientific world.
3. Gowers E. The Complete Plain Words. Baltimore: Penguin Books, 1970. An excellent paperback guide concerned with the choice and arrangement of words to get an idea from one mind and to another, as exactly as possible.
4. Hewitt RM. The Physician Writer's Book. Philadelphia: Saunders, 1957. A gentle overview on how to put thoughts and ideas into manuscripts and papers—a classic for many years.
5. Huth EJ. How to Write and Publish Papers in the Medical Sciences. Philadelphia: ISI Press, 1982. A small paperback published by the Science Information Service that is well annotated, and full of helpful ideas about writing and submitting papers and the review process.
6. King LS, Roland CG. Scientific Writing. Chicago: American Medical Associations, 1968. A sophisticated, small paperback that assists the expert in organization, the subtle use of words and phrases, opening sentences, and avoidance of clichés. It extends the basic English of Strunk and White into the world of science.
7. O'Connor M, Woodford FP. Writing Scientific Papers in English. New York: Elsevier/Excerpta Medica, 1976. A small volume filled with information about writing scientific papers for authors whose first language is not English. It covers the review and editing process as well as the construction of manuscripts.
8. Strunk W Jr, White EB. The Elements of Style, 3rd ed. New York: Macmillan, 1979. A small paperback that has been a classic for more than 30 years. It gives excellent advice about how to eliminate redundant words and phrases, construct clear messages, and achieve a clear, graceful prose style.
9. Research: How to Plan, Speak and Write About It. Hawkins Fliffor, and Sogi, Mario, eds. Berlin-Heidelberg-New York-Tokyo: Springer-Verlag, 1985.
10. Graves R, Hodge A. The Reader Over Your Shoulder: A Handbook for the Writing of English Prose. New York: Random House, 1979.
11. Fowler HW. Dictionary of Modern English Usage, 2nd ed. New York: Oxford University Press, 1965.
12. DerSimonian R, Charette, LJ, McPeek B, Mosteller F. Reporting on methods in clinical trials. N Engl J Med 1982;306:1332–37.
13. Emerson JD, McPeek B, Mosteller F. Reporting clinical trials in general surgical journals. Surgery 1984;95:572–79.
14. Snedecor GW, Cochran WG. Statistical Methods, 7th ed. Ames: Iowa State College Press, 1980.
15. Colton T. Statistics in Medicine. Boston: Little, Brown, 1974.
16. Mosteller F. Writing About Numbers, In: Medical uses of statistics. Bailar, JC, Mosteller F, eds. Waltham, MA: N Engl J Med, 1986.

Additional Reading

Eger II EI. A template for writing a scientific paper. Anesth Analg 1990;79:91–96.

Evans M. Presentation of manuscripts for publication in the British Journal of Surgery. Br J Surg 1989;76: 1311–15.

46

What to Do When You Are Asked to Write a Chapter for a Book

B. Lewerich and D. Götze

When you receive an invitation to contribute a chapter or section of a book, allow yourself 10 minutes to feel flattered. Then, read the letter again and try to figure out exactly what the editor or senior author wants you to do. Most invitation letters are rather vague because, for understandable reasons, the inviting editor does not want to give away too much information about the project before gaining a prospective author's agreement to participate. Before you answer the invitation, ask yourself a few specific questions and try to answer them honestly.

Do I really have the time to take on another obligation?
Is it likely that I will be able to complete the required work by the stipulated deadline?
Do I want to write about the topic suggested, or will the editor permit me to alter it in some satisfactory way?

Accept the invitation only if you are able to answer "yes" to all these questions.

A good friend may feel offended if you reject such a request, but your friendship will suffer much more if you have to ask for repeated extensions beyond the deadline. Be aware that experts in delaying contributions soon earn a "special" reputation among editors and publishers.

Before you agree to write a chapter for a book, make sure you ask the inviting editor the following questions, at least:

What kind of readership do you want to reach?
What is the complete outline of the book like? (Ask for as much detailed information as is available.)
How many pages will the publisher allow for your chapter?
How many figures and how many tables are you allowed to use?
How many references are allowed?
Do you have to prepare camera-ready figures?
Is the use of color figures permitted?
Has a sample chapter been prepared, which would help to clarify any further questions?

Since some editors feel that their job is finished when the outline of the book has been drawn up and the authors have been invited, ask your editor for a detailed explanation of how your chapter should be structured.

The more detailed the editor's advance instructions are regarding your chapter, the less difficulty there will be in incorporating your contribution into the book and the fewer revisions you will have to make. As indicated above, an editor is well advised to send participating authors a sample chapter at the beginning to give them some idea of what their work should look like. It can be taken as a general rule that, the less specific and the less strict a book editor is in approaching authors, the less acceptable the book will be.

When you have received answers to all the foregoing questions, start work as soon as possible. Good authors have many demands on their time and energy. Do not postpone writing the article until two days after the deadline. The excuse that you can work only under pressure is a very bad one. Grapes and cheese produce excellent results when put under pressure, but brains behave differently.

There are several things you can easily do as soon as you agree to prepare a contribution:

Develop your own manuscript outline and check it with the editor(s) to make sure you really understand your assignment.
Start a bibliographic search and collect relevant reprints. Speak with other experts for fresh ideas or recent work you are not aware of.

Look into other books on the subject to see whether a similar contribution has been published before.
Find out what could be done better.
At an early stage, start developing sketches of the figures you are going to use.
If you want to use figures that have already been published, seek permission for their reproduction from the author or publisher, now.
Obtain author's instructions for the preparation of manuscripts from the editor or publisher to avoid inconsistencies of format within the book as a whole.

Technical Considerations

Type the text of your contribution double-spaced with broad margins on both sides to allow space for the editor's and the copy editor's corrections. The compositor will have fewer difficulties when your text is not crammed together too closely.
Most authors produce their papers using word processors, and some books are produced by turning authors' diskettes over to a conversion company, which uses computers to print the material, rather than the labor of compositors. If the publisher has not already sent you information as to whether diskettes are to be used for typesetting the book, you should ask them which programs their printers prefer. Some publishers have designed special software to make your secretary's work easier.
Attach figures, diagrams, and tables on separate sheets—these parts are handled separately in the production process, and doing this will make things easier for the compositor or printer.
Make sure that each page and each figure carries your name. It may happen that some figures will get mixed up, but yours never will.
See that all your figures and tables are cited in your text by numbers. The book editor may change the numbering, if necessary, but your material can always be identified.
Be sure that the way you cite references complies with the instructions given by the publisher. Be even more careful about giving correct page numbers, volume numbers, and publication years.
See that all the references listed at the end of your chapter are mentioned in the text, and vice versa. Make sure that all references are complete, with names of all authors, title, publication date, volume, and pages. If books are quoted, supply authors' names, editors' names where appropriate, book title, pages referred to, publication date, and publisher's name and location. Ask your editor or publisher which citation system you should use (e.g., Vancouver or Harvard guideline for the preparation of manuscripts). Regardless of how the references will appear in the printed book, in your manuscript they must be double-spaced, like the rest of the text.
No one else can verify the sources you have used as well as you can. Readers who order a reprint of a paper you have referred to will be anything but pleased when they receive a photocopy of an article on water pollution, when your article was about surgery of the pancreas.

A final important rule to be heeded when you are involved in the writing of a book is this. **Do not tell the readers what you know about the subject; tell them what they should know about it.**

When you have delivered the complete manuscript to the editor or publisher, you are not quite clear of your commitment, yet. Your manuscript will be checked by the editor and publisher for its content, consistency, completeness, and clarity. You may get your manuscript back, marked with queries and flags. Even if you consider the queries inappropriate, try to answer them as clearly and positively as possible. If someone has misunderstood a point, do not attack the messenger; accept the opportunity to explain the point more lucidly. In most instance, this will improve the book's readability, promote readers' understanding, and facilitate production. Make sure to adhere to the deadline set for the return of the revised manuscript. The manuscript that comes in last sets the pace for the whole publication.

When the final copy-edited manuscripts of all contributors are in the hands of the publisher and everything is ready for composition, the publisher will notify you of the date on which you can expect to receive galley and/or page proofs so that you can plan your time for proofreading. If you will be unable to do the proofreading at the indicated time (you may be on holiday, at a congress, etc.), let the publisher and editor know immediately so that an alternate date can be arranged.

When you receive the proofs:

Check them carefully for correct spelling, completeness, correct structuring (headings, sections, paragraphs), and optimal arrangement of text, figures, and tables.
Respond to *all* queries even if you think some of them require no comment.
Do not add new material (text, figures, or tables), since this may necessitate a complete new

"paste-up" of the whole book. This will not only delay publication but probably will cause you to be billed for the extra costs so incurred.

Return proofs by the requested time (usually 48 hours after you received them). Publishing a book is a team effort that involves not only the author(s), editor(s), and publisher, but also the less visible and equally important compositors, printers, and binders. If anyone's work is not delivered on time, the schedule of everyone else is disrupted, progress comes to a halt, publication is delayed, and costs soar, sometimes astronomically.

Summary

Do not agree to contribute to a book unless you honestly believe you will be able to complete the task by the stipulated deadline. Moreover, do not agree until you have received, from the editor, a detailed outline of the planned book, as well as sufficient information about the intended readership and the type of material desired. Write exactly what you have been asked to write. Show understanding toward your readers and mercy toward your coworkers in the production of the book.

47

How to Review Manuscripts

C.M. Balch, M.F. McKneally, B. McPeek, D.S. Mulder, W.O. Spitzer, H. Troidl, and A.S. Wechsler

Reviewing a journal manuscript makes a vital contribution to the peer review system and gives the reviewer an opportunity to develop a perspective that will improve his or her skill in writing manuscripts for the scientific and medical literature. Unless your other commitments preclude it, always accept an invitation to review a manuscript on a topic within your field of expertise.

Responsibility of the Reviewer

When you accept the task of reviewing a manuscript, you are also making a commitment to fulfill several important obligations.

1. You will review the manuscript in a timely manner—usually within 2 to 3 weeks—according to instructions from the journal office.
2. You will provide a meaningful review because you understand the subject material.
3. You will review the content of the manuscript using fair, consistent, and objective criteria.
4. You will keep the contents of the manuscript confidential and will not cite its original work without obtaining direct permission from the editors.
5. You will not communicate directly with the authors or disclose their identity without prior editorial consent.

You may be unable to accept a particular request to act as reviewer because of time constraints, insufficient knowledge about the subject, or a personal conflict with the author that might compromise your objectivity. In such circumstance, return the manuscript immediately and provide any help you can to the editorial office by suggesting other individuals who might review it.

Criteria for Review

The best interest of a quality journal's *readership* is the primary criterion set by its editorial board for publication of manuscripts. Consequently, you will be asked such questions as "Does this work add new and important insight into the field?" and "Does the message reported increase our understanding of the problem?" and "Is the topic appropriate for the readership of this journal?"

The principal criteria a manuscript must satisfy, in approximate order of priority, are:

1. Credibility.
2. Originality.
3. Clarity.
4. Relevance.

Credibility

Credibility is the most important criterion for acceptance or rejection; it is strengthened by reproducibility within the author's experience, reproduction in an animal model, confirmation by the related experience of others, and appropriate and convincing statistical analysis. You will be reassured about the credibility of the data if they have been analyzed by conventional, understandable, and convincing statistical techniques. A lucid discussion of the design elements, and the power of the study to detect an effect when it is present, or its absence when it is not, are potent strengthening features.

Originality

Originality is concerned with what new information, bearing directly on a particular area of knowledge, is being reported. To be certain the information presented is new and original, you must rely on your knowledge of the field, on the indexes of relevant current journals as guides to references on the same subject and, to a much lesser extent, on textbooks. If the results and conclusions duplicate those in an earlier publication, you will be much less inclined to recommend acceptance of the paper, even if the quality of the work is excellent. It is your responsibility, as a reviewer, to know the literature well enough to resolve this matter.

Although the technique or observation reported may not be entirely new, a manuscript may increase understanding of a field by providing a unique analysis, a reformulation of a problem, or a thoughtful analysis based on the author's reflection on his or her own observations and the published literature. The clarity and wisdom of the author's view of a subject, already reported in a different form, can be a valuable contribution. While it would be unusual to recommend publication solely for this reason, the presence of such insight weighs heavily in favor of accepting a solid piece of work despite its similarity to something already in the literature. In like manner, confirmatory studies may qualify for publication because they broaden the understanding of a subject previously reported in a less complete form. The authors of such papers should clearly state how their work strengthens and clarifies understanding of work already published.

TABLE 47.1. A checklist for reviews.

1. Is the work scientifically sound? Is the experimental question valid and clearly stated? Is there a hypothesis that was tested?
2. Does the title accurately and concisely describe the theme and content of the manuscript?
3. Does the abstract properly summarize the pertinent points of the manuscript?
4. Is this the most appropriate journal for publication? Is it understandable by the readership and germane to their concerns?
5. Is the manuscript well written and well organized? Does each section of the manuscript have an appropriate length? If not, what specific sections or sentences should be deleted? Are there major typographic or grammatical errors?
6. Are the tables and figures clear and relevant, and the critique adequate? Is each one necessary and complementary to the text?
7. Does the manuscript contain original and reproducible results that are properly analyzed and presented? What are the important contributions?
8. Does the paper differ significantly, in content, from earlier reports by the same author(s), and is adequate reference made to the work of others?
9. Are the interpretations and insights appropriate, balanced, and relevant? Are there any ambiguities that need clarification or omissions that are critical to interpreting the results?
10. Are the conclusions warranted (from the data presented), and do they give appropriate credit to previous work by the authors or others?

Clarity

Clarity of language, tables, photographs, and other illustrations is a very important criterion when you are judging a paper's acceptability; it greatly influences the decision of many reviewers. A clearly written manuscript about a trivial subject is not acceptable, but neither is one containing many original and interesting observations if it is too difficult, or impossible, to decipher the message its text and illustrations are trying to convey. Too often, authors present a lot of data, some of it extraneous, without any synthesis or interpretation of their results in the form of a concise and understandable set of conclusions.

Relevance

Relevance is concerned with the interest the subject matter holds for the readers of the journal to which it has been submitted, or its significance in relation to what is already known. The manuscript may be highly creditable, original, and well written, but more suitable for another journal directed toward a different, more appropriate audience. Its level of significance to the literature is another matter. This is a "judgment call" that will be made by the journal's editor(s) in the light of the individual responses of you and your fellow reviewers to the same manuscript.

Assembling the Review

Make a duplicate copy of the manuscript on which you can write your comments, because you must return the original manuscript to the editorial office, unaltered. An approach to reviewing a manuscript that often makes the task easier, is to read it several times, to focus each reading on a different aspect of your evaluation (e.g., scientific content, validity of the results, writing style). Jot down your comments and criticisms in the margins of your copy of the manuscript, make notations on a separate sheet of paper, and assemble your critique when you have completed the various elements of your review. Some of the criteria we use for each component of the manuscript are listed in Table 47.1 Examples of reviewer's forms from several journals are included in Appendix 47.1.

Writing "Advice to the Authors"

This section of your review contains the written comments the journal editor will usually convey to the author, whether the final editorial decision is to accept, reject, or request revision of the manuscript. Your advice should be constructive, polite, and considerate . . . something you would want to receive as an author. If possible, start with a brief positive comment about the strengths and inherent value of the manuscript, and avoid harsh or personal tones in your critique.

The format usually consists of one or two paragraphs describing your interpretation of and conclusions about the manuscript, including an overview listing the strengths and weaknesses of the manuscript's content. It is usually not appropriate to recommend that the author perform additional experiments; the manuscript should be judged on the basis of the data submitted and the conclusions drawn. It may be appropriate, however, to suggest additional controls, inclusion of other data that might enhance the validity of the results, or consideration of alternative interpretations of the results.

Following the overview, provide a list of specific comments in numbered order, so that the author can offer comments or rebuttals regarding specific items of your critique. Begin with the most important areas of criticism and be as specific as possible regarding the areas needing clarification, amplification, or correction. General statements like "this discussion should be reduced by half" are not as helpful as pointing out specific sentences or paragraphs that should be deleted. Include specific comments about figures and tables, if necessary. Finally, note any major errors in grammar or style, but do not rewrite the paper to correct typographic or grammatical errors; your job is to evaluate the paper according to the criteria already discussed, not to edit it.

Do *not* to make a statement about whether the article should be accepted or rejected in the section of your review that will be sent to the author. That decision belongs to the journal's editor(s).

Writing "Advice to the Editor"

This is the place to make your recommendation regarding the manuscript's acceptance, revision, or rejection according to the instructions you received from the editor (see Appendix 47.1). State the major reasons underlying your recommendation in a concise comment to the editor; it will not be sent to the authors. Finally, you will be asked to indicate an overall priority for publication, usually by marking an appropriate box.

Editors usually request reports from two or three reviewers for each manuscript. If the reviewers' recommendations coincide, an editor usually will accept the decision the reviewers advise and will enclose the collected "comments to the authors" with the letter conveying the editorial verdict. When recommendations conflict, editors usually resolve the problem by making their own decision or by asking for an additional review.

Additional Reading

The *Journal of the American Medical Association* devoted a special issue to editorial peer review in biomedical publication. See JAMA 1990;263:1317–1441.

Appendix I

Examples of reviewer's forms that must be completed as part of the manuscript. Reprinted with permission of the publishers, Archives of Surgery, Oakland, California.

ARCHIVES OF SURGERY
Comments for Editorial Office

Reviewer Name ______________________________ Date ____________

Title: ______________________________

Author/s: ______________________________

Ms. No. : ______________ No. Pages: ____________ Enclosures: ____________

Special Instructions to Reviewer:
Your opinion and suggestions are solicited for the suitability of this manuscript for publication. Please do not mark the manuscript. It is a **privileged communication and should not be copied**. If you are unable to review the manuscript within two weeks (__________), please return it without delay.

Please check the appropriate boxes:

Recommendation	***Quality***	***Priority***
☐ Accept as is	☐ Superior	☐ Fast Track
☐ Accept if suitably revised	☐ Good	☐ ASAP
☐ Revise and reconsider	☐ Fair	☐ Routine
☐ Reject because	☐ Poor	
☐ Poorly written		
☐ Of insufficient importance		
☐ Conclusions not justified by the data		
☐ Subject adequately covered in the literature		

General comments for the editor. This page will **not** be sent to the authors; however, portions may be paraphrased or excerpted. (Please type.)

____

This paper should be reviewed by a statistician. ☐ Yes ☐ No

If acceped for publication, should a commentary accompany this article ? ☐ Yes ☐ No

Date: ______________ Signature: ______________________________

RETURN TO

Archives of Surgery • 1411 E. 31st Street • Oakland, CA 94602

1 2 3 4 5

CANCER RESEARCH

REVIEWER'S COMMENTS ON ORIGINAL MANUSCRIPT

PLEASE RETURN THIS MANUSCRIPT TO ________________, ASSOCIATE EDITOR,
IF YOU ARE UNABLE TO REVIEW IT **WITHIN TWO WEEKS.**

DATE SENT:________ TO BE RETURNED BY:________

Dear Dr.____________________

The Editors would appreciate your opinion concerning the suitability of the enclosed manuscript for publication in *Cancer Research*. Please type your comments on this form (and additional sheets as needed) in a manner suitable for transmittal to the authors. Kindly return a signed original and three unsigned copies of your comments.

MS #:__________ AUTHOR:____________________
TITLE:____

RECOMMENDATION
__ 1. Acceptable
__ 2. Acceptable with revision
__ 3. Not acceptable in present form
__ 4. Unconditional decline

PRIORITY RATING
Please circle:
(HIGH) (LOW)
1 2 3 4 5

COMMENTS:

NAME (Please print)____________________ SIGNATURE____________________
DEPT. & INSTITUTE____
FULL ADDRESS____
TELEPHONE NO. ( )____________________

R5a

SURGERY

EDITORIAL REVIEW

Date ______________________

The following manuscript is sent for your review:

TITLE ____

____

AUTHOR ____

Reviewer ______________ **Ms. Pages** ______________ **Illustrations** ______________ **Tables** ______________

Please make your comments in the space provided and indicate your suggested disposition. This must be accomplished within one week of date of receipt; prompt action is only fair to the authors. If you are to be unavailable during this period, please ask your secretary to return it to us un-reviewed immediately.

Comments:
(use back of page if necessary) **PLEASE DO NOT WRITE ON MANUSCRIPT**

Summary:

1. Accept ______________________

2. Revise ______________________
   (be specific)

3. Please indicate priority:

   High Average Low

4. Reject ______________________

   Not new ______________________

   Poorly written ______________________

   Unwarranted conclusions ______________________

   Minor significance ______________________
   (explain in detail)

Thank you for your review and comments.

Return to:

48

Audiovisual Support For Scientific Presentations

P. Steele, M. Siminovitch, D.M. Fleiszer, and D.S. Mulder

This chapter focuses on planning and preparing audiovisual materials to enhance the communication of ideas. It describes the basic requirements necessary to prepare audiovisual materials for the support of both written and verbal presentations. After studying this chapter readers should be able to:

1. List various media available.
2. Describe media selection criteria.
3. Compare relative production costs and requirements.
4. Evaluate audiovisual support materials.
5. Identify and find resources required to produce audiovisual materials.
6. Develop, using the tools and information provided, effective artwork for a variety of media.
7. Work more effectively and efficiently with audiovisual production professionals.
8. Handle the legal and ethical considerations involved in producing audiovisual materials.

The old adage "a picture is worth a thousand words" has been capitalized on by advertising executives, television producers and good speakers to attract our interest during presentations and to alter our behavior. Levie and Dickie[1] stated:

> Learning is facilitated by increasing the number of relevant cues and reducing the number of irrelevant ones in terms of the concept to be learned. When a presentation involving a media form can be reduced in complexity so that only the factors that directly contribute to accomplishing the tasks (like realism, color, motion, picture detail) are included, learning will be more predictable and reliable.

Educational psychologists believe we retain 20% of what we hear and 30% of what we see. However, a written or spoken message augmented by a visual image more than doubles retention.

Today we see revolutionary advances in the number, variety, and complexity of audiovisual media available to support scientific presentations. Only our imagination and budget restrict us. Most hospitals and universities have an audiovisual department able to provide varying degrees of skilled help. Investigate the resources in your own institution and establish an effective collaboration with the professionals in your audiovisual department. Greater complexity may demand the use of external commercial production facilities.

Define the Communication Objective

Defining the communication objective is your first step in planning effective audiovisuals. It identifies what you want your audience to know after viewing the presentation or the audiovisual. Listing the five to ten key points that the audience should be able to do or know after the presentation keeps objectives clear and keeps you on track when designing a presentation. Each audiovisual should have a defined communication objective: What should the audience do, ask, or feel after seeing or hearing this audiovisual? The outline at the beginning of this chapter is an example of a statement of a communication objective.

The importance of keeping presentations simple and succinct cannot be overemphasized. Clear identification of the objectives for the entire presentation and individual audiovisuals helps ensure that the presentation and communicates your message effectively.

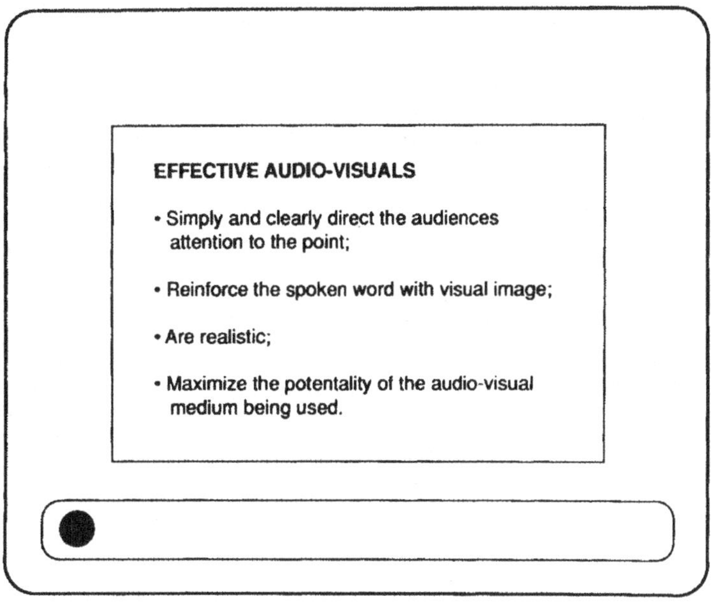

FIGURE 48.1. Characteristics of effective audio-visuals.

Media Selection

Next, identify your intent or how you wish to affect the audience. Do you want to present new scientific data and facts, to teach a skill, or to elicit an emotional response? This information will influence the tone, pace, and approach of the presentation. It will have the greatest influence on the selection of audiovisual media. Graphs, charts, and illustrations have more effect on the cognitive domain. Moving images (film or video) and realistic drawings or illustrations tend to have a greater impact when dealing with subjects in the affective domain, and for demonstration of skills or new techniques. Tables 48.1 and 48.2 identify the options, advantages, limits, and relative costs of producing two types of audiovisual material.

Message Design

You can convey the same message in a variety of ways. Two major considerations in selecting an approach, media, and content, are your audience and your resources. A variety of factors influence perception, including level of education, culture, language, and degree of special training. A clear understanding of your audience in these terms will help to ensure that your message will be perceived in the way that you intended. The resources available in terms of prepared material, time, budget, manpower, delivery systems, and the location of your presentation further define your audiovisual requirements. When you know your communication objectives, statement of intent, audience analysis, and resource analysis, your content should be relatively easy to map out. You may find it helpful to consult audiovisual professionals (medical artists, photographers, planners, etc.) at any one of these stages. You and the audiovisual professional must have a realistic time schedule to achieve mutual satisfaction.

Options

Available technology will allow the novice presenter to dazzle even the most sophisticated audience. Use audiovisuals to attract and direct the audience's attention to the point, simply and concisely. Audiovisuals developed for scientific and educational purposes need not compete with commercial productions. Carefully planned and executed audiovisual material will always enhance your presentation. Yet, poorly produced audiovisuals may distract the audience's attention and ruin an otherwise excellent presentation.

There are four principal audiovisual options.

1. **Still images**: The most commonly used forms of this medium are the overhead transparency and the 35 mm slide (see Tables 48.1 and 48.2). These two modalities can be used to present

TABLE 48.1. Summary of characteristics of 35 mm slides.

Best Uses:	Problems:
• To explain cognitive subjects. • For realistic reproductions of original subjects. • Effective dealing with affective subjects especially if accompanied by a sound track.	• Slides can get out of sequence, upside down or backward. • Room setup may not be adequate. • Heat from lamp may burn film. • Slides may get stuck.
Advantages:	Techniques:
• Camera equipment and processing services widely available. • Quality slides can be produced by novices. • Shows realistic pictures or artwork. • Variety of techniques available to highlight certain points. • Can be used for large audiences. • Flexible presentations possible. • Presenter can control when and how long visual is projected. • Presenter can back up or advance. • Slides can be designed for progressive disclosure. • Various projection equipment available allows for projection in a variety of room sizes. • Equipment allows for multimedia and multi-image capabilities.	• Consider where and how the slide will be projected when deciding on the type of mount to use. • Use a remote control or an assistant to change slides. • Set up a lighted lectern for notes. In a dark room light yourself. • Rehearse entire presentation. Use an average of 15–20 seconds per visual. Prepare audience for what you will be presenting. Use buildup slides (progressive disclosure) to keep interest and to show relationships. • Limit the uses of special effects like dissolves between slides unless there is a specific purpose for special effects. • Plan carefully especially when using multi-image presentations.
Disadvantages:	Cost:
• Requires some skill in photography. • May require special equipment. • Artwork must be specially prepared. • Long lead time necessary. • Room lights must be dimmed and controlled.	• Variable. Inexpensive (the cost of film and processing) too expensive depending on the complexity of the artwork, specialized equipment and process involved. • A commercially produced slide could easily cost $30 or more.

TABLE 48.2. Summary of characteristics of overhead transparencies (OHTs).

Best Uses:	Problems:
• To explain cognitive subjects. • To supplement lectures or discussions. • To summarize. • To present data.	• Positioning in the room. • Keystoning. • Burned out bulbs. • Glare.
Advantages:	Techniques:
• Can be produced by a variety of simple methods. • Sophisticated methods are available to produce 35 mm slide quality results. • Can use overlays. • Useful with large groups (a variety of projectors are available to accommodate projection distances ranging up to 100 ft.). • Can be easily edited and revised. • Allows speaker to face audience and control the pace. • Are portable. • Projector is easy to operate. • Can be used in normal room lighting.	• Mount transparencies in frames and label them. • Reveal information as it is being discussed (use overlays or progressive disclosure). • Point to information on the surface of the projector rather than on the screen. • Can use 2 or more screens to project complementary images. Cost: • Could be the cheapest of all media to produce. • More sophisticated OHTs cost as much or more to produce as 35 mm slides.
Disadvantages:	
• Meeting location may restrict use. • Quality may be less than with other media. • Transparencies are more difficult to store.	

TABLE 48.3. Summary of characteristics of video and film.

Best Uses: • To treat affective subjects. • To demonstrate procedures and processes that call for a continuous sequence. Advantages: • To provide exactness of detail and color. • Can vary speed of motion for closer analysis of detail. • Growing library of films and tapes available. • High credibility. • Relatively maintenance free. Disadvantages: • Difficult and time-consuming to produce; • Specialized equipment and expertise required for production; • Limited speaker control;	Problems: • Tape may not be properly cued. • Equipment may not be properly connected. • Duplicated tapes may be of poor quality. • Copyright laws on commercially produced tapes may restrict uses. • Standard size monitors not appropriate for large groups. Techniques: • Prepare audience in advance; • If long, show only portions relevant to the presentation; • Pause film or tape or have pauses edited in to allow for discussion. Cost: • Expensive (it is reasonable to expect to spend a minimum of $1000 per minute of finished product to have a video produced professionally).

graphs, charts, tables, and x-rays. Photographic, computer, and fiber-optic technology is now so advanced that virtually anything we can see can be photographed, reproduced on paper, or shown as a transparency or computer image. We can capture hand-drawn originals, computer-generated plottings, graphs, charts, tables, and drawings. We then transfer them to black and white or colored slides, photographic-quality transparencies, or hard copy for publication.

2. **Models**: Consider real-life models like pathologic or anatomic specimens, or reconstructed images from a microscope, angiogram, or x-ray. Computerized tomography and magnetic resonance imaging make available the three-dimensional construction of images from virtually anywhere in the body, such as the central nervous system or the heart, or the cross-sectional anatomy of any body region. This new medium will ultimately play a greater role in clarifying and amplifying basic scientific and clinical presentations of all kinds.
3. **Moving images**: Include videos or films of operative procedures or clinical examinations (Table 48.3). We frequently use moving images in the education realm, although on occasion they augment a scientific presentation. The creation of a video or motion pictures is a major subject and will not be discussed in this chapter.
4. **Audio recordings**: We can use audio recordings to supplement either a still or moving image in many innovative ways. Most commonly we use a soundtrack for a movie or video to narrate the contents of the visual presentation. Many authors use a combination of slides and a soundtrack to augment the presentation of scientific data and as an effective teaching device.

The list above provides investigators with a framework for planning audiovisual requirements. This chapter emphasizes the use of still images and models, and introduces the reader to the use of computer technology for the production of audiovisuals. This wide range of options, with increasing levels of complexity, reinforces the need for an early consultation with the audiovisual department in your hospital or university. Experienced photographers, artists, and instructional designers will always assist you in the selection of appropriate media, as well as in preparing audiovisual materials. Many commercial companies in the computer and photographic industries have useful resource booklets and brochures to help in preparing audiovisual material and to acquaint you with the latest audiovisual technologies. Ask your audiovisual department or call the manufacturer directly.

Planning and Preparation of Audiovisuals

Careful planning of the audiovisuals required for your scientific presentation, in conjunction with an audiovisual professional, will greatly enhance your presentation and eliminate last-minute scrambling for changes in slides or drawings. "Good, fast, cheap – choose any two," is the response you are likely to get to the question "How long will it take to prepare and how much will it cost to produce audiovisual materials?" Thus, after establishing

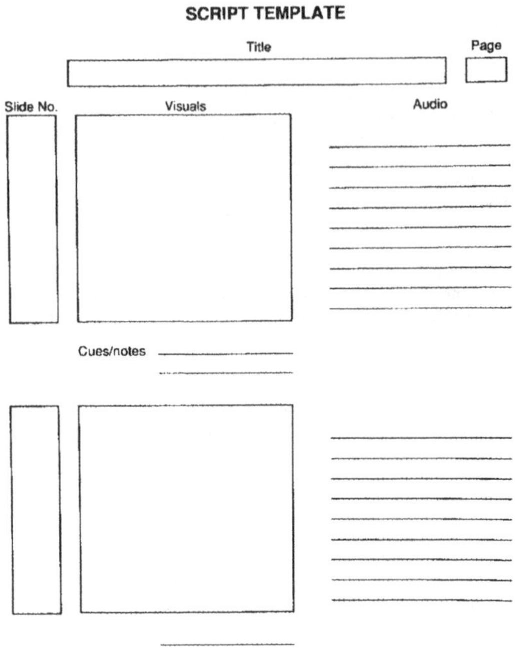

FIGURE 48.2. An example of a script writing form defining areas for descriptions of narration, accompanying visuals and sequencing.

your communication objective, draw up a careful timetable that respects your time and that of the audiovisual person collaborating with you.

Start by developing a script for your talk or scientific presentation. The old advice KISS (Keep it simple and succinct) is the key to successful audiovisuals and presentations. Your visuals will supplement your text and serve as a visual guide for you. Your text will direct your audience's attention to the message in the visual. A good slide should be self-explanatory. The script is the detailed blueprint of what you want the audience to see and hear. The same principles apply whether working on a script for a lecture, a slide–tape show, a videotape, or a film. The script will document the narration, the visuals, and any other special effects you wish to achieve.

There are many ways to develop a script for a talk. Do not copy the contents of a previously written abstract or scientific presentation for publication. The spoken presentation of scientific data should be specially prepared with simplified visuals rather than simply photographing the tables used for a previous publication. Some authors write a script in narrative form and then take the basic document and break it into words and picture segments using a script writing format (Fig. 48.2). The boxes on the left-hand side of the page contain information about the visual elements of the script. The corresponding narration appears on the right. Indicate cues and special effects in the script. An alternative method to develop a script is to construct a storyboard prior to the presentation of visuals (Figure 48.3). A storyboard consists of a series of cards that detail the visual and verbal components of the script. Each segment of your presentation appears on one or more cards. Separate cards may be used for titles or special cues. Standard cards such as 3 × 5 inch cards are commonly used with the narrative in the bottom portion of the card and the text of the visual on the top. Once you have finished the storyboard, prepare the script. Other authors dictate a talk and insert the graphics or visuals in the appropriate position in the typewritten talk with a numerical cue for each slide.

When you have completed the script, you will have very definitive requirements for picture taking, artwork, or photographic needs. Now sit down again with your audiovisual consultant and prepare reasonable time guidelines for each visual required for this particular talk. The workload in the medical illustration department will influence the timetable. You may have to send special or more complex needs out of the department. Most visuals require between two and three weeks for production. Remember the concept: "Good, fast, cheap—choose any two."

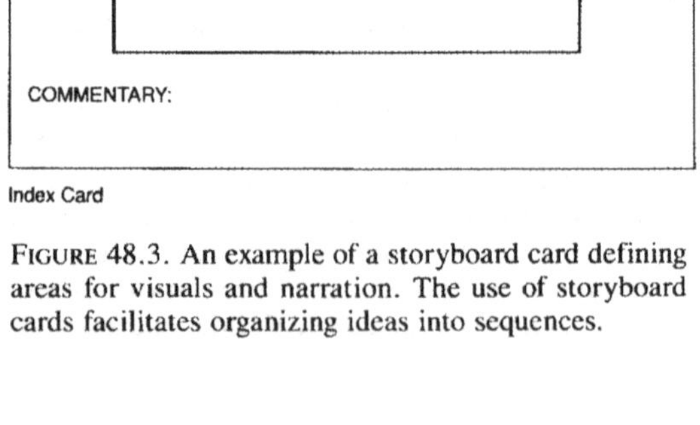

FIGURE 48.3. An example of a storyboard card defining areas for visuals and narration. The use of storyboard cards facilitates organizing ideas into sequences.

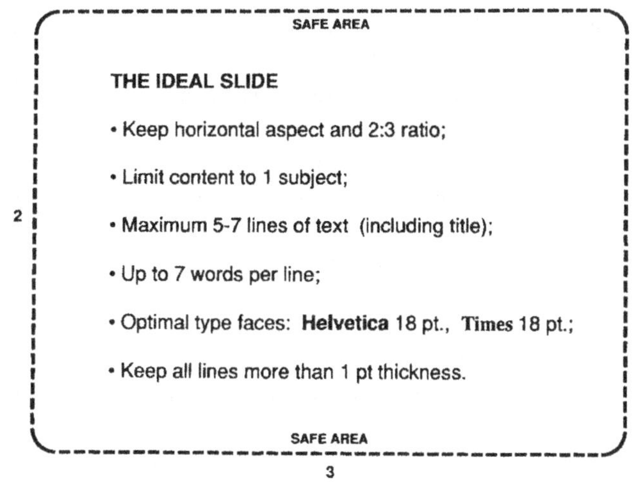

FIGURE 48.4. A scale model of an ideal slide. The text is written in the area of maximum visibility and is a summary of graphic considerations.

Production of Graphics and Camera-Ready Artwork

Whether you prepare artwork or graphics for illustrations, photographs, slides, overhead transparencies, or posters, the same design principles apply. A word of caution—artwork prepared for one medium may not work for another. Charts, graphs, or diagrams designed for publication in a scientific journal are not suitable for motion pictures. Their size, format, tonal contact, and detail are usually not appropriate for direct conversion to other media. They presume that the reader will have considerably more time to analyze the data presented, in contrast to the simplicity needed for a 15 to 30 second exposure of a 35 mm slide.

Artwork Standardization

Figures 48.4, 48.5, and 48.6 show scale-model templates for use when preparing graphics for slides, overhead transparencies, and artwork for television. These templates can be enlarged, reproduced on paper or acetate, and used to prepare your own slides or artwork. These templates include line and lettering guidelines for each format, to ensure legibility. Note that each template has a horizontal aspect. The technical restrictions of the recording or projection equipment dictate these proportions. Failure to respect these guidelines will result in audiovisual material that is inferior in quality, and perhaps unusable. Note that all television screens have similar proportions and horizontal orientation.

Design and Layout

When designing and laying out graphics, use such visual tools as line, shape, color, texture, and space to create simple, balanced visuals and to add emphasis where required. Again, simplicity is the key. A picture may be worth a thousand words, but it may take all those thousand words to explain a picture that is unclear or cluttered. Limit each visual to the presentation of one idea or concept. Generally speaking, the fewer elements into which you divide a given space, the more effective and aesthetically pleasing it appears.

Use bold, simple drawings that contain only key details. Use heavy and distinct lines around key elements. Add details with thinner lines or symbols. Remember you want to direct attention. Don't distract with too many embellishments.

Use tables, including bar graphs or column charts, to compare different results from different study groups. Limit them to a maximum of five columns or contrasting bars per graph. Space the columns or bars to accentuate the differences. Most medical artists have unique ways of differentiating the bars one from another. Use a bold print title to reflect the differences being shown (Figs. 48.7A,B and 48.8A,B).

Pictograms use symbols to show qualitative relationships. Symbols used in pictograms should be simple and easily identifiable (Fig. 48.9A,B).

Line graphs are the most commonly used format for the presentation of numerical data. Limit the number of lines in a graph to three or four. Use easily distinguishable designs for each line and make sure that all lines are thick enough to be seen from a distance (Fig. 48.10A,B).

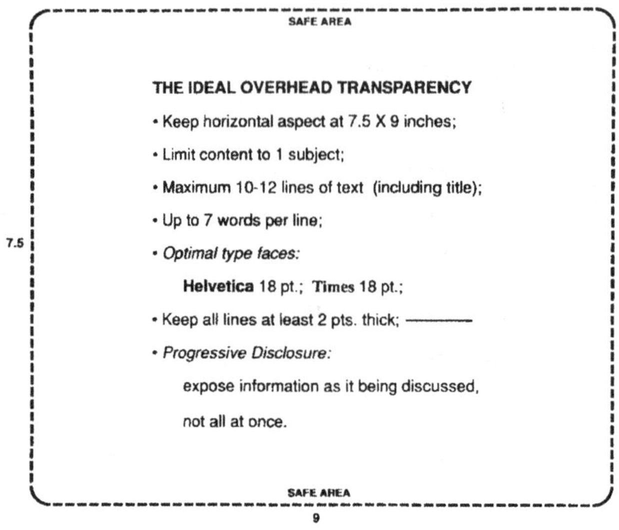

FIGURE 48.5. A scale model of an ideal overhead transparency. The text is written in the area of maximum visibility and is a summary of graphic considerations.

Use pie charts to illustrate components of the whole study group. Limit the number of slices to four or five; use a code to differentiate each component of the pie chart. For examples of good and bad pie graphs see Figure 48.11A,B.

We commonly use photographs to complement a scientific presentation. A photograph may reflect a scene in the operating room, but make sure the photographer understands the orientation and the anatomy to be illustrated in each photograph. Carefully prepare the surgical scene with clean drapes and assure that the surgeon and the assistants have clean gloves and instruments. A carefully prepared operating room photograph will always enhance your presentation. A poorly oriented, badly prepared, or blood-splattered surgical scene will detract from your presentation. You can photograph x-rays, but you must highlight the feature to be illustrated. Do this by marking a radiological feature with an arrow or by cropping the x-ray film in such a matter as to accentuate the radiological findings.

In all graphs be careful to label axes clearly. Stick to the fonts and size range recommended in Figure 48.12. Divisions along axes should be clear and well spaced. Do not clutter axes with too many

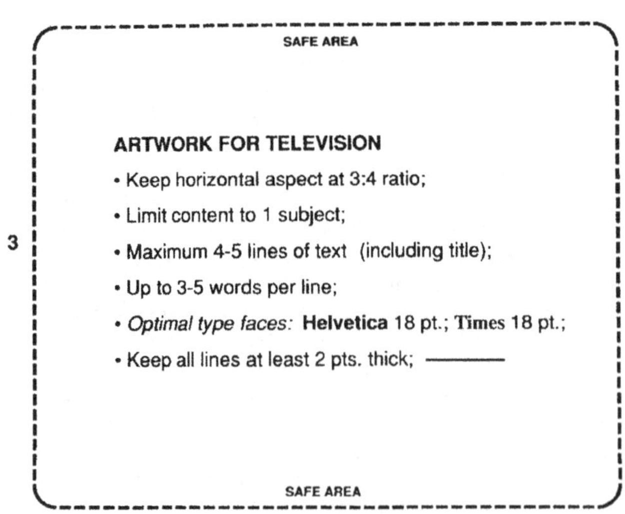

FIGURE 48.6. A scale model of artwork for television. The text is written in the area of maximum visibility and is a summary of graphic considerations.

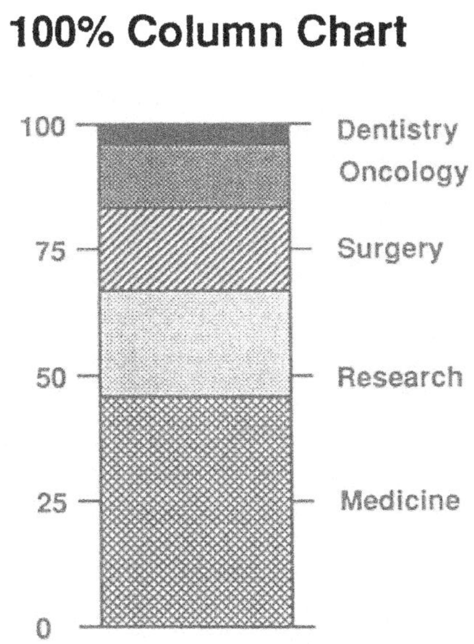

FIGURE 48.7A. An example of a good column chart.

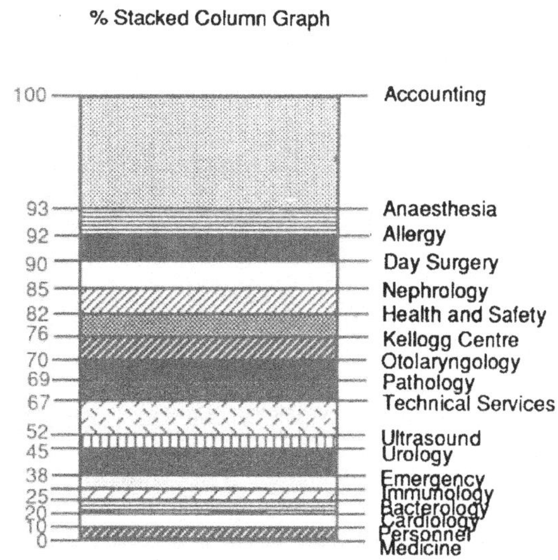

FIGURE 48.7B. An example of a bad column chart.

Too much information for this type of graph (i.e., should consider using line graph or regular bar graph;
Title should be more visible (larger);
Numbers and sub-titles should be larger;
Textures too confusing.

subdivisions. Select lettering of all graphics for simplicity and comprehensibility. We generally recommend sans serif lettering styles. Again, limit the number of lines as shown in the examples (Figs. 48.4, 48.5, and 48.6). Limit the number of words on a projected image to 15 to 20. Avoid a change in lettering styles in a visual or in the same series of visuals. Computers can produce a variety of fonts and sizes of lettering, which greatly improves the completed image. (Fig. 48.13). provides a template to help you determine the minimum image size required for visibility in relation to screen size and the audience's distance from the screen.

Try to use *color* as an element in a visual presentation. It presents a direct emotional appeal to the senses. It stimulates interest, attracts attention, and emphasizes special elements of a visual. Again simplicity is the key. Select colors to complement, not compete. Remember that some members of your audience (as many as 8%) will be color blind and will miss important elements of your presentations if the color combinations are too complicated. We often specify black lettering on a white background for the presentation of scientific data. This allows for a brighter room and facilitates note taking by the audience. Lettering on a blue or diazo background comforts the eyes. When designing color artwork for television or video, review the artwork both in black and white and in color. Be sure that color contrasts and separation of tones are suitable for telecast.

Know and respect the guidelines of the scientific journal to which you are submitting a manuscript or the scientific society at which you will present your work. Each scientific journal has guidelines for their publication of graphs, tables, photographs, and x-rays. A careful review of these requirements prior to the submission of your manuscript will help to prevent rejection of your manuscript or delay in publication. Some of these general principles have been published in the *Canadian Medical Association Journal*.[2] When your abstract is selected for presentation at a scientific meeting, the organization will send you a series of instructions that include requirements for audiovisuals involving graphs, tables, operating room photographs, and pathology specimens, as well as technical details regarding the format of 35 mm slides. They will ask you to complete a form detailing your requirements for presentation, particularly if you are going to augment your talk with a video or motion picture.

The success of many audiovisual materials is attributed in large measure to the quality and effectiveness of the artwork and related graphic materials. Quality results do not require a professional background; rather, they are achieved

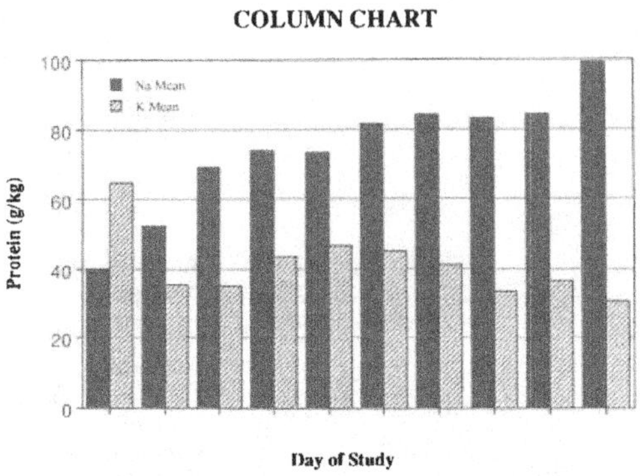

FIGURE 48.8A. An example of a good bar chart.

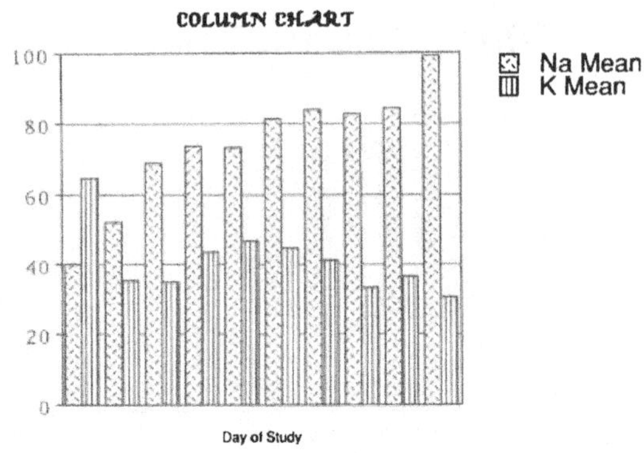

FIGURE 48.8B. An example of a bad bar chart.

Should be more difference between textures;
Legend too large (overpowering);
Title and sub-title type styles should be consistent;
Sub-titles should be of same size;
Numbers should be of same type style as sub-titles;
Bars are too close together;
Graph could be stretched-out horizontally to differentiate between bars;

through organizing your thoughts carefully, effective planning, and the application of appropriate techniques. Whether you are preparing artwork for slides, for overhead transparencies, for posters, for film, or videotape, the same basic principles apply.

Technical Features in the Preparation of a Slide or Overhead Transparency

Many investigators, using a 35 mm camera and/or a computer, can generate all the slides or transparencies they require. Many "do it yourself" systems using the Polaroid technique or automatic copiers will generate slides or transparencies in a few minutes. Most authors, however, depend on an audiovisual professional in their hospital or university to produce their visuals. Undoubtedly the greatest advance in the recent past has been the development of computer-generated visuals. Again, these may be generated on your own microcomputer and slides produced with your own equipment, or your computer-generated slide may be transmitted by a network of microcomputers to an audiovisual department or outside contractor for final production.

Consider some important features of slides. By far the most popular slide used today is the 2 × 2 inch, 35 mm slide. You find them mounted in many different formats. Paper mounts are inexpensive but may bend or fray at the edges and present difficulties with projection. Plastic mounts are light, fit most of today's projectors, and project better than cardboard mounts. Glass-mounted slides, required for high-intensity light source projectors, to prevent melting, are recommended when projecting on very large screens or for television. Glass-mounted slides are prone to crack during transportation or projection. This can detract from a presentation.

The majority of presentations in North America use a standard 80-slide carousel. Always load your own carousel and review with the projectionist any fine details for an effective presentation. Some European slides will not fit a North American carousel, and vice versa. The presentation of slides may occasionally involve a linear tray for projection. Loading is similar to the carousel, but you must carefully review the apparatus before presentation. Be aware that rear screen projection systems require the reverse insertion of your slides. Very rarely, one is asked to make a presentation with the old 3¼ × 4 inch glass lantern slides. This will demand special preparation by your audiovisual professional and probably will take longer.

Each of your slides should be carefully labeled using a system you understand that conforms to conventional requirements for presentation. A red dot usually appears in the lower left-hand corner of the slide as one is viewing it on a lighted box. This dot will be in the upper right-hand corner as the slide sits in the carousel or linear tray. Most speakers find it useful to number the slides as they occur in the script or presentation. Include a brief written summary of the slide contents or the major topic when storing the slides. Chapter 52 discusses

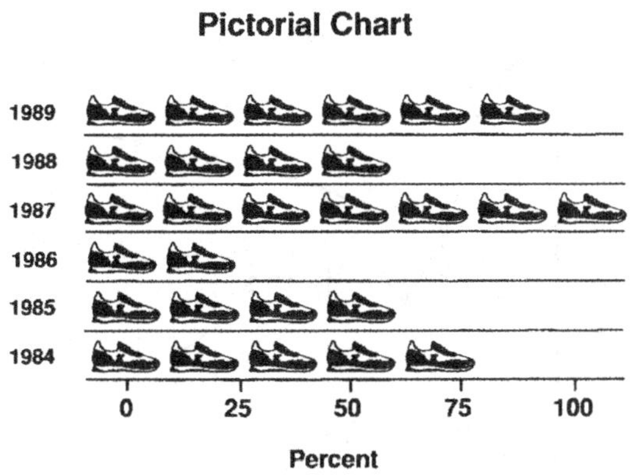

FIGURE 48.9A. An example of a good pictorial chart.

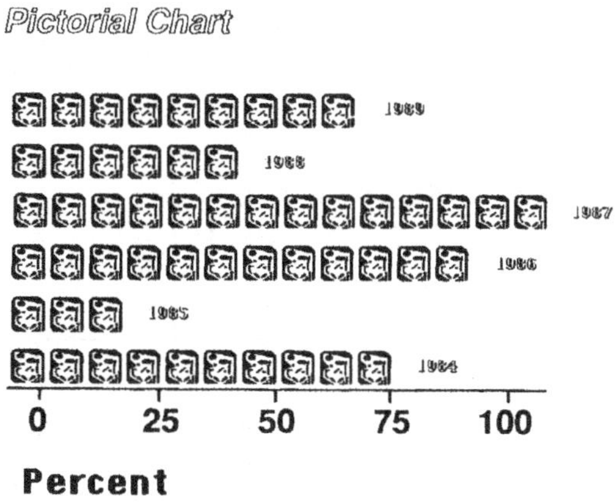

FIGURE 48.9B. An example of a bad pictorial chart.

Title, sub-title and numbers should be of same type style and centered;
Years should appear before symbols (clarity);
Numbers on X axis should be smaller;
Pictograms (symbols) should be clearer (simpler and more identifiable);
Bold and confusing.

in further detail the storage,[3] transportation, and sorting of slides.

Room Setup

Rarely will you have the ideal physical setting for your presentation. Make a point of checking the room beforehand and seeing to the arrangement of furniture and equipment to suit *your* needs. You want your audience to *see* and *hear* your presentation comfortably. In the standard classroom or conference room, the screen is mounted in the middle of the front wall. Do not be accept this or any other setup that may be inadequate for your presentation. A variety of portable screens and equipment can be obtained to create the desired effect. Figure 48.14 shows good and bad examples of screen placement.

Check for power outlets and be sure that there are enough extension cords to connect your equipment. It is possible to connect slide projectors, video cassette recorders, and monitors so that the same images can be synchronously projected on different screens or monitors.

When showing visuals to large audiences, obtain special equipment to project larger, brighter images.

Check both the view and the sound from the front and the back of the room. This is especially important in very large rooms, where glare or echo can reduce the quality of your presentation.

When planning your presentation, consultation with a technician from your own audiovisual department will help you identify your options and requirements. Do this as early in the planning stage as possible. Occasionally, you may need a duplicate set of slides or overhead transparencies. It is much cheaper to make duplicates at the time of production. Furthermore, the technician can provide you with information, training on the equipment, assistance in setting and presentation, and any necessary adapters and connections you may need.

Presentation Checklist

- Check the room.
- What audiovisual equipment will you use?
- Are your audiovisuals in the right format for the equipment?
- Do you know how to operate the equipment for your needs? (Can you change slides, pause videotape, do simple troubleshooting, focus, and adjust color?)
- Do you know how to connect the equipment?
- Does the equipment work?
- Do you have all the extension cables and adapters you need?
- Do you know how to operate the microphone?
- Where are the light control switches?
- Do you need or will you have assistance from an audiovisual technician?
- Have you spoken to that audiovisual technician?
- Will an audiovisual technician be available if problems arise during your presentation?

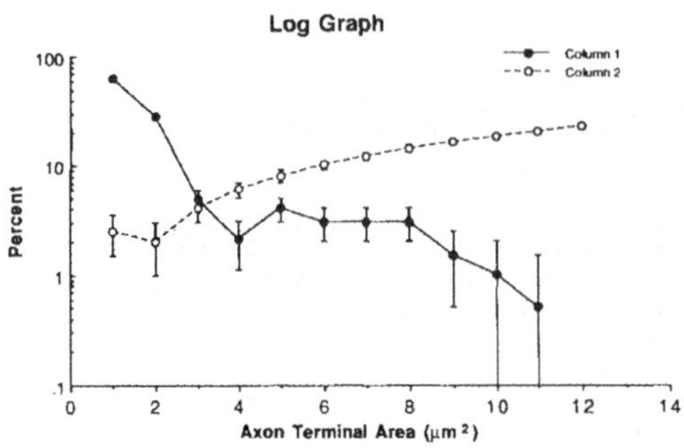

FIGURE 48.10A. An example of a good line graph.

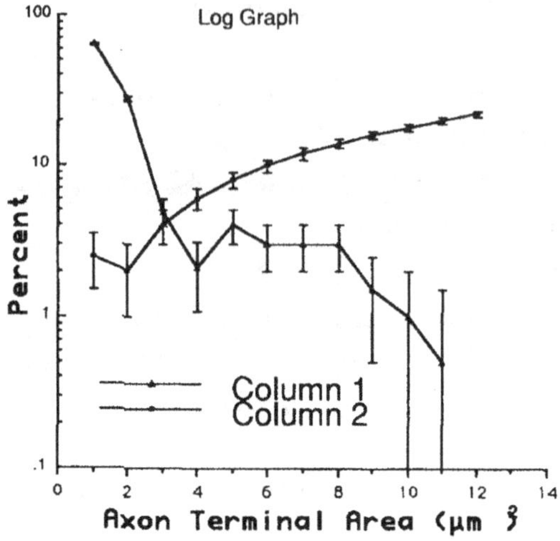

FIGURE 48.10B. An example of a bad line graph.

Graph much too cramped, should be stretched out;
Legend too large, and should appear outside of graph;
Title is too small;
Sub-titles should be farther away from axis, and should be of a clearer typeface;
Axis numbers are too small;
Symbols are not visible enough;
Lines should differ more.

Computer-Generated Slides

Most audiovisual departments now use computer-generated graphics to produce slides or overhead transparencies. Many recent publications document the successful use of various computer systems for desktop publishing and graphics production.[4,5] Each of these has essential components.

1. **Input device**: This is simply a mechanism for entering your data into a computer. It may be as simple as a keyboard, or you may require a graphics tablet or scanner.
2. **Central processing unit**: This is the basic computer, and there will be many important variables to consider such as the global access memory, speed of working, size and scope of the storage system, and basic costs.
3. **The display unit**: This is the "monitor" screen on which your image is displayed. The many factors to be considered include size, black and white or color, and other types of graphic enhancement adapter.
4. **Output device**: Information prepared in the software package can be fed to a variety of output devices such as printers, plotters, cameras LED units, etc.
5. **Software**: There are many programs; software devoted to creating and structuring slide shows, graphic art and desk top publishing for both computer systems. There are also programs which allow data imputed in one computer system manipulated in the other—this requires quite sophisticated software and computer literacy.

A greater variety of graphics programs and presentation programs are available for the MacIntosh environment. When selecting the software package that you will use you should consider 1. Availability of the system; the type of output you require, userfriendliness of the software; its ability to manipulate data as you need it.

Often presentation software can be combined with, or is part of, a graphics package. These programs allow you to organize the sequence of slides (be they text, graphs, or illustrations) and thus have the computer present them in whatever order you choose. This is similar to sitting down with the projector and slides, deciding the order of the slides, and practicing a presentation. Often it becomes evident at this stage that a particular slide needs some modifications or that an extra slide is necessary to produce a better flow for the presentation. Such changes can be made quickly and easily in the graphics program, and the sequence again previewed. No slides need be produced until the author is fully satisfied with the presentation. This

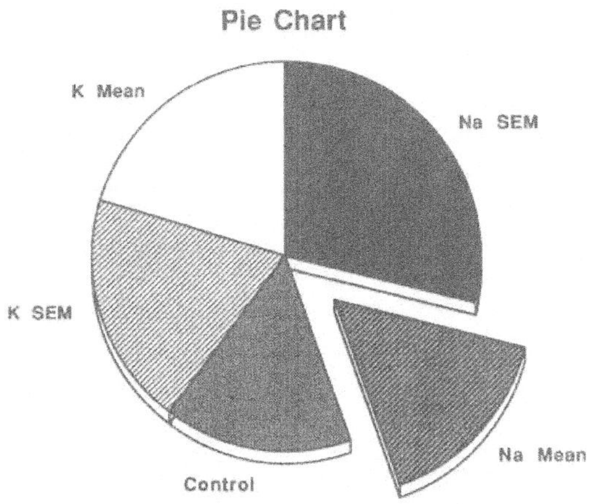

FIGURE 48.11A. An example of a good pie chart.

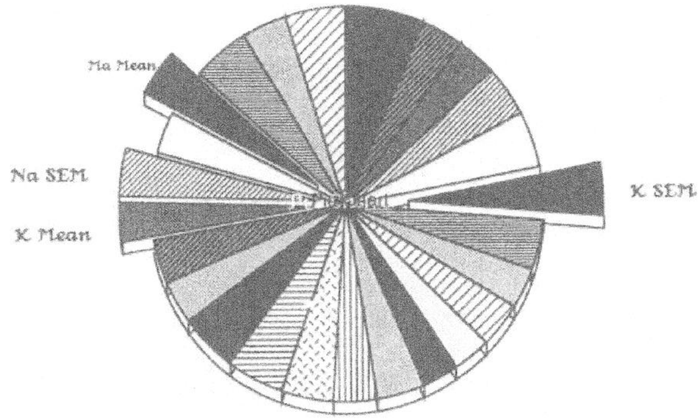

FIGURE 48.11B. An example of a bad pie chart.

Pie chart not a good choice—too much information;
Too many different textures— confusing;
Title should appear at top of pie chart (not in the center of it);
3-D effect not necessary;
Pull-out wedges should be limited to one or two.

avoids delays while waiting for extra slides, which in turn facilitates the quality of the work and reduces the cost of making unnecessary or marginally acceptable slides.

The microcomputer industry is changing rapidly, costs are decreasing, and the potential for producing graphics is virtually unlimited. Collaboration with your computer department and your medical illustration department will help, particularly if you wish to link into an existing microcomputer network. This may allow the convenience of preparing a slide in your office and having the image quickly produced in the medical art department.

Interactive videodisc is a computer technology that promises exciting opportunities in the near future. The videodisc is a device similar to the currently popular compact disk (CD). A videodisc can store enormous qualities of photographs, 35 mm slides, videotape sequences, diagrams, text, and soundtrack. The computer can access any of these images and sounds in any order you wish. You can superimpose line drawings and labels on complicated pictures for explanation purposes. You can demonstrate various surgical maneuvers using videotape or line drawings with movement presented in a "cartoon" fashion or even superimposed on the videotape. Tutorial presentations can be produced, and clinical simulations can be set up. The computers can test user performance and provide instant feedback. Decision points can be presented to the student and, if an incorrect decision is made, the computer can choose and present the appropriate complication. This particular technology is still quite expensive, although prices are rapidly falling and the equipment is becoming more widely available. Only one's imagination limits the presentation of information with this medium.

The Poster Session

The poster session is a relatively new method for the visual presentation of an investigator's data. It usually takes the form of a 4 × 8 foot poster that summarizes the scientific data presented. Poster sessions generally run concurrent with other scientific sessions and allow for the investigator to stand by the poster and explain or amplify the material presented. Many scientific organizations now require the submission of an abstract in a specific format for a poster session. Other program committees will select some abstracts that were not accepted for the regular oral-presentation scientific program for presentation at a special poster session.

Preparation of a poster should follow standard guidelines for presentation of an abstract or a scientific publication. Begin with the title, followed shortly thereafter with the abstract or the hypotheses or question proposed. The experimental methods should be well outlined and should include all important experimental design or materials. The results should then be presented in

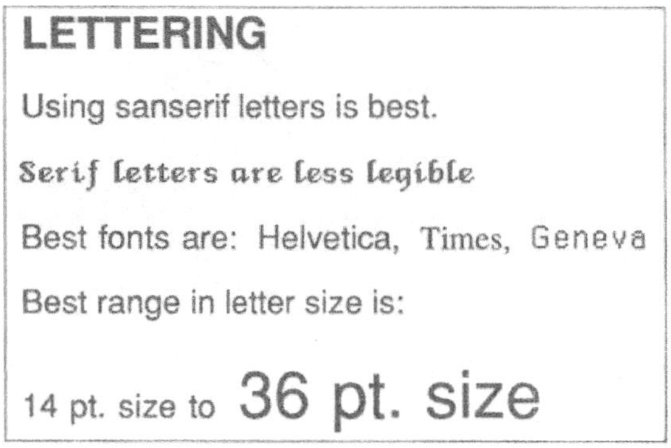

FIGURE 48.12. A summary of recommended lettering styles and sizes for audio-visual.

a central position, supported by graphics appropriate to the scientific data. Here again visuals are critical to successful presentation. You can clearly present scientific data using charts, tables, and graphs in considerably more detail than is possible using a 35 mm slide. In many cases the detail you would insert in a scientific publication can be duplicated in the visual aid. With a poster, interested observers will have considerable time to study each chart and graph. Schematic drawings and graphic presentation of scientific data are more effective than words or complicated tables. Many poster sessions now provide a written manuscript or handout at the time of the session.

Most posters are made of a heavy cardboard that can be rolled for transport and subsequent display. Here again, it is important to collaborate with your audiovisual professional so that photographs, text, and tables are all mounted in an appropriate and eye-catching manner. The audiovisual consultant will provide useful advice on the thickness of the mounting paper, method of application on the poster board, and protective devices for transportation.

A carefully prepared poster session is often more satisfying for an interested observer than a 10-minute scientific presentation. The presence of the knowledgeable investigator makes this a mutually satisfying means of communicating scientific data and exchanging ideas.

Evaluation

There are three times when evaluation should be undertaken in planning and producing a presentation. The first is prior to starting. This evaluation

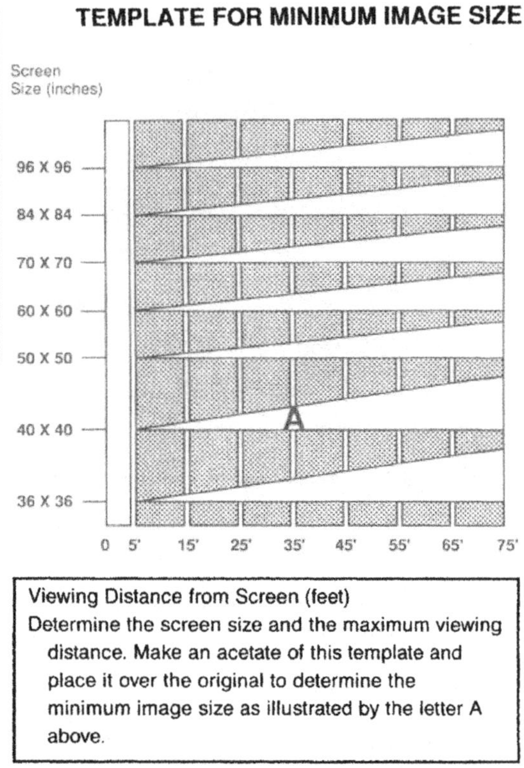

FIGURE 48.13. A guide to determine the minimum image size required for visibility in relation to screen size and the audiences' distance from the screen.

consists of establishing the communication objectives of the investigator and relating them to the audience in terms of their background and level of comprehension. The second evaluation comes after preparation of the script. This helps ensure the accuracy and necessity of each content element and of the approach. It will verify that each visual and each section of the narration clearly communicates a necessary point. Question each element: What does it communicate? Is it necessary for the communication objectives? Next, test the script out on a subject matter expert. Perhaps you can use a sample of individuals "like" the target audience. Many departments allow the presentation of preliminary data at departmental rounds or a laboratory meeting. Do this early enough to allow time for revision to the script and to the visuals.

A final evaluation occurs after the presentation. The results of this evaluation can assist you in subsequent presentations. It may be based on structured feedback from the audience; it may also take

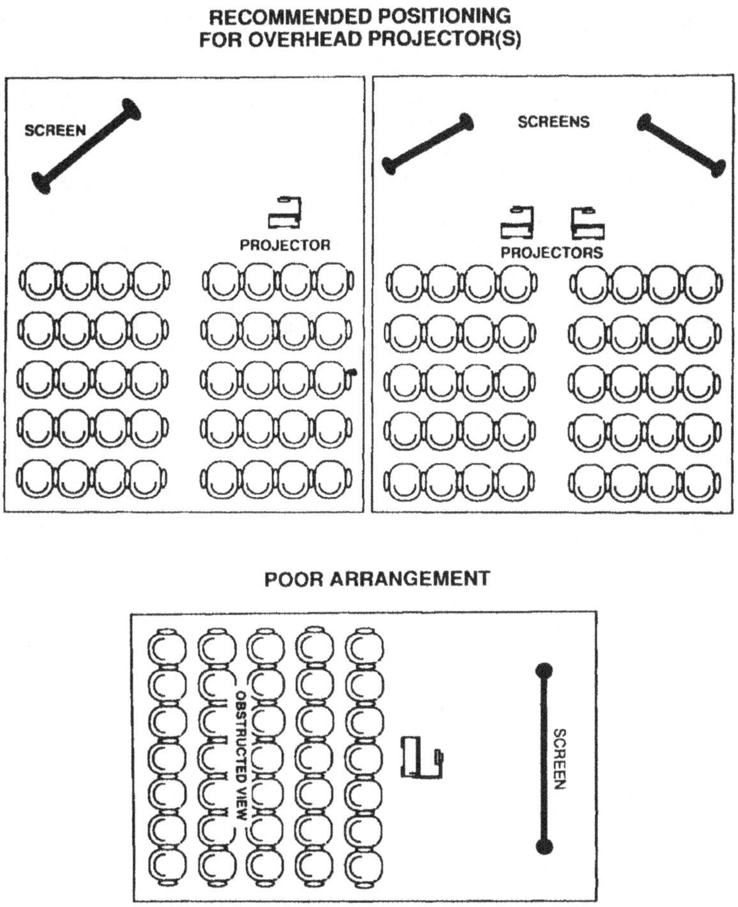

FIGURE 48.14. Recommended room layouts for viewing projected images.

advantage of a lively discussion period or questions after your formal presentation.

Ethical and Legal Considerations

Each investigator must take care to avoid graphical misrepresentation of data. Camera angle or misorientation in the operating room can create an optical illusion that might support an inappropriate conclusion. Graphic demonstration of data may create trends that are not really present. Work closely with the medical artist or audiovisual professional to prevent this type of inaccuracy in line drawings, graphs, tables, or slides.

Each scientific journal has specific copyright requirements on the manuscripts submitted for publication. These vary from journal to journal and must be carefully respected, particularly when using material for future publication in another manner. Most authors will be asked to sign a specific copyright agreement prior to the publication of the manuscript.

Most videotaped telecasts and motion picture film programs are copyrighted. These copyrights limit the way programs can be used in the future. Many postgraduate educational programs have attached copyrights applicable to the material presented and that specific educational setting.

There have been several well-written papers on the ethics, confidentiality, and copyright of graphic material.[6] Each hospital and university has guidelines in terms of confidentiality and release forms required for the publication of hospital data, particularly photographs of patients, operating scenes, or pathology specimens. Carefully respect these in any publication.

References

1. Levie HW, Dickie KE. The analysis and application of media. In: Second Handbook of Research on Teaching. Skokie, IL: Rand McNally, 1973.
2. Squires BP. Illustrative material: what editors and readers expect from authors. Can Med Assoc J 1990;142:447–49.
3. Eaton GT. Proper storage of photographic images. J Audiov Media Med 1985;8:94–8.
4. Williams R. Networked personal computers for desktop publishing and graphics production. J Audiov Media Med 1988;11:41–8.
5. Lacey A. IBM's great AT slides. J Audiov Media Med 1987;10:7–11.
6. Cull P. Aspects of confidentiality, copyright, and accreditation. J Audiov Media Med 1988;11:8–10.

Additional Reading

Tufte ER. The Visual Display of Quantitative Information. Chester, CT: Graphics Press, 1983.

Tufte ER. Envisioning Information. Cheshire CT: Graphics Press, 1990.

49

The Longer Talk

B. McPeek and C. Herfarth

A good friend and colleague has invited you to come to London to present the results of your research. You are honored and flattered at the invitation. But what do you do? How do you respond?

First, consider the invitation. A wise and gracious host will tell you about the audience and the occasion. He will tell you what he has in mind, the purpose of the talk, and any suggestions he may have regarding the topic. Pay close attention to these three issues. If you are contacted by letter, it is a good idea to telephone your host to be certain you understand the audience and occasion, the specific purpose of the talk, and your host's ideas about the subject. If the invitation comes in person or by telephone, be sure the discussion does not end until you are certain you understand the setting, purpose, and proposed subject.

A good talk reflects not only your interests and enthusiasm but also the interests, concerns, and limitations of the audience who will hear it. To speak *to*, rather than *at*, any group, you must analyze the audience. From your host, you will learn about the expected size of the audience; its composition in terms of age, sex, and professional and educational status; and the scope of its interest in and knowledge of your subject. Analyze the occasion also. In what setting and what circumstance will you speak? What will precede and follow your talk? What rules or customs prevail? What is the room or auditorium like? How is it equipped?

What is your host looking for in the talk? Is it a detailed presentation for specialists familiar with your work in the field, or are you to introduce new concepts to a younger audience? Is a presentation for scientists or clinicians from other fields intended? Should the talk be specific and concrete, or more general? Should you stress the clinical aspects or the more theoretical scientific applications? Is your host committed to a specific subject, or have you been given a more general invitation to "come and tell us about your latest work"?

You will want to give great attention to selecting your subject. The audience and occasion ordinarily determine the purpose of the talk, and the purpose will influence your subject.

If you are lucky, you know your subject and have recently spoken on it. You may have a talk almost ready to deliver. You know what has worked well in the recent past, with what kinds of audience and occasion and you have appropriate visual aids prepared. Only a little refining is necessary. Perhaps you will want to make some new slides, or cite fresh examples keyed to the new audience.

Frequently, there is more to do. Although your knowledge of the subject is sound, you may not have given the talk before. Or, if several years have passed since you last talked on the subject, you will need to gather additional information to bring your talk up to date.

A rare unhappy soul finds that a research job must be done after he has committed himself to speak on a subject.

Before you accept the invitation, be brutally realistic about the request. Do not let your pleasure at being asked to speak, or the honor of the occasion, carry you away. Only you know the other demands on your time. Your host may have an overly optimistic view of your knowledge. Consider what you know about the topic and how much preparation will be required before you can speak on it. Be prepared to suggest an alternative topic, or topics, suitable to the audience and occasion and congruent with your host's purpose for the speech. Remember, only *you* know what you can do with the material and time you have available. Many speakers prefer not to respond to an invitation immediately, but to take a day to be sure they are not being asked to agree to something they cannot carry off well and comfortably.

The longer talk differs from a written paper or a 10-minute presentation of research. If readers start to read a paper in a journal, they can leave it if they do not like it. A 10-minute oral presentation may be painful to some in the audience, but it will be over in a short time.

After you have agreed to speak on a specific subject, you must construct your talk. Many speakers start by carrying a notebook around with them and, as ideas occur—perhaps at random—they jot them down. Make sure you note down all ideas. Many of the ideas that occur while you are getting up in the morning, at lunch, or going to bed at night will be good, but most of them will be lost if you don't write them down as soon as they come to you.

Next, you will want to rank your ideas in terms of their importance and start to develop an outline. Then, assemble the available materials from your own previous work or from the work of others in the field. Perhaps you need a library search to make sure you have not missed a recent paper. You may want to telephone colleagues who are working in the same area. They may know of new work you have missed, or may have a fresh suggestion you can incorporate. You will want to graciously acknowledge their assistance when you give your talk.

At this time, make a preliminary list of the ideas to be included and indicate their arrangement. Wait until you have gathered necessary supporting material before making a complete outline or final speech plan. Keep the plan flexible, and continue to make adjustments as you go along. Only when you are sure you have the basic material in hand do you arrange the points you expect to make in their final order.

A talk generally has an opening or introduction, a main body, and an ending or closing. Most speakers start by working on the body of the talk.

Remember, you want the audience to grasp and be able to recall important data and ideas about the subject. A talk is not the opportunity to parade your own knowledge, nor should you try to see how much ground you can cover in a given time. Rather, your efforts should be focused on securing your listeners' understanding and on presenting material in such a way that it will be recalled.

Speakers should consider the following guidelines:

1. Keep the principal ideas few in number. If masses of data are given too rapidly, your audience will become bewildered and will catch only an occasional point here and there. In particular, when you are discussing a new or complex topic, do not try to deal with too many major ideas or pass over any of them too quickly. Select the data and the concepts that are essential to understanding your subject. Then, through the use of appropriate visual aids or supporting material, hold each topic in the minds of your audience until you are sure it has been absorbed.
2. Define unusual terms. Frequently, in science, there is a specific meaning for a word that has a different or more general meaning in ordinary usage. Stop to define a strange or ambiguous term before you go ahead. Sometimes the meaning of a word is clarified by telling the audience what it does not mean.
3. Present information at an appropriate rate. Pace your delivery so that the talk keeps moving forward at a speed calculated to ensure understanding, but avoid becoming boring.
4. Wherever possible use concrete illustrations. Don't be too abstract. Frederick Mosteller[1] reports that he learned an important idea for presenting new material from a friend, Professor E.K. Rourke. Rourke calls his idea "P-G-P." The letters stand for *particular, general, particular.* Rourke believes that a difficult concept is best presented by a *particular* example to motivate the listener and clarify the technique. The *general* refers to a broad, necessarily more abstract treatment of the idea or technique you present. Rourke then drives the whole thing home with a second *particular* example. The point of your effort is to have the information retained after the talk.
5. Clarity is almost as important as accuracy of detail. Try to present statistics in round numbers: say "about half" rather than "48.92%." Be honest, but try to avoid explanations that are so extensively qualified that the central point is lost in a mass of details. Visual aids help with data presentation. After a mass of data has been presented, a slide can sometimes drive home the major point.
6. Relate new material to something the audience already knows. Listeners want to put new information in context. Help them by showing how your work developed from previous work. For example, in speaking about a new or innovative treatment, compare the new treatment to standard practice.
7. Be easy to follow. Make transitions explicit. As you pass from one point to another, make clear to the audience that you are leaving one aspect and moving to another. Let them know where you are going and how your new point relates to the preceding one.

Once you have the body of the talk in hand, think about the beginning and the closing. First and last impressions are important. We are likely to make up our mind about a speaker on our first impression, though we may change this opinion later. We generally carry away from a talk, and remember for some time, the last things the speaker says.

The beginning of a talk requires special consideration because it sets the stage for what follows. It may be impossible to cancel the bad impression made by a poor beginning. The introduction of a talk depends in part on the occasion and the audience. Speakers need to win the attention of the audience and prepare them for the ideas they are to hear. You may wish to refer to the occasion, extend a greeting to the chairman of the meeting, and thank your host. You want to make clear the specific topic you are going to discuss and lead the audience easily and naturally into it. Some speakers ask a rhetorical question, cite a vivid example, or offer a startling opinion. Speakers should attempt to tie their own experience or interests to those of the listeners.

Absolutely the last thing you will do is begin by undermining the audience's confidence in your ability. Don't begin by saying, "I'm not quite sure why I was asked to speak on this topic" or "I wish I were a better speaker." If you aren't worth listening to, the audience will quickly discover it.

The ending of a talk should be both a finish and a summing up. You want to focus the thoughts of the audience on your central theme. You want to bring your important points together in a condensed and unified form to sum up their overall significance. Tie your talk together so that the pattern of your presentation comes to an end. Deliver a strong concluding sentence and then stop.

After you have a final outline in hand, develop the wording of your talk. Either speak it through or write it out. Generally, it is best to start by reading the detailed outline to fix major ideas in your mind. Then, "give" the talk to an empty room several times. Word your sentences in different ways until you discover the most effective. The first several times you will need to hold the outline, but put it aside as soon as you can.

This is a repetitive process. With each repetition, you become increasingly sure of yourself. Don't try to fix the exact words you will use at the time of your final delivery. Just now, you want to master the ideas, not the language.

After you have finished wording the speech, you will want to practice for fluency. Deliver the speech to an empty room, aloud, several times from beginning to end. If you plan to show slides, introduce them at this point. If you plan to use a blackboard, have a blackboard in your room and write or draw on the board the way you will when you actually speak. Have a friend listen and time you so that you know how long you take.

After you have practiced awhile, use a tape recorder to record the talk exactly as you hope to say it. Remember, *don't read* it, *speak* it. Use the recording to make a typescript of the talk.

Some speakers like to use a typescript at the time they given the talk. For an important talk, we use a triple-spaced typescript in a loose-leaf binder. We can mark the appropriate points for slides or other visual aids on the typescript in pencil. Today, almost no one reads a talk verbatim from the manuscript. Only a polished actor should try to commit a talk to memory and recite it like a part in a play.

Many speakers don't like to have a manuscript with them. They prefer to speak from the outline or from a set of notes, perhaps on small cards. Other authors fear they might stumble on the way up to the lectern, drop the cards on the floor, and scramble their thoughts, their talk, and their self-control.

By now, you have your talk well in hand; you have a manuscript, or an outline, and you will be comfortable about speaking it.

At this point, step back. Look the talk over carefully with a cold eye. Rank-order your individual points to see exactly which part of the talk is the central one. If you had to shorten the talk drastically, say to 15 minutes from your expected hour, what points would you really try to make to the audience? Occasionally, there are last-minute changes in a schedule, and you will want to be able to react to these. To shorten a talk, the only thing you can do is to omit whole sections of it. Do not even think about trying to speak faster. An attempt to delete extraneous sentences will not gain you more than a few minutes. Lay out a careful plan as to how you would shorten the talk if you had to. This exercise is worthwhile.

Lengthening a talk is no problem. In the first place, audiences are always pleased when a speaker does not take quite as long as expected. How many times can you remember that ever happening? If you do find that you have a great deal more time available than you have material for, restrain yourself. Do not add filler. Don't take up time with long-winded stories; simply move ahead and give the talk you have, crisply and carefully. Audiences almost always like more time for questions, and when good questions come along you can expand on the points they raise.

Again, practice with your tape recorder. The greatest value of a tape recorder is to help you appreciate weaknesses you might otherwise miss. Use the tape recorder systematically, not like a toy. Play the recorded talk back. Do this once or twice to get the overall sound of it, then take paper and pencil in hand while you play it back again. This time, look for a monotony of voice and note the places at which this defect was most noticeable. Now, replay the tape and look for repetitions or for hemming and hawing—note them. By this repetitive process of playing and replaying the talk over and over, each time listening for a single fault, you can completely transform an average talk and improve it beyond recognition.

If you really want to become a master speaker, look to an even newer method. Technologic advancements have brought the cost of small television cameras and video cassette recorders so low that they are increasingly available in universities and hospitals as well as the homes of individuals. The newer cameras and video recorders are reliable and easy to use. Many universities and scientific societies offer workshops that allow faculty to videotape themselves while giving a lecture.

Most speakers, even well-known lecturers, are appalled when they first see and hear themselves on the television monitor. Yet, by looking at themselves, by seeing and listening, they uncover weaknesses in delivery; identifying weaknesses is the first step toward fixing them. Speakers who want to improve platform performance use the camera and video cassette recorder repeatedly, employing much the same tactics as those just recommended for the tape recorder. The visual image, however, has much greater impact than sound alone. Speakers study and modify dress, body stance, bizarre bobbing and weaving movements, facial expression, and the use of gestures. With remarkably little effort, a wooden, toneless, monotonous delivery soon becomes lively and interesting. Bad habits melt away, replaced by an effective platform manner. Both excellent and poor speakers routinely find this technique helpful.

Remember that, as a speaker, your appearance is important. Consider, carefully, what you will wear. Inquire beforehand about the degree of formality expected. If anything, dress a bit on the conservative side. This will almost never offend your audience, whereas if you err on the side of informality, the effectiveness of your message is undermined.

Stage fright affects us all to a greater or lesser degree. Many years ago, the famous surgeon Professor Edward D. Churchill gave his personal treatment for stage fright—Churchill was well known as an effective speaker. Each time he got up in an auditorium, he would stand silently for a few seconds in front of the podium and do two things. First, he remembered he was the speaker and was in charge of the occasion. Second, he looked out over the assembly and, in his mind's eye, tried to visualize the members of the audience dressed only in their underwear. He reported that the technique never failed and that the second step was particularly effective when facing a front row of distinguished professors.

At the time you agreed to speak, you learned something about the room or auditorium. Now that the talk is almost prepared, telephone your host and confirm the program. Make sure you understand what facilities are available, what the room is like, where the speaker stands, and where the audience sits. After all, things might have changed.

At this time, with a week or so to go, develop a strategy for handling disasters. What will you do if the projector gives out in the middle of the talk? Think about your slides. What do they really show? If you had to select only two or three, which are the crucial ones? What are their main points? Could a blackboard sketch substitute in a pinch. Don't scare yourself silly, but think in advance about how you could repair a variety of problems.

When traveling a distance, it is a good idea to have a copy of your talk and an extra set of slides in another piece of luggage. Sometimes airlines lose bags, and you would not want the world's only copy of your talk and slides to be mislaid.

On the day of the talk, arrive at the room you are going to use early so you have a chance to look over the auditorium for yourself. Usually, the podium is fixed, but sometimes you can move the lectern to one side so that you can more easily see the slides and use a pointer without turning your back on your audience.

You must be prepared for the possibility of surprises. Perhaps there is no chalk, or no eraser, or maybe not even the expected blackboard. Try out everything in the room. See that you can turn the lights on and off. If there is a projector, have someone plug it in to make sure that it works and your slides fit. Focus it. Make sure there is enough light at the lectern for you to see your notes. Locate the pointer. If there is a microphone, try it out. Find out how far you should stand from it. Have some water near by in case your throat dries up. You may feel embarrassed about all these preparations, and a lecturer testing a microphone always feels silly, but you will look even sillier fumbling around during the talk. Strange things happen, be ready for them.

Professor Mosteller[1] offers the following suggestions:

1. You find the door locked or the room occupied. Relax. Let your host work it out. Introduce yourself to people waiting around and chat with them. Don't complain.

2. The room is too small. Already you are a great success. Don't apologize. Say how happy you are to see such a large audience.
3. Sometimes only two or three people show up. Go ahead with your talk as though you hadn't noticed. See it as an opportunity to share your work with those who are really interested. You may decide to turn the talk into a seminar with a lot of audience participation.
4. Sometimes at the last minute, the schedule must be changed. Perhaps a previous speaker ran over his time limit and used some of your time. Your talk is now too long. If you have prepared your speech as described above, you know exactly which 20 minutes of your talk are the most important. Tell the audience what is important, then stop for questions. Try not to let anyone suspect that you had expected to have more time.

Finally, don't feel bad when some of these things happen. They happen everywhere. Someday you will be host and it will happen to one of your guests.

You will be a great success. You have purposely and systematically set about preparing and delivering a great talk. You have selected a good topic, gathered the material, and rehearsed thoroughly.

After the talk is over, you are pleased that your planning and forethought have paid off so handsomely. The delivery and the audience's response were just as you had hoped. Nothing went wrong, but you knew that you were prepared to cope with the unexpected, and this only added to your poise and confidence. You felt good up there. Your host is delighted, and so are you.

Checklist

1. Consider the invitation.
   - Analyze the audience by size, professional status, age, and interest in or knowledge of subject.
   - Analyze the occasion. What is the setting? What are the customs? What precedes and follows your talk?
   - Determine whether the host envisions a presentation for specialists, a basic introduction, a theoretical discussion, or a clinical focus.

2. Should you accept? Is your own knowledge up to date? Are there other demands on your time? Consider suggesting an alternative topic.

3. Start working on the body of the talk.
   - Keep principal ideas few in number.
   - Define unusual terms.
   - Use concrete illustrations. Don't be too abstract.
   - Clarity is almost as important as accuracy of detail.
   - Relate new material to something the audience already knows.
   - Be easy to follow.

4. Once you have the body of the talk, work on the beginning and the closing.
   - The beginning of a talk sets the stage.
   - The ending of the talk focuses on your central theme.

5. From your final outline, develop the wording.
   - First, master the idea, not the language.
   - Use a tape recorder to hear how you sound.
   - Don't read your talk, speak it.
   - Practice, practice, practice.

6. If you had to cut the talk in half, what points would you try to make to the audience?

7. About a week before the talk, telephone your host and confirm the program, the facilities, what the room is like, etc.

8. Develop a strategy for handling disasters.
   - What if the projector gives out?
   - Could a blackboard sketch substitute?
   - Take an extra copy of your talk and a spare set of slides with you.

9. The day of the talk, arrive early so that you can see the auditorium for yourself. Anticipate surprises.
   - If you need a blackboard, is there chalk and an eraser?
   - Make sure the projector works and your slides fit.
   - Try out the microphone. Locate the pointer.

10. If anything goes wrong, don't complain, don't apologize; proceed as if you hadn't noticed.

Reference

1. Mosteller F. Classroom and platform performance. Am Stat 1980;34:11–17.

50

Presenting Your Work at International Meetings

T. Aoki and J.-H. Alexandre

The Advantages of International Exchange in Science

Scholars, particularly those near the beginning of their research careers, find that presenting their research results personally at international academic and research meetings imparts a special impetus to learning how to communicate their findings concisely, lucidly, and effectively to their peers. Such presentations provide on-the-spot opportunities for substantial and stimulating discussions of the significance and implications of your work.

If you are a young investigator, preparing to make the results of your research public, you should take part in repeated prepublication discussions of your work at academic and research meetings with the leaders in your field. Such discussions serve to clarify the procedural and analytical methods of your study, as well as the pertinency of your conclusions and their relation to other related and future issues. If the points generated from these discussions can be included later in your published article, it will likely receive a higher evaluation than material submitted before adequate deliberation.

The basic purpose of presenting research at meetings is the same for domestic and international gatherings. "Free-paper sessions" have increased recently because conference hosts would like to see an increased number of participants, and researchers do not want to participate in discussions unless they are given the opportunity to present their own research. When these free-paper sessions do not provide enough time for discussion because of overcrowding, the clarifying and defining functions of effective scientific exchange are frustrated.

When problems in the management of the meeting result in inadequate time for discussions, be prepared to shorten your presentation for the sake of having a full discussion.

International meetings obviously provide more opportunity for discussion from a global perspective than domestic meetings. Non-native speakers of the language used at international meetings must give careful thought to the words they select to express scientific facts. This exercise often leads to new insights, and realizations that were previously only vaguely understood or grasped by the author in his mother tongue. The greatest disadvantage of international meetings is the language barrier. There is a real possibility that adequate discussion of your paper will not be possible after you have presented it. Try to prearrange some discussion to "break the ice." There is a possibility that errors may arise in the understanding of scientific "facts" as the result of misinterpretations of your presentation or your answers to questions, caused by language problems. Discussion slides prepared in advance to answer questions you anticipate can help prevent this problem.

Extra effort is required to exploit the advantages gained from international exchange. It is particularly important for young researchers to learn to reach out across the language barrier for these rewards.

The accurate expression of facts presupposes our recognition that language, itself, is a science. Our deepest understanding of science is realized in the context of its translation into foreign languages, the meanings of each of their words, and the nuances behind their usage. The scientific element of research is heightened when the researcher gives careful thought to what kind of facts should be expressed under what circumstances and with which words. This helps us experience the common language of all researchers, which is science itself, in a much richer way.

One significant benefit of attending international meetings is the stimulus it gives to mastering the multilingual approach to thinking—the approach that ultimately trains your mind to think in the scientific mode. Young scientists are advised to seek language education aggressively, to acquire the minimal level of language ability needed for the communication of basic facts.

Suggestions for Speakers

Presenting a paper at an international meeting calls for strict discipline in facing many handicaps, meeting specific requirements, and analyzing what is appropriate for a given situation.

The Subject

Most often, ideas, personal experiences, or the results of advanced research are presented and are likely to be compared to the ideas and results of related team research in other countries. More and more meetings focus on very precise themes, so you may find that your paper is almost identical to the presentation that precedes or follows it. Don't let this destabilize you. Compliment the other speaker, and proceed. Emphasize, if you can, the details that make your research methods, approach, perspective, or future studies different from the others.

The Speaker

An international gathering eagerly awaits you. If you are famous, the audience will want to attach a face to your name; if you are unknown, you have an opportunity to contribute your new information or perspective to what has been published. You must take advantage of this chance to gain the interest of an international audience. Speaking with ease, clarity, and conviction will add more weight to the information you have come to present.

The International Audience

Because they are accustomed to attending similar conferences, many members of your audience will be very demanding as far as style, content, and adherence to time restrictions are concerned. For some, the language of your presentation will be a problem. English is now the most commonly used language at international meetings; Spanish, French, German, and Japanese are used less often. When the program indicates the possibility of simultaneous translation, appropriate preparation is required. A few specific cases merit consideration.

English as the Only Language

If English is your mother tongue, you must remember to speak slowly, pronounce each word clearly, and pause frequently for your Japanese, French, German, and Spanish listeners. If at all possible, use bilingual slides with English on the left side and the language of the host country on the right.

If you are asked to make a presentation in English and your mother tongue is German, French, Japanese, Spanish, etc., your preparation may be long and difficult. You will have to rehearse your presentation a number of times in front of a critical audience or with a tape recorder to be sure that you will remain within your time limit (10 or 15 minutes). Under no circumstances should you expect an extension of the allotted time because of the language difficulties. You must prepare a 2-page manuscript, typed double-spaced, from which you can read the introduction and the conclusion of your paper. Your slides, which are best committed to memory, must parallel the talk and may contain a maximum of 20 clearly visible words. If speaking in English is a struggle for you and you have complex slides to present, it is accepted practice to read your presentation. You must, however, read slowly, take time to face your audience, look straight at a third or fourth row listener, and frequently scan the room.

Simultaneous Translation

When simultaneous translation is available, your presentation will have to be slow-paced to give the translator a chance to keep up with you. Pause when you are presenting visual material, and be sure to provide the translator with a copy of the manuscript and slides well in advance. If possible, visit the auditorium ahead of time to assess where you will be in relation to your audience, the chairman, the moderator, and the projection screens. If two projectors are available, you may be able to judge which material would be best projected on the right or on the left.

On Stage

Before you begin to speak, sit down in front of the room near the podium so that you will not have to run to the stage, trip over a wire on the way, or have to catch your breath when you get there. Be sure to note how close the microphone is and to face your listeners—you must not turn your back to them. You must remain standing without waving your arms or walking about. Keep an eye on the time.

Four important points to remember are:

Take a big breath before you start to talk.
Speak slowly and loudly.
Enunciate clearly.
Be confident in yourself.

When you and your presentation are well prepared, your audience will be hanging on your every word.

As the timer goes off, you must finish the sentence you are in and go directly to your concluding three sentences. By then your information has surely been conveyed, and everyone knows that you cannot say everything in so short a time. The discussion period will allow some time for relevant questions, and the hallways are there for the exchanges of addresses and reference. Your extra effort to make a clear, concise presentation will help your own research, and will win the respect of your international colleagues.

51

Strategies for Coping with Jet Lag

E.N. Brown

Malaise following a long transmeridian flight is an all too familiar condition to many transoceanic and transcontinental travelers. Known as jet lag, this condition refers to the general fatigue, insomnia, gastrointestinal distress, and inability to concentrate that often result from crossing several time zones within a short period. The severity of symptoms depends on the number of time zones crossed, the crossing time, and the direction of travel.

One component of the ill-being associated with jet lag is simply fatigue from the demands of taking a trip. Research on circadian physiology suggests that the more significant features of this disorder may be attributable to a dissociation between time according to the body's internal clock and time in the external environment at the traveler's destination. Appreciation of the mechanism underlying jet lag makes it possible to devise strategies to help transmeridian travelers reduce, if not avoid dyssynchrony between the time setting of their internal and local external clocks.

A review of some basic principles of circadian physiology makes it easier to understand how these strategies are formulated. Chronobiologists—scientists who study the timing of biological processes—have long recognized that even though humans live in an environment organized around a 24-hour day, the intrinsic cycling period of the human biological clock is slightly longer than 24 hours. Indeed, when an individual lives for an extended period shielded completely from external environmental time cues, his internal clock exhibits a period of approximately 25 hours. To remain "in synch" with time in the external environment under normal conditions, the internal clock must be advanced one hour each day. Environmental factors, such as the timing of the individual's sleep–wake schedule, the scheduling of meals, and social signals from other provide cues that facilitate this daily time advance. Within a single 24-hours period, the human internal clock can be advanced 1 to 2 hours, or delayed 2 to 4 hours; so that shifting to a longer day of 25 to 28 hours is easier than moving to a shorter day of 20 to 22 hours. This asymmetry in the clock's propensity to be reset is believed to arise because a delay requires the clock to shift in the direction of its intrinsic period while a time advance moves it further away.

These factors help explain the difficulty transmeridian travelers have adapting swiftly to time zone changes greater than one to two hours. Moreover, adaptation following easterly travel is harder than adaptation following westerly travel across a comparable number of time zones since the former requires an advance of the internal clock whereas the latter requires a delay.

These basic biological facts suggest strategies for easing the adjustment to a time transition between the points of origin and destination. Suppose you are taking a nonstop flight from New York to Paris. The 6-hour eastward trip usually begins around 9 P.M. New York time. The time difference between the two cities in the winter is also 6 hours. Your 9 A.M. arrival in Paris corresponds to 3 a.m. on the New York setting of your internal clock and raises the difficult task of making a quick 6-hour advance to close the difference between your internal time and the new external time. Because eastbound travel requires a phase advance of your internal clock, the most you can make up during your first day in Paris is 2 hours.

You will exacerbate the problem if, upon arrival in Paris tired from your journey, you go straight to your hotel, shut yourself in your room, go to sleep, and lose the impact that light, social cues, meals, and appropriate scheduling of your sleep–wake cycle can have on your adaptation. At 3 A.M. according to your internal clock, you are at the circadian nadir of your mental alertness and should avoid making any important decisions.

One way to help yourself adjust to the change in time zones is to start advancing your internal clock prior to departure. Suppose that on your normal sleep–wake cycle you sleep from 12 A.M. to 7 A.M. every day. Three days prior to your departure, start going to sleep and waking up an hour earlier each day (i.e., on the first day, sleep from 11 P.M. to 6 A.M.; on the second, from 10 P.M. to 5 A.M.; and on the third, from 9 P.M. to 4 A.M.) You can use the time cues given by rescheduling your sleep–wake cycle to advance your internal clock by 3 hours. When you leave for Paris on the fourth day, you will have already adjusted to 3 of the 6 hours of time change required, and need to make up only another 3 hours after you arrive in Paris. You can easily make a shift of 1 to 2 hours during your first 24 hours in Paris, and the remaining 1 to 2 hours during the following day. You can further facilitate your adaptation to Paris time by making every effort maximize your exposure to Parisian time cues.

Similarly, if you are flying westward from Paris to New York, you can ease your adaptation to New York time by making phase delay adjustments in your internal clock prior to departure. The flight from Paris to New York leaves at 2 P.M. Paris time and arrives in New York at 2 P.M. New York time, which is 8 P.M. in Paris. If you stay up only 4 more hours and go to bed at 12 A.M. Paris time–6 P.M. New York time–expect difficulty in adjusting to the time in your new environment. Suppose, once again, that you normally sleep from 12 midnight to 7 A.M. and you delay your bedtime 1 hour on each of three successive nights prior to your departure; when you fly from Paris to New York, you will need to make up only 3 hours. This 3-hour adaptation is within the amount you can expect to make up in 24, hours since your internal clock shifts more easily in the delay direction. By forcing yourself to stay awake as long as possible after your arrival, you can probably make up all the remaining difference between the time in New York and the partially preadjusted setting of your internal clock.

The same principles can be used for easing the adaptation of your internal clock when you make longer journeys by the insertion of an extended intermediate stop. If you are flying from New York to Sydney, Australia, make a one-week stopover in Hawaii to adapt to the time in Hawaii and reduce the time adaptation on the second leg to Sydney.

A strategy for reducing the effects of jet lag on a shorter trip is to maintain the schedule you follow at home. If making a two-day trip to California, you may be able to maintain your normal internal New York time schedule while conducting your business in California. This includes keeping your watch on New York time so that there is no time shift to be made by your internal clock during the trip.

A third approach to jet lag has been suggested by the work of Charles Czeisler and his research group at Harvard Medical School.[1,2] Czeisler recently demonstrated that the human internal biological clock can be systematically shifted to any point in its cycle by properly timed exposures to light of an intensity of 7000 to 12,000 lux for 4 to 5 hours on each of three successive days. In a subsequent study he showed that shift workers could be made to adapt more quickly to changes in their work schedule with appropriately timed exposures to bright light.[3] Therefore, one strategy you may be able to use in the future is to expose yourself to bright light of a specific intensity and duration on the days prior to your departure on a transmeridian flight. This would enable you to advance or delay your internal clock as much as needed according to the direction of your travel. You would still want to maximize contact with the environmental time cues on arrival at your destination. Although this work is still in the experimental stage, it appears very promising.

A fourth approach suggested for treating jet lag is with various pharmacologic agents since a wide range of drugs have been used to shift the internal clocks of lower organisms. In an attempt to apply these concepts to humans, several investigators have looked at the ease with which transmeridian travelers treated with benzodiazepines or melatonin[4] adjust to the internal–external time dyssynchrony of jet lag. These studies have not established any widely accepted guidelines about the amount and timing of benzodiezapine dosage required to induce a shift of the internal clock by a specific number of hours in a specified direction.

A recent investigation by Moline and colleagues suggests that the highly publicized jet lag diet may be of no benefit in helping travelers avoid the disorder.[5]

You can use the basic principles of circadian physiology[6] to facilitate the resetting of your internal clock to the prevailing time at your destination and reduce, or avoid, the frequently annoying effects of jet lag.

Summary of Strategies for Coping with Jet Lag

1. For easterly travel, begin advancing the traveler's internal clock by advancing the sleep– wake cycle on the three to four days prior to departure.
2. For westerly travel, begin advancing the traveler's internal clock by delaying the sleep–wake cycle on the three to four days prior to departure.
3. Upon arriving at the destination, maximize contact with and abiding by such time cues in the new environment as exposure to outside light,

social contacts, and the scheduling of sleep, meals, and other normal daily activities.

4. For short trips, the traveler should maintain if possible, his external time schedule relative to his point of origin so that there is no need to shift the internal clock.
5. For long trips with an extended intermediate stopover, the traveler can facilitate synchronization of his internal clock to time at his final destination by adapting first to time at his stopover point.

References

1. Czeisler CA, Kronauer RK, Allan JS, Duffy JF, Jewett ME, Brown EN, Ronda JM. Bright light induction of strong (type 0) resetting of the human circadian pacemaker. Science 1989;244:1328–32.
2. Czeiseler CA, Allan JS, Strogztz SH, Ronda JM, Sanches R, Rios CD, Freitag WF, Richardson GS, Kronauer RK. Bright light resets the human circadian pacemaker independent of the timing of the sleep–wake cycle. Science 1986;233:667–71.
3. Czeisler CA, Johnson MP, Duffy JF, Brown EN, Ronda JM, Kronauer RE. Exposure to bright light and darkness to treat physiologic maladaptation to night work. N Engl J of Med 1990;322:1253–59.
4. Arendt J, Marks V. Jet lag and melatonin. Lancet 1986;2:698–99.
5. Moline ML, Pollak CP, Wagner DR, Zendell S, Lester SL, Salter CA, Hirsch E. Effects of the "jet lag diet" on the adjustment to a phase advance. Second Meeting of the Society for Research on Biological Rhythms 1990;77.
6. Moore-Ede MD, Sulzman FM, Fuller CA. The Clocks That Time Us. Cambridge, MA: Harvard University Press, 1982.

52

Organizing Your Slides

C. Troidl

Slides are the most common medium for oral communications of scientific information. An active investigator may accumulate hundreds or even thousands of slides over a period of years. When you are preparing a talk or lecture, access to the information contained in your slides can become increasingly difficult unless you have a system of organization that is specific to your needs. Recently, I conducted a survey among 32 investigators who lecture frequently; 65% of them were not satisfied with their slide filing system. They estimated that the mean time required to retrieve a specific slide was 2 minutes, and to assemble a scientific presentation, 60 minutes. Faster and easier access to specific slides is vitally important if busy investigators are to maximize the efficient use of their time and prepare better quality presentations.

This chapter describes three specific aspects of slide organization: storage, assembly, and transportation. Because there is no single approach that works for everyone, several different approach "modules" are described; you can assemble a combination that suits your particular needs.

Storing Your Slides

Slide storage has two components:

1. *Easy access to specific slides* includes visualization of slide content by good backlighting and the ability to view an array of slides about common medical or scientific subjects. The access system should be expandable, to permit slides to be added to each storage location.
2. *A cataloguing system* permits storing slides according to topic and subject.

Storage Devices

A variety of storage devices are available in each country. The factors determining the type of storage device you choose include its cost and the space available for housing it. Examples of such devices are shown in Figure 52.1. The one you choose should permit fast and easy access, with good background lighting, for a panel of slides dealing with the same topic; the simplest cataloguing of slides for retrieval and storage; and easy expansion of the system.

Other helpful devices include a magnifying glass to read the content of each slide during your selection process, and a horizontal light box adjacent to the slide storage device for assembling the slides for a talk. Horizontal light boxes are available commercially, but some people find that an old x-ray viewing box placed horizontally on a table is quite satisfactory.

As your collection grows, you may find it necessary to separate the slides into two groups according to how frequently you use them. Put the slides you use often in the most readily available system, and those you use infrequently, but don't want to throw away, in a separate storage area. Keep in mind that a waste basket is a third option for poor-quality or never-used slides. If you hoard all your slides, over the years they may become so numerous that you can't retrieve those you really need.

Some investigators find it useful to keep a separate filing system for the hard copy of each slide. This provides a backup for making duplicate slides or for identifying lost slides; it also allows you to update or modify old ones on the hard copy without starting over.

Another principle is to make duplicate sets—to guard against loss of slides that are difficult to

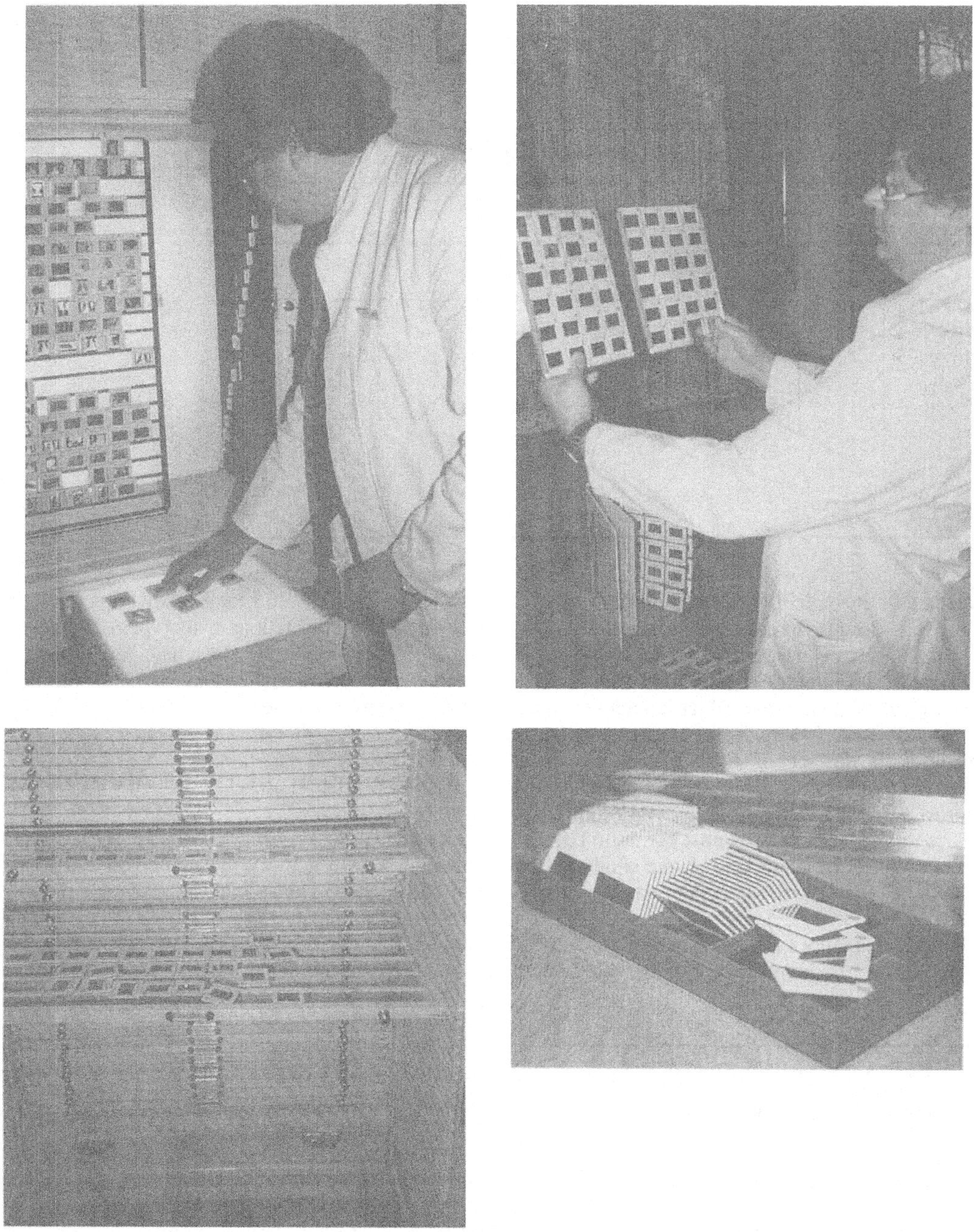

A C D B

FIGURE 52.1. Examples of slide storage devices: three very effective (A–C) storage devices and one (D) that is very uneffective.

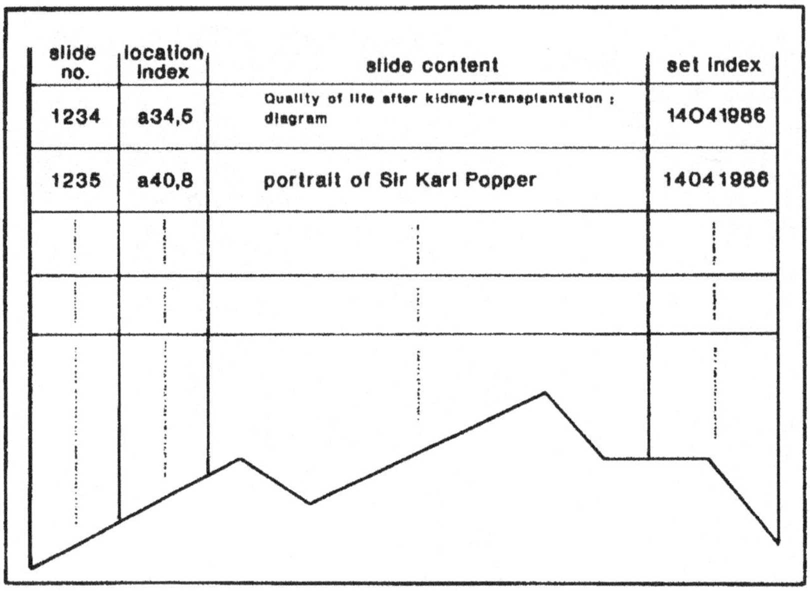

FIGURE 52.2. Sample arrangement of a slide catalog.

replace, or to permit storage under several categories. Because of concern about possible loss or damage during transport to a presentation in another city, some investigators like to keep a separate set of their most valuable slides in their own department. Others prefer to carry duplicate sets in their luggage or briefcase to avoid the tragedy of losing or misplacing these materials just prior to a major presentation. Finally, some want to have duplicates for their most common talks so that one set can be kept together in a single folder, while the duplicates are filed under various subject headings.

Some investigators have a separate section for slides that are common to all their talks. These generic slides are useful for interspersing the various subjects of your talk in many types of presentations. Slides displaying "results," "experimental methods," "conclusions," or a list of investigators or coworkers are examples.

LEVEL 1	⟶	RESEARCH FIELD
quality of life	—	Ringbinder 2
LEVEL 2	⟶	DIAGNOSIS
lung cancer	—	Chapter 3
LEVEL 3	⟶	OUTLAY
curve	—	Page 35

FIGURE 52.3. Examples of different elvels of organization of a slide collection or catalog.

Cataloguing and Coding Your Slides

Your cataloguing system should make it easy to put slides back into a location where you can easily find them again. The system should be sufficiently understandable to permit one or two other individuals (e.g., your secretary) to work with it; but remember that allowing several people to handle your slides may cause confusion, or misplacement or loss of slides.

A new slide should be coded as soon as it is made; doing this can be a simple matter, or quite complex. The simplest systems use colored dots, letters, or abbreviated titles. More complex coding systems involve formal indexing or entry into a computer (Figure 52.2). The simpler system will work with a relatively small slide collection or when your storage device allows you to view a large number of slides simultaneously, with a background lighting system (Figure 52.1A).

You may prefer a catalog system that lists all your slides according to different topics or subjects. The system you design must accommodate the number of slides and the diversity of your subject material. Adopt an organizational system whose sophistication for slide retrieval and storage increases as your slide collection grows. Relatively early, think about the ultimate goals for your system, to avoid having to make a major overhaul later.

A sophisticated indexing or cataloguing system will let you cross-file slides according to different topics or levels of organization (Figure 52.3). Slides are coded by numbers, letters, symbols, or colored dots (e.g., Fig. 52.4), and a formal catalog can be logged on hard copy or, ideally, in a computer. In the survey of investigators mentioned earlier, the majority organized their slides around medical headings, although a number organized them according to particular presentations (Figure 52.5). Some had duplicate sets of slides organized both ways.

Establishing a slide catalog requires considerable time and effort, especially for a manual system. More and more investigators use computerized systems; some are commercially available, and it is not too difficult to program a computer to meet your unique needs. An automated system allows you to assemble your talk in the computer

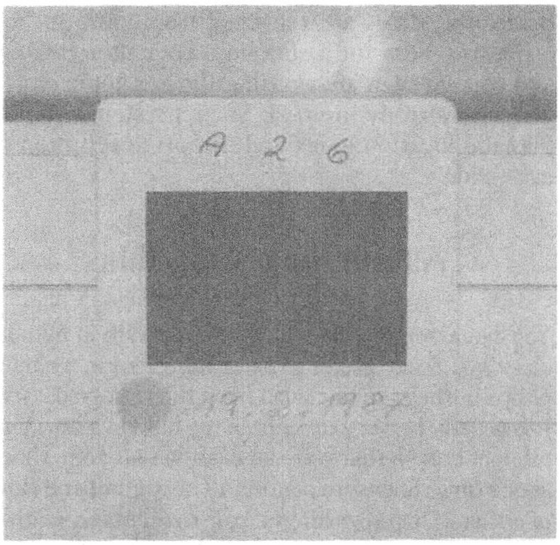

FIGURE 52.4. Proper marking of a slide: a location index on top, the date of production and a sticker bearing a color code at the bottom.

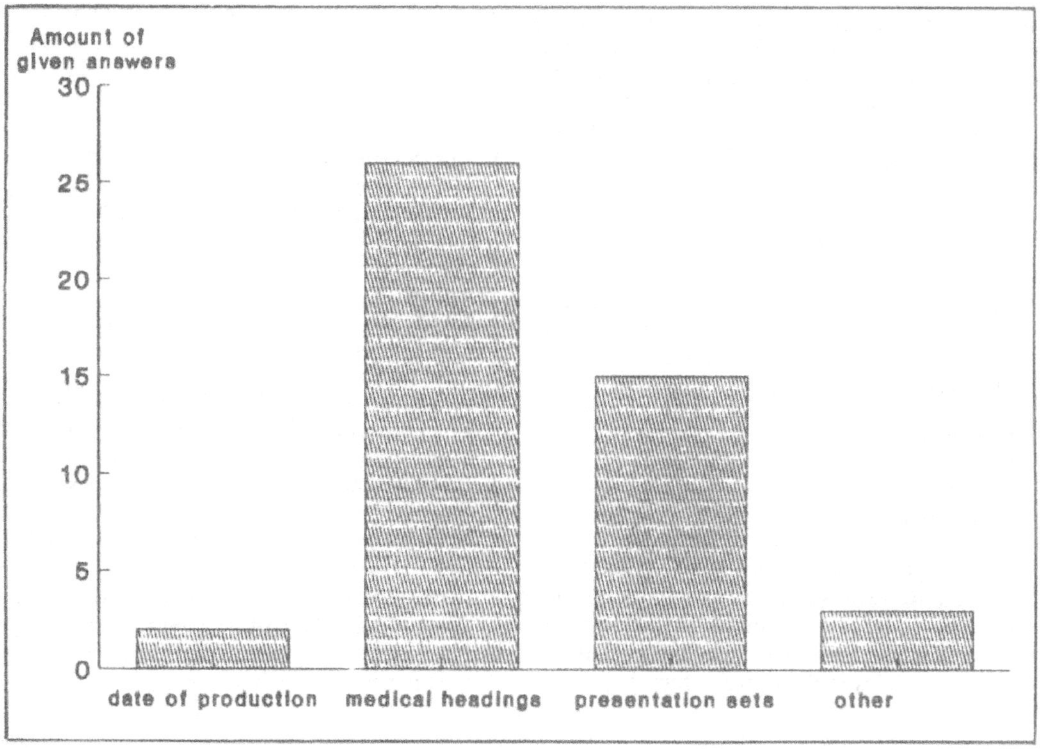

FIGURE 52.5. Results of a survey on slide organization (December 1988) that queried respondents on the ordering of their slides. (Total responses exceeds 30 because some participants cited more than one category.)

before the slides are retrieved from storage. You can also search for a slide in a computer catalog, and sort through slides using the key topic words you have already inserted. Such a system will display the location index and a short description of each slide.

Assembling Your Talk

You can assemble the slides for your talk in numerous ways. Some prefer to place the slides in a binder or box as they are retrieved from the storage device. It is usually better to assemble the talk on a horizontal light box so that you can examine all your slides at one time, to ensure continuity of content and flow of ideas. This also allows you to intersperse title slides as you introduce new subjects, and quickly scan the content of your talk from beginning to end. A magnifying glass helps you to confirm that you know what each slide contains and to examine each one for the clarity of its message.

In more sophisticated computerized catalogs slides can be arranged in sequence on the computer without pulling a large number of slides from the storage device. You can search through all the slides on a given topic to be sure you have retrieved a set that encompasses the information you wish to convey. A computerized system also lets you recover a list of previous presentations on the same or similar topics and retrieve the same slide sets without starting from scratch.

Transporting Your Slides

When you take your slides to a meeting, carry them personally. Do not send them ahead or put them in the luggage you will check at the airport.

Products for transporting slides include:

Slide binders.
Slide trays.
Slide boxes.
Slide carousels.

Binders let you take a quick glance at the slides when you are reviewing your presentation. Slide trays or boxes are more useful when you are carrying a large number of slides. Some individuals like to transport slides in their own carousel, to avoid having to arrange them on the airplane or at the hotel, or the possibility of getting someone else's broken carousel at the meeting. If you keep your slides in presentation sets, number each one according to its position in the set. Otherwise, you may have reassemble them if, by accident, any drop out of your slide box, binder, or carousel.

Before your presentation—especially at international meetings—be sure your slide frames fit in the slide projectors available for your talk. Arrive early enough to check the projector and the type of carousel being used. Put your slides in the carousel personally, and review them ahead of time to ensure that they are correctly oriented and in the right sequence.

Conclusion

Slides play an important role in the communication of scientific and medical information. Try to develop a system of organization that will meet your particular needs in this area of your professional activities. If your system provides easy access to your slides and lets you put them back where they belong without difficulty, your ability to give excellent presentations will be enhanced.

Checklist

1. Check efficiency of storage device for (a) fast and easy access on every slide, (b) sufficient view on a large group of slides with the same medical or scientific topic, and (c) the possibility of adding slides at any location of your collection.
2. Check the internal order of the slides, which should make it possible to have a rough overview on your slides.
3. A catalog system should make it possible to find every specific slide in your collection. It can be either a computer program or a handwritten list that tells you almost immediately the position of the slide you want.
4. Mark every slide immediately after its production.
5. Do not produce too many slides. Think carefully about the necessity of each slide you produce.
6. Put slides that have not been in use for a very long period of time into storage.

53

Organizing Meetings, Panels, Seminars, Symposia, and Consensus Conferences

M.F. McKneally, B. McPeek, D.S. Mulder, W.O. Spitzer, and H. Troidl

Just as they communicate ideas by writing and lecturing, academicians conceptualize, plan, and organize scientific meetings throughout their careers. Planning and organizing a meeting, especially a new one without an established format, is a major challenge that requires a systematic approach as well as scientific creativity.

Why Are We Meeting?

When you are called upon to plan a meeting, panel, or conference, maintain a clear vision of the *purpose of the meeting* as you choose the venue, program, size, and time of the session, and the relationship of your meeting to others whose rationale and content might otherwise be overlapped or duplicated.

Meetings of large surgical organizations like the American College of Surgeons or the German Surgical Society have several purposes which are simultaneously achieved.

1. They provide a *forum for the presentation of new clinical and scientific information*.
2. They *update the education of practicing surgeons* through postgraduate courses in clinical care and through formal and informal peer interaction.
3. They provide an opportunity for the membership to *inform the leadership* of their views and for the *leaders to present policy recommendations and reports* to the members.

The answer to the question WHY, the rationale for the meeting, has an important influence on the choice of a final product to be derived from the meeting. Progression toward this goal should be part of the planning of the meeting and will influence its structure significantly. For example, a meeting to establish an organization will put more emphasis on a final banquet and the establishment of a bylaws committee. A meeting intended to document the state of the art in a field emphasizes the production of a publication based on the material presented, and will expend resources for recording and editing the discussions. A meeting called to move an idea forward may terminate in a press conference.

Meetings designed primarily for postgraduate education in North America must be planned to meet continuing medical education (CME) requirements as dictated by a sponsoring university. The accrediting agency will require the proposed program, faculty, length of meeting, budget, and pre- and postsession evaluation formats. To ensure that registrants receive appropriate continuing medical education (CME) credit, which may be required annually by provincial or state licensing bodies, this planning process must be completed well in advance.

How To Do It

Organizing a meeting is a pleasant and interesting diversion for surgeons and their staff. However, as the complexity and size of the meeting increases, and the day-to-day pressures of clinical and research activities continue unabated, the resources required to ensure a successful meeting may be depleted. Professional organizations are available to assist with scientific meetings of every size, just as they are available to assist with social and business functions. Large organizations of 500 members or more may retain a professional business manager to plan and organize meetings at the direction of the executive council. The experience and skill of the organizer in dealing with international guest lists, arranging visas, accommodating audiovisual requirements and translation systems, and supervising program preparation, publicity, and social functions, far outweigh the additional cost to the organization. *Professional management companies* minimize confusion over submission of abstracts, preparation of manuscripts, and deadlines in preparing for publication in a journal. The professional management group adds continuity and stability to the organization and to the planning for any meeting. Professional management companies are experienced in negotiating for facilities and supplies for the meetings. Their involvement in the budgeting process and their ability to identify sources of revenue is very helpful.

International meetings present special problems and opportunities. They are more difficult and costly to organize because of differences in language and travel distances, but they contribute to the shrinkage of the world in terms of dissemination of surgical knowledge. An international meeting may be designed to fulfill any of the functions of meetings described above. International meetings entail certain specific considerations, such as jet lag or time zone changes, which should be factored into the scheduling of international speakers. Language problems should be anticipated in the development of panels. A clear policy must be delineated from the outset regarding the choice of language for the meeting. Arrangements for international meetings may be complicated by poor communication, even with the availability of telefax. Time zone changes, local holiday schedules, and imperfect distribution systems for information demand a much greater lead time. Telex is useful, as are international couriers, and even diplomatic pouches when the mail and the telephone will not do the job.

Some common features of the organization of a surgical meeting include the *organizing committee*, which should meet well in advance to plan the topics, speakers, chairmen of sessions and panels, location, time, and size and length of the meeting. As previously discussed, the objective or rationale for the meeting provides the guidelines for the decisions of the organizing committee.

A meeting that is primarily directed at the collection and dissemination of new scientific knowledge usually requires a request for abstracts. Plan enough lead time for the abstracts to be submitted and screened by a *program committee*, which will ultimately determine the final program for the meeting. Many scientific meetings request that each speaker produce a paper for publication to be delivered to the recorder at the time of presentation. This document must meet the publication requirements of the sponsoring journal or publisher of the symposium. It is imperative that a decision regarding manuscript preparation be made and communicated well in advance. Attempts to record oral presentations and turn them into a permanent record of the meeting are notoriously difficult. Meetings developed to promote a specific idea or new surgical concept often include investigators with a special interest in the concept or technique, who have a leadership role and interesting data to present. Other investigators with a more traditional or different approach are invited to present an opposing viewpoint. This may take the form of sequential short presentations followed by discussion, chaired by a carefully chosen moderator. Small group discussions carefully spaced between formal presentations enhance discussion and allow for the definition of a position paper based on the available data. Publications of the proceedings of these meetings may well require recording of discussions as positions evolve during the course of the meeting. It is important that an editorial committee take on the responsibility of collating and editing the manuscript and subsequent discussion.

Business Meetings

Surgical organizations generally hold a business meeting in conjunction with their scientific meetings. These should provide a well-organized opportunity for introduction of new members and committee reports, as well as allowing direct communication between the leadership and the members. Committee reports and controversial agenda items should be well prepared. To avoid lengthy floor discussion, major decisions, such as changes in bylaws or policies, are sometimes presented in writing at a preliminary meeting at the onset of the congress.

Where to Meet

The location of the meeting and the associated social program enhance free exchange of ideas. A degree of isolation in a resort setting increases attendance at the scientific sessions and facilitates informal discussion in a relaxing atmosphere. The degree of isolation, however, should not preclude relatively easy access for busy surgeons. The overall length of the meeting should be realistic, as should the length of the scientific session. Group discussions lasting longer than an hour usually become nonproductive. A change in format or a diversion from the topic at hand will increase overall productivity.

Paying for the Meeting

Careful thought must be given to the *financing* of any meeting, particularly an international meeting. Professional organizers are helpful in developing and strengthening funding. The meetings associated with a scientific organization are usually supported by the membership through annual dues or the levy of an attendance fee. This may include the cost of all social functions, or it can be designed to cover the cost of the entire meeting, minimizing the subsidy required by the organization. Surgical meetings designed to promote a concept or develop a consensus usually require the support of a surgical organization, a hospital, or a university. In many cases, the funding can be augmented by obtaining support from the many companies representing the surgical–industrial complex. To be certain that the sponsors' expectations for publicity or endorsement are not unrealistic or unmet, specific guidelines must be established at the outset and administered uniformly.

Format

The format of the meeting varies with its purpose. Small breakfast sessions, fireside chats, or meet-the-professor sessions give participants informal access to leaders in the field. Motion pictures provide a venue for exchange of technical information in a relaxing format. Fun is important, and opportunities to swim, hike, and participate together in sports or other physical activities enhance the attractiveness of a meeting.

The *social program* should be interesting, diverting, and appropriate to the interests of the participants, their spouses, and guests. Educational programs about the interesting features of the setting for the meeting provide common and stimulating diversion, which can increase the energy and enthusiasm of the scientific portion of the meeting. Many successful scientific meetings are carefully programmed to allow substantial periods for relaxation and social activity, which increase absorption and reflection on the scientific material presented. A dense program of continuous scientific activity reduces creativity and responsiveness of the participants.

Panels

Panel discussions have been particularly popular and successful in the United States for many years, and they are now widely used in most other countries as well. There are two common formats. One is the combined half-hour panel discussion as a joint question-and-answer period following several individual formal presentations. The other format is a true panel discussion, in which the panelists take their places on the platform at the outset. The moderator offers brief introductory remarks, and each panelist speaks for not more than 5 to 8 minutes on a particular aspect of the main theme. An open discussion follows to illuminate what the speakers have said. Panel discussions are informative in an authoritative and emphatic way because of the participation of several experts who are able to offer well-based opinions on any issue that may be raised. Properly handled by the moderator, such a group can provide a lively and entertaining exposition of the subject under consideration.

For variety, the moderator may pick a controversial clinical problem and have each of the speakers present their views on the optimal management in a short, formal, illustrative talk. The moderator then presents a clinical case to the panel. The results of key investigative studies are progressively revealed when they are requested by a member of the panel or prompted by a question from the audience. Surgeons with opposing views are asked to defend their positions in relation to the particular problem. This leads to a stimulating discussion in which the audience can participate by written or spoken questions.

Panels are popular with audiences because of their informality and variety, and because they offer the opportunity to hear and contrast different points of view. Listeners particularly enjoy the opportunity to participate in the interchange of ideas through questions or comments. This aspect of a panel discussion, though sometimes technically difficult or inconvenient for the moderator and the panel, is an important one and is well worth the effort required to make it successful.

The success and productivity of a panel depends on the expertise, tact, and wisdom of the chair, the specialized knowledge and communication skills of the participants, and the care and thought put into the planning and organization of the panel.

The Choice of Speakers

The best speakers for a panel may differ somewhat from those who would be ideal to address a congress, as the panel requires a greater degree of spontaneity and interactive skill.

Panelists should represent fairly both sides of any controversial issue. The ideal panelist is an accepted authority who is expert at expounding his ideas and engaging in debate. At international meetings, panels can be very challenging. If a common language is chosen, it is usually English. Many doctors whose native language is not English have a good command of the language during a prepared talk, but few are up to a brisk, hard-hitting panel discussion that is not in their mother tongue. It is particularly difficult to transmit humor across the language barrier, since it so often depends on subtle nuances. As a consequence, panel discussions in English with multinational participants tend to be rather humorless, in sharp contrast to the spirit that pervades a first-class discussion in which an element of humor is an important, if not indispensable, ingredient. The use of simultaneous translation at international meetings, despite the immense skill displayed by experienced interpreters in translating complex ideas extemporaneously, inevitably slows and occasionally confuses the process of discussion. It also tends to suppress attempts to enliven the proceedings.

The person responsible for the selection of participants and their invitation should be certain to include the names of all other panelists, the anticipated composition of the audience, a request for a current curriculum vitae to assist in introductions, and an indication of the method of reimbursement of travel and expenses, and whether there will be an honorarium.

The Moderator

The key to a successful panel discussion, the moderator should be a good speaker whose knowledge and credibility in the field allow firm and positive intervention, reasonable discipline, and the maintenance of an agreed timetable and agenda. A good moderator has a sound overall knowledge of the subject, but need not be familiar with its more abstruse aspects. A moderator who is well known as a strong protagonist of certain controversial beliefs must allow and encourage the expression of contrary views, controlling the expression of personal convictions. Biased moderators are like defense or prosecution lawyers who are elevated to a judgeship. To be effective, they must assume an impartial attitude appropriate to the higher office. When planning a meeting, it is useful to know the personality and style of the candidates for moderator, based on previous performance in similar situations. Some individuals have rightly earned reputations as superb moderators and are widely sought after for this role.

A good moderator brings out the strong points of each member of the panel by skillful questioning. This is best done in an atmosphere of cordiality and good humor. A moderator who knows the panelists well can foster such an atmosphere. *At the close of a panel, it is useful to have a closing statement from the moderator, which can be developed from notes taken during the course of the discussion.*

At the end of a panel discussion, the speakers and audience should feel that the moderator has exercised firm control, has maintained a reasonably objective stance, and has given all the members of the panel a fair opportunity to express their views. This will not happen as a matter of luck or even of considerable skill, if exercised only during the meeting. To ensure success, the moderator will need to get in touch with the speakers before the meeting to define the limits of their discussion very clearly and to obtain outlines of what they intend to say.

Every attempt should be made to start and finish at the appointed hour. Mechanical timers are helpful in controlling brief presentations. Time discipline can be maintained with tricks, such as gavel pounding, placing a samurai sword, a water pistol, or a rose on the table in front of the moderator (leaving the intended use of such objects to each speaker's imagination), or announcing that a trap door will open or the lights and microphones will go off at the end of the assigned time. If an inconsiderate speaker fails to observe the time requirements, the moderator should walk to the podium, gently taking the microphone to share the problem of time pressure with the speaker and the audience. The moderator may then invite the speaker to continue the discussion during a subsequent part of the program, which may never materialize.

Prediscussion Planning

The moderator is responsible for making certain that the topic to be discussed is well covered. The success of the panel depends on the moderator's explicit instruction to the panelists to be sure that the main theme is covered without overlap. *A carefully written mandate to individual speakers from the moderator well in advance of the panel discussion is the only effective method of preventing duplication and ensuring adequate coverage of the chosen topic.*

Briefing

Most successful moderators hold a preliminary meeting with their panelists the day or the morning before the discussion is to take place. If you have been chosen to act as a moderator, use this occasion to explain your thoughts on how the discussion should be conducted, and briefly review the presentation of each speaker. Some rather surprising things may be learned at such meetings. For example, a speaker who has been instructed to present an 8-minute summary of his subject may announce that he has carefully budgeted 30 minutes of formal discussion with 60 slides. The preliminary meeting is the time to clarify what will happen in the conduct of the panel; refine general strategy; change the order of talks, if necessary, to make them more effective, and deal with technical problems to ensure that the formal presentations go smoothly.

The panel members can decide who is best equipped to handle particular questions, and panelists can be prepared for pre-selected questions to lay the groundwork for a lively debate. Occasionally, it is impossible to arrange a preliminary meeting of this kind, and the moderator may have to rely on the second-best arrangement, which is a telephone conference. The third choice is correspondence; this is usually the least satisfactory. Use whatever means are required, but do not omit the preliminary meeting.

Questions

The classic method of securing audience participation is to invite written questions. Cards are distributed to the people in the audience so that they can write down their questions during the formal presentation. Preprinted question cards should indicate to whom the question is directed and the name and address of each individual raising a question. The question cards are collected by assistants who stroll the aisles. There is often a break for coffee between the portion of the symposium allocated to the presentation of papers and the subsequent period assigned to the panel discussion. This convenient interval is available to look through the questions before the discussion begins. If there is not a break, time pressure makes the sorting of questions difficult. An assistant and some planned questions will help you through this difficult period. It is always best to have two people available for sorting questions. If the moderator is sorting while asking questions, the panel discussion may get out of control.

For foreign guests, very clear questions prepared in advance may avert the problems inherent in participating in panels when there is a language problem. Know the communication skills of your panelists and prepare them for the questions they will be asked. There are some very interesting and pertinent questions that should be asked about the topic under discussion. Even if you intend to collect questions from the audience on question cards, it is perfectly reasonable to have a prepared set of questions that will focus the discussion, and to forewarn your individual panelists. This reduces spontaneity only slightly and helps the panelists compose their thoughts about some questions. You can enliven boring sessions by altering the age or setting of the clinical problem presented by the audience. The discussion can be controlled effectively by grouping submitted questions into topic areas that fall within the expertise of particular panelists. If you make up three questions for each speaker from your own knowledge of the topic and choose three additional questions from those submitted by the audience, an orderly and interesting discussion can be anticipated.

The alternate way of obtaining questions from the audience is to allow them to use microphones strategically placed about the conference room. This provides spontaneous and direct contact with the audience, but it suffers from several disadvantages. Some people are inhibited by the equipment itself. Floor microphones sometimes have technical problems. The most serious problem is that the microphone takes control of the discussion away from the moderator. Floor microphones should be monitored, and a technician should be on duty to activate and deactivate a microphone on the command of the moderator. Turning off the microphone is an effective way to deal with audience members who present lengthy statements or arguments instead of questions. If discussion from the floor is to be recorded for transcription, the moderator must assure that the discussant's name and city are clearly stated.

Seminars

Seminars are usually small group presentations in which the seminar leader serves as a facilitator, eliciting participation of the audience. Skillful direction of a seminar is a fine teaching art; the keynotes are informality and participation. The purpose of the seminar and the general rules for its conduct should be clearly stated. Since an enthusiastic audience may use up all the available time, it is important to announce the subheadings of the seminar clearly through an outline on the blackboard or a transparency; this allows the discussion to progress through the full range of the topics scheduled for review.

Seminars may serve to expose students to the thinking of the seminar leader or visiting professor. Case presentations or research project presentations by the students provide an excellent format for accomplishing this purpose. Slides tend to reduce the spontaneity and creativity of seminars; they should be used sparingly.

Consensus Conferences

A consensus conference is a formalized way of seeking advice. It is usually called by a policy maker, such as the minister of health, or science and technology. The convening authority seeks the advice of the conference members to deal with unresolved scientific, medical, or social problems when a summary of the current state of scientific knowledge in the field is required for the development of a new course of action. The policy recommendations may relate to treatment of patients or to assignment of resources to fund research. Consensus conferences almost always attempt to reach an agreement among experts as to exactly what is known about the specified topic, what issues are settled, and what issues are still open to debate. It usually tries to focus the attention of the convening authority on areas of potentially fruitful research.

Participation in a consensus conference is almost invariably by invitation. The sponsor wants advice that cannot be successfully assailed or discredited. Members of consensus conferences are sought from a wide spectrum of scientific backgrounds, and representation of minorities, political groups, and partisans is emphasized. The attempt to ensure that the whole process will be perceived as thorough, complete, inclusive, and honestly executed may lead to an inconclusive, bland position paper that displeases no one.

Consensus conferences have proven to be useful for translating evidence from research studies into professional policy. Consensus conferences should emphasize scientific evidence and attempt to minimize the impact of unsupported personal opinions of panel members, no matter how senior or prestigious they may be. The National Institutes of Health in the United States have used consensus conferences to integrate considered opinions of recognized experts in many controversial areas.

If you are asked to chair such a conference, be fair, but take a position. Seek the support of a very skillful, informed scientific secretary to take notes during the deliberations and to write a clear account of what has happened, so that the report of the discussion will reflect the true consensus faithfully. *It is extremely difficult to chair a meeting effectively and take notes at the same time.* With a scientific secretary it will be easier for you to develop a report that avoids introducing your own biases more heavily than is warranted.

Summary

Maintain a clear vision of the purpose of your meeting.
The location, social program, and format influence the scientific productivity of a meeting.
Publication of the proceedings and presentations from a meeting requires more lead time and much more forethought.
Professional management provides continuity, stability, and knowledge.
Successful panels require explicit mandates to the speakers and careful briefing.
The ideal panelist is an engaging, spirited debater.
Humor is an important, if not indispensable, ingredient of panel discussions.
Question periods are inconvenient but very engaging for the listener.
Consensus conferences guide policy through carefully balanced summaries of the current state of knowledge.
Fairness and representativeness may lead to bland, inconclusive consensus. "Be fair, but take a position."
The keynotes for successful seminars are informality and audience participation.

Checklist for Organizing a Meeting

Develop a time table: Call for Abstracts/Program Deadline.
Develop Budget–Seek Sponsorship.
Assess adequacy of Site: Conference Rooms, Banquet Facilities, hotels, transportation.
Reserve Adequate Space for Scientific or Industrial Exhibits.
Select Hotels.
Develop a Promotional Schedule–Advertising?
Travel Arrangements–Appoint an Experienced Travel Agency.
Social Program–Final Banquet, Spouse Tours–Appoint an Experienced Agency.
Scientific Program–Publication of Abstracts, Recorder at Meeting, CME Certification.
Audio Visual Requirements–Microphones, Projection (slides/video), Translation, Professional Projectionists.
Appointment of Guest Speakers–Honoraria, Plaques.
Press Conference.
Administrative: Staff for Registration, CME Credits.
Recognition: Certificates for Participants, Gifts for Support Staff and Special Guests.

Acknowledgments. The authors are grateful to Mr. William T. Maloney of Professional Relations and Research Institute, Inc., 13 Elm Street, Manchester, MA 01944, for helpful advice and review of the manuscript.

Additional Reading

Hoaglin DC, Light RJ, McPeek B, Mosteller F, Stoto MA. In: Data for Decisions. Cambridge, MA: Abt Books, 1982.

McPeek B. Consensus conferences: seeking advice. Theor Surg 1989;3:169–70.

Neugebauer E, Troidl H. Meran Conference on Pain After Surgery and Trauma. A Consensus Conference of Various Clinical Disciplines and Basic Research, 10–14 May 1988 in Meran, South Tyrol, Italy. Theo Surg 1989;3:220–24.

Professional Meeting Management, 2nd ed. Birmingham, AL: Professional Convention Management Association, 1990.

Section V

International Perspectives on Surgical Research

This book was born in the course of a series of consultations about barriers to surgical research, unattained but attainable goals for investigators, and training opportunities for aspiring academic clinicians.

The informal and enlightening international pilgrimage of one of the editors, described in the introduction to the first edition, progressed to a more formal consultation in a planning conference convened at Eppan in the Italian Tyrol. There was no intent or pretense that the planning process could involve an extensive representation of nationalities. However, the architecture of the book was adopted at this conference, and the book has subsequently been written for the international community of university surgeons and their scientific partners. The preceding sections dealt with the methodological and practical aspects of clinical research; this section is a "tour d'horizon" of real-life settings in which the principles of surgical research can be and are being translated into research accomplishments. In many ways, this is the "soul" of the book. Reports from academic surgeons in 10 countries are presented. The status of surgical research is presented from the individual viewpoint of each author, not as a summary of all available information from each country. We did not impose a rigid format on each chapter, nor did we attempt to standardize the language. Instead, we have preserved the unique style and flavor of each contribution within the limits of translation requirements.

In Chapter 65, the editors have pooled some of the information supplied by the authors to allow more direct comparisons to be made between the postgraduate educational programs in surgery. Data on the funding of research from the Harvard School of Public Health, presented in this chapter, help establish a framework for comparison of the level of interest and accomplishment in biomedical research.

54

Surgical Research in Canada

D.S. Mulder

This chapter reflects the personal experience and observations of the author and makes no attempt to be a comprehensive discussion of the contribution of every university department in Canada.

The science of surgery has made tremendous strides in Canada since Sir William Osler stated in the late 1880s: "The physic of the men who are really surgeons, is better than the surgery of the men who are really physicians; which is the best that can be said of a very bad arrangement."[1] Since that provocative statement was made, surgery at McGill University has evolved quickly, primarily on the basis of clinical activities. The personality, wisdom, and forward thinking of George Armstrong, Thomas Roddick, James Bell, and Edward Archibald brought high clinical standards to surgery at McGill by the late 1930s.

Dr. Archibald made monumental contributions and was influential in the establishment of the American Board of Surgery in 1937. In addition to his efforts in graduate surgical education, he had a life-long interest in promoting both basic and clinical research. He led in the investigation of gastric, biliary, and pulmonary physiology, and more importantly, inspired and encouraged several young surgeons to obtain additional training in laboratory science. He was instrumental in sending Donald R. Webster to work on gastric physiology with Boris Babkin in 1928.

The tremendous advances in surgery during World War II set the scene for rapid developments in clinical and basic laboratory surgery in Montreal. Dr. Fraser B. Gurd established the McGill residency training program and developed the Department of Experimental Surgery and the Donner Building laboratories on campus. These were the beginnings of laboratory research in surgery at McGill University.

In Toronto, Professor Gallie was a leader in establishing a training program that placed academic surgeons in most university centers across Canada.

Wilder Penfield established the Montreal Neurological Institute on a solid base of clinical and surgical research. His basic surgical investigations led to the current surgical management of epilepsy and the training of several generations of neurosurgeons who have assumed positions of academic leadership throughout North America and the world.

William Bigelow in Toronto, Fraser Gurd, and Lloyd D. MacLean in Montreal, and Walter McKenzie in Alberta, led the development of research in university surgical departments in Canada.

Bigelow's innovations in the use of hypothermia and the development of effective cardiac pacing were landmarks in the progress of cardiovascular–thoracic surgery. The observations of Gurd and MacLean in the area of shock and low-flow states led to improved nutrition in the surgical patient and to an objective assessment of patients' immune status in many surgical illnesses.

The development of surgical science in Canada has been greatly influenced by the proximity of the United States. The opportunities afforded to Canadians to participate in the scientific forums of most major U.S. surgical societies was invaluable in the development of surgical science in Canada. Exposure to such giants in surgery as Blalock, Ravdin, Graham, Wagensteen, Francis Moore, and Gibbon left their mark on many of the young Canadian surgeons who have become today's surgical leaders.

It is paradoxical that virtually every university department of surgery in Canada conducted significant basic and clinical research in the 1980s, and concern for the status of surgical research in Canada reached a peak. This was reflected in three studies of research grants to clinical scientists. A research committee established by the Canadian Association of General Surgeons held a retreat in 1985, to examine the problems confronting surgical research in Canada and the possible solutions. On the basis of a preliminary questionnaire sent to university departments of surgery in Canada, Dr. John Duff was able to identify requests for $2 million to support research that was not approved for funding by granting agencies and applications for a further $500,000 for projects that were approved by peer review although funds were not available. The acute lack of research funds on both the federal and provincial level, identified at the Canadian Association of General Surgeons' research conference, was attributed to a general shortage of biomedical research funds and a particularly pronounced decline in the funds specifically allocated to surgical research.[2]

Twenty-five scientists identified five problems facing surgical research over the next decade.

1. *Failure to recruit the most scholarly individuals into surgical programs*. "Universities are not actively encouraging the most scholarly students to consider surgical careers. Instead, application for surgical training tends to be left to the individual, and those who might accomplish the most outstanding research results do not always apply."
2. *Training programs are not designed to train the surgical scientist*. "Cooperation from universities and department heads is necessary to ensure that provision is made within surgical training programs to encourage research and to train researchers."
3. *Surgical investigators are not held in high esteem by clinical surgeons*. "Practicing clinical surgeons, in general, do not yet realize the importance of surgical investigators to the profession as a whole, or to their own day-to-day work."
4. *A critical shortage of adequate funding of research and researchers*. "If more funding is not made available for surgical researchers in Canada, not only will general surgery be deprived of the new findings it needs to meet the patients' requirements, but Canada will lose its research talent to other countries, particularly the United States."
5. *Demands of research, teaching, and practice produce time constraints that cannot always be resolved*. "In Canada, research funding does not permit the researcher to devote his full-time attention to his investigations. This places a great limitation on research productivity, and makes it more difficult to acquire the excellence that can only be developed through sustained research activity."

In 1982 Dr. Pierre Bois established a second joint Task Force of the Medical Research Council (MRC) and the Royal College of Physicians and Surgeons of Canada [(RCPS(C)] to examine the apparent continuing decline in the number of clinicians engaged in research. This followed a similar study by Dr. Robert Salter[3] in 1981, whose committee emphasized the need for clinician–scientists and noted the problems in attracting, recruiting, training, and supporting them. Salter's study recommended an overall increase in funding for biomedical research and particularly for the support of M.D. scientists. It also urged the RCPS(C) to increase its emphasis on, and recognition of, the research component of specialty training.

An earlier MRC subcommittee, under the chairmanship of Dr. David Sackett,[4] had drawn attention to the need to improve the clinical application of new scientific knowledge. Sackett identified the lack of human and financial resources required for epidemiological studies and clinical trials as one of the most important barriers to the application of new knowledge to clinical care. Such expertise is almost nonexistent in Canadian departments of surgery.

In 1984 the joint task force, chaired by Dr. Henry B. Dinsdale, made several important recommendations.[5] The task force defined the "clinician–scientist as an M.D. who is engaged, both in research and patient-care" and noted that the amount of patient-care and responsibility will vary between individuals and disciplines, and may change during any one professional career. The task force emphasized the importance of continuing exposure of medical students to research and suggested an evaluation of the impact of summer research traineeships on the subsequent development of M.D. holders as basic researchers following graduation from medical school. Research training following the M.D. degree was also carefully assessed.

The Medical Research Council Fellowship program has been a major source of financial support for research training in Canada. Figure 54.1 shows the number of M.D. and Ph.D. applicants for MRC fellowships. The low success rate of 50% in the 1980s is undoubtedly a factor in encouraging medical graduates to consider a direct route to full-time practice. The task force stressed the importance of post-M.D. fellowships for research training remaining a high priority program for the Medical Council. It also recommended that MRC consider the establishment of a program to augment research training for all M.D.'s considering careers as clinician–scientists, which would include salary support for fellowship training and initial faculty appointments (5 years).

FIGURE 54.1. MRC fellowship applications.

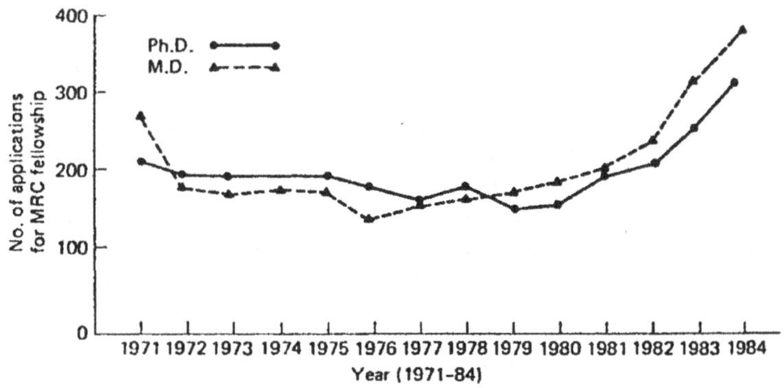

This generic program, designed to stimulate and encourage the development of clinician scientists in Canada, is now a reality. Its two phases are support during appropriate research training and salary support during the critical initial period of getting established as an independent investigator. This fellowship program requires a major commitment by the sponsoring university department, including a faculty appointment and an institutional guarantee of office and laboratory support, and protected time to allow the successful candidate to spend not less than 30 hours, or 75% of the investigative time, on research. (See Appendix II). This MRC program offers support similar to the training grants of the U.S. National Institutes of Health and will be invaluable to all Canadian departments of surgery.

The Task Force felt that the RCPS(C) must assume greater responsibility for encouraging research training in all medical and surgical specialties. It recommended that the accreditation of specialty training programs be made conditional on satisfactory levels of research activity and that all disciplines be encouraged to include at least one year of research training in their specialty training requirements.

The research committee of the Canadian Surgical Chairmen (Jean Couture, John Duff, and David S. Mulder) has recently completed a study on the level and funding of research activity in Canadian departments of surgery.

This study demonstrated a significant increase in the number of surgical residents completing formal research training. Fifteen candidates completed a Ph.D. in 1986–1987 compared to 3 in 1980; 30 surgical residents achieved an M.Sc. degree in 1986–1987 compared to 12 in 1980. Much of this increase in research training was in clinical epidemiology.

Funding for surgical research remained stable, with an increase from university and private sources, and a decrease from MRC. Surgical investigators received an estimated 4% of the global MRC budget, in 1981–1982, but only 2.2% in 1985–1986. Nonsurgical investigators (Ph.D.) in surgical departments increased in number and in their level of financial support.

The conclusions of this in-depth study of surgical research in Canada, compared to those of a similar study in 1967, are as follows.

1. There has been a global increase in the number of surgeons involved in research. Eight of sixteen departments of surgery do not have sufficient staff involved in research to support an optimal student learning experience or to meet minimal RCPS(C) standards.
2. Research training by surgical scientists has increased and improved in caliber.
3. The disparity of resources for surgical research continues among Canadian departments of surgery and also between surgical disciplines.
4. Levels of training for research fellows, in both basic and clinical research skills, have improved.
5. While global funding of surgical research has remained stable, funding by the MRC has declined over the past 5 years.
6. Clinical research by surgeons is still neglected in Canada—surgical epidemiology remains "the last frontier" of clinical epidemiology.

This report received the support of all the departments of surgery and all the surgical societies in Canada, and led to the formation of the Canadian Conjoint Council on Surgical Research at the Royal College meeting in Edmonton, in September 1989. Its objectives and mission statement are provided in Appendix I. This council will maintain a continuing inventory of surgical research activity in Canada and a special plenary session on "Training the Surgical Scientist" will take place during the Royal College meeting in 1990.

The Medical Research Council does not have a separate surgical committee; all grant applications are submitted to standing committees for adjudication of their scientific merit. The desirability of creating a separate surgical committee to review all grants submitted by surgical scientists has been debated for a long time, but the consensus, to date, is that all medical surgical scientists should compete solely on the basis of scientific merit. However, Pierre Bois, president of the Medical Research Council, has responded positively to a recommendation by the surgical chairman and has been most helpful in encouraging more surgical scientists to sit on MRC review panels. This increase in surgical representation on the various scientific committees will improve the peer review process for surgical grants.

Another source of concern is that, while surgical research is proceeding at varying levels of effectiveness in every department in Canada, current fee schedules, particularly in Quebec, exert growing pressure on surgeons to increase clinical productivity at the expense of research and teaching. Maintaining an environment for effective surgical research is the major challenge facing any surgical department chairman.

Attitudes

Canadians have a very positive attitude toward medical research in general. Public knowledge and understanding of specific advances in surgical research are increasing rapidly, quite apart from such dramatic developments as heart and liver transplantations. The public interest in biomedical research is convincingly demonstrated by its voluntary contribution of $77 million to biomedical research in Canadian faculties of medicine between 1985 and 1988. Well-organized lay groups not only participate in fund raising and volunteer care of patients, but also donate their expertise in management, budget control, computer science, etc. This type of support is invaluable, particularly when governmental health care funding is constantly being reduced.

Surgeons' attitude toward surgical research has changed dramatically over the past 10 to 15 years; surgical research is now significantly more important in the eyes of most practicing surgeons and trainees in surgery. The development of outstanding role models in every university department of surgery has been a highly significant factor in bringing about this change of attitude. To be such role models, surgical scientists have to maintain a high level of excellence in the clinical arena, provide research leadership, and be productive surgical investigators.

Funding of Surgical Research

Biomedical research expenditure in Canadian medical faculties from 1979–1980 to 1987–1988 has been documented in a study by Ryten[7]. Table 54.1 is a summary of the essential data, which confirm that the financial support of biomedical research comes mainly from federal or provincial governmental agencies. The Medical Research Council of Canada is the major funding agency at the federal level; the FRSQ (Fonds de la recherche en santé du Québec) functions at the provincial level in Quebec.

Ryten also emphasizes that the level of MRC funding, corrected (or indexed) for inflation, has been significantly eroded over the past 5 years, although it has been offset by increases from provincial sources. Private industry has also augmented its contribution to funding of biomedical research in Canada greatly over the past 5 years

TABLE 54.1. Expenditures for biomedical research by Canadian faculties of medicine (1980–1988) (thousands of Canadian dollars).

Source	1979–80	1981–82	1983–84	1985–88
Federal government	68,000	94,000	118,000	176,000
Provincial governments	15,500	43,000	63,000	92,500
Charitable agencies				
National	29,000	38,000	46,500	69,500
Provincial	7,000	6,000	6,000	8,000
Private industry	2,500	4,700	8,000	24,000
University sources	3,000	10,700	15,800	20,000
Foreign sources	8,200	10,750	9,700	25,500
Miscellaneous	8,400	5,600	12,000	4,500
	141,600	212,750	279,000	419,500

Modified with permission from Ryten E[7] (1989).

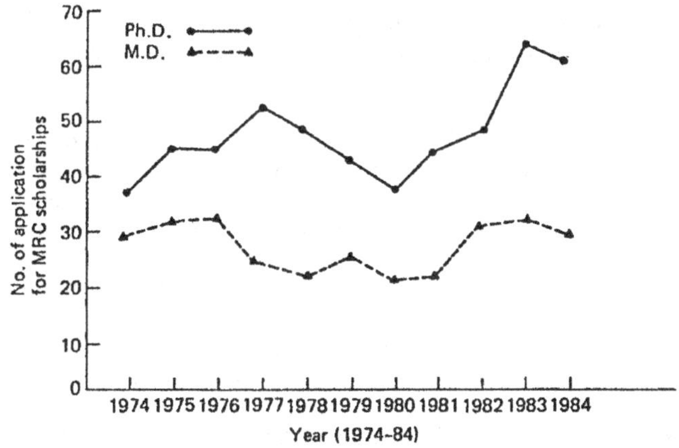

FIGURE 54.2. MRC scholarship applications.

(Table 54.1). (A surgeon was added to the MRC Committee on Committees in 1988–1989, and it is intended to add surgical scientists to all appropriate MRC standing committees.)

Overall, Canada spends approximately 0.11% of its gross domestic product on biomedical research and development.

MRC provides personnel support for research training through its fellowship program and for new and established investigators through its scholarship program (Fig. 54.2). The FRSQ provides similar support in Quebec. Operating grants, awarded by the MRC on the basis of annual competitions, usually provide for a 3-year period of support during which annual progress reports are required. The low success rate of applications for operating grants (25%) often discourages young surgical investigators and leads to interruptions in valuable research programs or a return to full-time clinical surgery.

Monies voluntarily donated by the public are channeled through such organizations as the Canadian Cancer Society and the Canadian Cardiovascular Society or their provincial counterparts. In addition to supporting basic and applied research on a competitive peer-reviewed basis, these organizations actively educate the public about the importance and results of biomedical research.

The funding of biomedical research by private industry in Canada comes primarily from the pharmaceutical sector. Much of this (relatively meager) support takes the form of "contract research" for specific clinical studies on the efficacy of particular drugs or antibiotics organized by university departments of medicine or surgery.

Virtually every department of surgery is provided with space and other indirect financial support for research activity that is channeled through hospitals and universities. These sources have grown in importance, particularly in the province of Quebec. Such support is frequently administered through the establishment of a research institute closely associated with a university teaching hospital. University salaries are an important but shrinking means of support for full-time clinician-scientists in every department of surgery in Canada. Identification of the precise level of support for research is often difficult because clinical activities, teaching, and research are so often blended in the daily lives of clinical scientists.

The MRC is the principal source of funding for research training for surgical residents, and its program is directed at individuals who wish to pursue 2 or 3 years of research training culminating in a Ph.D. So far, provincial ministries of health have not provided funding for shorter periods of research training during surgical residency.

A significant level of financial support for surgical research is generated by virtually every surgical department through the "excess earnings" of its full-time university staff, or donations made by individual academic surgeons. These funds are important to the chairman because they provide "seed money" for launching research projects and travel expenses for surgical residents and surgical scientists who present papers at scientific meetings. The current low fee schedules in Quebec have considerably reduced this form of financial support for surgical scholarship.

The Royal College of Physicians and Surgeons of Canada provides limited funds for research training in the form of scholarships, travel grants, and research awards. The Canadian Association of General Surgeons has established a scholarship program for surgical research and intends to generate funds to support surgical research in Canada, but the level of support currently available is small.

The Education of the Academic Surgeon

Most doctors who intend to be surgical residents now proceed through a straight internship following graduation from medical school at about age 25. The straight internship, combined with a variety of surgical rotations in the second year, constitutes a 2-year core training period that is designed to include exposure to the basic principles and techniques common to all surgical disciplines. On successful completion of this 2-year period, the candidate is eligible to write the examination in basic science in surgery set by the RCPS(C). This training meets the requirements for virtually every surgical discipline.

The McGill training program in general surgery is 5 years in length. The weekly schedule of the clinical surgical service is outlined in Table 54.2. A sabbatical-type year of surgical scholarship is encouraged following the 2-year core training. This year may be spent in the basic surgical laboratory, in a basic science department on the university campus, or in another hospital department such as the Department of Pathology. It allows the surgical resident time, not only to read and reflect, but also to acquire some of the methodological skills common to all research, such as statistical analysis and experimental design. Some surgical residents are extremely productive during this year, but the basic purpose is to ensure their active involvement in laboratory research and to give the program director an opportunity to select potential candidates for more intensive research training or Ph.D.'s in basic science disciplines.

Residents become eligible, after 2 further years of senior surgical responsibility, to try the written and oral examinations in general surgery of the Royal College. Successful candidates are allowed to become consultants in general surgery in community-based or university centers. University-based surgeons tend to acquire additional skills

TABLE 54.2. Weekly schedule of a general surgical resident (Montreal General Hospital).

	Monday	Tuesday	Wednesday	Thursday	Friday	Saturday	Sunday
06:00 07:00		Ward rounds Structural literature					
07:00 08:00	Ward rounds	Review	Ward rounds	Ward rounds	Ward rounds		
08:00	Outpatient clinic	Operating room	Operating room	Operating room	Operating room	Ward rounds	Ward rounds
11:00 12:00	Endoscopy	↓	Oncology rounds		Oncology rounds		
14:00 15:00	GI rounds, service chief rounds, ward work	↓	↓	Teaching afternoon: Formal ward rounds and all staff Informal case presentations Combined pathology, radiology rounds	↓	On call for all emergencies every third night and every third weekend	
16:00 17:00		Attending staff rounds	Mortality & morbidity rounds		Attending staff rounds		
17:00 18:00	Surgical Research seminar						
18:00			Basic science seminar				
19:00			Monthly practice oral examinations				

in more specialized areas of surgery or more research training in areas of particular personal interest. The certificates of special competence in vascular or thoracic surgery, recently approved, usually require 1 or 2 additional years of specialty training. Specialization in cardiovascular-thoracic surgery requires a minimum of 2 additional years of training beyond completion of the requirements in general surgery.

Every surgical trainee is required to participate in historical or prospective controlled clinical research studies under the supervision of a staff surgeon. Virtually every university department of surgery in Canada is well supported in terms of library facilities, computerized literature searches, and audiovisual aids.

Ample opportunities to present the results of studies are provided at surgical meetings throughout North America. Canadian surgical residents can present their research findings at the annual meeting of the Royal College or at any of its subspecialty meetings. The most prestigious achievement for a surgical resident is to have a paper accepted for presentation at the American College of Surgeons' forum on fundamental surgical research. Most surgical training programs sponsor an end-of-the-year surgical residents' day, to give recognition to both the clinical and basic research performed by residents during the preceding academic year. The considerable variation in the quantity and quality of research usually reflects the attitudes of the faculty in the various surgical discipline.

Few privileges and responsibilities can be greater than being the research adviser of a budding surgical scientist. A close one-to-one relationship develops during the period of at least a year when the research adviser is not only a role model but also the principal source of guidance in the formulation of a problem and how to undertake its rigorous investigation. Advisers must create an environment that is conducive to research by providing adequate laboratory facilities, effective personnel support, and advice on how to obtain operating funds and choose suitable didactic courses to supplement the research activities. It is imperative that, in the process of giving such support and guidance, the research adviser still allow the candidate sufficient flexibility to branch off into his or her own independent research.

Legal and Cultural Considerations

Although opposition to animal experimentation is growing in Canada, as it is elsewhere, public education has been effective in convincing most citizens of the value of basic surgical research and the direct contribution made to it by animal experimentation. Emphasis has been placed on the humane care and attention given to every animal used in a hospital laboratory. The rigid standards enforced by hospital research institutes and by Medical Research Council accreditation visits have done much to improve the standards of animal care throughout Canadian laboratories. The care of animals of virtually every university department of surgery is supervised by a veterinarian.

Interest in clinical trials in surgery is increasing in Canada, and the urgent need for improvement in the quality of such studies is evident. Sackett has drawn attention to the deficiency of basic epidemiological and statistical techniques in most Canadian clinical trials.[4] Canadian surgeons are awakening to the need to acquire such skills to enhance their success rate in competing for MRC grants. Most university hospitals now have well-established clinical trials committees that carefully examine the ethics of any human study. The value of clinical trials carried out in intensive care units, wards, and surgical operating rooms may be one of the most underdeveloped areas of academic surgeons in Canada. The unique opportunities these areas present for studying cost effectiveness in the delivery of surgical care have received minimal attention in Canada.

Conclusion

Surgical scholarship has made great progress in Canada since Osler's assessment in 1880. Basic surgical research has blossomed in many university centers since World War II, but disparities in the quality and quantity of surgical research in Canada's 16 medical schools is still cause for concern. As many as two-thirds of the university departments of surgery fail to meet the level of research activity required for accreditation by the Royal College of Physicians and Surgeons of Canada. Studies carried out by the Canadian Association of General Surgeons and the chairmen of surgical departments have identified a serious inadequacy in the funding for training in surgical research and the insecurity of personnel support for young surgical scientists.[7] Implementation of the recommendations of the MRC/RCPS Task Force (1984)[5,8] would go a long way toward guaranteeing the continued growth and development of surgical research and would allow the production of the individuals needed to fill the depleted ranks of surgical scientists.[9]

References

1. Cushing H. In: The life of Sir William Osler, Gryphon, ed. Birmingham, AL: The Classics of Medicine Library, 1982.
2. Cohen M. Chairman of Canadian Association of General Surgeons Research Committee. Personal communication.
3. Salter RB. Report of the Medical Research Council Committee on Clinician Scientists in Canada. MRC, June 1981.
4. Sackett D. The application of biomedical research to health care. MRC, December 1980.
5. Dinsdale H. Medical Research Council Royal Joint Task Force on Clinician Scientists. MRC, 1984.
6. Frederickson DS. Biomedical research in the 1980s. N Engl J Med 1981;304:509–17.
7. Ryten E. Financing the research of Canadian faculties of medicine: comparison and trends. Assoc. Can. Med. Coll. Forum (1989)3:1–11.
8. MacBeth RA. The present status of surgical research in Canada. Ann R Coll Phys Surg 1968; 1:296–302.
9. Roncari DAK, Salter RB, Till JE, Loey FH. Is the clinician scientist really vanishing? Encouraging results from a Canadian Institute of Medical Science. Can Med Assoc J 1984;130:977–79.
10. Mulder DS. Entre Amis. Presidential address, 45th Annual Meeting of the Association for the Surgery of Trauma, Boston. Published in the Journal of Trauma, 1986.

Appendix I
A Proposal to Establish a Canadian Conjoint Council on Surgical Research

The goal of this council is to enhance the quality and quantity of surgical research in Canada and thus improve the quality of care provided to all surgical patients.

Founding Organizations

1. Canadian Surgical Chairmen.
2. All national surgical societies as defined by the Royal College of Physicians and Surgeons.

Mission

1. To foster the development of research as an essential and valued activity of university departments of surgery.
2. To develop an appreciation of the importance of surgical research within our medical schools, provincial and national granting agencies, provincial and federal government agencies, and the public in general.
3. To establish an inventory of the current status of surgical research in all surgical disciplines in Canada using the recent questionnaire of Canadian Surgical Chairmen as a base.
4. To develop methods to improve *research training* at the basic and applied level in each surgical discipline.
5. To support the peer review systems of MRC and the other granting agencies and ensure that there is appropriate surgical input into policy development and implementation.
6. To establish educational programs designed to improve the quality of surgical grants.
7. To promote development of clinical research in all surgical disciplines, including multicenter clinical trials with appropriate methodological design.
8. To encourage development of surgical research related to health care policy and delivery (e.g., quality assurance and outcome analysis).
9. To identify other mechanisms to increase the present level of funding for surgical research and to continue to encourage innovation and creativity in all surgical disciplines.
10. To create an inventory for sources of both personnel and operating funds that would be accessible by all departments of surgery and all surgical disciplines.
11. To encourage the research committee of each surgical discipline to identify and prioritize specific problems for investigation.
12. To promote development of a national reward system for excellence in surgical research at the undergraduate and graduate education levels.

Liaison with Other Organizations

1. The Royal College of Physicians and Surgeons of Canada. (Formal request for a position on the RCPS Research Council.)
2. The Conjoint Council on Surgical Research in the United States which has become a standing committee of the American College of Surgeons (Education and Research). (Canadian representation on this ACS Committee named in 1989.)
3. The Medical Research Council (the need for a surgical scientist as part of the permanent staff).

Appendix II: Medical Research Council of Canada Clinician–Scientist Program*

290. In order to stimulate and encourage the development of clinician–scientists in Canada, [the Medical Research] Council [of Canada] offers a new program with two phases: research training and the initial establishment of the clinician scientist as an independent practitioner–researcher. The program is a continuous one whereby a successful candidate receives support for research training to be followed by salary support. One important aspect of this program will be the strength of institutional support provided to the candidate throughout. This program is offered in addition to other existing MRC programs in order to address the special needs of clinicians prepared to make a substantial commitment to research.

Description

291. The Clinician–Scientist award is offered to highly qualified and motivated clinicians who have been identified by a Canadian medical school as having strong potential to become clinician–scientists. At the time of application, the candidates will have recently completed their specialty clinical training (or will shortly do so), and are undertaking, or intend to undertake, research training followed by a career as a clinician–scientist.

Commitment of the Nominating Institution

292. The nominating medical school or affiliated institution must offer successful candidates a faculty or equivalent position as a clinician–scientist at the completion of the training, subject to satisfactory performance in the research training period. This commitment is required at the time of the initial application and with each subsequent request for the renewal of support. The institution must be prepared, at each renewal stage, to confirm a plan concerning their commitment of a full-time faculty position for the clinician–scientist. During the second phase, when the Council provides a contribution to the salary support, both the candidate and the institution must make a commitment that not less than 30 hours per week (75% of the candidate's time) will be spent on research).

Eligibility Requirements

293. A candidate must hold an M.D. degree and be within one year of completing specialty training. The candidate may also hold a Ph.D. degree but this is not a requirement.

Duration of Support

294. During the first phase of the award, the candidate must undertake training, and will be supported for a minimum of 3 years and a maximum of 6 years.
295. During the second phase, the candidate will receive 3 years of support, renewable once for a total of 6 years of support. Support is designed to recognize the needs for clinical and research activity, bearing in mind a 75% time commitment to research.

Location

296. In the training phase, the award is tenable in Canada or abroad. The recipient is encouraged to seek training in more than one location. The salary support phase award is tenable in Canadian medical schools or their affiliated institutions.

New Applications

297. Candidates must use the application package MRC 36. Candidates being nominated for the award must collect and submit all material required to complete the application package which consists of (a) forms MRC 36 and MRC 18, (b) official transcripts of the candidate's complete academic record, (c) supporting letters from at least four sponsors, and (d) a supporting letter from the dean of the faculty of medicine of the nominating university.
298. Candidates may be called upon to present themselves for an interview by the review committee.

Closing Date for Applications

299. The closing date for receipt of complete application packages is November 1. Late or incomplete applications will not be considered.

*Excerpted from the *MRC Grants and Awards Guide.* (Applicant instructions for a government grant applications form.)

Renewal Applications

300. Renewal applications are required at 2-year intervals throughout the training phase.
301. When applying for the continuation of a contribution to salary support, candidates must provide information on their research and clinical expertise and on their research plans. In addition, the nominating institution must provide details of the facilities and equipment to be provided, the measures taken to protect the candidate's research time, and the efforts made to enhance the candidate's clinical and research activities.
302. Although it is not a requirement, the candidate may establish contacts with a research mentor to assist him or her through the initial phases of a research career. Plans by the institution and/or the candidate to develop contacts with such a mentor should be described in the application.
303. Renewal for a further 3-year period will be based upon satisfactory research progress.

Closing Date for Renewal Applications

304. The deadline date for receipt of renewal applications is November 1. Renewal application forms will be sent to the awardees by the MRC as required.

Stipends

305. The value of the training phase of the award is related to the amount of experience of the applicant since obtaining the professional degree. Internships and residencies are taken into consideration but not time spent in private practice. Stipends are paid in Canadian dollars and are subject to income tax.

Contributions to Salary

306. In the salaried phase, the recipient will receive a contribution to his or her salary consistent with the MRC Salary Scale for Independent Investigators.

Research and Travel Allowance

307. A research allowance for $3350 is provided for each year of the training phase of the award. This sum is made available to supervisors, through the institution concerned, to be used at their discretion for the purchase of materials and supplies, for travel to scientific meetings, or to meet other research costs incurred by awardees. These funds cannot, however, be used to pay course fees on behalf of the awardee.
308. For the first 3 years of the second phase, the MRC will provide a research allowance of $40,000 per annum.

Earnings from Other Sources

309. Awardees during the training phase are allowed to undertake up to 10 hours per week of clinical work during their research training, and to receive reimbursement. The clinical work must be at defined times, and never "on call." This, however, is the only other remuneration the awardee may receive. No other major scholarship or stipend support may be held at the same time as the MRC award.
310. During the second phase the awardee may receive local remuneration for clinical work in amounts consistent with institutional policies.

Transfer of Award

311. The second phase of the award cannot be transferred to another institution within the first 3 years. Subsequently, applications for transfer must be made in the form of a letter to the Council from the awardee stating the reasons for the transfer and the opportunities presented. Accompanying the letter should be support from the new institution detailing its commitments to the awardee. A letter from the current institution acknowledging the transfer is also required.

55

Contributions from France

J.-H. Alexandre

Surgical research in France is carried out principally at the largest university-affiliated hospitals. Most of the major French surgical departments have active research programs. The results of research activities in the surgical specialties are the mainstay of national meetings and international conferences conducted in France under the sponsorship of European surgical associations such as the *Association Française de Chirugie* (3000 members), the Plastic Surgery Society, the National Vascular Surgery College, the Bone Surgery Study Group, the Hand Study Group, the International Organization for Statistical Studies of Esophageal Disease, and the Research Group on Abdominal Wall Studies (GREPA). Each surgical department organizes at least one convocation annually for the presentation of the results of innovations and surgical accomplishments.

Since 1960, experimental surgery chairs associated with anatomy and physiology departments have been created as an adjunct to surgical services at the teaching hospitals. Most hospital-based surgeons complete a rotation in the Department of Anatomy during internship, comprised of lectures to medical students, cadaver dissections, and fundamental research in surgical anatomy. I followed this path in my training, and eventually became professor of anatomy as well as professor of surgery.

In addition to collaborative research with anatomists and other basic scientists, surgical research projects are carried out in our community in conjunction with biostaticians, radiologists, ultrasonographers, and other clinical scientists.

Surgical research provided the basis for Lortat-Jacob's successful completion of the first right hepatic lobectomy, Dubost's replacement of aortic aneurysm by prosthesis, and Henry's successful completion of a cardiac transplantation in a recipient still alive 20 years following surgery. The development of cardiac valve bioprostheses by Carpentier and hip prostheses by Judet and Merle d'Aubigné, and the transplantation of the kidney by de Gaudart d'Allaines, heart by Cabrol, liver by Bismuth, and pancreas by Dubernard are among France's contributions to surgery that arose from research programs. Surgery by laparoscopy, born in France in 1970, is now taught as an alternative to classical pelvic and biliary tract surgery.

The Surgeon's Curriculum and the Role of Research

Internship has a somewhat different meaning in France from its traditional understanding in many Western countries. The internship (*internat*) lasts 5 years, somewhat like a general surgical residency program in North America. A typical week for a French surgical resident is outlined in Table 55.1. It is followed by 2 to 6 years as an assistant to the chief of the surgical department, as occurs in the German, English, Swedish, and Japanese systems, among others. This latter category may soon be replaced by the designation *praticien hospitalier*, a more permanent position achieved after 6 years of internship and successful completion of examinations, subject to the approval of the chief of service.

Candidates for surgical training are selected for the residency on the basis of their standings in highly competitive examinations taken by candidates between the ages of 22 and 27 years, and after 4 or 5 years of medical school. From the beginning of the residency, the surgeon-in-training finds a place on a research team on a voluntary basis and commits one or two afternoons a week to attending a laboratory in experimental surgery, transplantation or, less frequently, anatomy, immunology, or physiology.

TABLE 55.1. Weekly schedule for a French surgical resident.

	Monday	Tuesday	Wednesday	Thursday	Friday	Saturday	Sunday
08:00	Ward rounds	Oncological study group (discussion) of neoplastic cases	Ward rounds	Report meeting Discussion of new cases New schedule	Ward rounds	ICU ward rounds	ICU ward rounds
08:30	Grand rounds (60 beds)						
09:00						Student teaching Lectures by assistants or chiefs	
10:00		Special outpatient clinic			Special outpatient clinic		
11:00	Operation						
12:00	Schedule meeting with students, nurses, etc.	Operations	Operations	Operations		Gastroenterological conference, once a month	
	Emergency operations					Emergency operations	Emergency operations
14:00	Surgery teaching techniques Film discussions, etc.				Special outpatient clinic		
15:00							
16:00	Mortality conference						
17:00				Meeting with other hospitals, once a month			
18:00		Bibliography meeting					
19:00	ICU ward rounds	ICU ward rounds	ICU ward rounds	ICU ward rounds	ICU ward rounds		
20:00			Emergencies–Consultations and operations				Rounds

Approximately one out of four residents seeks further, more concentrated training in surgical research. The future cardiac, hepatic, or transplantation surgeon has a higher probability of linking his training directly to research. Because of the unresolved technical and biological problems in these fields, there seems to be tangible benefit for the candidate's future practice and career if he achieves proficiency in research.

Residents who do not pursue training in surgical research may choose programs leading to a university certificate of proficiency in statistics, anatomy, or legal or occupational medicine. For those who pursue a career in research, original experimental or basic scientific publications definitely promote the advancement of their academic careers. The quality of the work, the number of publications, and the reputation of the journals in which results are published are important considerations in advancement.

The amount of time spent on research during surgical training has been variable in the past. In 1985 a general decision was reached that each surgeon who seeks to be a hospital physician will dedicate one full year of his residency to surgical research. Those who envision a university career may spend a longer period leading to a specialized diploma. A resident must spend at least one year of his surgical training in research to learn how to set up a project, including formulation of the original idea, obtaining financial support, assembling a research team, and learning to work both as a team member, and competitively in the field. Statistics and other related skills should be developed during this period, which should be between the third and fourth year of the residency. It seems desirable that the researcher be exempted from clinical work for this period. When integrated into a clinical unit, the surgeon who has received adequate training in surgical research can devise other projects and will be sufficiently competent in the research process to direct a team or supervise it personally one or two afternoons a week.

In my opinion, a steady commitment to research should be maintained throughout the university surgeon's academic career—that is, during residency and assistantship, and later as head of a surgical department. This commitment need not be as binding for those destined for community hospitals or private practice.

There were approximately 4500 surgeons in France in 1989, among 170,000 physicians in a total population of 55 million. Sixty percent of surgeons work in the private sector, 15% work part time in hospitals, and 35% are full-time hospital surgeons. The majority of full-time hospital surgeons are university surgeons who are committed to a career that includes surgical research, teaching, and patient care.

Although surgical research is theoretically possible in a large number of hospital centers in France, it is really the prerogative of university centers. These centers have the staff and equipment needed to conduct surgical research, such as laboratory facilities, support personnel, and access to computerized data bases of the medical literature, to assist in the accumulation of a bibliography of French and foreign articles.

The surgeon-in-training in surgical research has the opportunity to present his work at the French Surgical Association's Annual Research Forum. There are a variety of other annual meetings in France and Europe where research data can be presented after appropriate committee review. Nearly all these meetings use English as the common language, even now in France. Accordingly, a foreign exchange program appears highly desirable for the surgeon training for a university career. We consider it mandatory that a French researcher spend at least 6 months in a country where he will be able to perfect his mastery of English.

The conclusions of a recent (1990) consensus conference about a European surgical curriculum have been presented to a European Economic Community committee. The goal is to establish the same internship in all EEC countries, beginning with an M.D.—same schedules, stages of the same duration, same controls, and possibilities for exchange. The training would be divided into two parts: general surgery (3 to 4 years) and specialization (2 to 3 years with 6 months in surgical research).

Animal experimentation is conducted in French laboratories under ethical surveillance. The public is sensitive to animal suffering, but for the most part accepts the need for experimentation on animals. The advantage of using animals for development of proficiency in surgical procedures is well illustrated by the Amphithéâtre d'Anatomie des Hôpitaux de Paris, Fer à Moulin directed by Professor Cabrol in Paris. This special institute for teaching surgery and anatomy provides the setting for learning advanced techniques in surgery from films, videos, demonstrations, and direct personal experience performing new surgical procedures on experimental animals. Through this mechanism, new advanced techniques of surgery can be made available to the population at a high level of efficiency through effective use of a surgical research laboratory. For example, the techniques of replacement of the ascending thoracic aorta with coronary reimplantation, and the regimen of immunosuppression currently used throughout the world for cardiac transplantation, were developed in the experimental surgical laboratory in France by Cabrol and his colleagues in Lyons and Marseille.

Research institutes offer the only full-time research opportunities for surgeons. Nearly all surgical researchers are paid by hospitals or universities as full-time university hospital employees to fulfill the threefold objective stated in the Debre law of 1960: caring for patients, teaching, and conducting research. Research objectives and funding are determined by national granting agencies, such as the National Scientific Institute for Medical Studies and Research (INSERM), which provides some limited funding for surgical studies, and the National Center for Scientific Research (CNRS), which is more oriented toward basic science.

Funds are also awarded from the 24 universities in France, and from municipalities through public assistance. For example, some of the support for surgical research at my hospital comes from the Public Assistance of Paris—an organization employing more than 90,000 people, which supervises the management and funding of 50 hospitals in Paris. At *Assistance Publique de Paris* a special department of research has been created, with a budget: a foundation collects money from industry and private sources, and funds are awarded to a selection of the best research projects.

Detailed research proposals are submitted to these bodies for support of research through an established research institute such as Gustave Roussy in Paris-Ville, the Curie Institute in Paris, the René Huguenin Cancer Center in Saint-Cloud, or the International Center for the Fight Against Cancer in Lyons or Montpellier. The choice of a research subject for the young surgical researcher depends, somewhat, on the availability of funding from the research institutes and on the chief of service, who serves in a supervisory role, assisting and establishing research goals, and obtaining research grants, work spaces, manpower, and help in the analysis of data and presentation of results. The chief of service can oversee a number of researchers involved in several projects and is responsible for the quality and quantity of the work performed. The government has proposed a more complex integrated structure to combine autonomous surgical units under large surgical departments, whose chief and departmental council will determine policy and report to the university dean to ensure that the goals of teaching and research activity are attained.

Funding for Surgical Research

Overall, France spends approximately 0.18% of its gross domestic product on biomedical research and development. Government funding is responsible for the bulk of research in France, but the allocation for surgery remains a very small fraction of the research budget. In addition to the CNRS, INSERM, the Ministry of Welfare, and the Ministry of Education, municipal governments allocate money for research. It is noteworthy that 20% of the research budget allocated by the City of Paris is set aside for surgical research projects.

Certain university departments or hospitals receive private, anonymous donations for research, but the funds from these sources are relatively limited compared to their counterparts in the United States. Some pharmaceutical companies have participated increasingly, since 1985, in research projects involving their products (e.g., anticoagulants, antibiotics, analgesics) when the substance under evaluation will be the object of upcoming marketing campaigns. Most funding from pharmaceutical companies goes to their own research departments or to departments of internal medicine, because surgeons use only a few highly specialized drugs.

Some surgical research units have been forced to develop private sources of funding to support scientific projects and travel to scientific meetings.

In some hospital centers, academic surgeons or professors are asked for personal donations to create bursaries to support research. Curiously, tax credits are not allowed for such gifts. Funds or facilities for foreign surgical researchers to visit French laboratories are minimal. The Ministry of Research plans to establish a system of bursaries for exchange programs.

French surgical research, though embattled for priority and funding, has a proud record of accomplishment and a prospect of continued contribution to the advancement of surgical science.

56

Traditions and Transitions in Germany

H. Troidl and E.A.M. Neugebauer

This description of surgical research in the Federal Republic of Germany is the expression of the authors' personal views, rather than a survey of all institutions. It is mainly based on the experience of the senior author (H.T.) during several years of training at three different university surgical departments (Munich, Marburg, and Kiel) and as the incumbent of the second chair of surgery at the University of Cologne.

Brendel[1] describes three levels of surgical research.

1. Basic research that attempts to gain basic knowledge without regard to its applicability to man.
2. Applied research that explores possible new treatments using all the available methods of research.
3. Clinical research, the goal of which is to extend our knowledge of disease and to test new methods of diagnosis and treatment.

Surgical research is conducted at all three levels only in university departments of surgery, but not always in each of them. In West Germany, including West Berlin, university departments retain the old, traditional structure, generally with one responsible chairman heading the entire department. These university departments provide surgical care for patients and engage in teaching and research. The chairmen of such departments usually hold their positions for as long as 25 years and play the important and indispensable role of bridging all three commitments.

The chairman or "Ordinarius" is expected to operate almost every day and to have a wide-ranging practical knowledge of surgery.[2] To be selected for a chair requires broad training in all aspects of operative surgery and a reputation for both surgical skill and scientific activity. In the final selection process, a candidate must demonstrate practical abilities by performing surgery—sometimes in front of a commission. Consequently, a narrow focus in clinical surgery is not desirable for academic surgeons-in-training. The chairman is also expected to have the administrative skills required to run a large department, even though his previous experience generally provides little preparation for such responsibilities. The German Association of Surgeons (Berufsverband) has recently responded to this need by implementing management courses in hospital administration, personal guidance, and teaching for incoming surgical chairmen.

German surgeons qualify for an academic appointment through a process called "habilitation" derived from the Latin word *habilitas*: aptitude, ability. The requirements for habilitation include

1. An academic thesis on a surgical subject, often with the collaboration of a basic scientist or department of experimental surgery.
2. A general reputation in the field covered by the thesis, documented by a significant number of publications in peer-reviewed international journals and invited lectures.
3. General ability to perform surgery at a high level of technical excellence.

All of this is evaluated by the chairman of the Department of Surgery, who has the full responsibility for the candidate.

Because the traditional chairs have such extensive responsibilities, some have established more or less independent theoretical or experimental units to strengthen the traditional research responsibilities. The universities of Munich, Cologne,

Heidelberg, and Marburg pioneered the development of this approach to surgical research in Germany. The head of the theoretical or experimental division has usually had special training or basic education in a biomedical science, such as biochemistry or physiology. In addition, the research director has a special program of education in human medicine to fulfill departmental needs and to address broad issues of surgical research from preoperative risk analysis to postoperative follow-up.

Occasionally, the small size and relative independence of these experimental surgery units make it difficult for clinical surgeons to pursue their own research ideas. As a result, some surgical chairmen have established their own experimental groups in addition to the existing surgical research divisions—sometimes without any help, sometimes in cooperation with scientists from such fields as anatomy, pathology, chemistry, and biochemistry. This approach has not satisfied most surgeons, because cooperating scientists are not primarily interested in solving principally clinical problems.

One solution to this dilemma has been the so-called Marburg Experiment in Surgical Research, a new concept of surgical research started in 1970 by creating a Division of Experimental Surgery and Pathological Biochemistry at the Surgical Clinic in Marburg and then developing it into an Institute of Theoretical Surgery[3] (see Section I, Chapter 6). In this novel concept, clinical surgeons and basic scientists work together by *integration*—not merely by cooperation—in small working teams on a long-term basis to undertake joint exploration of scientific and clinical problems. "*Theoretical surgery*" is defined as a system for nonoperative decision analysis and for clinical and basic research support for surgery. It is established in only a few universities.

The attitude of the German population toward surgical research is somewhat indifferent or skeptical. Much of the public has no idea that surgical research exists, except when a sensational surgical event, such as the implantation of an artificial heart, attracts media coverage. There are virtually no spontaneous or organized financial campaigns to support surgical research. The outstanding exception is the *Deutsche Krebshilfe*, a public initiative founded to raise money for cancer research, treatment, and rehabilitation.

Information on surgical research in the media is rather scant and naive. In this atmosphere, clinical trials must be carried out very carefully, if at all. We must deal with the suspicion that we are "experimenting on the patient" by devising ways to inform patients about planned treatment or research without increasing their anxiety. There is a tension between patients' wish to be fully informed and their not wanting to be frightened by undesired detail.

Some surgeons are suspicious of clinical trials and mock them, because of the requirement that there be an explicit expression of doubt concerning the best choice of medical treatment. The admission by a surgeon of any element of doubt in his decision making is regarded unfavorably. "A surgeon should always know everything!" is the traditional expectation of the general public. But, only God is omniscient!

Even in universities, surgical research is not as highly valued as surgical practice. Scientists in other disciplines take a critical view of surgeons as researchers. The chance of acceptance by a university of an academic thesis about purely clinical issues in everyday surgery is severely limited or nonexistent! For a thesis to be acceptable, the young surgeon must spend a lot of time in a theoretical institute, sometimes only to add a "scientific veneer" to the thesis project.

Even in university departments of surgery, the attitude toward surgical research may not always be enthusiastic. Many professors of surgery think of surgical research as a major part of their responsibility, have done serious work, and are keenly interested. Advancement depends more on numbers of papers and presentations than on original ideas and their careful analysis and validation. Sometimes, interest in research ceases with the acquisition of the title of professor. In spite of their administrative burdens, masses of students, and persistent struggles with administrations, most chairmen remain enthusiastic about new ideas and aware of the worldwide influence Germany continues to exert in such areas as gastric surgery, orthopedics, vascular surgery, and endoscopy.

Surgical research certainly does not rank first in the minds of practicing surgeons. "Practical experience" and "excellent technique" are at the top. As a result, German technical standards are very high in any comparison among countries. This applies to the smaller hospitals, the universities, and the larger community hospitals.

Outside the university departments, the academically oriented surgeon is regarded with some suspicion and frequently encounters the view that if he is scholarly, he may be able to analyze surgical problems, but unable to operate! Stelzner summarized this attitude as: "The nightingale doesn't win a prize at the poultry competition." It is important to recognize that there can be excesses in either direction, including the possibility that some practical surgeons may employ the best techniques but perform the wrong operations.

TABLE 56.1. DFG grant history of general surgical departments.

Year	Grant applications submitted n (DM)	Grant applications approved n	Grant applications withdrawn n (DM)	Percentage of requested sums approved
1983	36	26	1	
	(5,593,100)		(115,496)	50.7
1984	46	32	3	
	(5,160,355)		(49,225)	51.4
1985*	28	22	3	
	(4,754,137)		(12,758)	52.7

*January 1, 1985–August 31, 1985.

The attitude of German surgical residents toward surgical research is not different from those in other Western countries. Few enter a university surgical department to carry out research exclusively; most choose a department on the basis of its ability to teach them good surgical practice. If, along the way, they are given an opportunity to take part in a research program, they gladly embrace it because research productivity leads to an academic title and the possibility of a better position later on.

Research Funding

Overall, the Federal Republic of Germany spends approximately 0.28% of its gross domestic product on biomedical research and development. After the prosperous 1960s, financial support for research began to diminish slowly in Germany. General availability of resources is exemplified by what has been happening in our department at Cologne.

The university provides each surgical chairman with an annual budget derived from a grant from the provincial (Bundesland) government to carry out teaching and research. The amount of such budgets varies considerably among different provincial governments and universities. This annual amount is independently managed by the chairmen to support research and teaching activities. The experimental unit of the second chair for surgery in Cologne comprises 5 academic professional research colleagues and 14 assistants employed on a full-time basis for research. The annual provincial budget of 60,000 deutschmarks means that only DM 12,000 (U.S. $7500) per investigator per year is provided by current university funding. Flexible research funds are even less, because of the general administrative responsibilities of the departments. This example shows how small the basic budget for surgical research is, and how important it is to raise additional money from federal and private sources.

Except for university grants, and some industry and private money, funds are awarded on the basis of competitive research grant applications for the support of specific research projects. Most are reviewed by a commission that requires progress reports at defined intervals during the grant period and for competitive renewal. From 1975 through 1985, the German Research Foundation (Deutsche Forschungsgemeinschaft: DFG) received from 38 to 51 grant applications from surgical departments; approximately 50% of the requested sums were approved and funded (Table 56.1).

Local conferences and workshops are financed by the surgical societies (e.g., the Lower Rhine–Westphalian Surgical Society) from their membership dues with additional support from industry, or exclusively by industry. Private donations are a rare source of research support.

Local community budgets for hospitals provide no money for research; they cover patient care only. Travel expenses to conferences inside and outside Germany must be financed personally or by seeking sponsors from industry. As an investigation of a provincial ministry found out, there has been remarkable variance in the allocation of university-distributed federal research money to different colleagues at the seven universities of North Rhine–Westphalia ranging from DM 27,000 to DM 6000! It might be interesting to correlate these allocations with a citation or productivity index.

The same analysis could make interesting international comparisons—for example, funds per researcher per entry in the Citation Index, number of doctoral theses, number of supervised Ph.D.'s, or number of publications in respected journals.

Training

The educational programs for a clinical surgeon and a surgeon with scientific ambitions are outlined in Table 65.1 (see Chapter 65 below). In West

TABLE 56.2. Weekly schedule.

Time	Monday	Tuesday	Wednesday	Thursday	Friday	Sat/Sun
A.M.						
7:00	Ward Rounds	Ward Rounds	Ward Rounds	Ward Rounds	Ward Rounds	
7:30	Report/Meeting	Report/Meeting	Report/Meeting	Report/Meeting	Report/Meeting	
8:00	I.C.U. Ward Rounds	I.C.U. Ward Rounds	General Surgery Research Meeting	I.C.U.	I.C.U. Ward Rounds	Ward Rounds
8:30	Operations	Operations	Operations	Operations	Operations	Report/I.C.U.–Ward Rounds (9:15)
	Special Out-Patient Clinics	Special Out-Patient Clinics	Special Out-Patient Clinics	Special Out-Patient Clinics	Special Out-Patient Clinics	
P.M.						
2:00		Chief's Ward Rounds				Non-elective Operations
2:30	Operation–schedule mtg.		Operation–schedule mtg.	Operation–schedule mtg.	Operation–schedule mtg.	
4:30	X-Ray mtg.		Lectures and Grand Rounds	X-Ray mtg.	X-Ray mtg.	
5:00	Report of Op/Gen. mtg.			Report of Op/Gen. mtg.	Report of Op/Gen. mtg.	
5:30	Interdisc. Angiology Conf.			Journal Club & Case-F Conf.		
6:00	I.C.U. Ward Rounds	I.C.U. Ward Rounds	I.C.U. Ward Rounds	I.C.U. Ward Rounds	I.C.U. Ward Rounds	I.C.U. Ward Rounds
6:30	Interdisc. Gastroenterology Conference					

Germany, there is no uniform concept for the training of an academic surgeon. The ideas vary from university to university, within a single university at any time, and from time to time. There is no universal agreement about when surgeons should obtain research training, and whether they should do only experimental research, only clinical research, or a combination of both. We prefer that a young colleague spend 1 to 2 years in a basic scientific discipline before becoming a resident at a surgical university department. It is certainly advantageous for the assistant to be able to communicate in an additional language, such as English or French.

Young residents in our surgical university clinic often join an ongoing research project in the Department of Theoretical Surgery as a member of a small working team. They devote a limited amount of time during the week's routine to it, and gradually progress under the guidance and the help of the Department of Theoretical Surgery to their own projects—which may eventually lead to habilitation.

Time Management

Adequate time is an essential precondition for research. The schedule in our department is fairly typical for Germany (Table 56.2). The need for efficiency in patient care leaves little time for research; our calculations indicate that we need two more assistants to staff our clinical program without including time for research! After a 6-hour operating day and taking care of a ward, a surgeon has difficulty in changing his focus of concentration from a bleeding gastric ulcer or a difficult anastomosis to the planning of an experiment or discussion of scientific problems with freshness and enthusiasm. The toll of night duty, usually twice per week, is another problem surgical residents must cope with. In addition, there is the German compulsion to master surgery from head to toe. Possible solutions to these problems include arranging days without an elective operating list, providing a larger number of residents, granting some residents a complete exemption from clinical obligations for some period of months, and a combination of these, with the establishment of an experimental unit adapted to the local situation. Setting aside an additional day without operations will require a reduction in the bed occupancy, which, in our country, would bring a reduction in budget and in surgical personnel. On the other side, an increased number of residents reduces the ratio of cases per surgeon and prolongs the length of residency training because a resident needs a defined number of operations to take the examination for certification as a surgeon.

Debate continues in Germany about the ideal way to combine research and surgical training. Some believe that surgeons should be out of daily clinical practice for a year or two to carry out their research projects. Others argue that surgeons, and especially junior surgeons, need constant surgical practice to develop and maintain their skills. This need is comparable to the situation of a serious athlete who must work out continuously to "stay in shape."

A novel approach to this dilemma is offered by the Marburg Experiment, which allows integration of the clinical surgeon's skills and clinical knowledge into a small working team with a theoretical surgeon for continuing scientific collaboration (*integration concept*). In Munich, Berlin, Freiburg, Würzburg, and Heidelburg, departments of experimental surgery or surgical research utilize a different model; they normally run their own research projects, but offer the surgeons a "work bench" where they can work on their own research project for a certain amount of time (*cooperation concept*).

What is specific about the Marburg Experiment? *Integration* is the key word because, without it, a gap generally develops between clinical surgery and research. The legitimate independence of the theoretical or basic scientist does not always lead to greater efficiency in surgical research. Professor Heberer, who established the Cologne surgical research department, commented on this in 1974, as follows: "The contact of the researchers with the clinic can be loosened by institutionalization. As a result, special fields can become the primary foci to the extent that creative impulses arising from clinical practice are not accepted any more."

Surgeons look for other collaboration if there are no receptors within their own surgical research department. This has the effect of isolating the researchers from the clinicians. The Marburg Experiment requires the basic scientists, as theoretical surgeons, to accept responsibility for participation in medical decision making, even for individual patients. They are permanent partners of the clinical surgeons and are involved in everyday clinical questions. The theoretical surgeon must help to answer such questions as "How important is a gastrin assay for the patient in this bed?"

Recent advances in experimental methodology are brought into the department by the theoretical surgeon, such as methods of medical decision making for diagnosis and prognosis of diseases, design and conduct of controlled clinical trials, meta-analysis, different methods of clinimetrics (risk and causality analysis, technology assessment, assessment of postoperative quality of life and pain, etc.), and the application of computers in surgery for documentation and quality assurance. The theoretical surgeon in the Marburg arrangement also assumes a major responsibility for administration of both clinical and experimental research. A diagram with the different tasks of the theoretical surgery department established at the Second Department of Surgery in Cologne is shown in Chapter 5, Fig. 5.3.

The "small working team" is an essential feature of the Marburg Experiment. We demand the fullest exchange of ideas and integration of clinical and basic research, not only until surgeons achieve a habilitation degree, but for life. The "small working team" is characterized by the following:

Purpose: integration of clinical and theoretical research on the basis of long-term, personal, and practical cooperation.

Composition: one theoretical surgeon, one or two clinical surgeons, one technical assistant, one or two students.

Assignments: a weekly meeting; planning and discussing experiments; systematic follow-up; special clinical examinations; conduct of experiments; special services or projects for the department.

The discussion and exchange of information gleaned from the literature form part of the planning and discussion of experiments. The "small working team" jointly examines patients included in clinical trials for systematic follow-up. The rapid exchange of ideas that develops between the clinicians and the theoretical researchers makes it possible to carry out effective basic and clinical research. The relative smallness of each group does limit its capacity to cover all aspects of research work, but the main research areas of a department of surgery must be covered by a theoretical surgery department. In Cologne, we have established seven small working teams with different topics, but slightly overlapping research areas. Seventy-five percent of all surgeons in the department (all academic surgeons) are members of "small working teams."

We feel that fulfilling the role of an academic surgeon as an active, effective clinical surgeon and as a researcher is challenging but achievable. The first and most important qualification is genuine concern and compassion for patients. The second is practical, technical ability to perform operative surgery well. The academic surgeon should not be perceived as a biochemist or statistician with surgical training, but as a surgeon. The Marburg model clarifies this definition of the clinical surgeon. Third, but essential to the successful performance of surgical research, is a fascination with ideas and the ability to develop, analyze, and validate them. Finally, the academic surgeon must be physically strong, energetic, and psychologically resilient. The Marburg model facilitates and supports these endeavors through the stimulation and guidance of the theoretical surgeon.

References

1. Brendel W. Medizinische Forschung: Mensch und Tier. Gesundheitsforum SZ 1985;154:8.
2. Troidl H. The general surgeon and the trauma surgeon binding wounds: an old-fashioned German general surgeon's solution to structuring trauma care in West Germany. Theor Surg 1990;5:64.
3. Lorenz W, Rothmund M. Theoretical surgery–a new specialty in operative medicine. World J Surg 1989;13:292.

57

Surgical Research in Italy

N. Cascinelli

Scientific surgery in Italy dates back to the first century A.D. when Celsus summarized the advances in surgery after Hippocrates and described new operations, such as hernia repairs, extraction of urinary bladder stones, and eye surgery. Celsus was the first to use ligatures to stop bleeding.

In the medieval period, Constantine the African, working at Monte Cassino (Naples), translated Arabic works into Latin. Toward the end of the thirteenth century, William of Saliceto at the University of Bologna revived the use of the scalpel over cauterization and stressed the importance of anatomical knowledge for surgeons. In the late fifteenth century, Antonio Benivieri of Florence described pathological anatomical changes in more than 100 patients. In 1543 Andreas Vesalius, Professor of Anatomy at Padua, published the brilliantly illustrated *Fabrica* which overcame the Galenic doctrine of anatomy. Also in the sixteenth century, anatomical dissections received a great impetus from the studies of Leonardo da Vinci.

In the sixteenth and seventeenth centuries, the use of firearms caused more severe wounds, and surgeons became indispensable for an effective army; yet throughout Europe, except in Italy and in Holland, they were excluded from universities. In this period, European families developed specific operations and new instruments, the knowledge of which was secretly transmitted from one generation to the next. In Italy, the Branca family specialized in plastic surgery of the nose, and the Norsini family in hernia repairs.

Professor Antonio Scarpa, at the University of Pavia, published an illustrated textbook of surgical anatomy in the late 1700s. A milestone operation for modern surgery was described in the late 1800s by Eduardo Bassini, Professor of Surgery at Pavia. In more recent years, Italian surgeons have contributed to technical advances in surgery in many areas. A major scientific contribution to academic surgery is the clinical research in surgical oncology pioneered by Umberto Veronesi. Professor Veronesi has made significant contributions to surgical research as director of the National Cancer Institute in Milan. He and his colleagues used the randomized clinical trial methodology to advance the understanding and management of breast cancer. He has used this approach for more than 20 years as director of the World Health Organization Melanoma Group through a series of randomized clinical trials involving investigators from countries throughout the world.

Funding of Surgical Research

Surgical research in Italy is actively practiced at university hospitals, scientific centers, and general hospitals; it covers a wide range of activities from basic research to prosthetic replacement and bioengineering. The funds are made available by the state through the National Council for Research (CNR), by industry, and by private associations or foundations. The CNR and industry finance specific research projects aimed at achieving results in the short and medium term, while private associations and foundations give grants to young researchers to acquire experience in widely different fields to complete their education as academic surgeons of the highest professional qualification. The funds allow a period of study at both national and foreign centers.

In most cases, funding from the CNR and industry is managed by a responsible researcher who is usually the chief of the division or department, or a senior staff member at a surgical center. There are no special advantages or disadvantages related to these sources. In theory, funds from industry—

whose final aim is oriented toward industrial products—might introduce a bias, but industry and the scientists it sponsors are sensitive to this danger. A positive aspect of industrial funding is the review of the research process; it is closer and more frequent because of the sponsoring organizations' policies of keeping the projects brief and reviewing them before deciding to go ahead to the next phase.

Public funding is less susceptible to bias from the point of view of the desired result because the state agency is not profit oriented. The review of research progress is usually less pressing. The scientific stature of the responsible investigator and the objective interest of the research question justify the choice made by the public funding agency and guarantees the quality and the punctuality of the research. Italy devotes 0.14% of its gross national product to research, but it is impossible to estimate what percentage of this money goes to surgical research because of the overlap with other fields ranging from immunology to electronics.

Limited facilities are available for foreign surgeons to perform surgical research in Italy. The Ministry of Foreign Affairs, Department of Cooperation and Development, provides funds for foreign investigators who wish to come to our country for a period of study within the framework of bilateral agreements between Italy and many other European and non-European countries. The National Council for Research sponsors visiting professors for periods of 1 to 12 months. The Italian Association for Cancer Research awards grants for research to be carried out by European investigators at Italian centers.

There are no plans for formal training in basic research in the schools of surgery in Italy, because their aim is to train skilled clinical surgeons who are able to solve the practical problems arising in community practice. Young surgeons who choose practical surgery as a career have no motivation to gain personal experience in surgical research, and forced involvement in research would be nonproductive. Young surgeons who choose academic surgery should enter research programs as early as possible in the residency period. The ideal consists of progressively increasing levels of responsibility in research and clinical practice—not breaking the linkage between the two, yet maintaining an emphasis on the practical application of scientific knowledge.

Italian surgeons do not expect their academic leaders to cover the broad range of knowledge from molecular biology to daily clinical practice. They favor the model of an academic surgeon who is paired with a surgical scientist who participates equally in the planning of research and enjoys an equal level of dignity and respect within the department. The dependence of the surgeon on the clinical scientist is particularly well appreciated in studies of tumor-host relationships, transplantation, host reactions to prostheses, and the multidisciplinary therapy of surgical diseases.

Cooperation between clinicians with different specialties who combine their treatment modalities in research protocols presents few problems because of the similarity of the investigators' backgrounds and the time available for research. The multidisciplinary clinical research programs between surgical and medical oncologists in breast cancer are an outstanding example. These studies brought together the excellent unidisciplinary research skills and clinical expertise of surgeons whose primary interest was early breast cancer, and medical oncologists whose primary interest and expertise was in disseminated disease.

The interaction between clinicians and basic science researchers is more complex because of the difference in the rhythm of their research. The time axis for laboratory research is generally far shorter than that of clinical research, and clinical data are accumulated slowly. The rapid turnover of hypotheses and results in laboratory research can lead to deeper and deeper penetration of avenues of research, which can be misleading if they do not relate to the practical problems observed in patients. Close linkage is necessary to achieve balanced understanding by both partners in this exchange. Expertise in both laboratory research and clinical research is extremely infrequent in a single investigator in Italy.

The Training of a Surgical Investigator

The young academic surgeon should begin with intensive clinical experience to develop a surgical mentality. This may not take more than a year or two and is not intended to bring the surgeon to a high level of technical skill, but to allow his professional growth to develop with a surgical approach to scientific problems. The acquisition of this mentality is extraordinarily important. Subsequent research experience should be developed without losing touch with clinical practice, so that young investigators will not lose sight of their long-term goal.

The motivation of academic surgeons to pursue research is an intrinsic philosophical need to look beyond the surface phenomena of daily clinical activity, and to critically evaluate the underlying mechanisms and the results achieved. Critical thinking in research requires periodic verification and modification from the critical review provided by other surgical and nonsurgical specialists. We evaluate young academic surgeons on the basis of their scientific productivity and individual maturity. Intellectual growth is certainly the more important but, unfortunately, there are no objective criteria for its evaluation. The research adviser's observation of the young surgeon's behavior as he interacts with his colleagues and patients, his openmindedness to biological or fundamental discussions of surgical interventions, and his caution in introducing research results into daily practice constitute the basis for evaluation of an individual's maturity. The younger academic surgeon may be impelled by enthusiasm to stress the superiority of his own innovation or line of research. This may lead to the danger of overinterpretation, prevarication, or anxiety to introduce insufficiently consolidated results into daily practice.

Youthful enthusiasm is normal and a very positive finding in the early years of training. A final judgment on the potential of an academic surgeon is usually possible after 4 to 6 years of training. The young academic surgeon must show excellent manual skill and diagnostic insight, as well as expertise in perioperative care. At our institution, 90% of surgeons are engaged in research activity. Research training is regarded as extremely important to prepare the new generation of surgical leadership with comparable strengths in research and surgical practice.

The young surgical researcher should be given freedom to choose a research project that fits into the overall strategic research plan of the department of surgery, after a preliminary research proposal has been accepted by the department. New long-term research lines are rarely initiated by residents, but the incentive of testing one's own ideas one day is a strong stimulus to all members of a research group.

Research is not a compulsory part of graduate surgical education, but basic scientific methodology is taught well enough at the undergraduate level to provide sufficient understanding of the quality of scientific papers. Computerized literature searches make use of international networks to allow review of scientific books and journals.

Meetings

Several surgical societies in Italy organize annual congresses with sessions reserved for young surgeons to present the results of their research. The format includes oral presentations of projects considered to be of wide enough interest to stimulate discussion of a general nature. Poster exhibits are used for specialized messages that might be of interest to a limited part of the audience, needing more extensive individual discussion. These scientific meetings require that results be presented as an opportunity to test the investigator and provide constructive criticism that may be extremely useful in the progress of a given research project.

International discussion is considered to be essential, and a good knowledge of another language, usually English, is indispensable.

Ethical Considerations

Research, as a whole, is well accepted in Italy, but there is growing opposition to animal experimentation. The Ethical Committee at our institute evaluates ongoing research and allows animal experiments only when an incontrovertible rationale for their use is presented and a guarantee provided that only the minimum number of animals required to answer the research question will be used. It is also expected that the research will be carried out personally by the responsible investigator.

There is wide consensus about support for research in human subjects. In addition to verifying the rationale of a clinical trial, the Ethical Committee carefully checks to make sure it is "dedicated to the exclusive interest of the patients." Written informed consent is not always required, but the prerequisite discussion between the investigator and the research subject must be verified.

58

Japan's Integration of Eastern Values and Modern Science

K. Hioki, T. Aoki, and T. Muto

Japan is a small nation comprised of many islands and populated by 120 million people. There are nearly 150 physicians per 100,000 population, and the number of physicians continues to rise. They are concentrated in the larger, populous cities. The remote mountainous regions and outlying islands still have few doctors. The country has well-developed science and biomedical research programs. It is now generally accepted in Japan that research is absolutely necessary for the advance of medicine and surgery. Japanese surgeons recognize that clinical practice and surgical research are equally important, like the wheels of a car.

Research projects are formulated in each surgical department, and sometimes by a cooperative team formed with other clinical and academic departments in the university. In most universities, there are several research groups in a surgical department, and each surgeon generally belongs to one of the research groups.

Despite heavy clinical commitments, many full-time surgeons are able to find time for surgical research because they belong to a group of two or three surgeons who share the responsibilities for treating their common patients. Some senior residents can spend a period doing full-time research. This generally occurs in the third year of surgical training, when the resident is 26 to 32 years old.

History of Surgical Research in Japan

From the seventh to the nineteenth centuries, medicine in Japan was based on Chinese medicine. In the midnineteenth century, Western medicine was introduced.

The government invited scholars from Germany to establish the national medical colleges and dispatched young doctors to Germany to study medicine. As a result of this policy, Japanese medicine became completely German, from the academic system and facilities to the methods of diagnosis and treatment. This continued even after Japanese physicians assumed the leading professorships. The Japan Surgical Society was founded in 1897, and German surgery completely predominated until 1945.

Just after the end of World War II, American surgery, together with American culture, became the prevailing influence, replacing the German approach to medicine, with its emphasis on theory. The American approach emphasized empiricism and innovations in practice. A change was observed in surgical research, from the European style to a mixed style including American methods, with particularly obvious progress after 1950.

Advances in anesthesia, including excellent equipment imported from the United States, England, and Germany, facilitated the gradual spread of general endotracheal anesthesia. Major improvements were made in operating room equipment, instruments, and the equipment and techniques for pre- and postoperative management. More invasive surgery became possible for malignant tumors; the survival rates in operations for cancer of the esophagus, stomach, rectum, lung, pancreas, and liver improved. Dramatic advances occurred in the specialized fields of thoracic surgery, especially in open heart surgery, in microsurgical techniques of neurosurgery, and in pediatric surgery.

Advances in both clinical and laboratory research were achieved through cooperative efforts among scholars in all areas of medicine, including pathology, physiology, and biochemistry.

Although Tatsu Ohsawa, at Kyoto University, reported successful resection of carcinoma of the esophagus in 1933, following the work of Torek and Kirschner, it was Komei Nakayama at Chiba University who established the effectiveness of resection of the thoracic esophagus through his large experience. Shigetsugu Katsura, at Tohoku University, made important contributions to surgical research on operative methods of thoracic esophagectomy and perioperative care of the patient. Nakayama and his students, through their surgical research, lowered mortality while enhancing resectability and survival rates. To attain this, they studied pathological physiology and nutritional management. They emphasized the importance of staged operations and examined the significance of preoperative irradiation. Nakayama was famous for his rigorous instruction in clinical research. Most of the present Japanese leaders in this field were his students.

Ichio Honjo (1913–1987), at Kyoto University, successfully performed a total excision of the pancreas in a case of pancreatic cancer for the first time in Japan in 1949. In the same year, he performed a right hepatic lobectomy for metastatic liver cancer following an operation for rectal cancer, the first successful case of its kind in the world. Research by Honjo and his students elucidated the pathophysiology and treatment of diabetes following pancreatic resection. They carried out experimental and clinical research on hepatoenterostomy in cases of inoperable cholangioma and interruption of the hepatic artery and branches of the portal vein in inoperable liver cancer. They carefully conducted animal experiments to resolve questions arising from their clinical research. Their specialized knowledge of pathology, physiology, and biochemistry was indispensable.

Tamaki Kajitani, honorary president of the Cancer Institute Hospital in Tokyo, established systematic lymphadenectomy for gastric cancer through investigations in the pathology laboratory and the operating rooms. He conducted this research over a period spanning 47 years while he was on the surgical staff of a hospital affiliated with the Cancer Institute, a private foundation for cancer research. Many foreign surgeons visit his hospital to observe surgical procedures and many university surgeons in Japan have been his students.

Japanese surgical research developed endoscopic diagnosis and treatment of diseases of the airway and digestive tract. This has revolutionized surgical treatment throughout the world.

Current surgical research in Japan is focused primarily on:

1. Elucidating such *general problems* as wound healing, mirocirculation, fibrin glue, and the chemistry of fibronectin.

   Nutrition includes home hyperalimentation, infusion of branched-chain amino acids or eicosopentanoic acid, and new methods for nutritional assessment.

   The pathophysiology and treatment of endotoxin **shock**, surgical infection, and disseminated intravascular coagulation are among the major research projects.

2. Research aimed at elevating the level of success in *cancer treatment* or eradication.

   Hepatectomy for liver cancer, a major problem in Japan, requires development of improved surgical techniques for intraoperative diagnostic evaluation and postoperative care.

   Composite resections and **reconstruction** problems in advanced cancers of the airway, lung, and esophagus including extensive lymphadenectomy.

   Techniques for early detection and treatment of lung, esophageal, gastric, and hepatic cancer.

   Adjuvant therapy such as chemotherapy, hyperthermia, or immunotherapy.

3. Research in the field of *organ transplantation*.

   Kidney transplantation in Japan is established to a degree comparable with other advanced countries; however, *heart* transplantation and *liver* transplantation are markedly delayed. Due to strong religious feelings, public debate continues on the determination of death. Liver transplantation candidates are currently sent overseas for treatment. In 1968 Professor Wada performed a human heart transplant operation. Strong public feelings about the definition of brain death were aroused, and strict criteria were developed by a commission of the Ministry of Health and Welfare.

   In 1989 partial liver transplantation from a living donor was performed at Shamane Medical University. Though the judgment of brain death has been permitted by the Japanese Transplantation Society and the ethics committees of some universities, there is no public consensus. For this reason, partial liver transplantation from living relative donors will be the standard. In the near future, the performance of transplantation of organs from patients with brain death is anticipated, whereupon major organ transplantation will develop rapidly in Japan. Meanwhile, scholars are busy performing basic research in transplantation laboratories.

Research During Residency Training

The residency system has been adopted in only a few medical institutions in Japan. Graduates from medical school obtain a medical license for the first time when they have passed the national examination, but they can practice only after a training period of 2 years. Only medical institutions authorized by the government may provide this training. Most candidates for surgical training, after passing the national examination, enter the hospital associated with the university from which they graduated. In some cases they must pass an additional entrance examination. These young surgeons-in-training may enter research after 2 years of basic surgical training. Research may lead to the title, Doctor of Medicine, a special academic title held by fewer than 30% of medical graduates in Japan. During the pursuit of the M.D., the candidate serves as an unpaid assistant at the university and, indeed, pays tuition for the "postgraduate course in surgery." To provide for living expenses, most young surgeons work part-time in private hospitals, assisting in the operating room.

There are two possible tracks to become an "M.D." in a surgical field:

1. Following completion of 2 years of clinical training, the candidate attends a postgraduate course, after passing the school entrance examination, and starts surgical research. It takes 4 to 5 years for a candidate to publish a research thesis to obtain the "M.D." In this track, the fresh M.D. then receives clinical surgical training.
2. After 4 to 5 years of clinical training, the candidate enters surgical research under the instruction of the chief professor, and publishes an M.D. thesis 8 to 10 years after graduation. Young surgeons are motivated to carry out research, in part, to obtain the title "M.D.," which is required or advantageous for gaining a teaching staff position in a medical school or a position as chief in another medical institution, or even for the purpose of operating a private clinic.

Since surgical research is carried out to resolve questions encountered in daily clinical situations, we think it best that the research training be started only after at least 2 years of surgical training. Young surgeons who embark on research at this time are motivated by a desire to solve clinical problems, to advance their surgical careers, or to advance a career in clinical surgery. We estimate that more than 75% of young surgeons enter surgical research for at least a brief period. However, it may be disadvantageous for them if the period of research training is too long or if the training lacks opportunities for clinical surgical experience. Ideally, young surgeons should choose their own research problems. However, when an institution cannot fully provide the required staff or facilities for a particular project, residents are sometimes exchanged with another institution; otherwise they must limit the scope of their research to what their own institution can accommodate.

In Japan, the chief professor usually selects research topics for residents. In most institutions, young surgeons chosen to enter research are free of clinical responsibility during the day for at least 2 years, but share night duty with the other residents. During research training, young surgeons do not always stay in one department but may move to another department or even to another institution, if necessary.

Although it is disadvantageous for young surgeons to be isolated from clinical surgery training for two or more consecutive years, this is considered an inevitable consequence of choosing research training in Japan. During clinical training, it is difficult to find time for research. In our institution, only young surgeons involved in research with the aim of acquiring the "M.D." are relieved of clinical responsibility. No exemption is made for other surgeons doing research, in order to maintain the cooperative arrangement of cross-coverage among the staff. The typical week for a Japanese resident is outlined in Table 58.1.

General Comments About Research

In the private medical school in Osaka Prefecture, each department maintains its own research unit. There is also a larger, general research facility furnished with equipment, and technicians are available to every scholar. It is possible to collaborate with other clinical or basic science departments if more specialized knowledge or techniques are necessary.

Most university surgeons participate in research. Their clinical work and teaching responsibilities force them to allocate time for research in the early morning or at night. Research training varies widely in Japan. Community hospitals generally provide only clinical training. Young surgeons who seek academic careers generally return to the

TABLE 58.1. Weekly schedule for a Japanese surgical resident.

	Monday	Tuesday	Wednesday	Thursday	Friday	Saturday/Sunday
07:30	Resident's ward rounds	Residents' ward rounds	Residents' ward rounds	Residents' ward rounds	Residents' ward rounds	Residents' ward rounds
08:00	Preoperative patient conference			Preoperative patient conference		
09:00	Elective surgery / Care of ward patients / Out patient clinic	Grand rounds: Walking rounds with professor of surgery / Out patient clinic	Care of ward patients: Endoscopy, Radiology, Hepato-biliary conference / Out patient clinic	Elective surgery / Care of ward patients / Out patient clinic	Grand rounds: Walking rounds with professor of surgery GI conference Care of ward patients / Out patient clinic	Care of ward patients / Out patient clinic
10:00						
11:00		Chest conference case study conference death conference				
12:00						Departmental staff meeting
13:00	Out patient clinic					
14:00	Special out patient clinic for follow-up studies		Special out patient clinic	Special out patient clinic	Special out patient clinic	
15:00						
16:00						
17:00						
18:00	GI conference			Research work/emergency operations		
19:00						

TABLE 58.2. Budget for surgical research for a typical Japanese department of surgery.

Source	Amount	
	Yen	U.S. dollars
University funds	3,000,000	20,000
Ministry of Education	3,000,000	20,000
Ministry of Health	3,000,000	20,000
Pharmaceutical industry	5,000,000	33,000
Municipal government	2,000,000	13,000
Prefectural government	2,000,000	13,000
Private foundations	2,000,000	13,000
Total	20,000,000	132,000

university to do research after completing a few years of clinical training in community hospitals.

In Japan, literature searches are computerized by an on-line information system available in the library of each university. Each library stocks not only journals in Japanese but also foreign journals, most of which are published in English. Accordingly, it is an indispensable qualification for physicians to be able to read papers written in English. Most journals published in Japan are written in Japanese. Among them, the *Journal of the Japan Surgical Society* enjoys the largest circulation.

In the past, medical education was conducted through the use of German textbooks, and patients' medical histories were generally recorded in both Japanese and German, in mixed style. Recently, this custom has changed and most young doctors use English. Since the textbooks for clinical training and the references needed for research are written in English, skill in this language is important.

The time has come to introduce new and different ideas and methods in every field in Japan, Fellowships for residents from other countries to study in Japan are an important means for promoting this exchange. A few institutions, including ours, have put this into practice. We firmly believe that such exchanges will be beneficial to all countries involved. We all must support this important development in surgical education.

The Research Adviser

Many of the hospitals attached to research institutes are university affiliated and have a large number of research fellows. Since the acquisition of an M.D. or a Ph.D. degree is a basic requirement for obtaining a position or advancing academically, Japanese academic surgeons must have their own research programs and also serve as research advisers to their assistants.

One research adviser may be responsible for varying numbers of research fellows depending on the university, hospital, or department. The number may differ among individual advisors within the same department. On average, four or five fellows are attached to one adviser, but that number ranges from zero to 10. Research advisers usually provide guidance to their fellows throughout their careers. Advisers help assistants find sources of research funding and part-time jobs for living expenses. The overall group research program frequently proceeds with the adviser's work as its core, and each assistant undertakes projects related to the adviser's theme. The ability to look to the needs of others is a desirable characteristic for the ideal adviser in Japan. Research fellows prefer to be affiliated with the research group of an adviser possessing such qualities.

Funding

Government funds administered by the Ministry of Education are the main source of support for scientific research, including biomedical research. The national universities and research institutes depend exclusively on this source. Grants for research are awarded on the basis of peer review and are equally available to all public and private universities or institutes. Prefectural, municipal, and private universities may receive additional support for research from university or hospital funds and from pharmaceutical companies. Funds are also available from the Ministry of Health and Welfare for Health Services Research. Awards for Surgical Research funded from the National Government are reviewed by *surgeons* chosen to serve for 2 years as referees. A typical research budget for our surgical departments is presented in Table 58.2.

The allotment of the grants for scientific research by the Ministry of Education is announced annually in the "List of Research Subjects Adopted for Grants for Scientific Research by the Ministry of Education" by the Society for the Study of Scientific Research Funds. The *Japanese Scientific Monthly*, published by the Japan Society for the Promotion of Science, carries a survey of organizations supporting research, listing various foundations providing grants for participants in international conferences, and for scholarships. Surgeons have not participated extensively in these grants and scholarships, which are intended to cover a wide range of scientific domains.

The surgical societies do not provide financial support for research or travel to scientific meetings. Surgical researchers usually carry out clinical work and serve on the teaching staff concurrently; there is no institution at which a specialized scholar can receive a salary for research work only.

In surgical research, granting agencies rarely attempt to influence research activities themselves; however, grants obtained for specific research cannot be spent for any other project, and spending equipment funds for travel or salary is not permitted.

Legal and Cultural Considerations

The Japanese public attitude toward animal experimentation is rather positive. Consideration must be given to the improvement of cages for laboratory animals and the assignment of a specialized veterinarian to breed and care for the animals in response to appeals of certain societies for the prevention of cruelty to animals. Researchers, as well as the general public, think that developmental work through animal experimentation is an indispensable step before controlled study in healthy human volunteers.

The public attitude toward clinical trials is extremely negative—patients will not permit themselves to be used as "material" for clinical experiments. The reason for this attitude is a basic public consensus that a certain treatment should be applied to specific patients only after its efficacy has been fully confirmed through animal experimentation, and after the physician is fully convinced that it is the *only* and *best* treatment available. The precept that *giving to the patient what the physician believes best is the basis of the physician–patient relationship* is widely accepted in medical education. Therefore, physicians who acknowledge that they are incapable of judging what is the best for their patients may lose the confidence of both patients and peers.

As a natural consequence of the belief that humans should not be used for experimentation, it is very difficult to obtain consent from a patient for participation in a clinical trial using the accepted North American and Western European method. Our medical legislation does, however, grant a patient the right to have sufficient explanation about the treatment to be given, and requires informed consent before any surgical operation. In Japan, eligible patients are generally admitted to a clinical trial and allocated to a treatment. Consent for treatment is then sought without reference to the method of allocation.

The number of medical malpractice suits is increasing rapidly in Japan. In 1985 a "Declaration of Patient Rights" was announced by a group of volunteers, including lawyers. The physician– patient relationship is losing its traditional basis, and a new basis, requiring more direct communication of detailed medical information, is developing. Traditionally patients have been protected from the diagnosis of cancer and, under such circumstances, clinical trials in surgical research require thorough legal and cultural consideration by research advisers. Because the direct method of obtaining "informed consent," used in the United States, is still not generally accepted and might incur trouble in Japan, careful consideration is especially necessary.

In Japan, there are no organizations or courses of instruction in surgical research save for those developed in individual surgical departments or in cooperation with other academic departments of a university. A formal program of instruction for surgical research would be very useful; it might be provided on an international or national basis. A book on academic management for surgeons would be very useful. Most of the chairmen of surgical departments are concerned about future financial support.

The future of surgical research is brightened by the many young surgeons who have committed themselves to academic training. We anticipate that Japanese surgery will contribute innovative research solutions and future leaders to the international community of surgical scholars.

Acknowledgment

The authors thank Professor Masakatsa Yamamoto, director of the Department of Surgery at Kansai Medical University in Osaka, and Professor Emeritus Fusahiro Nagao, Jikei University School of Medicine in Tokyo, for advice and support during the preparation of this chapter.

59

New Initiatives and Ideas in Spain

P.A. Sanchez

Spanish medicine has shared in the changes that have characterized developments in Western medical communities since the 1930s—the introduction of a great deal of advanced technology, increasing and irreversible collectivization of health care services, deeper appreciation and extension of the concept of individuality within the framework of pathology, and prevention of disease and promotion of health.[1] As a result of marked social disparities, progress has not been uniform, and major differences in health care delivery have coexisted in different regions and according to social class until recently.

After the civil war (1936–1939), the devastation of many areas and a very poor supporting economy made the rebuilding of medical facilities costly and slow. Attention had to be focused on such urgent needs as coping with epidemics and alimentary problems. The personal efforts of doctors contributed greatly to the improvement of community health in the face of precarious conditions and a considerable degree of sanitary disorganization. Shortly thereafter, in 1944, the National Health Act established the underlying principles of the Social Security system, changed the organization of medical care delivery, and strongly influenced the subsequent development of medicine. Historical and political circumstances conditioned the birth and growth of the system, and some of the errors and pitfalls introduced in the initial phases are still with us.

Traditional public and private beneficence has slowly disappeared, to be replaced by the Social Security services. These have grown enormously and have generated a giant bureaucratic machine whose budget approximates that of the country. At present, the Social Security medical care program covers virtually all the 38 million inhabitants of Spain.

Primary care was incorrectly organized at the outset, and the consequences are still evident—overloaded outpatient clinics, poor medical care, and maldistribution of resources. Nevertheless, a good network of public hospitals has been built and, although its geographical disposition is not completely adequate, it has brought evident benefits to the population and contributed to the modernization of medical practice. Although teaching and research were not considered to be among the primary goals of the system, residency programs have been progressively incorporated in hospitals since the middle 1960s, with great success. Research has remained the "poor sister" of the system. Only a few centers have limited facilities, and financial support remained extremely poor.

The Social Security Health Service permeates the entire system and influences not only medical care but everything related to it, by virtue of the economic resources it commands—even a high percentage of the beds in private hospitals and other institutions is under its control as the result of certain financial arrangements. This brief outline of the weaknesses and successes of the health care system is a prerequisite to understanding the practice of medicine in Spain and the modest role played by research.

An acute problem that has a great impact on the present situation is the existence of more than 20,000 *unemployed*, or underemployed medical graduates. The number of medical doctors has been increasing over the past 25 years and reached approximately 140,000 in 1990. The resulting density of one doctor per 270 inhabitants is one of the highest in Europe, and it will be even higher within the next 6 to 8 years.

Political concessions allowed new medical schools to open during the 1960s and 1970s without any serious planning, in spite of a lack of necessary financial support for some of the existing schools—with the exception of the University–Clinical Medical School of Navarra, all medical schools belong to the State Administration. Budgets have been maintained at a very low level, much below the requirements of modern medical schools. As an example, only $630 (U.S.) per student was spent in 1982, in contrast to $4500 in the United Kingdom and $2500 in France.

The problem is not only economic, but organizational. Medical curricula remain anchored in the past; subjects like bioengineering, preventive and social medicine, electronics, and research methodology are not taught during the 6 years of medical school. Spanish universities have not kept pace with the deep changes within society. Locked up inside themselves, the universities have maintained rigid individualistic structures and have lost, with few exceptions, the beat of time. Newer surgical areas, like cardiac surgery or neurosurgery, have developed almost completely outside the university environment. Security of privileges, a closed atmosphere, and strong archaic corporatism have caused universities to turn their backs on reality in many instances. The result is a dangerous disconnection from society.

Only a few of the medical graduates in recent years have had access to residency programs (12.5% in 1985); official public posts as general practitioners are also scarce. The immediate future for thousands of young doctors is dismal. Numerus clausus was introduced in medical schools recently, but it was not drastic enough. Some 3000 new medical students continue to be admitted each year, and the effects of this administrative decision will not alleviate the situation appreciably until another decade has passed.

Political attention has been focused on solving such urgent and sometimes dramatic problems, but research remains in a deferred position. The enormous rise in health care costs, combined in many instances with inadequate management of the public sector, has led to real financial difficulties, which have had an obvious repercussion on the funding of research. "Brain drain," mainly to the United States, has been a constant fact of Spanish scientific life during the past 30 to 40 years.

Research has generally and traditionally been confined to isolated groups with little or no government help. Personal efforts have occasionally produced some continuity, and such splendid results as those achieved in histology and neurology by Ramón y Cajal's school. This has not been the general rule, and scientific research has had little influence in, or on, Spanish society.

The general population has been indifferent to research, including surgical research, and is unaware of its importance to the real progress and development of the country; only in a very few exceptional circumstances has a plea been made for greater support. Things have changed slightly in the past 8 to 10 years, not because of a change in the general attitude, but as a result of occasional collaboration by the mass media to emphasize the need for research. Through the media, the man on the street is beginning to be aware of the chronic absence of a coherent policy toward research. Some professionals and scientists (Ortega y Gasset and Marañón in the past; Ochoa, Grisolía, Mayor Zaragoza, Sols, Rof Carballo, and others, now) are trying to influence public opinion through the media, but their efforts appear to have evoked little or no response from the general population.

There are no facilities for research by community surgeons. Their daily efforts are devoted exclusively to clinical activities, and most of them have had no training in surgical research.

The small amount of surgical research that is performed is carried out only in university or large hospitals, to which patients are sent for special diagnosis and treatment. There are few facilities, and it is always difficult to find adequate funding. With few exceptions, research is not an obligatory part of departmental commitments, although it is partly necessary for a university career. Attitudes vary greatly from one department to another, and it is very difficult to make any generalizations.

In contrast to this negative research panorama, the quality of health has risen spectacularly during this century; the mean life expectancy was 73.4 years in 1980, compared with only 34.76 years in 1900. Spain currently has the lowest overall mortality of the European Economic Community (EEC) countries, and 11.3% of the population is over 65 years of age. Cardiocirculatory disease (45%), tumors (20%), and respiratory disease (8%) are the main causes of mortality. The mortality from intestinal infection, however, is three times higher than in other EEC countries and reveals deficiencies in the organization of the health system, as well as poor public education regarding sanitation and hygiene.[2]

Funding of Surgical Research

Spain's position as one of the least developed among European countries in terms of research funding contrasts sharply with its level of industrialization. The number of investigators is currently less than half of the mean for other O.E.C.D. countries. In 1988 only 0.072% of the gross national product went to research and development, and

TABLE 59.1. Main areas supported by the Health Research Fund (FIS).

Research
Biochemistry and molecular biology
Immunology and cellular biology
Microbiology, virology, and parasitology
Anatomy, histology, and pathology
Human physiopathology and clinical medicine
Therapeutics; clinical and experimental pharmacology
Physiology and experimental physiopathology
Surgery and experimental surgery
Public health and preventive medicine
Oncology
Sanitary technology and image diagnosis
Sanitation planning, management, economy, and information systems
Health education and promotion of health sciences
Health problems related to age
Toxic oil syndrome (SAT) and related materials
Training and education (fellowships)
Initiation into research
Research structure
Studies in foreign countries
Traveling fellowships
Scientific meetings
Publications
Collaboration with industry

14% of that was spent on the medical sciences. Contributions to research by the private sector are also very low–only 20%, compared to 55% or more in other industrialized countries. The technological import/export ratio is 10:1; and mean annual expenditures per investigator are substantially less than in other European countries.

To reduce the country's great dependence on foreign technology–almost 80% of medical equipment and supplies is imported–the State Administration announced some national programs, mainly in the field of services. These appeared to be directed more at covering some of the big deficiencies than at stimulating the creative capacity of young scientists–traditionally, more attention has been paid to the humanities than to the sciences. In 1986 the Act of General Promotion and Coordination of Scientific and Technological Research, called The Science Act, was promulgated with the aim of establishing a solid base for scientific research. It was followed by approval of the National Plan of Scientific Research and Technological Development which, in its second year of application (1989), started to show some good results: national funds amounted to $180 million (U.S.)–25% of it was devoted to personnel training and 20% to establishing the necessary structures for research.

This ambitious plan has inspired new hope in the scientific community, although the main criticisms against it have been its almost complete dependence on political decisions and the excessive rigidity of the bureaucracy. The Science Act was promulgated without the highly advisable consultations with experts and other political groups; it does not define investigation as a priority for the country and it does not clearly establish the different steps and periods for the delivery of the funds.[3]

Surgical research units are supported by the budgets of their own hospitals as far as staff and facilities are concerned, but grants to finance programs and fellowships are also available. The main sources of such funds are the Advisory Committee on Scientific and Technical Research, which is closely connected to the Ministry of Education and Science, and the Social Security Research Fund (FIS), which is an organ of the Ministry of Health. Both organizations support research programs, including fellowships within and outside Spain, after presentation of successful project proposals.

The FIS is a government funding program that, in the past, received considerable support from the pharmaceutical industry. Its resources came mainly from the complimentary discount granted by the industrial companies when they sold their products to the Social Security services. It also received specified amounts from the budget of the National Health Institute, and from private and institutional contributions. At present, the funds are assigned directly in the national general budget.

The main areas financed by the FIS are summarized in Table 59.1. The total budget in 1988 was 3160 million pesetas (approximately $29 million U.S.), an amount that is expected to rise progressively up to 10,000 million pesetas per year over the next 10 years. Almost 80% was spent on health promotion research programs, including funding of projects, personnel training, and traveling fellowships. Each area has a Technical and Scientific Advisory Committee, composed of experts in the field. They review the projects, but final approval is in the hands of the Administrative Committee.

The FIS's current goals include progressive increases in the annual budget and the number of investigators in relation to the active population, and changing the scientific approach to problems. The responsible managers and directors prefer to talk of investigation in the health sciences rather than traditional medical or biomedical research.[4] They emphasize that this is not only a matter of semantics, but a true reorganization of the system, giving priority to "research by programs" involving a wide spectrum of investigators. In spite of these statements of good intention, different experts have criticized the structure of the FIS,[5] particularly its administrative complexity, lack of clear objectives in many areas, lack of coordination and control, obsolete technology, and shortage of trained personnel, basic installations, and facilities.[5,6]

The major grants to research in the past have gone to the following hospitals: Clinica Puerta de Hierro, Centro Ramón y Cajal, Fundación Jiménez Díaz, Universidad Autónoma, and Hospital La Paz, in Madrid; Hospital Clínico and Hospital Santa Cruz y San Pablo, in Barcelona; Hospital La Fe, in Valencia. About 10% of the projects supported by these grants deal with surgical research.

The new health act considers prevention and research to be obligatory parts of medicine. Some steps were taken after its promulgation to better the poor prevailing atmosphere; one was the opening of new 200-bed hospital—Carlos III, in Madrid—dedicated to clinical research. Surgical investigation is not included among its first projects.

The main surgical research laboratories in Spain are those of Clínica Puerta de Hierro, Centro Ramón y Cajal, and Hospital La Paz, in Madrid; they have full-time research staff. The Hospital Gregorio Marañón, in Madrid, has a new surgical research unit, directed, at its beginning, by Dr. J. Barros. The Hospital Clínico, in Barcelona (Prof. C. Pera) and Hospital Marqués de Valdecilla, in Santander (Dr. D. Casanova), also have active surgical laboratories. Surgical units in university hospitals and in Social Security hospitals in different cities usually have part-time research workers, especially in microsurgery.

Very few private foundations specifically support surgical research. The National Council for Scientific Research does not have a section dedicated solely to surgical research. Industrial companies seldom make grants for biomedical research, and pharmaceutical firms are mainly interested in trials of new drugs. In recent years, there has been an increase in funds and awards for investigation supported by industry.

Surgical associations do not have enough funds to support research projects, although in recent years some of them have offered grants to cover travel expenses incurred by those who have presented papers at scientific meetings. Travel has also been supported by the pharmaceutical and biomedical companies.

Surgeons in Spanish-speaking countries in Central and South America can apply for financial support through the Spanish Agency for International Cooperation (former Institute of Iberoamerican Cooperation), an agency associated with the Ministry of Foreign Affairs. Several hundred Iberoamerican students and graduates receive financial assistance every year through the grants offered by this institute. Five percent of the positions offered in residency programs each year are reserved for Iberoamerican medical graduates.

A considerable number of students (mainly undergraduates) from Arab countries are also favored by special grants offered by the government. The National Health Institute and the Department of Cultural Relationships, a section of the Ministry of Foreign Affairs, are the agencies providing most of the funds for surgeons from other countries to study in Spain.

An increasing interchange of scientific programs within the Western European countries has taken place in recent years. The entry of Spain into the European Economic Community has opened new channels of international cooperation, especially in the field of high technology.

Achievements in Surgical Research

In spite of inadequate finances and an unsupportive atmosphere for research, the personal efforts of some surgeons have made possible the development of original contributions through the years. The work of surgeons was decisive in introducing European medical advances and experimental research into Spain in the last third of nineteenth century. The institution founded by the surgeon F. Rubio (1827–1902) provided a model that was widely imitated thereafter. The work of J. Cardenal, J. Ribera, and A. San Martín reached international recognition in the following generation.[7]

The worldwide recognition of the significance of Cajal's investigations in the early years of this century was an incentive to many institutions to integrate research into their curricula. The powerful influence of the Institución Libre de Enseñanza (Free Teaching Institution) on several generations of investigators, including a number of renowned surgeons, is particularly noteworthy. The tremendous trauma of the civil war interrupted the advance of research in a number of different schools, because many investigators disappeared or went into exile. During the reconstruction of the country, there were other more urgent medical needs, and research was again dependent on the determination of a few. Since then, a constant flow of young investigators to industrial areas (England, Germany, and mainly the United States) has taken place.

During the late 1950s and early 1960s, new surgical specialties needed the support of research for their clinical work. Interesting results were obtained in many instances, although experimental laboratories were rudimentary in structure and equipment. Neurosurgery expanded thanks to the pioneering works of Ley, Tolosa, Barcia Goyanes, and Obrador. Pallencephalography was one of the original diagnostic techniques described in those years,[8] as summarized by Obrador,[9] founder of the Institute of Neurological Science, where a considerable amount of the experimental surgery was carried out. In recent years, Rodríguez Delgado has continued the experimental studies in neurophysiology that he started while at Yale University; his collaboration in the field of functional neurosurgery has been significant.

In the early years of experimental cardiovascular surgery in Spain, surgeons had to improvise experimental laboratories to evaluate new techniques of extracorporeal circulation; in some units, residents rotated through them as part of their training. Important and original contributions were made by C. Gómez-Durán (homologous and heterologous cardiac valves)[10,11] and F. Alvarez Díaz (first low profile valvular prosthesis).[12] The tricuspid annuloplasty described by N.G. de Vega[13] had universal acceptance. Cardiovascular surgery has maintained a number of ongoing research programs; some of the best known results are flexible valvular rings,[14,15] the use of heterologous pericardium,[16] and some innovations in prostheses.[17,18] Interest is now focused on surgery for arrhythmias,[9] heart transplantation, and the development of new techniques for dealing with congenital heart problems.[20-23]

Clinical research has generated important advances in most surgical specialties. For example, Spanish contributions in ophthalmology (Barraquer, Arruga, Carreras, Murube, et al.) and in urology have achieved international recognition. In urology, the following are of considerable interest: S. Gil Vernet's investigation on the structure and morphogenesis of prostatic carcinoma[24]; A. Puigvert's demonstration of nonobstructive calyx dilatation, (now known as megacaliosis or Puigvert's disease)[25]; and L. Cifuentes' demonstration of vaginal epithelium in the trigonum vesicae, which undergoes the same changes as the vaginal epithelium during the menstrual cycle.[26] More recent contributions include those of Ruano-Gil[27] in embryology and of Páramo[28] and Vela Navarrete[29] on polycystic disease and the technique of constant pressure flow pyelography.[30] The outstanding studies on lithogenesis by L. Cifuentes,[31] the important innovations introduced by J.M. Gil Vernet in surgery of renal calculi and renal transplantations,[32,33] transverse ureterorenoscopy,[34] and the transection of spermatic vessels in carcinoma of the prostate[35] have also received general acceptance. At present, interesting research on an implantable artificial kidney is being carried out.[36]

In traumatology and orthopedics, clinical investigations have been carried out mairly in the areas of prostheses and transplants, arthroscopic surgery, electrical stimulation in consolidation and pseudoarthrosis, and immunological studies.[37]

The foregoing examples demonstrate our existing and potential capacity to open new paths, if the chronic organizational problems afflicting Spanish medicine are solved. A detailed description of all the achievements in surgical research in the different specialties is beyond the scope of this summary. A multidisciplinary approach has been noticed in recent years, and the first results of collaboration with basic science investigators are beginning to be seen in different fields. One example is the current increase in interest in organ transplantation research that has developed in centers with well-equipped experimental laboratories.[38-42]

Legal and Cultural Considerations

In general, animal experimentation presents no problem from a legal point of view. The public's attitude is indifferent as long as the proper setup is provided. So far, the antivivisection movement is feeble and has almost no influence on public opinion. The present legal void in this specific area is partly covered by the recommendations of the International Council on Animal Experimentation, as stated by the Spanish Society on Animal Experimentation.

Until recently, it was not difficult to carry out trials, and few legal controls were applied. Now, a committee in each hospital has to approve clinical trials, and the local or regional health authorities have to know about them. This is the theory, but in practice, there is a certain degree of general permissiveness.

Consent is now required for clinical trials, as well as for invasive procedures, etc. The new health act stipulates patient rights, including the right to be properly informed about diagnostic and therapeutic procedures. In general, patients' and families' attitudes toward the professional behavior of hospital doctors are favorable, but there is increasing resistance to the health care system itself. Criticism of the functioning of the Social Security system is featured daily in the press, and it has had the effect of turning public opinion against doctors, too. The outpatient clinics are a source of constant conflict, because of their huge size and primitive diagnostic and treatment methods. Although there is increasing dissatisfaction with public medicine, recent polls have revealed a growing appreciation of doctors' work, especially in hospitals. Although 98% of the population is covered by public medicine under Social

Security, many social sectors still prefer private consultants or use the services of private insurance companies.

Changes are now occurring very rapidly, but not all of them are in line with real progress and better quality. The long-standing disorganization within the complex health care system certainly requires improved management; but the State Administration—a giant bureaucratic machine, reinforced under the current socialist government—seems obsessed with exercising control at all levels, including such obviously independent areas as research. Politicians' distrust of the medical profession has grown to a dangerous point. Physicians are dissatisfied with their daily work and the way they have to perform it, and they fear the possibility of being turned into regular civil servants. Professional, economic, and social incentives are disappearing, and a great confusion about the immediate future has replaced the enthusiasm of past decades.

The process of socialization in medicine is irreversible, but no sincere attempts have been made to find constructive solutions to the problems posed by the transformation of the health care system. Medical associations' points of view are not taken into consideration, and an image of the physician as a nostalgic defender of outdated privileges is often offered to the public. In this "ceremony of confusion," embroidered with dangerous demagogic statements, a general politicization of medicine has taken place in recent years, even in daily practice. The temptation to complete the nationalization of health care with a consequent loss of freedom and independence hovers over the whole medical profession, in paradoxical contrast to the undoubted rise of freedom in public life.

Physicians working for the public health care system are bound to fixed salaries and regulated working hours, regardless of the quality of their work; professional activities are restricted or forbidden outside working hours; patients' choice of physician is strongly limited to geographical areas and certain health centers; political influence has a growing impact on the appointment of individuals to such responsible posts as hospital directors and members on research granting committees, etc.

Necessary deep medical reforms are now arriving after much delay, but they include the incorporation of some of the big mistakes made a long time ago in other Western countries.[43] Progressive "proletarianization" of the medical profession is going to affect the development of medicine negatively, from the doctor-patient relationship to the highest levels of research. The tendency to equalize, regardless of commitment and creativity, has started to operate, and its first consequences are already being felt.

Some of these problems do not belong exclusively to Spanish society, but an outline of them is essential to a better understanding of the poor situation of medical research. In spite of all the inconveniences and difficulties, investigation has grown in recent years. There were 50% more projects in the period 1978–1982 than in 1973–1977, and some areas, like biochemistry, have reached a high level of achievement. The lack of organized support for Spanish investigators produces an unfortunate lack of continuity.

Few hospitals have surgical investigators on the staff. They are usually part of the department of surgery, physiology, or basic sciences. If the research department is independent, conflicts occasionally arise because its surgical projects are not always of interest to the persons in charge.

Existing administrative regulations oblige hospitals to have a research committee. Most projects have to be submitted to this group for approval, but there is a certain flexibility outside pure experimental work.

The preferences of granting agencies exert considerable influence on general research activities, and the main lines of investigation—epidemiology, currently, for State Administration grants, hypertension in the case of certain drug companies, etc. Most surgical research depends on government grants.

The meetings of surgical societies are the usual places to present research data and results. Each society holds at least one meeting a year. The Spanish Society for Surgical Research, founded 10 years ago, has been steadily growing and currently has 320 members. The society has a journal entitled *Research in Surgery*. In 1989, "*Trasplante*, Journal of Organ and Tissue Transplantation" was founded. Both journals are published in English. Major surgical journals are listed in Table 59.2.

Language skills are considered to be a prerequisite for surgical research. More attention is now paid to their development at all educational levels, and the younger generations are better equipped in this area. As in many other countries, English dominates, particularly in the scientific literature, while French and German have dropped markedly in comparison with their use in the first half of this century. Research results are usually published in Spanish surgical journals, but authors try to get their best work published in prestigious international periodicals to achieve recognition and reach larger scientific communities.

TABLE 59.2. Main journals in which Spanish surgical research is published.

Acta Chirurgica Cataloniae
Acta Ginecológica
Acta Obstetricia y Ginecológica Hispano-Lusitana
Actas de la Fundación Puigvert
Actas de la Sociedad Española de O.R.L.
Actas Urológicas Españolas
Actualidad Obstétrico-ginecológica
Anales de Angiología
Anales del Instituto Barraquer
Anales de Cuidados Intensivos
Angiología
Archivos Españoles de Urología
Archivos de Neurobiología
Archivos de la Sociedad Española de Oftalmología Cirugía Española
Clínica e Investigación en Ginecología y Obstreticia
Gastroenterología y Hepatología
Medicina Intensiva
Neurocirugía
Neurochirurgia
Oncología
Progresos de Obstreticia y Ginecología
Revista Española de Anestesiología y Reanimación
Revista Española de Cardiología
Revista Española de Cirugía Cardíaca, Torácica y Vascular
Revista Española de Cirugía Ortopédica y Traumatológica
Revista Española de Enfermedades del Aparato Digestivo
Revista Española de Obstetricia y Ginecología
Revista Española de Ortopedia y Traumatología
Revista Iberoamericana de Cirugía Oral y Maxilofacial
Revista Iberoamericana de Fertilidad
Revista Iberolatinoamericana de Cirugía Plástica
Revista Latina de Cardiología
Revista de la Sociedad Española de Diálisis y Transplante
Studium Ophthalmologicum
Surgical Research
Toko-Ginecología Práctica
Transplante, Journal of Organ and Tissue Transplantation

Surgical Training and Research

Training in surgery and other medical areas was not well organized until recently. Certain hospitals maintained high standards in their residency programs, with requirements in time and quality similar to other Western countries, but this was not the general rule. In addition to the disparity among the different programs and the lack of control over them, the official title of specialist could be obtained in a shorter time, regardless of the training followed. In certain cases, a certificate from the head of a department or service was enough to allow a candidate to obtain the official title without any strict verification of appropriate training by the administrative health authorities. Medical associations opposed this practice and attempted to remedy the inherent confusion and injustice.

Some centers made considerable efforts to improve their residency programs, but the negative consequences of the inadequate quality control and planning led to exploitation of residents as a "cheap labor force." Their training was faulty, and the experience they received fell far short of the desired objective. Some medical and surgical specialties became oversaturated after a few years, and many specialists could not find a job in their field at the end of their residency training. This bitter situation has generated a great deal of frustration among young doctors, particularly in those who completed long and intense programs of study.

This situation has been greatly alleviated by the Medical Specialties Act of 1978. The law codified the requirements and content of postgraduate training programs, and it regulates access of physicians to residency training. Forty-three different medical and surgical specialties requiring basic hospital training were officially recognized, in addition to another six (hydrotherapy, space medicine, physical education and sports medicine, legal and forensic medicine, work or occupational medicine, and stomatology) that did not require hospital practice. Thirteen of the specialties are surgical.

Each medical specialty has a national committee, composed of certified specialists who represent the Health Ministry, the Education Ministry, the Medical Association, and the specialty societies. Each national committee sets the requirements for its specific area, selects and controls the teaching units, regulates the number of residents to be admitted each year, judges the final examination, etc. The title or certificate of the specialty is given by the Ministry of Education and Science. This certificate is required to take up a hospital position, but not for strictly private practice.

A regulation, approved by the National Council of Medical Specialties in 1989, established a classification of specialties based on generic trunks (medical, surgical, laboratory, and radiology). Under this regulation, surgical residency programs must provide a 2-year period of training in general surgery—maxillary; ear, nose and throat; and obstetrics and gynecology require only 1 year—followed by 3 or 4 years devoted to the specific area. Cardiovascular, thoracic, neuro-, and vascular surgery require 6 years to fulfill the program.

A general consensus has been reached to adapt the different programs to those of the Western European countries, although the latter are far from being uniform. Accordingly, the present can be regarded as a transitional period leading to more exacting training, and the desirable possibility of a common European certificate. Starting in 1992, the free circulation of professionals, including medical doctors, will be a fact within the EEC countries. The obligatory homology and convalidation of titles and certificates will require the development of common requisites and training.

The Medical Specialties Act of 1985, and its 1989 modifications, introduced flexible programs, higher standards for obtaining teaching credit, a tendency to unify programs and provide opportunities for broader training in basic medicine or surgery, and residents' representatives in the national committees. A populistic administrative concession to the resident's associations increased unrest, perpetuated some general failures (particularly in quality control), and eliminated the final obligatory examination to obtain a specialty certificate. Annual evaluations are supposedly done by the local teaching committees; in practice, this is equivalent to the automatic awarding of the specialist certificate at the end of the residency period, regardless of the quality of the training received.

Candidates for the residency programs are selected through a highly competitive national examination–more than 23,000 candidates in 1989 for 3000 residency posts throughout the country. Those who obtain the highest scores have a choice of specialty and center, opportunities diminishing according to rank order. The number of places was reduced in the mid-1980s, partly because of oversaturation in certain specialties and partly because of a decrease in the funds provided by the National Institute of Health. This number was increased again in the past 2 years, however, mainly to cover big deficiencies in community and family doctors and in certain specialties like anesthesiology, radiology, and psychiatry. Some major failures are recognized in the system, mainly those derived from the impossibility for many to select their desired specialty. Teaching and training capacity is obviously underused and is only partly taken up by foreign doctors.

Research is not an obligatory part of surgical training, except in a very few institutions. In these, residents usually spend part of their third or fourth year in the research laboratory. During this time, they maintain contact with the clinical section by taking calls, attending medical-surgical meetings, etc. Although the differences among institutions make it difficult to estimate how many receive such training, the percentage of surgical residents obtaining some training in surgical research is probably less than 5%.

Large hospitals usually have some research programs, particularly in certain surgical specialties. In general, surgical residents are more attracted by the practical aspects of the training program; those who wish to dedicate themselves to research careers are the exceptions. Although reluctant to spend any time in the research laboratory, many feel pleased that they did so. Most of them state that the experience they acquired will be of great benefit to them in their future careers as clinical surgeons. During the period of research, the resident is paid the salary previously established for his training, which is the same throughout the whole country without regard to the institution.

TABLE 59.3. Surgical specialties with training programs and official certificates (1989).

Angiology and Vascular Surgery
Cardiovascular Surgery
Ear, Nose and Throat Surgery
General Surgery
Maxillary and Facial Surgery
Obstetrics and Gynecology
Ophthalmology
Pediatric Surgery
Plastic and Reparative Surgery
Neurosurgery
Thoracic Surgery
Traumatology and Orthopedic Surgery
Urology

A resident can seldom choose his own research problem. Usually, he is engaged in the project that is currently in progress. In some rare instances, he is permitted to choose a subject within a general area followed by the department. When the research project is part of the requirements for a doctorate in medicine or in a basic science, he is freer to choose a particular problem, but he must always be under the supervision of a tutor. To obtain the degree of doctor of medicine, a written thesis is mandatory, but it does not always have to deal with an original research project; it can be dedicated to the review of a particular problem. For many physicians, this is the only time in their career they are in contact with research.

In spite of the tremendous lack of facilities, most surgical national committees recommend the inclusion of some sort of training in surgical research in their programs. It has been suggested that some qualified residents rotate through the centers that have research laboratories, but this is very difficult to accomplish in practice.

The availability of only a few research fellowships–usually poorly funded–hinders the dedication of some time to research at the end of the residency program.

The main motivation for a resident to obtain training in research is usually to advance a surgical career within the academic community. Unfortunately, much of the work done in the laboratory, even at university level, is aimed at reproducing, in animals, surgical techniques or variations used in humans. This is considered to be a way of getting experience and developing skill with a particular technique. Lack of proper basic science support precludes engagement in major interdisciplinary research projects.

Participation in research is mandatory if an academic career within a university is planned. Sadly, much of it is performed only to fulfill curriculum vitae requirements. Deep-rooted university corporatism makes it almost impossible for a surgeon, no matter how experienced or excellent, to get a high teaching position as a professor by working outside the university hospitals.

Surgical residents participate more often in clinical research. There are more facilities in this area, and many residents appear as coauthors of clinical papers published by a department. Such collaboration is an asset when they apply for a hospital position.

Possible Solutions

The same broad considerations apply to surgical investigation as to research in general. First, it is necessary to put aside utopian plans. With her present feeble economy, Spain cannot approach, in the short term, the expansion in research and development of the Western industrial countries. It is mandatory, however, to consider scientific research to be a national priority under present circumstances. "Since society and politicians do not realize that industrial development, quality of life, and professional standards depend directly on the national scientific capacity, it will be very difficult to get the means and stimulation that Spanish science requires."[44]

The lack of a true scientific atmosphere is a fact repeatedly expressed by scientists with an international reputation.[3,44-46] The solemn and frequently impressive official statements do not correspond with the social role assigned, in reality, to the investigators.[47] Full-time investigators' salaries are below the mean for state employees of the same level or category, and the possibilities of professional promotion are very scarce.

It is time to put aside the investigator's image as a hero or martyr within the texture of the social structure.[45] The ambitious National Plan of Science and Technology can become a frustration unless considerable efforts are directed to increasing the number of scientists and dignifying their position.[47] A social atmosphere propitious to research cannot be improvised overnight, nor can it depend exclusively on the existing available money: social leaders must be clearly aware of its real importance to the country's progress, and the need to open wide channels of participation to stimulate creative capacity at all levels. Present circumstances, however, seem to favor a certain degree of superficiality and mediocrity. Under these conditions, Spanish society will not only miss the train again, but also the plane of the immediate future.[46]

Amiguismo—the shameless favoring of friends and political allies—a chronic evil of Spanish society, has been dangerously potentiated by the present State Administration. Promotion to responsible posts is often based on simple political grounds. This attitude, which has a certain wide acceptance, must be banished from the social stage: ideological or political affinity should not influence the professional career in such important and necessary fields as health care and research.

Most Spanish scientists are agreed that one of the worst impediments to research is bureaucratic stagnation. A good basic structure is essential for future development, and the lack of a coherent organization is felt at all levels. This matter has to be put in the hands of persons with acceptable track records in research and with the capacity to find solutions without having to depend on obscure bureaucratic decisions. Obviously, responsibility in the administration of public funds should be a strict requirement. Better coordination of public and private financial agencies is also necessary. Free enterprise should not be regarded with suspicion by the State Administration. More financial support is desperately needed, but the promised 1% of the total health budget assigned to research had reached only 0.2% in 1987. Finding appropriate incentives to promote the expansion of research activity in the private sector, which at the moment is really minimal, is urgent. The recent science act is too ambiguous in this respect, although it envisages greater administrative flexibility. Private enterprises have to change their mentality and begin to look at research as a real investment with undoubted future benefits. The possibility of collaborating in EEC scientific projects opens new paths that should attract a greater private investment.

Along with such important organizational changes, biomedical research needs to make better use of the available resources, both human and material. Priorities should be fixed without stifling the enthusiasm and independence needed by the investigator to maintain the ability to perform valuable scientific work. Clinical research also needs better control and coordination which, at the first level, can be done by the hospital or center itself. Quality and productivity requirements have to be exacting, so that the number of nonproductive persons can be reduced. The present high costs of research require that the opportunities to pursue research careers be reserved for those who are really motivated and demonstrating a dedication to continuity in their work. In addition to reinforcing the existing centers, careful planning is required to ensure that anomalies and external pressures do not interfere with investigators' freedom and spontaneity.[44] Part of the budget should be dedicated to the maintenance of the infrastructure,[48] which is so often neglected in the Spanish system.

Access to medical schools has to be reserved for those who are really capable, rather than the disastrous political populistic concessions of the past. Contact and dialogue between professor and student must be reestablished. Otherwise, the medical school can turn into an officially designated office for the conferring of titles and certificates. The system for selecting faculty members is in need of renovation. A post should not be tenable for life if the quality of the work performed over a period of years is not at a high level.

Only a small amount of surgical research is currently performed in the universities. To recover its true path and rhythm, and to maintain its connection with the society it serves, scientific research must be one of the primary aims of each university. The abandonment of the ivory tower mentality is one of the first actions to be taken for a true transformation to occur.

Medical students should be taught the methods of surgical research. During their training period, residents must have contact with experimental surgery, must be seriously involved in clinical investigation, and must not be regarded or treated only as data collectors. The possibility for clinical surgical staff to dedicate some portion of their careers to research should also be contemplated,[48] even though the present rigid administrative schemes are a serious obstacle.

Certain state centers like the National Council for Scientific Research and the Carlos III Institute have been greatly favored in official financial support with detriment to the research performed in other hospitals. In addition, public hospital surgeons are harassed by excessive clinical obligations without time or the facilities for research. The endless waiting lists are the tip of the iceberg of structural disorganization. Each regional or national hospital should have its own independent research department and freedom to contract the personnel needed to establish a successful research program.[5] Although clinical investigation is at an acceptable level in certain specialties, basic research is practically nonexistent.[49] Hospitals are the ideal place to carry out multidisciplinary research that can have the continuity of clinical investigation. Central coordination must avoid the present paradoxical repetition of the same lines of investigation.

With few exceptions, the libraries of medical schools and hospitals need improvement. Modern systems of information retrieval are urgently needed to give trainees easy access to the international medical literature. A national center of biomedical documentation with a wide net of branches has been indicated as a primary need.[5]

Adequate salaries are unknown in public medicine today. An experienced surgeon working for the Social Security system earns less than a specialized worker. As a result, many physicians hold a second post or have to dedicate extra hours to find a supplementary income. Mental and emotional dedication to scientific research is not possible if a decent living is not guaranteed.

Physicians were not accorded any active role in the organization of the health care system and were hardly consulted about it. Distrust and resentment have continued through the years as reforms were introduced. Physicians are not good at organizing for the defense of their profession; trade unions and other organizations are filling the gaps even if they represent only a minority of the medical community. An improvement in financial support and working conditions affecting surgical research will not occur without constant pressure on the health administrative authorities and an effort to ensure that the public is properly informed.

Summary

In summary, the complexity of the present health care organization gives rise to enormous problems for scientific research in Spain that are different from those in many Western countries. They can be solved by abandoning the narrow political scientific vision[50] and expanding the spirit of investigation. If we do so, historians in the twenty-first century will not have to investigate why there was no investigation in the twentieth century.[51] Little surgical research is done at present, and the structural organization does not permit rapid change. A solid supportive research atmosphere has to be created within the Spanish society so that intellectual daring reappears.[52] Critical thinking, a sound methodological approach to research, and motivation for scientific endeavor will then be accorded appropriate recognition and many of our promising investigators will not have to abandon research or leave the country.

References

1. Laín Entralgo P. Historia Universal de la Medicina. Barcelona: Medicina Actual, 1964;vii–xvii.
2. Díez Domínguez P. España, una salud europea. El País Futuro, Dec. 12, 1985.
3. Gómez-Santos M. Interview with F. Mayor Zaragoza, UNESCO General Director. El Médico, April 1986.
4. Fondo de Investigaciones sanitarias de la Seguridad Social. Memoria 1988. Madrid, Ministerio de Sanidad y Consumo, 1989.
5. Ricoy JR. Fondo de investigaciones sanitarias de la Seguridad Social: pasado, presente y futuro (as summarized by C. Nicolas). El Médico, September 1987.
6. Editorial: Los puntos negros de la investigación sanitaria. El Médico, June 1986.
7. López Piñero JM, García Ballester L, Faus Sevilla P. Medicina y sociedad en la España del siglo XIX. Madrid: Sociedad de Estudios y Publicaciones, 1964:105.
8. Barcia Goyanes JJ, Calvo W, Barcia Salorio JL. Un nuevo método de exploración del encéfalo: la palencefalografía. Rev Esp Oto-Neuro Oftalmol, 1956: 83–84.
9. Obrador Alcalde S. Evolución de la neurocirugía española en los últimos treinta años. Neurocir Luso-Esp. 1977;17–75.
10. A method for placing a total homologous aortic valve in the subcoronary position. Lancet 1962;2: 488–89.
11. Binet JP, Durán CMG, Carpentier A, Langlois J. Heterologous aortic valve transplantation. Lancet 1965;1275.
12. Alvarez F, Rábago G, Urquía M, Castillón L. Eccentric mitral valve prosthesis with a rigid hinge. Experimental observation. J Cardiovasc Surg 1966; 7:226–31.
13. de Vega NG. La anuloplastia selectiva, regulable y permanente. Una técnica original para el tratamiento de la insuficiencia tricúspide. Rev Esp Cardiol 1972;25:555–56.
14. Gómez Durán C. Clinical and hemodynamic performance of a totally flexible prosthetic ring for atrioventricular reconstruction. Ann Thorac Surg 1976; 22:458–63.
15. Puig Massana M. Conservative surgery of the mitral valve. Annuloplasty on a new adjustable ring. In: Cardiovascular Surgery 1980, Bircks W, Ostermeyer J, Schultes HD, eds. New York: Springer Verlag, 1981;30.
16. Gallo JI, Pomar JL, Artiñao E, Durán CMG. Heterologous pericardium for the closure of pericardial defects. Ann Thorac Surg 1978;26:149–54.
17. Castillo-Olivares JL, Goiti JJ, O'Connor F, Nojek C, Téllez G, Figuera D. Válvula supra-anular de bajo perfil para reemplazaminto mitral. Rev Esp Cardiol 1977;30:23–26.
18. Montero C, Castillo-Olivares JL, Cienfuegos JA, Figuera D. Xenogenic cervical dura mater; a new anisotropic tissue for heart-valve prosthesis. Life Support Syst 1985;3:233–46.
19. Cabo C, González MA, Linacero G, et al. Acquisition, processing and stimulation system in cardiac arrhythmias surgery. Melecon 85, Madrid, October 1985.
20. Alvarez Díaz F, Hurtado del Hoyo E, de León JP, et al. Técnica de correción anatómica de la transposición completa de grandes vasos. Comunicación preliminar. Rev Esp Cardiol 1975;28:255.
21. Alvarez Díaz F, Cabo J, Alvarez A, et al. Nueva técnica cerrada de ampliación del tracto de salida del ventrículo derecho. Rev Esp Cardiol 1981;34:293.
22. Alvarez Díaz F, Cabo Salvador J, Cordovilla Zurgo G. Partial reconstruction of right ventricular outflow tract without cardiopulmonary by-pass. J Thorac Cardiovasc Surg (letter) 1982;83:149.
23. Arcas R, Herreros J, Llorens R. Nueva técnica quirúrgica experimental para la transposición de grandes arterias. XV Congreso Nacional de la Sociedad Española de Cardiología, Santander (abstract book), 1977:61.
24. Gil Vernet S. Enfermedades de la Próstata. Madrid: Ediciones Paz Montalvo, 1955.
25. Puigvert A. La Megacaliosis (Disembrioplasia de las pirámides de Malpighio). Rev Clin Esp 1963;91:69.
26. Cifuentes L. Cistitis y cistopatías. Madrid: Ediciones Paz Montalvo, 1947.
27. Ruano-Gil D, Coca Payeras A, Tejedo Mateu A. Obstruction and normal recanalization of the ureter in the human embryo. Eur Urol 1975;1:287.
28. Páramo P, Segura A. Hilioquistosis renal. Rev Clin Esp 1972;126:387.
29. Vela Navarrete R, Robledo A. Polycystic disease of the renal sinus. J Urol 1983;129:700.
30. Vela Navarrete R. Constant pressure flow controlled antegrade pyelography. Eur Urol 1982;8:265.
31. Cifuentes L. Composición y estructura de los cálculos renales. Barcelona: Ediciones Salvat, 1984.
32. Gil Vernet JM, Caralps A. Human renal homotransplantation: new surgical technique. Urol Int 1968; 23:201.
33. Gil Vernet J. New surgical concepts in removing renal calculi. Urol Int 1965;20:255.
34. Pérez Castro E, Martínez Piñeiro JA. La ureterorrendoscopia transuretral. Arch Esp Urol 1980;33:3.
35. Romero Maroto J, Nistal M, González Gancedo P, Bellas C, Aranas A. Transection of spermatic vessels (Bevan's technique): experimental study. J Urol 1983;130:1232.
36. Vela Navarrete R. Personal communication, 1989.
37. Jiménez Cisneros A. Personal communication. 1985.
38. Cuervas-Mons V, Maganto P, Cienfuegos JA, et al. Ectopic liver using dispersed liver cells as a support measure in acute fulminant hepatic failure. Hepatology 1982;2:183.
39. Eroles G, Maganto P, Pinedo I, et al. Development of an experimental model of cirrhosis and its treatment by syngeneic hepatocyte transplantation into the rat spleen. Eur Surg Res 1983;15:26–27.
40. Abascal J. Aislamiento, preservación e isotrans-

plante de islotes de Langerhans. Doctoral thesis. Madrid: Universidad Autónoma, 1981.
41. Casanova A. Estudio del autotrasplante del tejido insular pancreático sin aislamiento específico en el sistema portal extraportal en perros totalmente pancreatizados. Doctoral thesis. Santander: Universidad de Santander, 1982.
42. Golitsin A, Pinedo I, Cienfuegos JA, Chamorro JL, Ortiz Berrocal J, Castillo-Olivares JL. Study of the early rejection of the heterotopic transplanted heart by using 201-thallium. Experimental study. Eur Surg Res 1983;5:41.
43. Biörck G. How to be a clinician in a socialist country. Ann Intern Med 1977;86:813–17.
44. Toledo González J. Investigación contra burocracia. Interview with S. Ochoa, F. Mayor Zaragoza, A. García Bellido, E. Viñuela and D. Vázquez. El País Futuro, October 16, 1985.
45. Hortal M. Interview with M. Barbacid. El Médico, March 1986.
46. Ferrater Mora J. Perder el avión. El País, March 21, 1986.
47. García López E. La dignificación del científico en España, una asignatura pendiente. El País, November 13, 1987.
48. Mariño C. Interview with F.J. Rubio. El Médico, November 1985.
49. Zarco P, Cortina A. Diario de Congresos Médicos, no 197, December 1989.
50. Ochoa S. Política científica de cortas miras. Noticias Médicas, February 14, 1990.
51. Laín P. Aquí y ahora. El País, February 12, 1987.
52. Laín Entralgo P. La ausencia de osadía de la inteligencia. El País, July 16, 1985.

60

Orderly Evolution to a Better Future in Sweden

S. Fasth and L. Hultén

Surgical research in Sweden has a long tradition of excellence enhanced by the positive attitude of governmental authorities toward medical and surgical research during the past 40 years. Significant investments made during the 1950s created a solid foundation for rapid and extensive expansion in research during the 1960s, in parallel with industrial and economic development in Sweden. External contacts, particularly with Western Europe and the United States, flourished during the 1960s, along with the growth in international exchange of research information. The resulting increased awareness of international research activity had a significant impact on internal standards for research quality and validity.

Limitations on state funding of research were introduced in the early 1970s, and it was generally understood that society's interest in research had abated and had been replaced by suspicion, in some quarters. Fortunately, this was a temporary phenomenon and research is now generally accorded a positive and important role in the development of Swedish society. In the 1980s, Sweden spent about 0.25% of its gross domestic product on biomedical research and development.

Surgical Research Training

It is widely acknowledged that advanced surgical research must be based on an extensive and effective training program. A comprehensive analysis of research training made by governmental authorities, during the 1950s and 1960s, concluded that too little organized instruction and supervision in combination with excessive clinical workloads resulted in a lack of effectiveness. The lack of collaborators and the isolation of research fellows in surgery was particularly noted. The commission recommended that surgical research training programs be more structured, that they be of 4 years duration, and that they give research trainees the opportunity to produce four or five original papers with their supervisors or other collaborators. The papers should be published in international scientific periodicals with high standards and should be brought together and discussed in a thesis, for subsequent defense at a public dissertation. The choice of scientific subject should be open, and the topic of the dissertation need not be surgically or clinically oriented—it could encompass basic research in physiology or biochemistry or other related scientific disciplines. When the thesis is approved, the degree of "Doctor of Medicine in Surgery" is conferred on the researcher. The degree is analogous to the Ph.D. and makes the graduate eligible to apply for an appointment as a "docent" in surgery. The application is evaluated by a special board that reviews the candidate's clinical independence and competence, scientific ability, general character, and qualifications for such an academic position. An approved dissertation, including four or five original papers, is not sufficient qualification in itself. Other scientific publications must establish each candidate's breadth of knowledge and independence. Evidence demonstrating ability to teach and to supervise research trainees also is required.

A shorter training program (e.g., 2 years) is sometimes discussed because the present system gives only a small proportion of the total number of surgeons an opportunity to do research. Arguments against shortening the training period include the inherent dangers of lowering the quality and revising the general aims of research training. The current aims of surgical research training are:

1. To inculcate an in-depth knowledge of surgery, foster a systematic approach to work, and develop a capacity to think critically and creatively that

will characterize graduates as individuals capable of performing independent scientific work.
2. To encourage research that will contribute to the overall development of science.
3. To reinforce the establishment of international contacts between research scientists.
4. To meet society's need for highly qualified surgeons in key positions of surgical leadership.

Training in research can be initiated at three stages in a surgical career.

1. *During medical school.* Medical students who intend to become surgeons sometimes undertake research training in a biomedical science, such as physiology. Alternatively, a "docentur" in physiology can, after a few years of surgical residency and surgical research, be converted into a "docentur" in surgery. Those who follow this route usually embark on it between the ages of 20 and 24 years as the result of deciding to pursue an academic career in surgery in a university department.
2. *Immediately following graduation from medical school.* Embarking on research training at this stage has become uncommon because it puts the research fellow in the position of having neither clinical experience nor scientific education.
3. *After 3 to 5 years of surgical residency in a county hospital.* Those who choose this path start their research training at age 32 to 34 years. With recommendations from a chief surgeon at a county hospital, the young surgeon will be employed as a resident in a surgical department of a university hospital. Table 60.1 outlines the weekly schedule for a university hospital resident in Sweden. This is the most common choice, and probably the most appropriate, because the young surgeon will have the opportunity to assess the surgical techniques and management procedures he has been taught. A county hospital residency is an extremely important part of the fundamental training of a Swedish surgeon. The surgery performed in most university hospitals in Sweden is so highly specialized that common operations, such as hernia repairs and cholecystectomies, are usually excluded.

The Research Adviser

Teaching medical students and supervising research trainees are duties of all members of the surgical staff of a university hospital. The number of trainees supervised varies, but is generally limited to protect the quality of supervision. The importance of supervising research trainees in surgical subspecialties has gained increasing recognition in recent years, particularly in the selection of candidates for such positions as assistant professor or professor. The supervision of research trainees carries considerable responsibility, since it is the adviser's duty to discuss possible research topics, participate in designing individual plans of research training, and contribute to the development of research protocols. The adviser is supposed to maintain continuous contact with the research trainee to discuss the work in progress and offer constructive criticism, while taking care to encourage the trainee's independence and creativity. The adviser is responsible for ensuring the availability of adequate resources for the research trainee (from the host institution), and accepts ultimate responsibility for the design of the thesis, the quality of the dissertation, and the nomination of an appropriate opponent for the public dissertation.

Funding of Surgical Research

The Medical Research Council of Sweden usually provides support for the employment of research nurses or laboratory assistants in surgical research. Surgeons-in-chief apply to the MRC for funds and are scientifically and administratively responsible for their expenditure.

Pharmaceutical companies may provide funds for staff support, other than the salary of the surgeon, for projects of particular interest to them during a specified period. Insurance companies support research projects on traffic and occupational accidents, and other industries make limited contributions. Private foundations give significant support to surgical research by providing funds for the compensation of human subjects and the purchase of laboratory animals and supplies; medical societies usually administer the awarding of these funds.

Hospitals support clinical research, but basic research is regarded as the responsibility of the universities. Medical schools supply funds to research trainees for laboratory animals and materials and for the compensation of human subjects. The universities also arrange and finance research training courses. Significant national support is given directly to hospitals to reimburse them for the research and teaching performed by surgeons. The distribution of surgeons' time between research, student teaching and clinical work is not clearly defined, but 10% to 15% is probably devoted to research. Research trainees can usually perform part of their research in parallel with their clinical duties while receiving financial support from national funds.

TABLE 60.1. Weekly working scheme for a resident in research training in a Swedish surgical university department.

	Monday	Tuesday	Wednesday	Thursday	Friday	Saturday	Sunday
07:45 08:30	Staff meeting, x-ray demonstrations						
08:30 10:00	Ward rounds with the consultants		Ward rounds with the consultants	Ward rounds	Ward rounds with the consultants		
10:00 11:00							
11:00 12:00	Ward work	Operations	Ward work	Operations	Outpatient, clinical, and ward work		
12:00 13:00						Literature studies, preparing of manuscripts, etc.	
13:00 14:00					Meeting with the research advisers	On duty at the hospital every fifth Saturday or Sunday	
14:00 15:00	Research work		Out patient clinic		Research work		
15:00 16:00	Ward rounds	Ward rounds					
16:00 17:00	Research education course	Scheduled student teaching	Staff meeting	Research work			

The financial resources available to individual researchers are satisfactory. There is freedom of choice among many possible projects and, normally, no interference or control is exercised, provided agreed scientific and financial reporting schedules are respected. Surgical societies in Sweden provide some financial support for research projects and for participation in national and international conferences. They do not contribute to any research fellowships.

The Medical Research Council of Sweden provides scholarships and stipends for foreign researchers to work in Sweden, accompanied by their families. Researchers can use whatever resources and funds can be spared from their basic personal support for their projects. The Medical Research Council publishes periodic announcements of available awards and eligibility requirements, and distributes them to all registered research trainees; similar bulletins are issued by the medical schools and medical and surgical societies. The pharmaceutical industry advertises the funding it will make available in national scientific periodicals. No topic preferences or biases are expressed by granting agencies, with the exception of the pharmaceutical industry, which expects a direct or indirect economic return from a research project.

The Effect of Research Training on the Surgeon

The overall objective of research training for the surgeon is to instill an extensive knowledge of surgery, develop a methodical approach to work, and encourage critical thinking. Enhancement of personal creativity is normally noticeable after a year or two of concentrated scientific studies. Most individuals who undergo such research training will continue in some sort of clinical research after they have left the university hospital. A surgeon who has completed research training and achieved an appointment as "docent" has a high social status.

Research training, an approved dissertation, and a position as a "docent" are now prerequisites for a consultant position in surgery (e.g., a chief surgeon at a county hospital or any academic position at a university hospital). The paucity of private surgical units in Sweden makes the number of surgical appointments smaller than in many other countries and increases the competitive pressure on candidates.

In Sweden, combining research training with full-time surgical work has few disadvantages. Although students get an insight into scientific methodology during their basic medical studies, the high demands placed on scientific competence by surgical research make such introductory courses inadequate. No form of undergraduate scientific training could produce the level of scientific sophistication required for surgical research. A surgical resident in a county hospital who develops an interest in a particular surgical topic can apply to any university, or to any group of researchers with the same interest, for research training; the resident's choice of research field is completely free. Residents who want to undertake research training, without specific research topics in mind, are given an overview of the different projects in progress in their institutions to enable them to make choices. Formal research training usually requires 4 years, but its duration varies according to the nature of projects and the difficulties that may arising during their execution. Projects involving animal experiments can sometimes be completed in a shorter period than clinical projects involving patient follow-up.

Research trainees are usually employed as registrars or junior staff members and can use part of each day or week for research activities. Because time spent "on call" is compensated by a corresponding amount of time off, research trainees can take every fifth or sixth week off and devote part or all of it to research. Although research trainees can be relieved of clinical practice duties during limited periods of time, they normally dedicate a significant portion of their nights and weekends to research work that does not have to be performed in hospital (e.g., reviewing literature and working up results). University hospital surgeons have to provide clinical services, teach medical students, and conduct and supervise research. University regulations require the devotion of 30% of total working hours to research supervision.

Organization of Library Service

All county and university hospitals have well-equipped library facilities for literature review and ready access to most national and international medical periodicals. Swedish and Scandinavian surgical societies provide several opportunities each year for the presentation of surgical research results. Swedish surgeons participate frequently in other international surgical conferences.

Since Sweden is a small country, research trainees depend heavily on medical literature in English, French, and German. To fulfill the requirement to publish their work in highly reputable international periodicals, research trainees must have a good command of English and, to some extent, of German and French. Because English tends to dominate at most international conferences, research trainees must be able to present their results and conduct subsequent discussions in English.

Attitudes Toward Surgical Research

Permission to perform animal experiments has been restricted during recent years, in Sweden as in many other countries. Acute (nonsurvival) experiments and some chronic animal experiments can still be performed, provided the protocol has been approved by a local ethics committee that includes lay people. The regulations covering human experiments are clearly defined, and the public attitude toward such experiments is mainly positive. Informed consent is mandatory. The written information provided to individuals prior to obtaining consent must be approved by the local ethics committee.

Since the Swedish socialized health care system relieves the patient of any medical or surgical fees, it is comparatively easy to perform clinical research. A high level of continuity, with regular and frequent follow-up visits, makes it possible to carry out reliable studies with a low percentage of dropouts. A great number of randomized clinical investigations of the comparative merits of different surgical interventions for peptic ulcer, cancer of the colon and rectum, and inflammatory bowel disease have been performed in Swedish hospitals in recent years.

Although the public's attitude toward surgical research is generally positive, criticism has been directed at animal experiments for surgical or medical research. In contrast, patients who are asked to participate in research projects generally display a positive attitude, so that it is usually not difficult to obtain informed consent for clinical trials or to find "healthy control subjects" for research studies.

Most universities and scientific societies regard surgical research in the same light as research in physiology or biochemistry; collaboration between surgical and basic science departments is common. Surgical staffs in university clinics view research favorably because it ranks with teaching and clinical work as a prerequisite for appointment to university clinical positions.

Chief surgeons in county hospitals are, with very few exceptions, "docents," which automatically signifies that they have had extensive research training and have produced successful dissertations. The same is often true of their surgical colleagues in consultant positions, because research training is considered to be a prerequisite for appointment to such positions. As a consequence, residents in county hospitals are encouraged to perform such clinical research as follow-up studies to assess surgical results.

The attitude among residents toward continuing their research training at a university hospital to the "doctor of medicine" level is generally positive, but social and economic changes during recent decades tend to interfere. Residents' spouses often have full-time jobs, and moving from county to university hospitals may entail significant or insurmountable personal or financial problems. During the 1980s, a few residents obtained their main research training in county hospitals supervised by a "docent" and have subsequently maintained a keen interest in research work. There are successful dissertations, based on experimental research performed in county hospitals, on such topics as postoperative adynamic ileus and gastrointestinal blood flow dimensions, measured preoperatively. This approach to research training, adapted to meet changing social patterns, may become more common in the future.

Achievements and Prospects for Surgical Research

Pioneering contributions to vascular surgery were made early in the twentieth century by Professor Einar Kay at the Karolinska Hospital. Clarence Crafoord won an international reputation in cardiac surgery by developing a method for surgical treatment of coarctation of the aorta, and by introducing the use of heparin prophylaxis against postoperative thromboembolism. Professor Herbert Olivercrona made significant contributions to the diagnosis and surgical treatment of brain tumors. Lund's test for assessing the exocrine function of the pancreas, developed in 1952, is in worldwide use and is an excellent example of how collaboration between clinical chemistry and surgery can lead to the development of diagnostic tests of wide clinical importance beyond the bounds of surgery.

Professor N.G. Kock gained international renown in 1969, when he presented a method for the construction of a continent ileostomy. This advance could not have been made without the extensive experimental studies in animals that Kock initiated and performed in the Department of Physiology.

Investigation is now well established in all surgical subspecialties in Sweden, and generally meets high international standards. It encompasses basic and clinical studies carried out in collaboration with other clinical specialties and academic institutions. The very positive attitude toward surgical research expressed by governmental authorities during the 1980s indicates that it will probably retain its good health and high status for some time.

61

The Confluence of Private and Public Resources in Switzerland

F. Largiadèr

Switzerland's 6.5 million inhabitants live in an area of 40,000 square kilometers that is partially covered by high mountains. Medical care is of very high quality and is organized according to liberal principles. The current ratio of medical doctors to inhabitants is high at 1:300 and will become higher if the present trend continues.

The general attitude of the population toward surgical research is friendly, but unengaged. Although research is considered to be a natural part of university-based surgery and often is equated with publishing, the average standard is not very high.

Practicing surgeons have reservations about research in a country that tends to adhere to traditional values. A humanitarian attitude, strength of character, and surgical craftsmanship are still considered to be the most important characteristics of a surgeon. Practicing clinicians are inclined to regard surgical research as an activity that is incompatible with such personal traits. Most medical students expect an emphasis on practical medical work and have only limited interest in research. Nevertheless, the international ties of Swiss surgeon–investigators are stronger than ever before, and attendance at foreign meetings is a normal part of their academic life.

Achievements of Surgical Research

Because Swiss surgical research has always depended on the efforts of single individuals, it has lacked continuity, has developed differently in each university, and has received systematic support only since 1950. Although surgical research programs have been established by Lenggenhager and Maurice Müeller in Bern, Allgöwer in Basel, and Senning in Zurich, purely Swiss contributions to surgical research are difficult to identify because of the close collaboration between Swiss surgical researchers and those in neighboring countries.

The early surgical research of César Roux, in Lausanne, and of Theodor Kocher, in Bern, must be mentioned. Kocher was the only Swiss surgeon ever to win the Nobel Prize. Theodor Billroth, Ulrich Krönlein, and Ferdinand Sauerbruch, professors of surgery in Zurich, also made notable contributions. All were trained in Germany, and Zurich offered them the opportunity to work independently, and to pursue their own ideas.

The *Arbeitsgemeinschaft für Osteosynthese* has an international reputation for its research in bone-fracture healing,[1] and Zurich was one of the first centers in the world involved in the clinical and experimental investigation of pancreatic transplantation.

Institutions for surgical research are associated with universities except for a few privately funded laboratories, such as one in Davos and another in Bern. Controlled randomized studies and other clinical investigations in university departments are not separated administratively from the usual clinical routine and are not performed by specially qualified personnel. No university has a position devoted permanently and exclusively to clinical surgical studies.

Lausanne is the only university with an independent division for experimental surgical research; in the other four – Basel, Bern, Geneva, and Zurich – it is part of the surgery departments. The head of surgical research is not a faculty member and has the position of a *Leitender Arzt* in Zurich and Basel and of *Oberarzt* in Bern. He is in charge of one or two residents, two to four laboratory technicians, and two to six nurses. In Bern, the group includes a veterinarian; in the other places, veterinarians are in charge of the animal facilities. Most of the research in the laboratories is performed by surgeons who are clinical residents or in receipt of salaries from research foundations.

Funding of Surgical Research

Government funding for surgical research covers a small part of the costs in Basel, makes up half the budget in Bern, and is the principal source of funding (in the amount of 200,000 Swiss francs per year) in Zurich. Approximately 0.46% of the gross domestic product of Switzerland is devoted to biomedical research. Pharmaceutical firms and industries provide practically no money for surgical research; they concentrate mainly on trials of new drugs. Surgical fees are not an important source of research funding, and surgical associations are unable to finance research fellowships or travel to scientific meetings. Research supported by the *Arbeitsgemeinschaft für Osteosynthese* belongs in a special category, since it is funded by profits from the sale of materials for osteosynthesis.

Many private foundations administered by universities, industries, or private boards support medical and, to some extent, surgical research, but the grants they bestow are only in the range of SFr 5000 to 50,000 per project. Only incomplete lists of these foundations are available from the administration departments of the universities and from the *Schweizerischer Wissenschaftsrat* (Wildhainweg 20, 3000 Bern).

The Swiss National Foundation (*Schweizerischer Nationalfonds zur Förderung der Wissenschaftlichen Forschung*, Bern) is the most important federal institution for the support of research. It has a government budget, and the research projects it funds meet internationally accepted standards.

Research During Residency Training

Acceptance criteria for residency training in surgery are set by the Swiss Medical Federation (FMH) and accepted by the government. Approved residency programs require a curriculum of 6 years, including a portion in small surgical units, but most surgeons voluntarily prolong the residency period to 8 or 9 years. The catalog of required clinical and operative activities is very precise, but it does not include research. A typical work day for a Swiss surgical resident is outlined in Table 61.1. Board certification in surgery is possible after residency programs outside the university hospitals.

Experimental surgical research cannot be made mandatory in residency programs because research

TABLE 61.1. A normal clinical day for a Swiss surgical resident.

07:30	Morning conference	
07:50	Rounds on emergency patients	
08:15	Operations	
14:00		
15:00	Daily conference of the sections	
15:30	Departmental conference: review operations of the day, programs for the following day	
16:15	Rounds and ward work, followed by:	
	Monday:	Scientific conference
	Tuesday:	Student teaching
	Wednesday:	Mortality conference
	Thursday:	Postgraduate teaching conference
	Friday:	Grand rounds
17:30		

opportunities are not available even in the large nonuniversity hospitals. Although research training is offered to residents in all university hospitals, the number of positions and the facilities are limited. Research fellowships are tenable during the residency program in Bern or in Zurich, or at the end of the residency program, at the start of an academic career in Basel.

Surgical research is an indispensable part of surgery at the academic level, because it enhances the surgeon's ability to think scientifically and to develop new concepts and techniques. Only individuals identified as future academic surgeons should embark on surgical research, and the limited resources available should be reserved for them. Including research in the program of every resident has been tried, but the results were disappointing in relation to the effort and money invested. Motivating a surgeon to engage in research was rarely possible if he had not previously expressed the wish to do so. Candidates for the degree of doctor of medicine in Switzerland must write a thesis that is scientific in style, although not necessarily in content. This is sufficient for most physicians.

The prevailing view in Switzerland is that surgical research should be reserved for an elite. Scientific interest and the will to solve problems are important criteria in the selection of candidates; they usually coincide with ambition and the concept of using scientific work to enhance career development. Since these two motivations are almost inseparable, no effort should be made to separate them.

About 35% of Swiss surgical residents are selected according to the criteria just enunciated, and we expect them to become scientifically oriented surgeons with high technical skill. The selection process is continuous, and inept candidates are eliminated during their residency program; about

20% will complete their training, as planned. The curriculum for these specially selected surgeons includes 6 to 12 months devoted to research. During this period, they are not involved in daytime clinical routine, but they have to fulfill regular night and weekend duties. Since truly valuable scientific work cannot be completed in 6 to 12 months, these surgeons must do research in addition to their regular clinical duties during the remainder of their residency, in off hours if necessary. In Switzerland, the privilege of being selected for a career in academic surgery is considered worthy of such an extraordinary effort.

General Aspects of Research

The foregoing comments apply mainly to general surgery. In Switzerland, general surgery includes surgery of the abdomen, thorax—except the heart and great vessels—neck and mammary glands, peripheral blood vessels, and traumatic injuries. The demands of teaching and patient care make it impossible for general and cardiovascular faculty surgeons to commit more than 15% to 20% of their time to research. In the other surgical disciplines, which are organized as separate clinical entities that require additional time-consuming administrative work with less support staff, the percentage is even lower.

The international literature search instruments (MEDLINE, Datastar, based on the U.S. National Library of Medicine) are available in all academic institutions. The cooperative efforts of the university libraries make nearly all pertinent books and journals available within a short time. Only one journal still publishes original surgical research work in German (*Langenbecks Archiv für Chirurgie*). Other important international journals for Swiss scientific publications are *European Surgical Research* for experimental research, and *Theoretical Surgery*.

Research data can be presented at the yearly congress of the Swiss Society for Surgery, but the audience is so small that it gives speakers more opportunity to gain speaking experience than to diffuse their work. The Surgical Forum (*Chirurgisches Forum*) held at the yearly congress of the German Society for Surgery, in Munich or Berlin, is the only internationally recognized opportunity for making research presentations in German. Otherwise, original research work is usually presented at international meetings, conferences, and symposia.

No particularly useful reference book for surgeons engaged in research is available in German. It is obvious that a good knowledge of English is indispensable for a research-oriented surgeon. Fortunately, training in English is part of high school and college curricula.

Legal and Cultural Considerations

The mainly friendly but unenthusiastic support of the population for surgical research has been subjected to several negative influences during recent years. The pre-1965 baby boom has induced a rapid expansion of the universities and a popular concern about a possible surplus of graduates that has spilled over into research. The enormous rise in health care costs tempts many politicians to cut research funding. Such pressure, combined with general financial restrictions, has resulted in a significant decline in government funding for research.

The "antivivisection movement" is getting increasing attention, and opposition to animal experimentation is growing. Swiss citizens are probably the only people in the world who can vote on any amendment to the constitution proposed by 100,000 of them and, in the near future, they will vote on an amendment banning all animal experimentation. The fear of an affirmative vote has already provoked more restrictive legislation, and experiments on dogs and other larger animals are becoming rare. Research workers must now devote more time to completing forms and seeking permission than to laboratory work.

Problems and Opportunity for Surgical Chairmen

Courses on the management of big hospital departments are offered by a variety of institutions, including the Swiss Federation of Physicians, but not by the universities. Although such courses are not mandatory for future department heads, they are well attended. Training or organized courses in the management of research programs do not exist. It is felt that the only way of really getting experience in the management of research is to spend some time doing it, along with becoming personally involved in research programs.

References

1. Müeller ME, Allgower M, Willeneger H. Manual der Osteosynthese. Berlin/Heidelberg/New York: Springer, 1969. Second ed. 1977.
2. Largiadèr F, Baumgaertner D, Kolb E, Uhlschmid G. Technique and results of combined pancreatic and renal allotransplantation in man. In: Segmental pancreatic transplantation. Stuttgart/New York: Thieme, 1983.

62

Opportunities, Achievements, Problems, and Solutions in Surgical Research in the United Kingdom

R. Shields

As we enter the last decade of the twentieth century, surgical research in the United Kingdom is faced with immense, and somewhat worrying challenges. On the one hand, more surgical research has been undertaken than hitherto. There is substantial documented evidence that surgery is definitely a subject in which British researchers are greatly increasing their share of world publications and citations.[1] There is hardly a surgical trainee who is not engaged in some form of clinical investigation. It would indeed be rare for a trainee, devoid of any research experience, to be promoted to the senior ranks of the profession. Many surgical specialties have founded their own research societies and the main society – the Surgical Research Society – receives three to four times the number of abstracts it can possibly present at its twice-yearly meetings.

Yet, in the past decade, the resources to support surgical research have been greatly reduced. Britain spends less on civil research than all the other countries belonging to the Organization for Economic Cooperation and Development (OECD). While it spends more on medical research than France, it spends half as much as West Germany or Japan, and about a sixth as much as the United States. There is a wide perception that reduction in governmental funding has led, and is leading, to a decline in British science, irrespective of the performance indicators. There is a disturbing increase in the numbers of projects rated as alpha and alpha plus that cannot be funded by the Medical Research Council. Major changes in the National Health Service are before Parliament, and there is some concern that the needs of teaching and research may not be safeguarded. It would certainly be the case that many of the intrinsic costs of clinical research that have hitherto been absorbed into the clinical care budgets of the National Health Service will now be clearly identified and will have to be borne, for the first time, by grant awarding authorities.

Increased productivity in the face of reduced resources may, to a superficial observer, indicate higher efficiency. In fact, it conceals a disturbing state of affairs. Several elements of the situation may be unique to that of United Kingdom – for example, an economic performance not equal to the United States, West Germany, or Japan, and a government committed to reducing public expenditure. However, some underlying problems are shared with many other Western countries – manpower problems associated with the overproduction of doctors, especially surgeons, and a greater allocation of resources to the community, to the old, the mentally ill, and the mentally handicapped. It is calculated that, in Western countries, the annual budget for health care requires an annual increase of about 2% to 5% percent, merely to cope with an aging population and to keep up with advances in medical care. In most countries, these needs are not reflected in increased funding.

History of Surgical Research in the United Kingdom

Surgical research, as we recognize it today, began in the United Kingdom about 50 years ago. The names of Hunter and Lister stand out in the earlier pages of medical history as surgeons whose influence and contributions have saved the lives of countless millions; but before the twentieth century, surgical advances largely sprang from careful clinical observation and deduction. It had been appreciated by only a few that advances could originate from controlled observations, or modifications in physiological and pathological processes in man or in animals. In 1933 the Royal College of Surgeons of England established the Buxton-Brown Farm for experimental research. The surgical establishment had recognized that advances in patient care were dependent on research, not least on experiments in animals. At the same time, two departmental heads—Wilkie in Edinburgh and Illingworth in Glasgow—created environments in their departments that were conducive to rapid development in surgical research. They did this by encouraging trainees and pupils to develop, in the laboratory and at the bedside, attitudes of scientific discipline, of forthrightness, and of questioning of current surgical views. The scene was set for the rapid burgeoning of surgical research that took place in the immediate postwar years.

At the end of World War II, many highly experienced, but still relatively young, surgeons returned from the armed services wishing to participate in the rapid advances of surgical care they had seen during the war. In 1948 the National Health Service (NHS) was established, providing comprehensive medical care without immediate cost to the patient, and initiating massive development in hospital services, especially of teaching hospitals, whose previous financing had largely depended on charities. There was a great increase in the size of the medical staff, especially full-time specialists, within the hospital service.

The influence of the United States during this embryonic development of British surgical research cannot be exaggerated. The close links forged during the second world war, and easier travel thereafter, allowed many British surgeons to visit departments in the United States. Departmental heads returned from these visits and sought to establish similar departments devoted to surgical research. Countless numbers of young surgeons spent a year or so in American hospitals and laboratories. The clinical studies of Blalock, Wangensteen, Moore, and Dunphy, and the physiological research of Code and others, created a ferment among British surgeons, who returned with the ambition of advancing knowledge and developing new methods for the provision of surgical care. These surgeons were determined to see that surgery shared in the rapid development of clinical research that characterized the 1950s and 1960s in the United Kingdom.

The 1960s saw an unparalleled expansion in universities, following the publication and governmental acceptance of the Robbins Report, which advocated the provision of university education for all who were able to satisfy the entrance requirements and wished to be admitted. Medical schools shared in this expansion: new buildings were constructed, and the staffing of departments was expanded by the appointment of full-time academic clinicians who helped to provide a clinical service to National Health Service patients. They were not involved in private practice and could devote their energies to teaching and research.

In the past decade, because of the government's aim of reducing public expenditure and curtailing the costs of higher education and research, the funding of universities, whether directly or indirectly derived from the state, has been greatly reduced. Between 1981 and 1984, state support for the universities was cut by an average of 15%. The magnitude of these cuts and the precipitate manner in which they were introduced meant that the brunt was borne by the faculties (e.g., medicine), that traditionally had a high turnover of staff. The 26 medical schools in England and Wales lost almost 500 posts. Because clinical services and teaching had to be maintained, research posts in clinical departments were among the first to be sacrificed. Scientists in clinical departments constituted the main casualty of these cuts. Many posts, whose holders had underpinned the scientific endeavor of entire departments, were lost. Not surprisingly, Britain's share of publications in biomedical sciences fell (by 11%), as did its citation share (by 27%).

Since 1988, there have been revolutionary proposals for the financing of higher education and the resourcing of research. Hitherto, universities have received from the government an overall grant to meet the costs of teaching and research, and it was left to individual universities to decide, in broad terms, how the money was spent. However, the funding of both teaching and research would be radically changed. On two occasions, the research activities of each department or departmental grouping in each university in the United Kingdom have been assessed and placed on a five-point scale. Funding of research will be allocated to the parent university on this basis. Unfortunately, such clinical subjects as surgery and internal medicine have been contained in a large grouping of nearly all clinical departments in a medical school—more than 16 departments in some instances. Consequently, the assessments for the major clinical subjects have tended to come out as average on the selectivity scale, much to the disadvantage of first-rate departments of surgery. Second, the dual support system of university research seems to be on the verge of being abolished. The essence of the system is that the university provides a basic research capability in its departments (e.g., the funding of academic staff salaries, the provision of "well-found" laboratories), and that other bodies (e.g., research councils, charitable organizations, and industry), provide the funding for staff on short-term research contracts and funds for the purchase of special items of equipment, as well as research running costs.

In the near future, universities will no longer be funded for the overhead costs of research; such costs will be derived directly from the grant-awarding authorities. Superficially, such an arrangement seems to be attractive, but there is fear that a central organization will not be able to pick its way through the complexities of funding research, with the result that only established and powerful research groups will be funded, and exciting and important new initiatives may go unrecognized. There is a strong feeling that neither the University Finance Committee, which allocates money to universities for the government, nor the Medical Research Council understands either the complexities of the funding of medical schools or the difficulties of clinical research. It has been left to such charitable agencies as the Wellcome Foundation to provide the more imaginative initiatives in clinical research.

TABLE 62.1. Research classified as "Surgical research" in the United Kingdom.

Phase	Type of research
Preoperative	Indications for surgery.
	Preoperative monitoring and preparation
Operative	Technique
	Suture material; prostheses; instruments
	Results of surgery
Postoperative care	Hemodynamic and respiratory monitoring
	Metabolism Fluid and electrolyte balance
	Parenteral nutrition
Complications	
Immediate	Thrombosis and embolism
	Wound infection and dehiscence
	Cardiopulmonary and renal failure
	Intestinal dysfunction
Long-term	Malabsorption
	Metabolic problems
	Mortality

Reprinted with permission from Chetty U, Forrest APM[2] (1981).

What is Surgical Research?

Surgical research may be defined as research that is undertaken by surgeons and is directed toward improvement in surgical care. Some hint of what constitutes surgical research was given in the paper by Chetty and Forrest,[2] who examined the contributions over a 5-year period to the major surgical research societies of the United Kingdom and Europe. At the Surgical Research Society, which is the main generalist society for surgical research in the United Kingdom, 97% of the papers were presented by members of university departments of surgery, with the subject of gastroenterology predominating. Almost two-thirds of the papers were oriented toward clinical practice; one-third were rated as "surgical" (Table 62.1). At the sister society in continental Europe, the European Society for Surgical Research, 85% of the papers came from departments of surgery, with cardiac surgical topics being the more numerous. Fewer papers were dedicated to clinical research than with the Surgical Research Society, but more papers were devoted to surgical topics.

The scientific program of the Surgical Research Society tends to concentrate on gastroenterology, oncology, and vascular surgery because, for historical reasons, these have been the major interests of senior staff in university departments. However, because many younger surgeons now receive their basic training in molecular biology, immunology, etc., rather than in physiology and biochemistry, there is an identifiable swing away from surgical pathophysiology of organs to the alterations in the biology of cells and their constituents. Other surgical disciplines (e.g., urology, orthopedic surgery, otorhinolaryngology, neurosurgery) have established their own research societies. Certain multidisciplinary societies (e.g., the British Transplantation Society and the British Society of Gastroenterology) constitute the main national forums for surgeons undertaking research in these particular fields.

The main journal of surgical research in the United Kingdom is the *British Journal of Surgery*. For many years, this journal limited its publications to retrospective reviews and reports of interesting cases, but in the past decade, vigorous editorship, combined with strict peer review, has lifted this journal into the forefront of the major journals of surgery in the world. The journal is the official organ of the Surgical Research Society, and twice a year, papers read at the Society are published in full in the journal.

Opportunities in Surgical Research

The Surgical Resident

Although the primary aims of the surgical trainee are to develop his or her clinical acumen and to acquire and expand operative experience, many wish to have experience in surgical research. There is an obvious desire to participate in surgical advances and to improve the standards of surgical care. There are many who are excited by investigative work and enjoy the pleasure, and enhanced prestige, of the delivery or publication of a well-

TABLE 62.2. Milestones in a surgical academic career in the United Kingdom.

Ages	Post		
5–11	Elementary or primary school		
12–17	Secondary school		
18–23	Medical school		
23–24	Internship		
24–26	General professional education, including experience in accident surgery and 6–12 months in a basic science department (usually Department of Anatomy)		
27–29	Senior house officer–registrar		
29 (approx)	FRCS diploma		
30–33	Post-FRCS registrar		
	University medical school	NHS equivalent	Approximate U.S. equivalent terminology
33–37	Lecturer	Senior registrar	Chief resident-instructor
36	Senior lecturer		Assistant professor
		Consultant	
37	Reader		Associate professor or professor
38–40	Professor		Chairman

prepared paper. However, the fierce competition that now faces surgical trainees has become the major force in developing and maintaining surgical research in the United Kingdom. Market forces have been largely responsible for many surgical trainees developing an interest in research. Recent proposals and agreements between the profession and the government will lead to a considerable reduction in the number of trainees, to bring their number to a level in proportion to the opportunities for promotion to a consultant rank within the NHS. Inevitably, there will be fewer trainees to undertake research and, therefore, department heads will need to seek a new source of research assistants other than the "cannon fodder" of time-expired trainees.

The United Kingdom doctor qualifies at an earlier age than in some other countries (Table 62.2). The majority of those aspiring to a surgical career take the first step on the promotional ladder immediately after internship. The young trainee quite properly wishes to acquire a critical mass of experience in the wards and operating room, and it is therefore unusual for a trainee to become involved in surgical research before the age of 30, by which time he has passed the examination for the diploma of Fellowship of a Royal College (FRCS). The FRCS, it must be explained, is only an early milestone along the surgical road, indicating that the trainee has acquired a certain standard of knowledge of surgery in general. It is an entry qualification to the more intensive higher surgical training taken at the senior registrar–lecturer level. Usually, surgical research is undertaken by a trainee at the age of 30 to 33 in a post-FRCS registrar post.

At this time, the trainee encounters a severe bottleneck to further promotion to lecturer or senior registrar, posts in which he or she will receive higher surgical training. Generally, posts for higher surgical training cannot be applied for with any chance of success until 10 years after qualification and at least 5 years after obtaining the FRCS. For each post, there may be up to 60 to 70 applicants, of which only 5 to 8 will be short-listed for interview. A review of the successful applicants for these posts[3] shows that nearly all have experienced 1 to 2 years in full-time surgical research, published on average 6 papers, and made 10 presentations at research meetings. Almost all possessed a higher university degree [e.g., a doctorate of medicine (MD), mastership of surgery (Ch.M. or M.S.), or a Ph.D.—for clarification, it should be explained that the basic British qualification on graduation from medical school is Bachelor of Medicine and Bachelor of Surgery (M.B.,Ch.B.)]. At one time, these degrees and diplomas would ensure entry to a consultant post in a prestigious teaching hospital; now they have become common currency for appointment to a senior registrar (senior resident) post. Surgical research obviously benefits from these circumstances, but it is perhaps the only useful by-product of a wasteful and increasingly unacceptable system.

A recent survey of registrars undertaking surgical research in the United Kingdom has produced some surprising information.[4] The salaries of more than a quarter of the research registrars were met by the National Health Service, twice as many as by the research councils, indicating perhaps the relatively low level of funding of clinical research by the Medical Research Council. The individual's enjoyment of and success in research were related to the quality of supervision. More than half the respondents to the questionnaire spoke highly of the direction of the research, with the supervisor taking an active role not only in the concept, but also toward completion of the project. Research supervision is obviously critical because only half of those undertaking research had any previous experience or, indeed, previous interest in the subject of their research; for example, the choice of topic was dictated largely by departmental interest and facilities. The British Science and Engineering Research Council issued valuable guidelines for research supervision which have been taken up by most research-oriented departments.[5] Most of those questioned considered that the experience had been worthwhile, with a positive gain in logical and critical thought and increased awareness of scientific methods. The conclusion of the survey was that the majority of trainees enjoyed their time in research, had been adequately supervised, and would probably continue to undertake some form of research throughout their career. The fact that few wished to continue in an academic career suggests that the research had been used mainly for career advancement.

At present, it is unusual for the trainee to receive a training in surgical research at an earlier stage. However, some may have been introduced to research during their student days by intercalating a year of study, usually research oriented, to obtain a science degree. Others may, during the early years of their surgical training, take 1 to 3 years off service to obtain experience in a basic science subject, often to obtain a Ph.D. degree. These young surgeons are more research oriented and academically inclined than their colleagues and usually have been attracted to research by working in an academic surgical unit in whose projects they have become involved. It can be a difficult decision to embark on research at such an early stage in a career because of the understandable desire to pass the difficult examination of a Royal College and, more important, to become directly involved in clinical and operative work. There is, therefore, a conflict in career aims. Without doubt, this is an ideal time to enter surgical research because the young surgeon is usually bright, curious, and inquisitive, with his or her mind unfilled by surgical dogma. At this stage, surgical trainees must receive considerable support from their seniors to allay fears that their surgical promotion may be delayed. Such reassurance is readily given because these people are of the highest caliber.

TABLE 62.3. Timetable of university lecturer in surgery in Hospital A (United Kingdom).

Monday	
08:30–10:00	Clinical round with junior NHS staff
10:00–11:00	Bedside teaching of undergraduate medical students
11:00–12:15	Administration Discharge letters Arrange admissions Select patients for teaching
12:15–13:30	Grand round in hospital A
13:30–14:00	Clinical round with consultant
14:00–17:00	Outpatient clinic
17:30–19:00	Postgraduate surgical meeting (organized by university department)
Tuesday (24-hour emergency intake)	
08:00–08:30	Clinical round with junior NHS staff
08:30–13:30	Operating theater
13:30–16:00	Service-research sessions in gastroenterology unit, including endoscopy, esophageal manometry, etc.
16:00–17:00	Clinical round with consultant
17:00–18:00	Histopathology round
Wednesday	
08:15–10:00	Clinical round with consultant
10:00–11:00	Departmental surgical round
11:00–12:00	Departmental research meeting
12:00–13:00	Departmental radiology meeting
13:30–17:00	Outpatient clinic
Thursday	
08:00–08:30	Clinical round with junior staff
08:20–12:30	Operating theater
13:00–	Research
Friday	
08:30–09:00	Departmental business meeting
09:00–10:00	Grand round in Hospital B
10:30–11:00	Endoscopy clinic
13:30–15:00	Outpatient clinic
16:00–	Clinical round with consultant
Saturday/Sunday	
48-hour emergency intake every fourth weekend	
Morning clinical round alternate weekends	

Lecturer and Senior Lecturer

The holders of these full-time university posts have honorary contractual duties within the NHS. Equivalent in status to senior registrar and consultant, respectively, the lecturer and the senior lecturer fill key positions in university departments and represent the main source of research activity. In addition to heavy teaching commitments, they have to contribute a considerable amount of service work to the hospitals to which they are attached. They usually work 6 *clinical* sessions, approximately 6 half-days out of the conventional 11 sessions per week. Most university clinicians devote more than their contractual sessions to clinical care because their services may be much in demand on account of their expertise and because of the heavy clinical load that is a common feature of British hospitals. Such an arrangement affords a stimulating and satisfying professional life but, inevitably, time that the university clinician wishes to devote to research becomes increasingly eroded.

A typical timetable of a lecturer in my own department is described in Table 62.3. In general, in what seems to be a 70-hour week, 8 hours are spent in administration (for university and health service), 4 hours in teaching, 30 hours in research (mainly in the evenings and on weekends) and 28 hours in clinical service. Each month a lecturer personally performs about 30 operations, the magnitude of which depend on his or her clinical experience.

In British medical schools, a lecturer's post is generally a fixed-term contract of 3 to 5 years. During this time the lecturer is engaged in higher surgical training leading to accreditation indicating completion of formal surgical training. Experience of up to one year in surgical research in an approved center in the United Kingdom or abroad will be recognized toward accreditation. Training programs are, by their nature, restrictive, and the understandable desire of trainees to become accredited can make it difficult for lecturers, who should underpin the research activity of surgical departments, to move freely from one center to another, especially to work for periods in a basic laboratory department as part of their research training and experience.

Senior lecturers and readers work as consultants in the university hospitals and usually have independent clinical and research status. Many have their own funding from grant-awarding authorities and have formed their own research teams within a department. My own view is that this practice should be encouraged so that the capabilities of senior lecturers to generate research, and to develop and lead an effective team, are given every chance of flourishing and being assessed, because it is from their ranks that the next generation of surgical academic leaders will be chosen.

University surgeons often find themselves in a professional dilemma. They must engage effectively and fruitfully in research, because failure to do so can lead to reductions in resources and delays in career advancement. Yet, professional colleagues will not have high regard for a university surgeon whose clinical practice is meager and narrowly restricted and whose research is divorced completely from surgical practice.

Professors and Chairmen

Clinical professors—for the most part full-time employees of the university medical school—also have honorary clinical contracts with the National Health Service and so, like a senior lecturer, spend more than half their working week as hospital consultants involved with patient care and other NHS service commitments. In teaching hospitals, surgical staff are usually grouped into service units or "firms." The university staff usually form one service firm, consisting of junior NHS staff (e.g., registrars), lecturers, senior lecturers (or reader), and professor. The university unit may be one of three to five firms in the hospital providing an equal share of clinical service. The management and administrative tasks of directing the hospital firm, as well as the academic department, take up a good deal of the professor's time over and above his clinical service and therefore tend to encroach upon research. In general, clinical professors spend little time at the bench in the laboratory, but tend to direct their own research teams, for whom they have to obtain resources from the grant-awarding agencies and foundations.

University departments are expected to spearhead clinical research. Surgical trainees in the National Health Service look to the university department for a formal training in research. Lecturers require a good deal of supervision of their academic activities, especially in the direction of their research. Because of their relatively junior position, they look to the head of the department to advise on grant applications and, indeed, to obtain resources for research. The chairmen and other directors of research who are accountable to grant-awarding agencies must ensure that the research is well done; therefore they have to distinguish between those aspirants who are competent and curious, possessing drive and initiative, from those whose only interest in research may be to advance their career prospects.

In some medical schools, there may be other surgical departments apart from that of general surgery (e.g., urology, orthopedic surgery, neurosurgery, cardiothoracic surgery). The main departments of surgery, for historical reasons, tend to have their research and clinical interests mainly in the fields of gastroenterology, vascular surgery, oncology, transplantation, and endocrine surgery.

National Health Service Surgeons

The majority of surgeons work within the NHS and receive salaries as full-time or part-time consultants. The extent to which NHS surgeons involve themselves in surgical research must depend on individual opportunities and preferences. Although there are considerable opportunities for *clinical* investigations, the National Health Service does not allocate laboratory space for research. Accommodation usually must be found within the university department. The NHS clinician has equal access to the major grant-awarding authorities, such as the Medical Research Council. Devoting time to effective research and a busy NHS practice and, perhaps, private practice can present considerable logistical difficulties.

Many surgeons, especially in district general hospitals, have neither the time nor the facilities for prosecuting clinical or experimental research. Nevertheless, there is a general awareness among them that improvement in patient care will be achieved only by investigative work, and most are only too willing to join in collaborative research, as part of a multicenter trial, or to refer patients with problems to university units for further investigation.

Although there has been a marked increase in private practice in the United Kingdom, the bulk of clinical work is still carried out within the NHS. Hitherto, the British NHS, whatever its shortcomings—and many of these are shared by other health care systems—offered considerable opportunity for clinical research. Since patients do not have to bear the cost of their own treatment directly, and since pecuniary interest and financial competition are generally absent among clinicians, the referral of patients to surgeons with particular clinical and research interests is facilitated. Despite the heavy clinical load of surgeons, the general atmosphere, especially in teaching hospitals, is conducive to research. Indeed, it is often surprising how much support there is for research from the hard-pressed NHS health authorities.

There is usually a close relationship between university and NHS clinical staff: they work closely together in the same hospital, and each has responsibilities for teaching. In general, a considerable respect has grown between university and NHS staff for each other's abilities and dedication.

Current governmental legislation seeks to alter the ways in which the NHS is managed. Hitherto, each hospital was given a budget, calculated from complex formulas, to bear the costs of treating patients referred to it by general practitioners and by consultants in other hospitals. The system was relatively cheap to administer but, as with most health care systems, greater difficulty was experienced in coping with the increased costs of medical care, higher technology, and the aging population. It is now planned that general practitioners and health authorities charged with the responsibility of providing health care for a defined population will place contracts with individual hospitals who will inevitably be in competition with one another. For many of the hospitals, these contracts will be the only source of funds. There is some concern that in the highly competitive business of providing health care as cheaply as possible, the needs of teaching and research will be placed at a considerable disadvantage. How successful these innovations will be remains to be seen.

Attitude of the Public

As a result of the media—especially television and the popular press—the public has a very active interest in medical matters but, as one might expect, people are more fascinated by the glamour of surgical research (e.g. heart surgery and organ transplantation). Both television and the press have shown considerable responsibility in their presentation of research topics, so that the public possesses a remarkably broad knowledge of significant advances in surgery. Most people are not entirely clear who carries out research and how it is funded, but they expect that surgical research will be performed in major teaching hospitals, and they admire and respect those making major contributions.

For the most part, the medical profession in the United Kingdom enjoys the respect of the public and is rated highly for its integrity and dedication. This respect shows itself in an easy cooperation and collaboration by the public in research. Patients understand that research and teaching have to be carried out and very readily give informed consent for participation in trials of treatment and also in investigation in which they themselves may not be an immediate or direct beneficiary. This cooperation is sustained by the establishment, in each hospital, of ethics committees in which lay members of the public are involved.

Animal Experimentation

Major legislation has been established in the United Kingdom concerning the use of animals in experimental work. Animals cannot be used for research unless the investigator receives a certificate from the Home Office, the responsible government agency. A laboratory can be visited at any time by Home Office inspectors, who have legal right of access. All animals are inspected and current work is reviewed. Any breaches of the regulations can lead to withdrawal of a license and indeed, criminal prosecution. As far as surgical research is concerned, the current arrangements are, on the whole, satisfactory. Animals receive good care, and investigators have demonstrated responsibility.

Criticism of the use of animals for testing of cosmetics and protests among the self-styled "animal liberators" have led to legislation to tighten the regulations. Granting of certificates is now related more to specific projects than to individuals. This change has not greatly restricted surgical research.

Financing of Surgical Research

In the United Kingdom, surgical research is mainly financed, directly or indirectly, from governmental sources; a smaller but important contribution comes from grant-awarding foundations. Only a small proportion comes from legacies, donations, and private practice.

Within British universities, research has been funded through the dual support system already alluded to. One arm of the system is the provision by the universities of buildings, major apparatus, and senior staff. The other limb is the provision, by the Medical Research Council, of capital and recurrent funding for research.

For its buildings and senior staff, a university medical school is largely funded by government through the agency of the University Funding Council. The government makes an annual grant to the council, which decides on the allocation of funds to individual universities, each of which assigns a proportion of its resources to its constituent faculties for staffing, equipment, and recurrent costs. The allocation contains very little direct funding for research.

The government's main direct support of medical research is the Medical Research Council, which hitherto has supported two major institutions of its own, one for basic science and the other for clinical research. Surgical research is represented in neither. The Medical Research Council also supports research institutes and units in universities throughout the United Kingdom, but none is devoted to surgical research. The Medical Research Council does not see that it has a major role to pay senior tenured staff or to establish major research facilities in universities. The council expects to find, in the areas it wishes to support, well-equipped laboratories and highly trained staff.

A surgical research worker can hope to obtain financial support by a successful application to the council for a project grant that lasts for 3 years, or a program grant that lasts up to 5 years. The latter is more substantial, but over the past decade, only a few have been awarded for surgical research. As far as project grants are concerned, in the past 5 years only 6% to 8% of those awarded for clinical research were related to surgery.

Fortunately, in the United Kingdom there are several other bodies, mainly charitable foundations, which not only provide considerable funding for research but seem to be more sensitive to the problems that face clinical research workers. Chief among these is the Wellcome Foundation, which has responded to diminishing governmental support by increasing considerably its own allocation for research, considerably. It has also, with great foresight, identified the particular problems of surgical research. For example, a young surgical trainee who has shown an aptitude for research may not wish to commit himself or herself too early to an academic career and may be reluctant to apply for a lecturer post—indeed, may have neither the basic qualifications nor the record of publications to permit doing so. A Wellcome Surgical Fellowship allows a young surgeon at the level of a third- or fourth-year resident to spend a year or two to obtain training and experience in surgical research. A Wellcome Fellowship is one of the most prestigious awards a young surgeon can receive and is an important means by which he or she can take the first step on the academic ladder. There are other charitable foundations, especially in the field of cancer (e.g., the Imperial Cancer Research Fund, the Cancer Research Campaign) that support research in departments of surgery; but the scope of their support is limited by their terms of reference.

There are two other sources of funding, indirectly from the government, that deserve mention. In both cases, the amount of support is relatively small. Central government assigns funding to support medical research to each NHS region. Although these grants are meant to fund research that would not normally receive support from the Medical Research Council, in practice, teaching hospitals and university departments receive a substantial proportion because of their expertise and research orientation. Although this funding does not involve extremely large sums, it is sensitive to local initiatives and serves usefully as pump-priming for pilot research projects.

Another source of funding is endowment or trust funds derived from monies bequeathed or donated to large teaching hospitals before the establishment of the National Health Service in 1948. These sums have not been taken over by government agencies, nor can they be used for providing health care. These endowment funds held by teaching hospitals give them considerable flexibility in supporting various initiatives, including research.

Most departments of surgery also obtain funds to support research from legacies, gifts, etc. Some support can also be obtained from drug companies, but such support is usually related to a drug in which the company has a specific interest. Some departments of surgery also depend on an income from the treatment of private patients. Many patients, both in the United Kingdom and from abroad, seek private medical care from university staff because of their national or international reputation. There are usually two restrictions on private practice by university staff: it must be carried out within NHS hospitals rather than private hospitals, and the income earned must not be used for the personal remuneration of the staff member; rather, it is to be added to the income of the department, largely for use for research purposes.

Conclusions

The opportunities to undertake surgical research in the United Kingdom remain good. Among surgical trainees there is a greater realization that experience in research will be helpful to career advancement. Surgical trainees and senior clinicians appreciate that advancement in patient care will depend largely on clinically based investigations, but it is doubtful how long this situation will continue, given the sharp reduction in the governmental funding of the universities and the major changes proposed for the National Health Service.

Considerable dismay is currently being felt among clinical researchers. In the past, planning in the universities and the health service was largely based on an expectation of economic growth. Increased governmental emphasis on reducing public expenditure has thrown both the universities and the NHS into a frenzy of activity, based on a drive for increased efficiency. The current aim is to treat, teach, and research at the same level of activity as heretofore, with greatly reduced resources. Only time will tell whether this drive for efficiency will not produce irrevocable damage to medical education and clinical and basic research.

References

1. Smith R. International comparisons of funding and output of research: bye bye Britain. Br Med J 1988; 296:409–12.
2. Chetty U, Forrest APM, Surgical research: a survey. J R Coll Surg Edinb 1981;26:110–13.
3. Taylor I, Clyne CAC. Senior registrar applications in general surgery in 1982 and 1985. Br Med J 1985; 291:143–46.
4. Dehn TCB, Blacklay PF, Taylor GW. A survey of registrars undertaking general surgical research in the United Kingdom on 1st October 1983. Br J Surg 1875;72:668–71.
5. Christopherson D, Boyd RLD, Fleming I, et al. Research Student and Supervisor–A Discussion Document on Good Supervisory Practice. Swindon, England: Science and Engineering Research Council, 1982.

63

Research Challenges and Solutions in the United States

M.F. McKneally

In the United States, the knowledge and skills required for surgical research are acquired almost exclusively in university programs. While many of the 292 surgical training programs encourage residents to pursue a period of research, only a small minority require a research rotation, and very few have well-developed curricula that provide reliable training in scientific methodology, organization of research projects, funding, analysis of data, and publication.

Surgical research training is largely tutorial, centered around individual surgeons who are proficient at research and gravitate toward surgical departments with a strong emphasis on research. Such mentors are also sought by smaller departments to impart academic luster to otherwise largely clinical programs.

Surgical research was initiated in a small number of institutions under the strong influence of Alfred Blalock at the Johns Hopkins University, Evarts Graham at the University of Washington in St. Louis, Isidore Ravdin at the University of Pennsylvania, and Owen Wangensteen at the University of Minnesota. These surgeons and their students recognized and emphasized the importance of research for the expansion of surgical knowledge and the development of technical solutions to unresolved surgical problems. There was a significant increase in surgical research during World War II, especially on blood substitutes, wound care in general, and heart wounds in particular. This experience led to the development of heart surgery as a major American surgical research theme and contribution to surgical progress.

Following the launch of the Soviet space satellite *Sputnik* in 1957, a broad commitment of federal funds to support scientific activities led to an expansion of surgical research in many institutions. The public and the government recognized the need to keep American science abreast of scientific advances in other countries. During the past several decades, funding for scientific research, including surgical research, has become more difficult to obtain.

There has been a study section for surgical research within the National Institutes of Health, the principal U.S. agency for research support, since its formation in 1947; it provides separate peer review for grant applications in fields related to surgery. There are now two surgical study sections: the "Surgery, Anesthesiology, and Trauma" section and the "Surgery and Bioengineering" section; together they review 400 to 500 grant applications per year and fund approximately 20% of approved applications.

The public attitude toward surgical research has generally been positive. The success of surgical research in the development of techniques for cardiac surgery and organ transplantation has fascinated the public and the press. Surgical research enjoys less esteem within the university community, partly as the result of deficiencies in the scientific training of surgical researchers during the period of most rapid expansion. Preclinical scientists have been critical of the level of scientific rigor of much surgical research, particularly clinical studies conducted in human subjects, where a multiplicity of uncontrolled patient variables may confound scientific analysis.

The attitude of surgeons ranges from the denigrating view held by some that surgical researchers are "mouse doctors," to the high level of respect accorded to the best surgical investigators within the university surgical community. Surgical residents usually reflect the attitudes of their mentors. The majority of residency candidates regard training in surgical research as a delay in their progress toward clinical practice, but this period is becoming more readily accepted as the number of attractive postresidency positions for surgeons diminishes. The zeal of a minority of applicants for studying the scientific analysis of surgical problems prompts them to seek highly academic residency programs requiring a substantial period of training in a research laboratory, such as those at Duke University, the University of Minnesota, and Washington University in St. Louis. The introduction of mandatory surgical research rotations into predominantly clinical institutions is frequently associated with friction and discontent.

Achievements of Surgical Research

Surgical research in the United States began with empirical attempts to improve the care of surgical patients. American surgeons eagerly pursued the application of the new techniques of anesthesia and surgery to ease the pain and extend the scope of surgical operations. This period of activity was characterized by active surgical scholarship that emphasized the acquisition of knowledge by direct experience, spirited discussion, travel and study abroad, and observation of the techniques of other surgeons. Early in the twentieth century the French surgeon Alexis Carrel (1873–1944) emigrated to the United States to perform experimental surgery at the Rockefeller Institute in New York City. Carrel imparted a major impetus to the application of the scientific method to the solution of surgical problems. His animal experimentation on wound healing, vascular anastomoses, and transplantation provided a dazzling illustration of the contributions scientific surgeons could make, but it took almost a century for full appreciation of Carrel's work to penetrate and be applied by the surgical community.[1]

Alfred Blalock at Johns Hopkins followed the tradition of John Hunter in attempting to devise surgical solutions to naturally occurring problems by taking advantage of anomalies and variants seen in nature—for example, the creation of a patent ductus arteriosus to increase pulmonary blood flow in patients with pulmonic stenosis and tetralogy of Fallot.[2] The clinical application of Blalock's experimental work caused a revolution in the care of patients with congenital heart disease, and accelerated the development of laboratories in which large animal experiments could be conducted to familiarize surgeons with the techniques of cardiac and vascular surgery. Isidore Ravdin at the University of Pennsylvania and Francis Moore at Harvard University pioneered metabolic studies of the surgical patient that profoundly influenced the care of all critically ill patients.

Owen Wangensteen and his students at the University of Minnesota studied obstruction and decompression of the gastrointestinal tract,[3] as well as basic gastric physiology, in partnership with the Department of Physiology under the direction of Maurice Visscher. Visscher and Wangensteen devised a training program that required a year of surgical research in the laboratory and a year of more abstract preclinical research in the physiology department. The surgeons brought a refreshing vigor, a tendency to start the day early, and enthusiasm for expeditious completion of experiments to the environment of the physiologists. In exchange, the intellectual standards of the physiologists had a positive impact on the scientific thinking of the surgeons. Wangensteen's mandatory laboratory rotations provided the setting for very active participation by young residents in experimental surgery on the heart during the 1950s. The development of the heart–lung machine by Dewall and Lillehei at Minnesota and by Gibbon at Jefferson Medical College represents one of the highest accomplishments of surgeons working in the laboratory, and emphasizes the uniqueness of surgical research. Surgeons who attempted to suture the beating heart were acutely aware of the necessity of stopping its action to allow repair of complex defects. As a result, they worked tirelessly to develop a means of perfusing the body with oxygenated blood during periods of induced cardiac arrest.

Funding for Surgical Research

The federal government, through the National Institutes of Health, provided a total of more than $7.5 billion in 1990 for the support of original programs of biomedical research, of which approximately 81% supports extramural programs, awarded on a highly competitive, peer-reviewed basis.[4] Approximately 0.37% of the gross national product in the United States is devoted to biomedical research. It is estimated that 5% of this total is devoted to surgical research, although the overlap with other areas such as cancer, heart disease, and immunology makes this estimate uncertain.[5]

National foundations, such as the American Cancer Society, the American Heart Association and others supported by public solicitations provide major sources of funding (Fig. 63.1). Drug companies and firms in the biomedical technology industry contribute funds to research laboratories for the testing of new applications of patented pharmaceuticals or devices. Private foundations have recently given increasing financial support

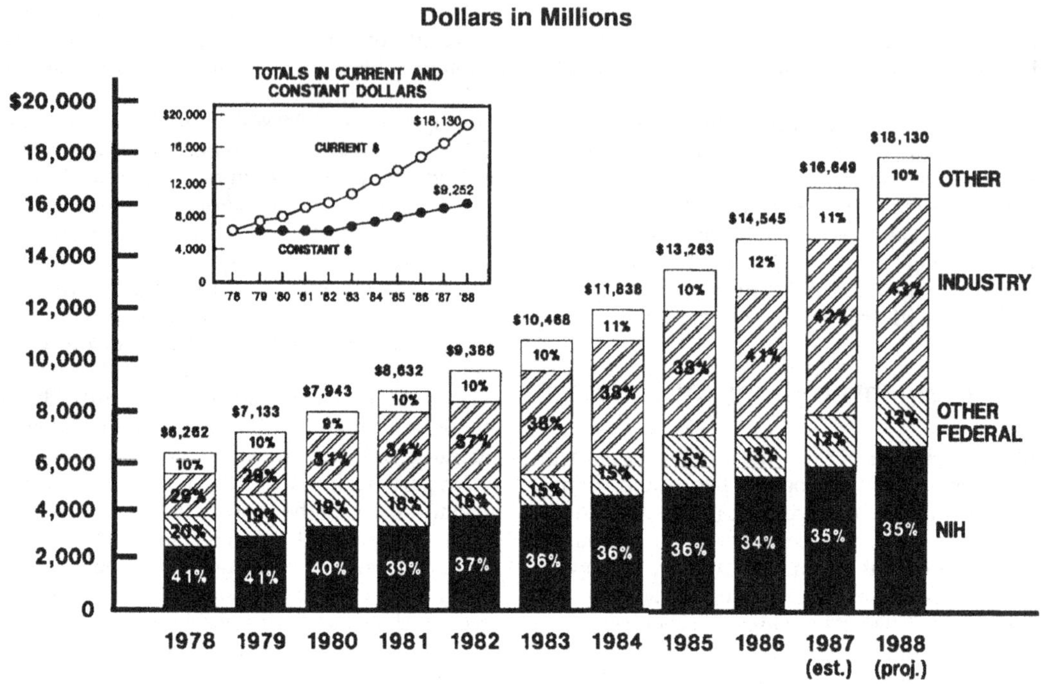

FIGURE 63.1. National support for health research and development by source, 1978–1988; fiscal year 1978 = 100; constant dollars based on Biomedical R & D Price Index. (From *NIH Data Book 1988*, U.S. Department of Health and Human Services, Public Health Service, National Institutes of Health.)

for scientific research and for the training of young surgeons in research techniques.[6] The U.S. tax laws are designed to encourage industry and private individuals to contribute to biomedical research.

Surgeons themselves have directly supported surgical research by paying for laboratory personnel, animals, and equipment from their surgical practice income. The creation of the Orthopaedic Research and Education Foundation (222 South Prospect Ave., Park Ridge, IL 60068-9962), supported by direct contributions from practicing orthopedic surgeons, is a highly significant development. This foundation allocated more than $2 million to residents and young academic orthopedic surgeons in 1990 to undertake research on problems targeted as appropriate areas for research activity. Such outstanding initiatives by surgical societies protect the young surgical investigator from the discouraging experience of competing unsuccessfully with full-time laboratory scientists for a shrinking pool of scientific research funds.

Some surgical departments make direct appeals for funds to support their research by mailings to postsurgical patients or by presentations to industry. This approach has the advantage of immediacy and gives the donors a sense of direct participation in the surgical research project. In some centers, faculty surgeons contribute a fixed percentage of their private practice income to an education or research fund for residents. Such funds provide important support for initiating research projects but are insufficient to run a surgical laboratory. However, they provide tangible evidence of senior surgeons' commitment to research and their concern for their juniors' careers.

Surgical societies provide scholarships for advanced residents or surgeons immediately out of residency training to spend time in laboratories where there is an emphasis on research. The American College of Surgeons supported four such awards in 1990 and administers two additional awards supported by industry. The American Association for Thoracic Surgery, the American Surgical Association, and several other surgical organizations initiated similar awards for North American applicants. Surgical societies generally do not support travel; this is regarded as the financial responsibility of training programs.

The Fogarty Fellowships, available through the National Institutes of Health, and the Graham Traveling Fellowships of the American Association for Thoracic Surgery, sponsor surgical research by foreign visitors to the United States. The American College of Surgeons provided seven International Guest Scholarships in 1990 to bring international guests to its congress and facilitate their visits to North American surgical centers. The College also administers the Armand Hammer Traveling Scholarship to support educational travel for a young North American surgical faculty member.

Career investigator salary awards are available in the United States from the National Institutes of Health for research in specifically designated areas, such as cardiovascular disease and cancer. Although they are not generically designated for surgeons, surgeons do submit applications. These awards substantially supplement the salaries of young investigators and require that they be relieved of clinical responsibilities while pursuing career development through research and educational projects. The National Institutes of Health also provide opportunities for surgeons to work as salaried members of the surgery branch for a training period of several years, or as career investigators. Scholarships for salary support during research training are provided by private foundations, such as the Clinical Scholars Program of the Robert Wood Johnson Foundation (College Road, P.O. Box 2316, Princeton, NJ 08543-2316).

Granting agencies emphasize particular areas in their selection of research programs for support, but they use the peer review system for awarding grants and do not interfere significantly with the conduct of the research. Drug companies and companies manufacturing medical devices tend to be more proprietary in their interaction with surgical researchers evaluating their products.

Surgeons in the United States, under the auspices of the American College of Surgeons and the leadership of William P. Longmire, formed the Conjoint Council on Surgical Research in 1985, to document the level and quality of surgical research in North America. The Conjoint Council developed because of concern about the diminishing success of surgeons competing with Ph.D. scientists for research funds at the National Institutes of Health level. This group defined surgical research as "research done by surgeons, but also research related to surgical diseases and perhaps, specifically, that form of research which benefits from a surgeon's recognition of a relevant clinical problem and the transition of knowledge into its solution." The Conjoint Council succeeded in securing grant support for a small number of model surgical research training programs. In October 1988 the Conjoint Council was incorporated as the Committee on Research and Education of the American College of Surgeons. The committee has facilitated the development of a Canadian counterpart and has fostered the growth of research in surgical departments. It is encouraging to note that NIH funding to surgical departments in the U.S. has increased steadily in recent years (Fig. 63.2) and that publication of experimental research may be increasing in surgical journals (Fig. 63.3). The committee plans to develop programs to support research following the model of the Orthopaedic Research and Education Foundation in order to catalyze this trend.

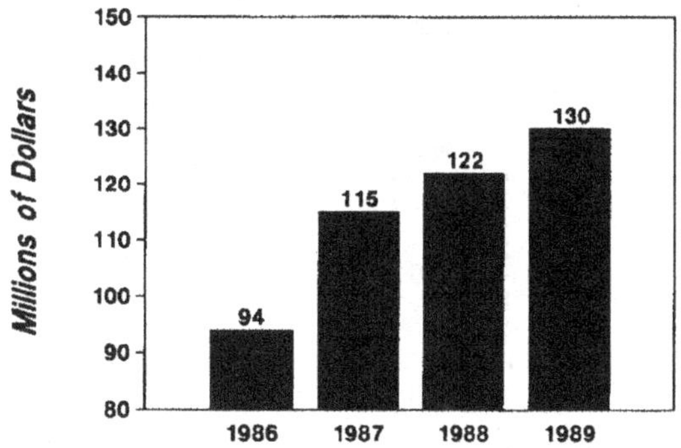

FIGURE 63.2. NIH grants and contracts to departments of surgery. (From NIH Office of Extramural Research, Office of Research Training and Resources, Blair C. Personal Communication.)

When viewed against the background of the diminishing rate of increase of federal support for all research[7] and declining American representation in leading clinical research journals,[8] it is imperative that surgeons provide energetic support for research through political action, fund raising and direct personal financial contributions. The NIH budget has remained fairly stable, but funding for AIDS research and the Human Genome Project has substantially increased, thereby reducing the availability of funds for the traditional RO-1 individual investigator grants in other areas and intensifying the competition for these monies.

Research During Residency Training

Residents who spend a significant period of time in research develop a more comprehensive knowledge of a specific area of surgical science, learn to appreciate the limits and pitfalls of data collection and analysis, master the rudiments of manuscript

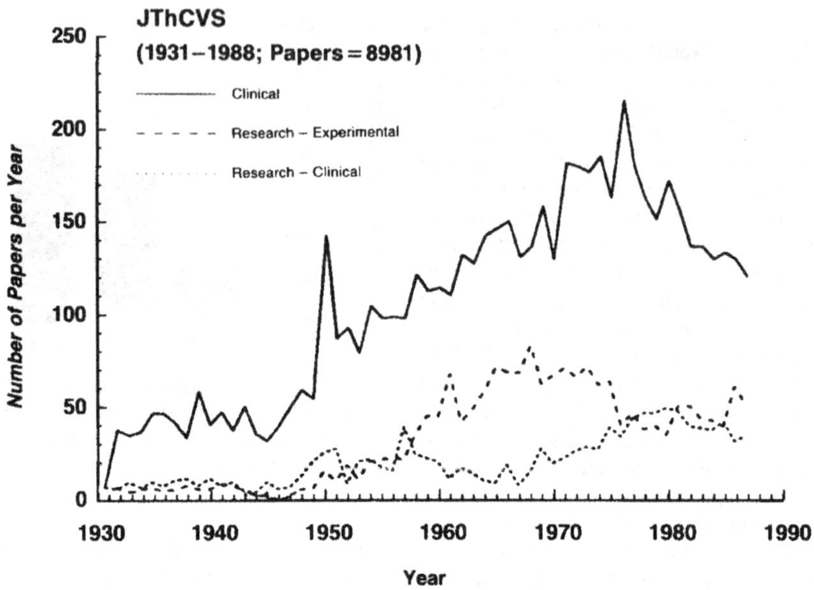

FIGURE 63.3. Number of papers published per year in the *Journal of Thoracic and Cardiovascular Surgery*, according to the nature of the publication. Reprinted with permission from Ebert PA. Presidential Address: A profile of thoracic surgery from the sidelines. J Thorac Cardiovasc Surg 1988;96:677.

preparation, add surgical publications to their resumés, and enhance the likelihood of obtaining a desirable clinical or academic position on completion of training.

During the 1960s graduates of research-oriented surgical training programs in the United States could readily find clinical and academic opportunities throughout the country. During the subsequent two decades, the demand for surgeons with research training decreased, except in rapidly developing fields, such as liver or heart–lung transplantation and surgical oncology. Surgical residents trained in the theoretical and practical aspects of these fields are highly sought. These and similar exceptions aside, most surgical training programs cannot afford to have more residents than are justified by postresidency clinical opportunities and hospital funding for clinical care. Consequently, inclusion of a research rotation in the surgical training program becomes a special consideration requiring careful integration of the needs of the resident, the surgical community, and society at large.

The salaries of residents during periods of surgical research were once funded fairly generously by the National Institutes of Health through training fellowships and research grants. Cutbacks in these programs have put severe constraints on this source of support. Special fellowships, such as the NIH Academic Surgery Training Program, need to be restored, to allow surgical departments to provide salary support for a resident who is not contributing to the generation of clinical income. Hospitals that depend on income from insurance payers or the federal government are feeling increasing pressure from these sources to stop allocating any portion of the health care dollar to the training of residents, even when they are performing exclusively clinical work. As a result, the hospital as a source of funding for the surgical trainee performing research is fast disappearing. In general, residents do not receive any special financial incentive to dedicate part of their training period to surgical research; the principal incentive is career advancement. Exposure to national meetings and scientific presentations at an early level in residency increases awareness and interest in an academic career.

Residents generally enter into a period of research after the 2-year core curriculum of surgical training, if research is to be an integral part of their training program. This seems to be an excellent time for participation in surgical research, as the resident is mentally prepared to see the potential surgical applications of research methods and has encountered many of the unsolved problems in surgery.

The research component of most training programs in surgery is generally a block period of one year; some academic programs allocate 2 years or more to research. Because the call of a patient in distress is an irresistible summons away from the research laboratory or library, isolation of the surgical trainee from clinical work has been a standard method of making time available for surgical scholarship. Complete isolation of the resident from clinical pressure for prolonged periods of research allows consecutive thinking, full concentration, and time to establish credibility and long-term, stable relationships with basic scientists. Block time in the laboratory completely isolated from patient care has definite advantages, but it tends to create the mistaken impression that research is incompatible with the daily life of a practicing surgeon and can be accomplished only in a sabbatical period.

The concept of devoting a part of each day or each week to research is foreign to North American surgical training programs, though common in France, Germany, and Japan. The development of a program incorporating research into the clinical work week before or after a block period of isolated research would teach residents how to integrate research activities into their subsequent careers as practicing scientific surgeons. Within the clinical context, the protection afforded to residents when they are assigned to the operating room for long surgical procedures is a good model. It is well established in the minds of colleagues, nurses, and patients that surgeons and residents must be cross-covered and protected to allow concentrated attention and consecutive thinking as well as sterility in the operating room during such periods. Application of the same principle in resolving the problem of how to perform research in the clinical setting seems highly desirable. At some institutions, the resident is advised to go to the laboratory to pursue research training after the residency is completed. This seems particularly unwise, because it disables the residents as clinicians, forcing them to reenter practice at an advanced level with inadequate immediate preparation.

Residents are motivated to pursue research careers when they perceive a positive effect of the knowledge and skills acquired in the laboratory on the performance and personal satisfaction of their clinical role models. Surgical researchers who are fumbling, incompetent, or impractical clinicians have a negative impact on the resident. Skillful surgeons who have a keen sense of the value of scientific research impart a powerful stimulus to residents to pursue research as a developmental step in their surgical careers. A positive experience in research training alters the practice of surgeons; it makes them more cautious about accepting folkloric remedies and authoritarian prescriptions of treatment, and kindles an enthusiasm for increasing knowledge in their chosen field of surgery.

Young surgeons who have learned the scientific approach to surgery through research and have published scientific articles are much more likely to secure attractive clinical and academic positions. This latter benefit is probably the most significant motivating factor in convincing residents to include a period of surgical research in their training. At our institution, residents who undertake training in surgical research are carefully selected on the basis of their promise, aptitude, and enthusiasm. Research support for the surgical resident during training is provided from clinical funds derived from patient care, and through a National Institutes of Health training grant specifically targeted at teaching surgeons basic scientific research skills in the physiology department.

The training required to make a surgical resident into a scientific surgeon is similar to what is needed to develop other research scientists. The usual undergraduate curriculum of medical students rarely includes exposure to the thinking process of the research scientist, or to reducing unsolved scientific problems to answerable questions. This qualitative difference is even more striking in medical school and residency, where the accumulation of factual knowledge and its clinical correlations are emphasized. Acquisition of the scientific expertise needed for the effective execution of research requires active participation in research; it cannot be obtained by reading about the accomplishments of others, talking to them, or replicating their experiments.

Part of the motivation to pursue research arises from the satisfaction derived from solving a personally formulated question based on one's own observations and thinking—a rare privilege enjoyed by only a small minority of scientists. Few scientists in industry are allowed to formulate their own research projects. Even medical research conducted in the more open milieu of the university generally follows broad outlines laid down by a seasoned investigator with proven competence to direct the expenditure of society's investment in research. It is generally unrealistic, and possibly frightening, to allow or force surgical residents to create their own research programs before they enter a research setting. Like all junior members of the scientific community, they tend to gravitate toward laboratories that are active in research areas of interest to them, and their training is enhanced if they are allowed to choose a component of the program that is most intriguing to them. When they have learned the methodology of science in such a setting, they often go on to develop and test hypotheses that are variants or logical sequels of the studies they participated in initially. The ability to choose one's own research problem and to defend the scientific approach adopted for its solution is generally a result rather than a prerequisite for research training.

The results of research by young surgical investigators are presented at the Surgical Forum of the American College of Surgeons, an annual research meeting introduced by Wangensteen in 1940 and generally regarded as the first choice among venues for the presentation of residents' work. The Surgical Forum attracts a fairly large international attendance and is accessible to residents and faculty members who submit their abstracts on a competitive basis. As many as 250 are accepted for presentation each year.

Other opportunities for the presentation of surgical research projects are offered by such societies as the Society of University Surgeons, the American Association for Academic Surgery, or the American Surgical Association. Regional and specialty organizations provide another category of local or specialized forums at which research-oriented papers are generally welcomed.

In training programs that lead to a Ph.D. in basic science, an acceptable level of knowledge of foreign languages is required in addition to successful completion of a thesis and course work in basic science. Statistics is occasionally allowed as an alternative to a foreign language. American surgical researchers often have difficulty in evaluating the accomplishments of those who publish their work in languages other than English. International exchange of research data and personnel would be greatly facilitated by an increase in the foreign language proficiency of American surgical scholars. If they are not proficient in English, foreign scholars studying in the United States are at a great disadvantage in securing positions and communicating with surgeons in the United States.

The Immigration Service of the federal government generally requires visiting researchers to return to their country of origin after a defined period of research in the United States. The likelihood of a foreign visitor securing a position to carry out research in the United States is usually enhanced if the applicant has an academic position to return to following the visit; this is a specific requirement of eligibility for the Graham Traveling Fellowship of the American Association for Thoracic Surgery.

Further information on scholarships, fellowships, and workshops may be obtained from the Committee on Research and Education, American College of Surgeons (55 East Erie St., Chicago, IL 60611-2797), and *The Foundation Grants Index*,[6] found in most libraries.

The Research Adviser

The surgical research adviser is responsible for providing perspective and insight in the selection of residents for research training. Some residents are best suited for a period of surgical scholarship that does not involve extensive experience at the laboratory bench. Research advisers feel privileged to participate in the scientific work of the residents who come under their tutelage, and they benefit from the residents' industry and intellectual energy in extending the advisers' own research, and in seeking answers to other scientific questions of mutual interest.

The number of fellows a single mentor can effectively advise depends on the time constraints imposed on the mentor. An active clinical surgeon with an active research program can rarely handle more than one or two research fellows. Research fellows can reasonably expect that their adviser will offer guidance and counseling during the period of research and in the months immediately preceding it. The research fellow is generally given an opportunity to participate in ongoing, productive research programs that involve exposure to the process of conducting research in a setting where many of the start-up problems have been solved. In addition to allowing the research fellow to step onto a "moving train" that is making progress toward a defined research goal, the adviser challenges the fellow to learn the basic process of developing new solutions to scientific problems. With rare exceptions, research advisers maintain a keen interest in the subsequent careers of their research fellows and facilitate their access to subsequent academic opportunities.

Legal and Cultural Considerations

The public attitude toward animal experimentation in the United States has become progressively more negative in recent years. Legislation, lobbyists, and very active protest groups limit the conduct of surgical experiments in domestic animals. Well-defined guidelines for the care of experimental animals are rigidly enforced by research institutions; compliance with these rules is an absolute requirement for funding by most granting agencies.

In contrast, open discussion of the potential benefits of participation in human clinical trials and wide publicity in the lay press about the knowledge gained through such trials have produced widespread and increasing acceptance of the controlled clinical trial. The trials of coronary surgery[9] and limited mastectomy[10] were particularly influential in this regard. Informed individual consent is a strict requirement for clinical research. Extensive documentation of the background for the clinical trial is generally incorporated in the informed consent document; a careful personal explanation of the purpose, risks, and gains of participation is mandatory and is generally regarded as the responsibility of the researcher. In practice, the required information and explanations are often given to the patient and family with the active participation of a research nurse or research fellow.

Most human clinical trials are conducted as two-armed comparisons between the best available treatment and a new treatment for which a reasonable scientific argument can be made that it may offer some improvement over standard therapy. Review boards composed of physicians, basic scientists, and laymen (e.g., such as clergy and lawyers) review proposed trials in human subjects at most institutions throughout the United States. It is the responsibility of these institutionally appointed review boards to protect both the participants and the institution from ill-conceived or unethical research.

Problems and Opportunities for Surgical Research Directors

Only a few organizations have courses devoted to instructing surgeons in the management of research programs. Such courses as are offered for the training of academic personnel in the management aspects of chairing an academic department generally emphasize contemporary management techniques. A unique program, specifically for training academic chairmen, is offered by Harvard University. A formal program of instruction for residents entering surgical research laboratories has been developed by the American Association for Academic Surgery. Excellent seminars on writing grant applications and on funding mechanisms are sponsored by the Committee on Research and Education at the annual congress of the American College of Surgeons.

The achievements of surgical research in the United States are the result of diverse, energetic, and devoted scholarly efforts at many levels in many centers. Despite the problems presented, we can celebrate the improvements in surgical care derived from the experimental laboratory and from controlled clinical trials in surgery. They warrant a firm commitment from our citizens to support and extend this productive enterprise.[11]

Acknowledgment. The author is grateful to Dr. William Longmire for thoughtful discussion and advice.

References

1. Carrel A. Results of the transplantation of blood vessels, organs and limbs. JAMA 1908;51(20):1622–67.
2. Blalock A, Taussig HB. The surgical treatment of malformations of the heart in which there is pulmonary stenosis or pulmonary atresia. JAMA 1945; 128:189–202.
3. Wangensteen OH, Wangensteen SD. Intestinal Obstructions. In: The Rise of Surgery: From Empiric Craft to Scientific Discipline. Minneapolis: University of Minnesota Press, 1987:106–141.
4. Justification for Appropriation Estimates for Committee on Appropriations, FY 1991, Vol 3, pg 32, National Institutes of Health. U.S. Government Printing Office: 1989:252–73.
5. Rikkers LF, Bland KI, Kinder BK, et al. Funding of surgical research: the roles of government and industry. J Surg Res 1985;39:209–15.
6. The Foundation Grants Index, 18th ed, Kovacs R., ed. New York: The Foundation Center, 1989.
7. Kennedy TJ Jr. The rising cost of NIH-funded biomedical research? Academic Med 1990;65:63–73.
8. Stossel TP, Stossel SC. Declining American representation in leading clinical-research journals. N Engl J Med 1990;322:739–42.
9. CASS Principal Investigators: Myocardial infarction and mortality in the coronary artery surgery study (CASS) randomized trial. N Engl J Med 1984;310: 750–58.
10. Fisher B, Redmond C, Poisson R, et al. Eight-year results of a randomized clinical trial comparing total mastectomy and lumpectomy with or without irradiation in the treatment of breast cancer. N Engl J Med 1989;320:822–28.
11. Thompson JC. The role of research in the surgery of tomorrow. Am J Surg 1984;147:2–8.

64

International Exchange for Surgical Education

A. Paul, J. Coleman, D. Marelli, E. Eypasch, and B. Bouillon

International exchange for surgical education has a long tradition. The development of the surgical residency program in North America is based on the Langenbeck-Billroth school of Germany and Austria. This is a direct result of William Halsted's postgraduate training in Europe, between 1878 and 1880.[1] At that time, Halsted was 26 years old and had just completed a surgical internship at the Bellevue Hospital in New York. During the years he spent studying abroad, Halsted gained experience in surgical techniques unknown to many North American surgeons. He formed close ties with a number of clinical and laboratory assistants and, in 1889, on becoming chief of surgery at the Johns Hopkins Hospital, adopted a training program for residents similar to what he had observed in Europe.[2,3] The knowledge and experience gained by Halsted was not only of enormous personal benefit, it also contributed substantially to the development of North American surgical institutions. This example of dual benefit should be held in the minds of those intending to join clinical or research surgical training programs abroad.

This chapter provides some guidelines for the surgeon who considers working abroad. Who is likely to benefit from a foreign program, how you should approach your stay abroad and what you should aim for on returning home are the areas covered. The ideas expressed here are based on the personal experience of the authors.

The Decision to Study Abroad

Ideally, the decision to study abroad should be linked with specific aims that may vary from gaining clinical experience to learning research techniques. Since the opportunity to study abroad will generally arise only once in your training, choosing the proper time to go is very important. While more junior residents certainly may benefit from experiencing another medical system, language, and culture, the maximum benefit will be gained by those with a minimum of 2 to 3 years of surgical experience. This background of basic surgical knowledge provides the framework for evaluating the new circumstances presented abroad. Sufficient lead time must be allowed, because language and funding require thorough preparation. Remember that there is always a reason not to go, and the ideal situation is infrequent.

Organizing Your Trip

When you are accepted into the program of your choice, you should begin to organize the paperwork outlined in Table 64.1. This takes a minimum of 6 months, and organizing adequate funding may take longer. Financial considerations can, potentially, impose limitations. Sources of finance may come from the host or from your own country. Surgical departments, traveling fellowships, local government grants, and industry are the usual sources. Although initial contact is usually made through the head of a department, early establishment of a relationship with a colleague at your own level will prove very beneficial. Prior contact with such

TABLE 64.1. Areas requiring early and thorough organization.

Funding
Work permit, visa
Medical license
Insurance
Accommodations
Travel arrangements

individuals will help you gain a more exact picture of the host institution. An initial "on site" visit is recommended. This allows you to gain an overview of the workplace, identify areas of expertise, and see the housing options available – most important if you have a family. From the point of view of the host, such a visit permits future colleagues and supervisors to discuss areas of interest, and leads to a more efficient coordination of activities for the incoming resident. Finally, such a site visit initiates the mechanics of obtaining visas, health insurance, and licensure equivalents.

The initial few weeks are essential for gaining acceptance and building relationships with colleagues. Trust the capabilities of the host institution and its staff, and recognize that there is more than one way to accomplish your goals and that your program will evolve in predictable phases (Table 64.2). Be realistic about your abilities and the opportunities available in your new work environment. *Plan* adequate time for observation, and construct a detailed schedule with your supervisor. If you travel to other centers, it is reasonable and far more effective to ask your primary host to facilitate travel and housing arrangements. Despite the best planning, a *period of frustration* will be endured as the result of problems with language, protocols, homesickness, and missing social contacts.

Stamina, initiative, team spirit, and a little luck will bring you to the *productivity phase*. This phase should be carefully controlled, to allow completion of your project. In experimental work, it is essential to have at least a first draft of work completed prior to returning home. Frequently, one miscalculates the spare time that will be available on returning to normal clinical duty for the completion of unfinished work. When the aim of the trip is to learn new techniques, adequate note taking, photo documentation, and reference literature collection are essential, because important specific details are quickly forgotten.

TABLE 64.2. Periods experienced while working abroad.

Period	Goals
Orientation	Establish contacts.
Planning	Establish exact time schedule.
Frustration	Do not resign.
Productivity	Initiative and cooperation. Have realistic goals.
Conclusion	Summarize your work; finish papers and thesis.

On returning home, continuity of research interests initiated abroad and introduction of new techniques learned will prove difficult. Critical evaluation of your experience with colleagues at home is vital for gaining help and support. Maintaining contact with the host institution will also help you integrate what you have learned into your home institution and will act as a basis for future academic exchange.

Concluding Comments

Studying abroad offers major advantages for the future academic surgeon. This part of the educational process should be planned and organized as effectively as possible. Halsted, in his time, set the example of maximum gain from international experience and established a precedent that we consider to be essential for the growth of the international academic surgical community.

References

1. Sabiston DC. A continuum in surgical education. Surgery 1969;66:1.
2. Carter BN. The fruition of Halsted's concept of surgical training. Surgery 1952;32:518.
3. Halsted WS. The training of a surgeon. Bull Johns Hopkins Hosp 1904;15:267.

65

Common Characteristics and Distinctive Diversity in Surgical Research: Some International Comparisons

M.F. McKneally, H. Troidl, D.S. Mulder, W.O. Spitzer, B. McPeek, C.M. Balch, and A.S. Wechsler

While there is general agreement that surgical research can make a substantial contribution to the education of surgeons, the care of patients, and the advancement of knowledge, there is considerable diversity in the approaches used to teach, conduct, and fund research in different countries throughout the world.

Time Management

Surgeons confront unique logistical problems when they are learning research methods and when they are attempting to practice research. Since excellence in surgery requires a high level of performance both in clinical judgment and technical application, the problem of integrating scholarly activities and clinical practice is usually more difficult for the surgeon than for academic physicians in other disciplines (see Section I, Chapter 4). Clinical investigators in medical specialties may spend 70% of their time in the laboratory and two or three half-days per week in the ward or the outpatient clinic. There may be only one or two months of rounding in a university hospital when the investigator must devote 100% of effort to clinical coverage of a medical service. Such a distribution of activities enables reasonably credible performance of academic internists and other physicians, both as clinicians and as scientists. A surgeon cannot retain clinical credibility without operating and caring for patients for an appreciably large number of working hours every week; yet success as an investigator requires a substantial investment of time and intellectual energy in "hands-on" research, especially during the first several years. The increasing complexity of hypotheses and methodology demands several years of nonclinical postgraduate education in basic sciences, statistics or clinical epidemiology, and even social sciences. A common denominator in many of the chapters of this section is the acute dilemma of the chairman, the investigator, and the trainee: how to reconcile the irreconcilable. For the established academic, the only solution advanced by implication in most countries is Osler's touchstone: Work . . . work . . . and more work. Generally, excellence seems to be reserved for those willing to do two full careers in one lifetime. For the trainee, the solutions involve not only the same magnitude of work, but greater risks in career choices, financial loss due to lengthening of the training period, and the need to master two or more disciplines to be able to achieve personal academic goals as bridge scientists.

Some of the patterns that have evolved in the countries surveyed may lead us to a better resolution. The early identification of a resident with a research team described in France, Canada, Germany, and Japan suggests that the awakening of awareness of the scientific method can begin early in clinical training. A period of full-time laboratory research without clinical responsibility is widely recommended after the second year of clinical training. The weekly research rounds for all surgeons at McGill provide a continuing stimulus for the clinical residents. Protected time in the laboratory during the clinical rotations appears to approach the ideal, but may require a larger number of residents to meet service needs. The manpower needed to staff research programs, without interrupting the residents' ongoing clinical responsibility, seems to be available only in England, Sweden, and Japan. The remarkable excess of doctors in Spain has not led to a glut of research manpower, but research program development and funding could not absorb more personnel there at this time. The increasing number of physicians and surgeons being educated throughout the world may lead to a queue of able candidates waiting for research posts in the future. At the present time, except for brief 6-month or 12-month electives in research, trainees must also fit their investigation into a busy service and didactic learning schedule. The examples of trainees' daily schedules show this clearly. Generally, research work is of subordinate priority in the eyes of service chiefs, service-oriented hospitals, and health agencies.

Financial realities do not explain the whole problem, but in all the countries contributing to this overview, resources are very important determinants of outcome in the clinical investigator's unending struggle to serve both the patient and science with insufficient time, and the disadvantage of competing for research funds with Ph.D.'s who have more extensive scientific preparation and are unencumbered by heavy clinical commitments. Interesting solutions to the time management problem of including surgical research in the schedules of busy academic clinicians are seen in the relatively independent experimental surgical departments in Munich and the more integrated "small research group" of the Marburg Experiment. A narrowing of the spectrum of clinical responsibility to coincide more easily with the research thrust of the investigator has been favorably reported from England, Sweden, and the United States but is apparently incompatible with German tradition at this time. The dilemma of restricted university funds to support research personnel, well presented in the German experience, is echoed by most other authors.

Investment in Research

Despite the universality of research and our desire to reap its benefits, there are marked differences between countries in the opportunities available for research. For many countries, there is scant information about the extent of research expenditures, perhaps due to peculiarities in reporting. For example, the U.S.S.R. has extensive research and development investment, but has published very little data on the extent or intensity of research efforts. So-called Third World nations perform little research, and rely on the more developed nations to pioneer science and technology. Some countries, like China, do perform research, but information about the extent of the effort does not appear to be collected and maintained in any central place. Available data are, therefore, largely confined to the industrialized Western European countries, Canada, the United States, Australia, New Zealand, and Japan. These countries are member states of the Organization for Economic Cooperation and Development (OECD). Yugoslavia participates in the OECD to a limited extent.

Even within the OECD data, sorting out medical research is difficult. For example, in Germany and Switzerland research budgets of pharmaceutical and chemical firms are pooled in a single category, because the large firms in both these countries produce industrial chemicals as well as pharmaceuticals. For them, such an aggregation makes sense, but it complicates comparisons of support for biomedical research between countries. Among international organizations, only the OECD seems to gather data across its member countries systematically. Despite some problems of definition, they appear to be the best available basis for comparison.[1]

The OECD defines biomedical research as the study of specific diseases and conditions including detection, cause, prophylaxis, treatment, and rehabilitation. This definition also includes the design of methods, drugs, and devices used for diagnosis or treatment; broad areas of scientific research undertaken to obtain a basic understanding of the life processes that affect disease and human well-being; and clinical trials and epidemiologic studies. Research in fields like health education is not included.

Figure 65.1 compares public domestic biomedical research and development (BMRD) funds per capita with gross domestic product per capita in 10 countries. The gross domestic product per capita is a standard indicator of national economic activity. The strong positive correlation we see demonstrates that, in general, biomedical research and development is funded at a higher rate in higher income countries.

Public domestic biomedical research and development, as a percentage of gross domestic product, also correlates strongly with gross domestic product per capita. Not only do the richer countries have more money to spend on biomedical research, they tend to spend relatively more of what they have.

In the data reported, the effects of inflation and differing national currency exchange rates are controlled by converting everything to 1975 prices and all funds to U.S. dollars using the 1975 exchange rates. Since exchange rates are based on supply and demand for internationally traded goods, one might expect the purchasing power of the constant U.S. dollar to be similar in terms of equipment. Salaries of research workers present a problem. The purchasing power is likely to be greater in countries with a lower per capita domestic product.

Data for the United States and for Switzerland were available for every year from 1970 through

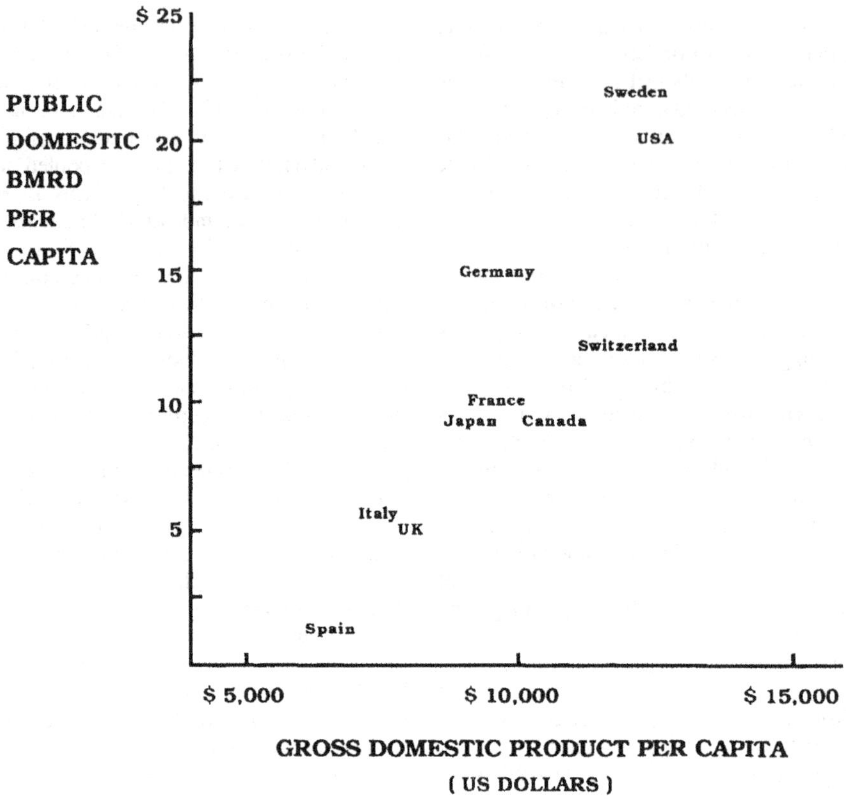

FIGURE 65.1. Public domestic funds for biomedical research and development (BMRD) per capita and gross domestic product (GDP) per capita. Reprinted with permission from Shepard DS, Durch JS[1] (1984).

1980. For other countries, data were available only for varying subsets of those years. For this reason, the reported data converted to 1975 U.S. dollars were fitted to an ordinary least-squares curve, and some of the values reported represent such smoothed data projections. The United States of America has the largest absolute funding for biomedical research development, yet the United States is only fourth highest in spending per capita. Switzerland is the highest per capita contributor to biomedical research and development. Overall, public funds generally account for half of the total. But for some individual countries, the private sector contributes the larger share. The most striking case is Switzerland, which has by far the highest private funding per capita, due in great measure to the presence of major pharmaceutical firms in a relatively small country. Switzerland's public funding level is only a little above the mean for the countries reported here and below that of Sweden, the United States, and Germany. Sweden leads in public sector funding.

A Comparison of Research Training for Surgeons

The general education of students who eventually enter a surgical career varies in the intensity of preparation for university studies. American and Canadian graduates of secondary schools generally enter the university for a 4-year premedical training program at age 18. At that point, they are approximately 18 to 24 months behind their European counterparts in terms of general and scientific education. Medical school begins earlier for European students and extends for a longer period of time. Table 65.1, prepared from the descriptions of the education of an academic surgeon in various countries, provides a comparative outline of the training programs. Research may be commenced in medical school and is required in some countries for an academic medical degree, but is not required for the practice of medicine. In Spain, Germany, Japan, and England, a doctorate in medicine is a

TABLE 65.1. Comparative outline of training programs.

Age[a]	Germany	Switzerland	Sweden	France
4	Kindergarten	Kindergarten		
5				*École maternelle*
6	Elementary school	Primary school		
7				Primary school
8			Comprehensive school	
9				
10	Gymnasium			
11				
12				Secondary school
13		Gymnasium		
14				
15				
16			Gymnasium	*Lycée*
17				
18				
19	Basic medical science (2 years)	Basic medical science (2 years)	Medical school	*Faculté* of Science (1 year)
20				*Faculté* of Medicine (4 years)
21	Clinical science (4 years)	Clinical science (4 years)		
22				
23				
24				
25	"Physician in training" (2 years)			
26		"Licensed physician" General surgery training (6–8 years, prolonged by intercurrent military service)	Compulsory health service (2 years including 6 months in general medicine)	"Certification" Internships – general medicine (2 years)
27	General surgery training (6 years)		General surgery training County hospital (4½ years)	Residency in surgery (5 years) (+ 1 year research for university career)
28	University hospital (research); or Community hospital			
29		University (research); or Community hospital		
30				
31				
32	*Oberarzt* (university); *Oberarzt* (community)	*Oberarzt* (community)		
33			Research training (5 years) Leading to doctorate in surgery	
34		*Oberarzt* (university)		*Professor d'Université*
35				
36				
37				
38	Habilitation			
39			Docent in surgery	
40	*Privat Dozent*	*Dozent*		
41	*Chearzt* (community)			
42				
43				
44				
45	Professor Ordinarius	Chief of Surgery	Chief of Surgery	Chief of Surgery
46				
47				
48				
49				
50				

[a] Where there is a range, ages given are generally minimums.

TABLE 65.1. *Continued.*

Age[a]	United States	Canada	England	Japan	Spain
4	Kindergarten	Kindergarten		Kindergarten	
5			Elementary school	Elementary school	Elementary education
6	Elementary school	Elementary school			
7					
8					
9					
10					Secondary school
11	Junior high school	Junior high school			
12			Secondary school	Junior high school	
13					
14	High school	High school			
15				Senior high school	
16					
17			Medical school	Medical school	University medical school(5 years); unlimited enrollment; high attrition
18	Premedical college	Premedical college		Premedical course (2 years)	
19					
20				Basic science (2 years)	
21	Medical school Basic science, 2 years	Premedical school (2 years)			
22			Internship	Clinical science (2 years)	Internship (license to practice)
23	Clinical science, 2 years	Clinical science (2 years)			
24			General surgical training (includes 6–12 months basic science)	Medical doctor, basic surgical training (2 years)	University or community hospital clinical assistant
25	Doctor of medicine (M.D.)	Doctor of medicine (M.D.)			Clinical apprenticeship (2 years with course work) Assistant
26	Surgical residency (2 years) core curriculum	Rotating internship		Postgraduate course (4 years) (2–3 years) research 1 year clinical training; or surgical training (6 years) (Senior course) may include 2–3 years research	
27	University hospital research (1 year) Community hospital surgical subspecialty (3 years)	Core training–surgery (2 years)			
28			Registrar		
29		Surgical scholarship (1 year)			Research 2–4 years Thesis leading to PhD in basic science General surgery (5 years) Self-arranged
30	Senior surgical residency (2 years)	Surgical residency; Senior clinical years (2 years)	FRCS diploma	Doctor of medicine Assistant doctor	
31	Chief resident	Chief resident	"Post FRCS Posts" University and NHS medical school	Doctor of medicine	Surgical assistant
32	Cardiothoracic. plastic residency				
33			Lecturer Senior registrar	Instructor	
34	Assistant professor	Assistant professor	Senior lecturer		
35					
36			Reader Consultant		
37					
38					
39			Professor		
40				Assistant professor	
41	Associate professor	Associate professor			
42					
43					
44	Professor of Surgery	Professor of Surgery		Associate professor	Chief of Surgery
45					
46					
47					
48					
49					
50				Professor of Surgery	

[a] Where there is a range, ages given are generally minimums.

special degree that requires a thesis based on research performed by the medical student. Residency in surgery begins as early as age 24 in England and as late as age 27 in Sweden, where a compulsory period of practice in the health service adds 2 years to the surgeon's overall training period. A 6-month rotation in general surgery is included during this period of service.

In Germany, Switzerland, and Sweden there is a clearly defined pathway for the education and certification of academic surgeons called "habilitation," which includes a requirement for extensive participation in clinical and experimental research, stringent criteria to qualify for examination by the faculty, and a clear designation as "docent" for the individual who has demonstrated this broad knowledge of surgery. The most rigorous requirements appear to be those in the German system, which demands about 25 publications, 15 oral presentations, and a clinical and experimental thesis defended in an oral examination. Only a small fraction of surgical residents pursue the lengthy pathway leading to full qualification for the academic life at approximately the age of 40 in all three countries. This course brings the candidate to a point that is approximately analogous to a publication and productivity record that would qualify an academic surgeon for promotion to the rank of a tenured associate professor in many North American universities.

The "habilitation" or thesis project in the German system may be started within the 6 years of general surgery training. It usually prolongs this period because it reduces the opportunity for the candidate to accumulate the list of surgical cases required to qualify for completion of the residency program. In German university hospitals, the assistant who is chosen to become an *oberarzt* or principal assistant to the chief, after 6 years or more of training, usually has completed the habilitation process and bears a responsibility for the day-to-day administrative management of the operating room and surgical floors considerably in excess of the administrative responsibilities of senior North American surgical residents. Four years following approval of the thesis and certification as a "docent," surgeons are eligible to be promoted to the rank of professor. They may then proceed up the academic ladder at the university hospital, or take a position as chief of surgery at a major community hospital.

Swedish residents may complete clinical training in county hospitals, where they have extensive exposure to the common problems of general surgery. Those interested in an academic career then return to a university hospital for advanced training in complex areas of surgery, such as transplantation. During this interval they prepare their dissertations, conduct research, and establish the publication record required to qualify for examination. The French system offers a shorter period of 5 years of residency training, without a chief residency at the end. Research is carried out intermittently during the course of the residency program; a recent modification of the French residency in surgery has been the addition of a dedicated year of surgical research at some institutions.

In the United States and Canada, medical students graduate and qualify for entry into surgical training at approximately the same age as their European counterparts. During surgical residency, some may spend one year in research as part of their general education in surgery. Residents who show a particular aptitude for an academic career select programs that offer one or more years of additional research to develop a solid foundation in clinical and basic science, including a knowledge of research design, and statistics, and familiarity with the methods of securing extramural funding for research. Research in North America is generally concentrated in a period of study isolated from the pressures of clinical surgery to allow the resident to concentrate on scientific development. This period of research is often placed after a 2-year core curriculum of surgery. Following the research rotation, the resident returns to the heavy clinical responsibilities of senior residency but may attempt to keep the research project going through a team of collaborators developed during the laboratory years. This period introduces the tension between research and clinical care that dominates the lives of most academic surgeons.

Residents who are entering surgical subspecialties leave the general surgery program after the core curriculum to specialize for 3 to 5 years in otolaryngology, urology, neurosurgery, or orthopedic surgery. Specialists in plastic surgery, cardiovascular and thoracic surgery, or vascular surgery complete the minimum of 5 clinical years of general surgery training before seeking further subspecialty training. Academic graduates of the North American programs generally finish their formal residency training at 32 to 35 years of age, depending on the amount of subspecialty training they pursue. At that time, they may be selected to join the faculty of a medical school and to serve on the surgical staff of a university hospital, where they usually begin their climb up the academic ladder as an instructor. In this role, they are analogous in some ways to the university *oberarzt*, but they do not stay in the hospital at night to take calls as they did during their residency. Academic rank, requirements for promotion, and the ages at which they are attained vary from university to university. The ages cited in Table 65.1 are approximate for the minimum at each rank.

In England, medical school graduates enter surgical training at a younger age than their counterparts in many other countries. Trainees are fully qualified for fellowship in the Royal College of Surgeons and for surgical practice by the age of 29. They may well have participated in research during residency training; because of a lack of opportunities to enter the practice of surgery, however, many registrars continue in a residentlike role in the National Health Service. While they contribute to patient care and research in the academic setting at this level, registrars may wait 10 to 20 years before the next advance in their academic careers.

Japanese academic surgeons enter the university for preclinical medical science at approximately the same age as their counterparts in Europe. After 2 years of basic science and 4 years of clinical science, they are eligible for certification as physicians at the age of 24. They may then enter surgical residency in a community hospital, where there is no opportunity to perform research or for academic promotion. Those who are interested in the academic track affiliate with a university hospital in the role of unpaid assistants or may enroll as postgraduate students of surgery, paying tuition to the university clinic in order to participate in the lectures and conferences of the university surgical service. Assistants support themselves by working part-time in the operating room at private hospitals for one half-day per week. This period of activity as a doctor-in-training or a "university clinic student" may last for 4 years or more. If an opening becomes available and these assistants have performed well, they may qualify for a position as "assistant doctor" in the university hospital. To qualify academically for this position, some applicants for the position spend 1 to 2 years in fundamental research in the laboratory.

At the age of 31, after a considerable period in the role of student, and 2 years in the role of laboratory researcher, the Japanese candidate enters a program analogous to a European or North American university hospital senior residency or assistantship. During this period the academic surgeon performs in a role similar to the role of senior registrar in England or instructor in North America. He may stay in this role until he is in his fifties, although successful candidates move up the academic ladder to the rank of assistant and associate professor and, perhaps eventually, to chairmanship. Assistant doctors and academic surgeons, in general, are not well paid and are expected to work one day per week in private hospitals to supplement their income. They may go into practice in the community if their prospects for advancement do not appear to be promising.

We asked our contributors to diagram a representative day or week in the life of a young academic surgeon. The time commitments for operating, outpatient care, ward rounds, research, and teaching are illustrated in several chapters. There was a striking difference in the time for research among the reporting countries. Because of the availability of funding for research, the large number of academic assistants, and the time schedule of the National Health Service in Sweden, a substantial amount of time is dedicated to research within the working day. In most of the other reporting countries, the dilemma of the academic surgeon is finding enough time to perform research.

Attitudes Toward Surgical Research

The attitude of the public toward surgical research seems to parallel the attitude of community-based and university surgeons, and is reflected by the legislative bodies in their level of funding for research in general and surgical research in particular. In general, public understanding about the benefits of medical research has improved in the past two decades. Information regarding surgical research has often emphasized spectacular high technology procedures, such as implantation of the mechanical heart or liver transplantation. There is a need for further public education in the area of applied clinical and health services research.

A survey from countries presented in this book reveals a wide spectrum of attitudes by the public and of surgeons toward research. In Spain, there has been little surgical research beyond technical exercises to develop the proficiency of clinical surgical teams in new surgical techniques. Formal scientific studies to analyze surgical problems are unusual at the clinical or laboratory level. This low level of activity in surgical research is not related to the number of physicians available to perform it, because Spain has a striking excess of physicians and surgeons, many of whom are forced to seek employment outside the medical community to survive. The intensity and organization of surgical research in Spain seems to reflect the attitude of the populace, which the author characterizes as indifferent. Only 0.072% of the gross national product of Spain is devoted to biomedical research; the atmosphere, support personnel, and organized programs of investigation have not been developed to allow easy access of surgeons to training in research. The mean for countries of the European Economic Community is approximately 0.16% of the gross national product. A fascinating funding mechanism for research exists in Spain, where a surcharge is added to each prescription drug and set aside for a medical research fund managed through the Social Security system.

The public's attitude toward research in Germany and France seems to be "positive but skeptical." That is, effective research programs that result in notable clinical success (e.g., cardiac transplantation) are beginning to reduce public skepticism about the application of the scientific method to the solution of clinical problems. Nevertheless, there is a strong residual feeling that the doctor, particularly the surgeon, should be an authority on his subject, able to prescribe and carry out appropriate treatment without any element of doubt. The success of the European Organization for Research and Treatment of Cancer (EORTC) in promoting randomized trials of cancer chemotherapy throughout Europe and the pioneering work of the National Cancer Institute in Milan, Italy, have increased public understanding of the application of the scientific method as opposed to authoritarian prescriptions for the resolution of clinical problems. A unique funding mechanism described by our French and Japanese colleagues is a specific allocation in the budget of some municipalities for the support of surgical research.

In the United States, Canada, Switzerland, and Sweden the application of the scientific method to the resolution of surgical problems is fairly well accepted within the general population and is regarded as appropriate by many physicians and surgeons. In these countries, as elsewhere, the position of surgical research within the scientific community is not as advanced as it might be. The precise level of funding for surgical research is difficult to isolate because of anatomic or disease-oriented panels that award and record funds without reference to specialty. There is a general feeling that surgical research, as illustrated by injury research, receives a low level of funding related to its importance as a health problem.[2] We need more accurate data on the funding of surgical research, a goal currently pursued by the Committee on Research and Education of the American College of Surgeons.

In Japan, scientific research is supported in the national budget at an increasing level each year. The solution of clinical problems by analysis of outcomes in groups of patients randomly assigned to a variety of treatments is still perceived as a culturally shocking, Western approach to patient care. Experimental trials of new treatments are generally characterized by low accrual when randomization is a requirement for patient entry. The attitude of clinicians toward surgical research, however, is positive.

The close relationship between levels of funding and public attitude demands that surgeons become involved in education of the public, governments at all levels, and granting agencies. Surgical leaders armed with data must develop a more effective interface with government, to assume an influential role in determining priorities and standards for the delivery of clinical care, as well as execution of basic and applied research.

Lessons Learned, Problems Identified, and Goals

The reports from the nations reviewed reveal the need for increased support among citizens of most countries for biomedical research, particularly clinical investigation. The crucial role research plays in improving the length and quality of patients' lives is not sufficiently understood. Everyone involved in clinical research, from world renowned scholars to first year registrars, must be involved in the process of public education to encourage better participation in research and more financial support through government agencies, private foundations, and individual gifts.

Funding for surgical research must be won in an increasingly competitive market. The issue of whether separate funds should be set aside by granting agencies for surgical research is unresolved. Improved instruments for quantifying the input and output of surgical research are required. It would be helpful in analyzing and justifying funding for research projects in surgery if the expenditure for surgical research per capita, or as a function of gross domestic product, could be related to outcome measures (such as published research papers in prestigious journals, citations, and impact on health care outcomes).

Academic surgical leaders must include among their responsibilities public education and dynamic personal interaction with the political process to protect their patient constituency, and to secure adequate funding for research education and the scientific analysis of the consequences of health policy changes. We recognize a special need for surgical leadership in health services research on problems of manpower, specialization, and health care organization.

The society that demands improvements in medicine and surgery, not just care for the sick, must get behind the effort in a tangible way. There is no more tangible support for research than willingness to be a participant in a clinical trial. Because the outcomes of surgical interventions are frequently manifest in the short term, surgeons, more than most clinicians, are keenly aware of the imperfections of their knowledge. Surgeons closely monitor their outcomes, by way of morbidity and mortality conferences and tissue committees. Instinctively, they wish to submit competing treatments in their armamentarium to rigorous scientific scrutiny. They are encumbered in their intent by the instincts of their patients, who want to consider their surgeon infallible and incapable of doubt. Such tensions are not easy to resolve in any society. They are especially troublesome in countries where the projected certainty of the doctor is considered to be an intrinsic part of the therapeutic maneuver. This task of public education by clinicians is facilitated by responsible journalism, which reinforces the benefits of patient participation in the development of improved treatments. Surgeons with access to political leaders and opinion shapers must exercise their responsibility to inform and judiciously persuade, whenever possible.

Our sample of opinions from academic surgeons in many countries identifies *time management* as a major problem in the training of surgical scientists and in the maintenance of operative skills to keep them competitive. Some of the solutions include:

1. The development of a *team* with sufficient clinical manpower to allow the surgical scientists to return to the laboratory and complete scientific tasks, unencumbered by clinical responsibility during defined periods of time.
2. The development of stable, long-term, productive relationships between clinical surgeons and basic scientists, focused on projects of mutual interest.
3. The integration of scientific collaborators into the surgical program, as in the Marburg Experiment, so that a surgeon's viewpoint is brought to bear throughout research on a problem even though the surgeon may not necessarily participate in hands-on laboratory execution of the research. The basic scientist partner, or theoretical surgeon in this relationship, has an extensive investment in the scientific validity of the clinical efforts of the integrated team, though not participating directly in hands-on execution of surgical practice.
4. Narrowing each surgeon's field of specialization sufficiently to allow intensification of scientific study of the field is an additional, useful mechanism for protecting surgeons from the overwhelming demands of a broad spectrum of responsibility. For example, concentration on pancreatic transplantation can facilitate the development of a focused clinical and laboratory research program that is highly interactive and intensive, yet the scholar is protected from the demand of covering the full breadth of general surgery. The development of focused programs of clinical and experimental research of this nature requires the collaboration of clinical colleagues and the support of the chief of surgery.

The rigid structure of training programs militates against an exchange of teachers and students among countries. We support attempts of academic and political leaders to correct such artificial barriers to progress. North Americans and others should emulate countries in the European Economic Community (EEC) who have started taking tangible steps to facilitate educational and research exchanges. By 1992 the member countries of the EEC plan to have common requirements for licensure and practice, enabling easy professional exchange across national boundaries.

We encourage program directors and chairmen to arrange adequate training in research for talented residents and registrars. At the same time, we recognize the importance of maintaining the credibility of surgeons as superb clinicians. We welcome and encourage the increasing trend for surgical scholars to seek methodological training in laboratory, clinical, and epidemiologic research. From such a process will emerge future leaders, independent bridge scientists, sophisticated collaborators in large trials, productive partners in laboratory inquiry, and knowledgeable contributors to health services research.

The development of increasing methodological skills among surgeons conducting research on surgical problems is illustrated by the well-designed and well-executed randomized trials of surgical versus medical treatment in coronary artery disease conducted in Europe[3] and North America.[4] Similarly, the definition of the role of surgical treatment and adjuvant therapy of breast cancer illustrates a happy combination of careful scientific methodology and disciplined surgical practice.[5] A surgeon who presents reliable data in precise and technically sophisticated statistical terms is a powerful new voice in surgery. The future surgical scholars must develop skills in writing and public speaking. Those who aspire to leadership in the academic world must work hard to communicate with scholars in other countries. Americans, especially, must study to overcome their lack of language skills, a major impediment to true international exchange. Surgical chairmen must remember that a surgeon with 1 or 2 years of experience in a sister discipline is able only to facilitate collaborative research, not to practice that other discipline independently. A half-trained statistician may be almost as dangerous as a half-trained surgeon, and a half trained molecular biologist cannot compete for research funding at the national level.

The universal desire of each of our patients is to get the best possible care. We can achieve the best standards if the leadership in academic surgery engages in research and focuses on problems that arise in patient care. If widespread involvement of academic surgeons in research is thwarted by review mechanisms that fail to give proper weight to the relevance of research questions put forward by clinicians, the review system requires revision to promote clinically related research. The success of the surgical study sections of the National Institutes of Health in the United States provides convincing support for this strategy. If funding mechanisms or local customs in any country fail to foster relevant research about problems that matter to surgeons and their patients, educational steps should be taken to correct the problem. For example, Japanese academic surgeons might insist that the medical curriculum include a strong orientation to scientific methods that have direct relevance to the choice of treatment for patients. Modern students must learn that decisions should be based on evidence and not on opinion, no matter how eminent the source. Students everywhere should learn how to weigh evidence from designs of various types and should know enough about statistics to be informed consumers of quantitative information, as well as judicious teachers of the public.

We have identified a small number of prominent issues that need to be addressed. Resource allocation for research must increase. Citizens must join with clinicians in taking responsibility to advance the knowledge that ultimately benefits each individual member of society. Clinicians and the public alike must learn how to deal with uncertainty, and clinicians must work to improve treatments, not pretend to know more than we do. In the short run, it means application of the highest order of clinical judgment and technical skill. In the longer run, it requires imagination, diligence, and excellence in the pursuit of new knowledge.

We can celebrate the fact that in spite of ostensibly insurmountable obstacles, the science of surgery advances and patients everywhere benefit from the achievements of those who will not be discouraged or defeated.

Each country can point to important contributions in recent years. Open heart surgery, pioneered in the United States, inaugurated a new era of effective intervention for a large number of disorders hitherto irreversible and often terminal. Investigators in France advanced both the surgical treatment of the aorta and laparoscopic surgery. In the United Kingdom, controlled trials were first applied in surgery by Goligher; and total hip replacement was introduced and rigorously evaluated, changing the lives of advanced arthritis victims. Spain has contributed technical advances in heart surgery, while Canadians made innovations in pediatric surgery, developed cardiac hypothermia techniques and cardiac pacemakers. Italian surgeons and physicians set a high standard for clinical trials of cancer surgery and adjuvant chemotherapy. Research in Switzerland enabled osteosynthetic surgery. The Swedes combined outstanding clinical investigation with rigorous population science to advance our understanding of the natural history of low back pain and to discriminate effective from worthless interventions in all stages of that disorder. Endoscopy was made possible in its present sophisticated modalities by Japanese research. In Germany, a combination of judicious program development and health services research established the world's exemplary prehospital trauma services for entire regions of that country.

We look forward to exciting new contributions in the closing decade of this century. We must study our problems together and work out joint solutions across disciplinary and national boundaries. The editors and authors of this text have had a stimulating and encouraging experience exchanging ideas about the solution to research problems. We look forward with enthusiasm to continued and increasing international cooperation and progress in this adventure.

The first step on the long road is excellence in methods. We have attempted to make it easier to take the first step for those committed to these goals, wherever they live and work.

References

1. Our data on research funding are adapted from Shepard DS, Durch JS. International comparison of research allocation in health sciences: an analysis of expenditures on biomedical research in 19 industrialized countries. Boston: Harvard School of Public Health, Institutes for Health Research, 1984.
2. Foege WH. Committee on Trauma Research. Commission on Life Science, National Research Council, and the Institute of Medicine. Washington, DC: National Academy Press, 1985.
3. European Coronary Surgery Study Group. Long-term results of prospective randomized study of coronary artery bypass surgery in stable angina pectoris. Lancet (8309) 1982;2:1173–80.
4. Kaiser GC, Davis KB, Fisher LD, et al. Survival fol-

lowing coronary artery bypass grafting in patients with severe angina pectoris (CASS). J Thorac Cardiovasc Surg 89;1985:513–24.
5. Fisher B, Redmond C, Legault-Poisson S, et al. Postoperative chemotherapy and tamoxifen alone in the treatment of node positive breast cancer patients aged 50 years and older with tumors responsive to tamoxifen: results from the National Surgical Adjuvant Breast and Bowel Project B-16. J Clin Oncol 1990;8:1005–18.

Section VI

Opportunities in Research

66

Future Horizons in Surgical Research

F.D. Moore

"... and a horizon is nothing save the limit of our sight."

To glimpse what lies beyond our horizon, it is wise to examine the terrain from whence we come. Since World War II, surgical research has functioned in four modes.

1. *Developing new procedures*. Examples of new procedures developed where none existed before include open heart operations using a pump oxygenator, organ transplantation, microsurgery of the brain and middle ear, laser surgery of the detached retina, direct arterial suture and repair (including aortic aneurysm), and prosthetic replacement of major joints.
2. *Building bridges to the basic sciences*. Bringing basic science directly to the bedside has resulted in advances in our understanding of the metabolic needs of surgical patients, intravenous feeding, the biology of convalescence, the use of anticoagulants and antibiotics, and the role of immunology in surgery.
3. *Collaborating with clinical colleagues*. The blossoming of cancer surgery into a multimodality collaborative treatment, improved orthopedic management of rheumatoid arthritis, and the use of pacemakers, ultrasound, and computed axial tomography are but a few examples of the effectiveness of collaboration between surgeons and other clinical colleagues.
4. *Improving existing procedures by surgical engineering*. The improvement of surgery is often triggered by self-examination and self-criticism. This time-honored practice by surgeons is now augmented by incisive research. The evolution of surgery for breast cancer, liver resection, prostatectomy, pituitary neoplasms, and fracture stabilization illustrates how surgical care has changed and improved through repeated performance and a clearer understanding of its own shortcomings. Advances in the evaluation of new procedures and technology assessment belong in this category.

Surgical research has two basic requirements.

1. *People, institutions*. The recruitment and academic support of young people interested in surgical research require the establishment of surgical laboratories and their expansion and integration. To accomplish this, collaborative bridges must be built with basic science departments, and the support of surgical research by boards of trustees, hospital directors, university deans, and science colleagues must be won. It also requires an adequate understanding of the significance of the mission of surgical research and its accomplishments in producing some of the most remarkable biomedical advances of this century.
2. *Financial support*. When young people embark on careers as investigators, they do not have bibliographies or research backgrounds that will command outside financial support for the pursuit of their ideas and their personal or family needs. Later, the full backing of home universities and nonsurgical faculties becomes a critical factor in successful searches for funds from large donors, foundations, and institutions, but it is, in some areas, very difficult to obtain.

Two questions have to be answered by each surgical department head about the surgical research in his or her department.

1. *What is the role of modern basic quantitative biology in surgical research?* Like their colleagues

in medicine, pediatrics, psychiatry, or radiology, very few surgeons are basic biologists. As the methods of modern science become progressively more challenging, fewer expert clinicians master them. Should there be more collaborating scientists in surgical departments?

2. *Where does health policy fit in surgical research?* Health policy research includes the role of surgical care in social rehabilitation, cost-benefit analysis, surgical manpower, the organization of surgical departments, the establishment of new procedures and practice patterns, law and ethics, the burden of malpractice litigation, and the application of highly technical methods to life support in critical illness. Since all the foregoing enter into the practice of surgery, these areas cannot be neglected by research, despite their not having been considered a part of surgical research in the past. If surgical investigators overlook or avoid them, critical decisions about surgery will be made by inadequately informed sociologists and legislators.

To have impact on the care of the sick, surgical research must be done *with or by surgeons or under their guidance. Whether the surgical investigator plays the key or a more modest role, the inspiration, driving force, and scientific and clinical insight of the surgical presence are essential for the success of surgical research.*

Now, within the same framework, we might take a quick glance—albeit not quite in focus—at the horizon.

New Procedures

In 1935 very few people would have predicted perfection of the pump oxygenator to support surgery on the open heart. Such a technological development and the transplantation of organs between unrelated individuals were termed impossible by the experts in 1952 and 1953, respectively. From the turn of the century onward, surgeons were taught that large foreign bodies in a wound were a sure recipe for disaster, to say nothing of artificial heart valves or such large plastic prostheses as new hip joints. Success in such endeavors is now the rule!

These examples illustrate the possible fate of negative predictions about new surgical procedures. One must be quite presumptuous to imagine what might be on surgeons' operating lists even 10 or 15 years hence.

I would guess that transplantation will be further perfected and extended to include additional organs and tissues. Although these operations will hardly be called "new," transplantation of the pancreas and long sections of small bowel are among the many unsolved challenges.

Head injury, whether inflicted by automobile or home accidents, child abuse, or military activity, remains the commonest cause of death from trauma. Microvascular operations for intracranial bleeding or for infarction caused by head injury might become a reality. The evaluation of head injuries to discern which might be remedied by early direct examination of the brain and its vasculature remains an important goal. New imaging modalities, such as nuclear magnetic resonance and positron emission tomography, may be crucial to success in this effort.

The development of artificial organs will surely continue for many decades. Such organs fall into two general categories.

First are the artificial organs that are physiologically outside the body, even if implanted under the skin. Extracorporeal pump oxygenators (the first effective artificial organ), pacemakers, artificial kidneys, and artificial pancreases belong in this group, although the first two are now in such wide use that we scarcely think of them as artificial organs.

The second group comprises those artificial organs truly incorporated in situ. The artificial heart is one example, although it currently suffers from a surpassing difficulty. In animal models, the tendency to cerebral microembolism may be masked by the inadequacy of our knowledge of the subtleties of animal behavior (speech, affect), or by actual differences in the coagulability of blood. In any event, microembolism, usually to the brain but possibly to other organs as well, has been a major complication in most of the patients in whom artificial hearts have been implanted. This unfortunate complication keeps this valuable, albeit expensive, bulky, and awkward form of life support, from providing a life of acceptable quality for patients.

The recent development of an endothelium-stimulating growth substance (fibroblastic growth factor or FGF) holds great promise. It seems reasonable to expect that implantable hearts and other left ventricular assist devices will eventually have endothelial linings grown within them to make them essentially physiologic as regards coagulation induction. If this becomes possible, the use of artificial hearts will be limited only by the awkwardness of the extracorporeal power source. The work of several investigators who are attempting to develop an electrical, magnetic, or nuclear implantable power source is important, and it should occupy the time and attention of several capable collaborative groups encompassing energy conversion, engineering, medicine, and surgery.

The human heart transplant requires toxic immunosuppressive drugs, the artificial heart implant capricious anticoagulants. The tradeoff has not been as simple as it appeared.

Will there be some new form of operation applicable to many forms of cancer? It could, conceivably, be an organ implant, such as lymph nodes or spleen containing "educated" lymphocytes to assault the tumor; a microfilter; or a microfilter containing gene-engineered microorganisms that synthesize diffusible substances such as interleukin 2 or antiangiogenin. Though these might not be new operations, they would basically be the application of new immunologic and genetic knowledge to surgical care.

When mastoidectomy yielded to antibiotics and polio reconstruction disappeared following the advent of the Salk vaccine, no surgeon objected! Indeed, all were elated. There are, however, other losses to surgical practice, such as ultrasound-guided deep needle biopsy, angiographic embolization in hemorrhage, percutaneous angioplasty, and colonoscopic polyp removal, where a steady surgical hand and the long-standing "field familiarity" of surgeons are still needed. Although surgery (*chirurgie*) is "doing with the hand" and can be learned by others, the surgeon should insist on participation, in some cases. Other new areas will require that the surgeon "keep a hand in" by mastering new techniques and learning new concepts from other fields, as has already happened in relation to the treatment of deafness and coronary disease.

Building Bridges to the Basic Sciences

Immunology looms large in this area, because molecular immunology should surely be applicable to cancer, to transplantation, and to surgical infection. Most immunologists who worked through the difficult decades of the '40s, '50s, and '60s readily acknowledge the stimulus they received from surgery, given that the growth of tissue transplantation, the description of the HLA groups, and enhanced understanding of the events of tissue rejection were all central to the rebirth of immunology and its movement from pragmatic clinical testing to basic molecular biology. Several Nobel laureates (Burnet, Baltimore, Medawar, Benacerraf) have worked on tissue types, immune competence, histocompatibility, and antigen genetics.

Many young surgeons are now selecting immunology as their basic science field just as they may select physiology, metabolism, neurology, microbiology, or biomaterials. Although, when viewed in the harsh light of the 1990s, molecular immunology has not yet revolutionized anything in surgery, my own scientific faith affirms its tremendous surgical potential.

Immune therapy for cancer seems, finally, to be on the verge of widespread applicability. The work of Rosenberg and his colleagues at the National Institutes of Health has an unmistakable ring of the future about it. Using their method, the patient's lymphatic system is stimulated by interleukin 2 (IL-2), as are also the patient's lymphocytes (in some instances from tumor infiltration itself). The combined treatment is very toxic, but it has produced some remarkable effects, such as the complete disappearance of some very large metastases of certain types of tumor, such as hypernephroma, lung cancer, and melanoma.

IL-2 treatment has been criticized as having an inadequate response rate but, in cancer treatment, the attention of the biologic and medical community should be focused on the nature and quality of the response rather than the fractional response rate. Although some tumors may, for example, display a response rate as high as 75% to certain chemotherapy regimens, almost all the patients die of their tumors without the tumors ever regressing completely. The response rate is high, but the quality of the response is very poor.

With IL-2 treatment, tumors have disappeared completely following immune intervention—an entirely new phenomenon in cancer therapy. The fact that some stay away while others return when the treatment is stopped raises the possibility of chronic immune therapy to maintain remission.

Immune modulation of this type will surely be applicable to other forms of cancer. By extension, some analogous form of immune treatment might become available for severe surgical sepsis and its attendant multiple organ failure.

Although our expanding knowledge of immunological processes seems to be establishing the basis for specific therapy, clinical case management has not yet altered much. It now seems clear that certain types of surgical trauma inhibit the production of immunoreactive globulins and may adversely affect the activity of specific lymphocyte subpopulations, possibly through an overload mechanism.

All clinicians are familiar with the phenomenon of sequential failure of several organs and death as a consequence of sepsis following trauma or surgery with multiple treatment modalities and successively changed antibiotics. These terminal events suggest widespread immune deficiency and raise the possibility that repair of the patient's immune system, were it feasible, might be lifesaving.

The 1940–1970 era may well go down in history as one whose prime characteristic was the mishandling of antibiotics. The adverse effects included immunosuppression from overdosing with antibiotics and the acquisition of antibiotic resistance by successive strains of organisms. Patients were converted into bacteriologically sterile but immunologically suppressed settings for the overgrowth of ordinary commensals, such as fungi and the cytomegalic virus. A better knowledge of the immune sequences in such complex cases may enable the surgeon to employ new agents more intelligently.

The induction of specific immunologic tolerance for transplant antigens from one organ source, without global immunosuppression, remains elusive. Significant as the replacement of azothiaprine by cyclosporin has appeared to be for many transplanted organs, particularly liver, cyclosporin is but another nonspecific immunosuppressive drug with neoplastic by-products.

Bringing basic science to the rescue of the surgical patient, through physiologic support systems, has several inviting possibilities. New knowledge about hormone mediators that translate peripheral injury into central organ damage, nitrogen loss, conversion of energy sources to lipid oxidation, and activation of the stress response holds much promise. The possibility that treatment modalities may exist in the endocrine area is brighter than ever. If, after severe injury, catabolic activity could be modified and necessary substrates could be simultaneously released from within the body, or be introduced, a more serene clinical course might be anticipated. Recent evidence suggests that glutamine may have specific nutritional functions for the GI tract and that human growth hormone may hasten recovery.

If such methods of stress modulation become available, their misuse and overuse can be predicted. It has been observed since the beginning of surgical metabolic research that healthy young men who show a very vigorous or brisk endocrine and catabolic response do very well clinically. The plentiful release of endogenous substrates for fibroplasia, leukocyte activity, and immune globulin production appears to be an obvious though unproven explanation. When some hormone becomes available to abate this response, the appearance of the vigorous young man with his "brisk and florid" endocrine response will rapidly be "mollified" to resemble that of a weakened old man having his fifth operation, totally devoid of physiologic response. The use of such potent and dangerous hormones, if and when they become available, will require a great deal of sophistication, but the dismal antibiotic record provides little assurance that a large group of surgeons and physicians will be able to use them intelligently.

Collaborating with Clinical Colleagues

The evolution of cancer treatment in the past decade has been one of the most spectacular examples of collaboration. Formerly limited to essentially "do or die" surgical operations whose effectiveness was based largely on early diagnosis, treatment now includes other modalities and often produces very good results. Nevertheless the net effect has often been overrated by the public media because of enthusiasm about their very existence. This is particularly true vis-à-vis chemotherapy for solid tumors and radiotherapy with supervoltage equipment.

Despite many disappointments and failures, cancer patients now have a better prospect than ever before of prolonged disease-free survival, with a good quality of life. This is due not to any single "breakthrough" but to noncompetitive collaboration in comprehensive cancer centers, where the welfare of the patient is more important than any specialty ambitions. When one visits such units, one can quickly discern whether the various and potentially competing treatment modalities and domains of sovereignty, such as surgery, radiotherapy, and chemotherapy, are truly collaborating for the welfare of the patient or actually seeking the enrollment of patients in their own "protocols" in order to get more money, more publicity, more patients, or a higher group income.

A professional is defined as a practitioner who places the welfare of the patient or client above the practitioner's own social, scientific, personal, or financial advancement. The availability of multiple cancer therapies and therapists has truly placed the professionalism of all physicians on the line. Although most multiple-modality cancer treatment centers demonstrate a high order of professionalism, it is evident that, in a few, research protocol enrollment rather than the welfare of the patient governs the outcome. Although collaboration now prevails in many fields, the psychology of professional interaction is an important component that remains to be analyzed.

Clinical and research collaboration promises many rewards for the surgical patient. The development of ultrasound and computed axial tomography are tremendous advances in surgical care. To appreciate them, one has only to reflect on the painful and uncertain procedures of encephalography and ventriculography to diagnose hemorrhage in the skull or disorders along the spinal column, and contrast them with the specificity and anatomic precision of tomographic scanning.

Nuclear magnetic resonance (NMR) and positron emission tomography (PET) hold great promise. Although NMR seems to have almost no adverse effects, current apparatus is expensive, cumbersome, and awkward, and does not lend itself either to the scanning of extremely ill patients or to any sort of emergency procedure. PET scanning has the unique feature of demonstrating areas of functional activity within the brain. The development of this type of combined engineering and its application to neurosurgery and various mental, behavioral, and psychiatric problems open a new horizon for neurosurgery.

It is possible to hope that these techniques, combined with very prompt attention, immediate and focal diagnosis, and microsurgery or CNS excision, will provide a way to save a few patients from that large group that now accounts for most of the mortality among civilian and military casualties.

Improving Existing Procedures by Surgical Engineering

While most of the quantum advances in surgery during the past century have come from university centers, gradual improvement and perfection of surgical procedures have often come via practitioners, clinical practicing groups, and community hospitals. As an applied form of biological science or human engineering, surgery improves with practice. The marked reduction in patient mortality and the tremendous increase in the fractional survival cf transplanted kidneys between 1965 and 1978, when there was no qualitative improvement in immunosuppression, is but one of many examples that demonstrate perfection by gradual engineering.

The same is true of open heart surgery, particularly coronary bypass operations. This formerly imposing and immensely complex surgery has become much safer, rather than more hazardous, with its widespread performance. The mortality over large areas of the United States is now around 1%.

Very few clinicians or scientists outside the field of surgery understand its remarkable capacity for self-improvement. Many adverse views of surgical operations are based on early results before surgery's in-built learning curve becomes manifest. Liver transplantation is one of the most difficult and complex of the frontier group of surgical procedures, but its perfection and the consequent improvement in morbidity and mortality have been spectacular. Liver transplantation should be undertaken only by a master surgeon with self-confidence and specific training. Within those limitations, its repeated performance has resulted in an improvement in results beyond expectation and highly challenging to the neophyte individual or hospital at the beginning of the learning curve.

Every hospital, clinical unit, group practice, or academic department conducting surgical operations in any quantity should periodically review its results in terms of immediate mortality and morbidity, and late survivorship and rehabilitation. While modern computer techniques render this very simple, there must be an established program that is adequately supported at the outset and periodically evaluated. This is a matter of pressing importance at the horizon of surgical research.

Hospitals that cling to old operations, such as radical mastectomy in breast cancer or subtotal gastrectomy for duodenal ulcer, should have the research fortitude, often called "discipline" or "guts," to examine their own results in the light of recent advances. If they can, indeed, document superior results with the time-honored procedures, they should be encouraged to do so and to stand up in the court of professional opinion to defend their view. The same principle applies to such frequently performed standard operations as prostatectomy, colectomy for cancer, heart valve surgery, laminectomy for disc removal, and arterial replacement of the aorta or in the lower limb. It should be an obligation of every surgical unit, wherever located, to know its own results, to compare them with those published by peer groups, and to set its house to rights if its results are inadequate. The support of research to do this should come from the institution itself.

The Two Basic Inputs: People and Support

We can say with perfect confidence that young surgeons devoted to a life in science will be as rare in the future as they have been in the past. The coercion of all young interns and residents to laboratory "projects" is positively unrewarding; it merely results in crowding the literature with trash. Nevertheless, the door to the laboratory should be open to all young surgeons so that, if their talents call them in that direction, they may give them a fair trial. The analogy with playing a musical instrument is too close to withhold: forcing every young person to practice 3 hours a day would produce only a large crashing of noise. And yet, one cannot learn to play by attending concerts: one must perform oneself and practice every day! The instrument—a laboratory—should be there, along with a teacher—the Professor—so that each resident in an academic unit can develop his or her talent, if it exists.

The backwardness of institutions in providing space for surgical research is depressing. Surgical research is not demanding of space, although animal facilities have sometimes been difficult to establish and maintain. Antivivisectionist pressures have been a problem for surgical research for almost a century. It is an obligation of the professor of surgery to convince the dean and the hospital director what the necessary components of surgical research are and to call to their attention that only where research thrives and inquiring minds are given scope, will the quality of clinical surgery be maintained at its optimal level and the hospital attract patients and residents.

Financial support for career development in surgery must come, increasingly, from practice income, although this has an ethical aspect that requires examination. If a practicing group, such as a private group clinic of the United States model (Mayo, Lahey, Crile), sets aside professional fee income for research, the problem of fee splitting must be considered. Patients, or their insurance companies, are being charged for an activity (i.e., research) they may be totally unaware of and unprepared to underwrite.

If such fee diversion becomes extensive, it is clearly unethical. This also applies when the dean or the university taxes practice income from academic clinicians. It is, in essence, a tax on the patient's pocketbook or on the insurance company, for the conduct of a medical school, which the patient may not feel is intrinsic to the treatment of her breast cancer.

This ethical concern is counterbalanced, however, by the fact that all enterprises in a free society require the diversion of some revenue to research and development. Given a proper explanation, even the most conservative patient would willingly make a reasonable contribution to the improvement of surgical practice.

Determination of what is a "reasonable" fraction must depend on the scene and circumstances, but somewhere in the region of 10% to 15% would seem to be appropriate. Some sort of notification should be included in hospital publications, or be given to the patient at admission, to make it clear that some of the professional charges incurred for his or her care will be devoted to assisting the research education of young surgeons. With that proviso, academic surgical group practices can provide fellowships and a few basic laboratory components for young people embarking on research careers. Although group practices can never supply the broadly financed support required by modern quantitative biology, they can play a critically important role by providing the seed money and the strong surgical supporting voice that the young surgeon must have to compete successfully on the national scene for continuing grant funds.

Where Does Basic Science Collaboration Fit?

Surgical research will, in future, involve a more searching appraisal of the role of basic science than it has in the past. The young surgeon embarking on research should spend a year or two acquiring the vocabulary, skills, and concepts of some area of basic biology, molecular immunology, genetics, or bioengineering and then have a period of collaboration with scientists holding Ph.D. qualifications. To make this happen, surgical departments must willingly give appointments in surgery to Ph.D. scientists. Medicine, pediatrics, and psychiatry have already assigned such appointments to scientists from other fields, but surgery has not done it very often.

Young people with the talents required to meet the mechanical, spatial, and operative challenges of surgery may not have the mental bent appropriate to thinking in terms of molecular interactions. The same limitation is found in medicine and pediatrics: as molecular biology becomes ever more challenging, an increasing proportion of total research funding in clinical departments is held by Ph.D. scientists. Surgery must do the same, if it is to move ahead.

Health Policy

Health policy research is one of the most interesting features of the surgical research horizon.

Surgical research has three phases: discovery, development, and delivery. *Discovery* covers the revelation of some important bioscience finding related to surgical care; *development* occurs during the period of surgical bioengineering improvement already discussed. *Delivery* is concerned with providing new modes of surgical care, and with the manpower, economic, and regulatory constraints within which surgery operates in every nation.

The manpower limitation in surgery is usually misunderstood by people outside the field and sometimes even by large national surgical organizations.

Because surgeons operate on specific disease entities, the requirement for surgeons is limited by the epidemiology and prevalence of those diseases. In many fields of surgery, 75% or more of the total operations performed may be devoted to a few disease entities. Thus, while the public "appetite" for family practitioners seems to be insatiable, that for surgeons is clearly limited. Failure to recognize this may lead to the training of an embarrassing and crippling excess of surgeons by postgraduate programs in the United States.

There is no point to expanding surgical training programs or recruiting additional people into surgery when the requirement for them is fixed and already met. Although many young people wish to enter surgery, boards of surgical examiners and colleges of surgeons must enforce strict and even "brutal" criteria to weed out everyone who cannot meet the highest standards. However, because it is not only uneconomic but also inhumane to cut people off at this late stage of their training, it is essential that potential incompetents be identified by in-house examinations as early as possible, and be counseled accordingly.

Malpractice litigation is a major disincentive to surgical practice in the United States and accounts for 3% to 5% of the total financial cost of medical and surgical care. The problem arises from the lack of any statutes of limitation relating to the care of children, judgments, and legal fees. Lawyers' concern for the welfare of the "victims" of incompetent physicians is rarely accompanied by an equal concern about the victims' receiving only a tiny fraction of the settlements awarded. Although there is a persisting need for high standards of quality assessment and constant surveillance of physicians for such damaging disorders as senility or drug and alcohol abuse, many crippling malpractice suits are launched against individuals who are delivering medical care of the highest quality. It is widely accepted in the press, with no basis in fact, that all malpractice judgments favoring the plaintiff reveal an incompetent practitioner.

The impotence of national surgical organizations in the United States in this area is largely the result of a lack of sound, relevant social research in collaboration with lawyers and judges. Other nations face, or will soon face, the same problem. Relief will come only from changes in public policy based on sound social research done by surgeons.

L'envoi

As we peer or peep over the horizon, we see many things promised and many challenges posed. On the basis of the past, many problems will be solved and many challenges will linger on.

It is my guess that two of the lingering challenges will be death from head injury and from widespread sepsis with multiple organ failure. In my own 50-year surgical career, to date, I have seen very little progress on either front. Such spotty advances as have been made have been overwhelmed, in some ways, by the larger number of early cases that have survived to show us the futility of existing modes of treatment.

Every professorial head of a surgical department should support an active research program that would, I hope, include health policy and the evaluation of clinical procedures used within the department and, most of all, a periodic assessment of the areas where injured or diseased patients still die despite our best efforts.

Our future failures will be those of blindness to the power of surgical research and of lack of focus in research. We will possess both vision and research focus if the surgical profession of each nation supports its own research establishment, and the leading departments of surgery take bold new initiatives in the outstanding salients of surgical mortality. Such new ventures will be far more rewarding than the pursuit of small details down some well-trodden path and will be inspired only by surgeons who study their own patients.

Index

About the Editors

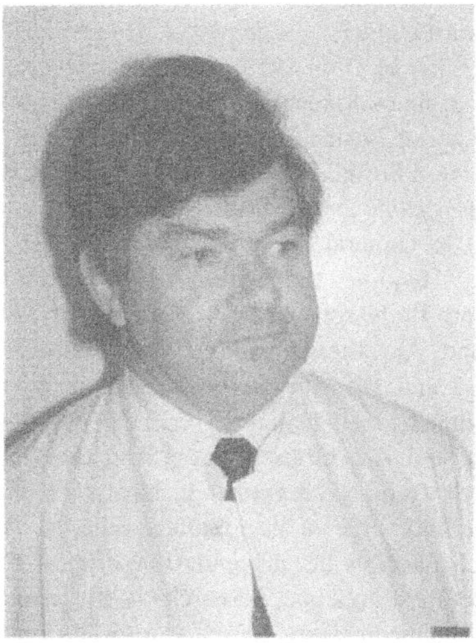

Hans Troidl graduated in medicine from the University of Munich in 1964. He became a licensed medical practitioner in 1967 and served as both clinical and research assistant in the Pathology Department of the University of Munich. From 1968 to 1969 he was a resident in the Surgical University Clinic of Professor Zenker and served as Zenker's private assistant. From 1969 he worked with Professor Hamelmann in the Universities of Marburg and of Kiel. He became professor in 1979.

In 1981 he was appointed Professor of Surgery and Chairman of the II. Department of Surgery at the University of Cologne and Director of the Surgical Clinic at Cologne-Merheim.

Professor Troidl's areas of interest are surgery of the lung, esophagus, colon, and especially the stomach as well as surgery of trauma. A pioneer in endoscopy and ultrasound, he currently performs cholecystectomies and appendectomies via the laparoscopy. In clinical research his main interests have been clinical trials and the development of innovative endpoints for the assessment of quality of life and pain as outcome measures. These endpoints are ones that concern most patients. Professor Troidl has published several textbooks in the field of lung, stomach, and colon surgery. He is author or coauthor of more than 300 publications and serves on the editorial boards of the journals *Endoscopy* and *Theoretical Surgery* as well as of *Surgical Endoscopy, Ultrasound, and Interventional Techniques*.

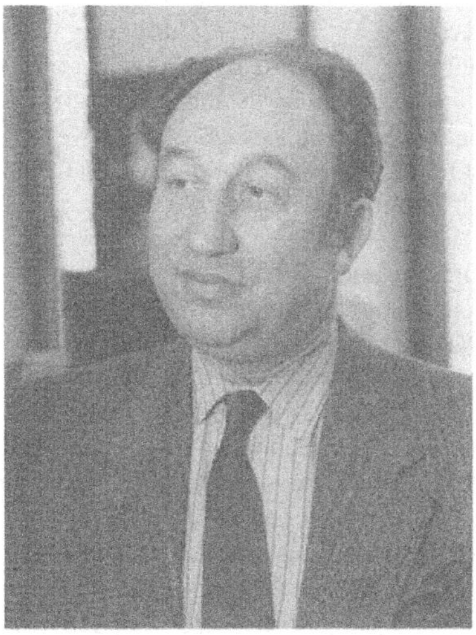

Walter O. Spitzer, M.D. was born in Paraguay, where his parents were missionaries. He graduated in medicine from the University of Toronto in 1962. He then completed postgraduate studies in health administration at the University of Michigan and in epidemiology at Yale University. He joined the Faculty of Biostatistics at McMaster University in 1969. In 1975 he was appointed Professor of Epidemiology at McGill University with cross appointments in Medicine and Family Medicine. He has been at McGill ever since and became Strathcona Professor and Chairman of his department in 1984. During his tenure at Montreal he was appointed National Health Scientist of Canada (1980) and elected to be a Member of the Institute of Medicine of the National Academy of Sciences of the U.S.A. in 1985. He has been Editor of *Journal of Clinical Epidemiology* since 1980 having also founded the Canadian medical journal *Clinical and Investigative Medicine* in 1979.

Professor Spitzer has published 72 original peer-reviewed articles in subject areas that include, clinical epidemiology, cancer epidemiology, health services research, the measurement of quality of life and pharmacoepidemiology. A keen interest, throughout his career in research and teaching has been the development of methods in clinical investigation and epidemiology. In recent years he has pursued his methodological interests in close collaboration with surgical colleagues focusing on measures of quality of life and other benefits of elective interventions.

Bucknam McPeek, M.D. has been a student and teacher at Harvard University since 1951. He received his A.B. in 1955, his M.D. in 1959, and holds the certificate in Health Systems Management from the Harvard Graduate School of Business Administration. After a year on the Harvard Surgical Service at the Boston City Hospital, he became resident in Anesthesia at the Massachusetts General Hospital under Professor Henry Beecher. He joined the faculty in 1962, and is currently Associate Professor of Anaesthesia at Harvard University, and Anesthetist to the Massachusetts General Hospital and Director of its Acute Pain Service. For more than 20 years he has served as Deputy Director of the Harvard Anaesthesia Center and the Anaesthesia Research Training Program. He has taught in Harvard College and three of its graduate schools. His major research interests lie in population studies of risk and postoperative outcome, research on the assessment of health and medical practices, and information gathering strategies for policymaking. He is co-editor of the journal, *Theoretical Surgery*. A previous book, *Data for Decisions*, is widely used in policy courses in graduate schools of government, business, and public health.

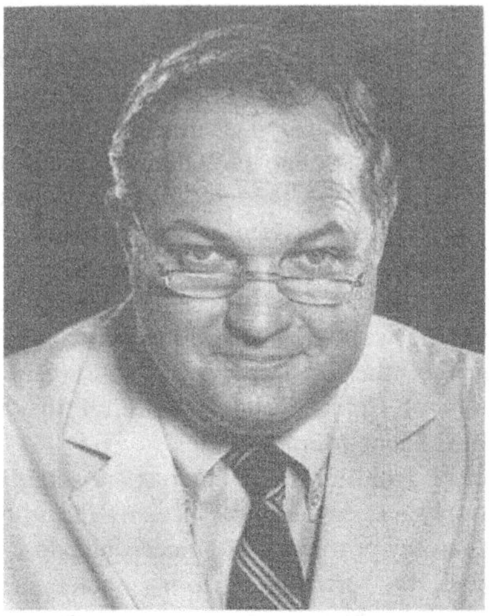

Photo by Karsh

David S. Mulder is a native of Saskatchewan where he received his M.D. from the University of Saskatchewan in 1962. He carried out a rotating internship at the University Hospital in Saskatoon prior to coming to The Montreal General Hospital and McGill University where he did his entire general surgical training under the direction of Dr. Fraser N. Gurd. This was followed by training in cardiovascular thoracic surgery at the University of Iowa under the direction of Dr. J.L. Ehrenhaft. He then returned to the McGill University Department of Physiology where he completed a further year of research training under the supervision of Dr. David Bates. He received an M.Sc. in Experimental Surgery in 1965 for a thesis on "The Use of Percutaneous Left Heart Bypass in Hemorrhagic Shock."

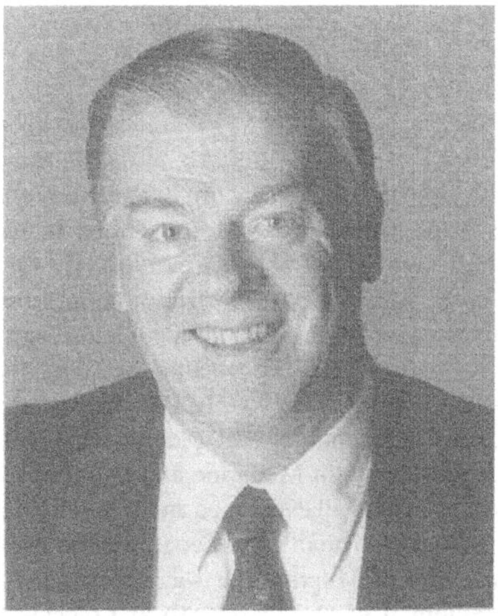

Dr. Mulder was appointed to the staff of The Montreal General Hospital and McGill University on July 2, 1970. He was appointed Surgeon-in-Chief at The Montreal General Hospital on January 1, 1977, and continues to serve in this role. He was named Professor of Surgery at McGill University in 1978 and served as Chairman of the McGill Department of Surgery from 1983 to 1988.

Dr. Mulder has been President of The American Association for the Surgery of Trauma, The Trauma Association of Canada and is presently Honorary President of the Pan-American Trauma Association.

Dr. Mulder's scientific interests have been in the field of cardiovascular surgery and trauma. His major research interests include basic investigations into the adult respiratory distress syndrome following hemorrhagic shock. This has more recently continued as basic investigations in the differentiation of pulmonary sepsis and acute rejection following lung transplantation. Studies in trauma have included laboratory and clinical investigations in airway trauma, peripheral vascular injury and thoracic trauma. He has also been interested in improving the organization of trauma care in Canada and the United States, and has worked actively as a member of the Committee on Trauma of The American College of Surgeons.

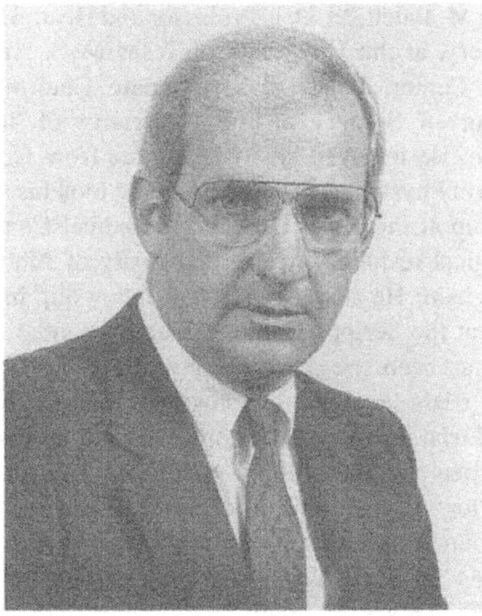

Martin F. McKneally received his M.D. from Cornell University Medical College. He completed general and cardiothoracic surgical training at the University of Minnesota in 1968 and received his Ph.D. in Immunology there in 1970. He established an active academic, clinical, and research program focused on general thoracic surgery, with a special emphasis on the treatment of lung cancer, at the Albany Medical Center in Albany, New York. He was Professor of Surgery and Chief of the Division of Cardiothoracic Surgery at Albany Medical College of Union University from 1983 until 1990. He is currently Professor of Surgery and Head of the Division of Thoracic Surgery at the University of Toronto and the Toronto Hospital. He has been principal investigator for several NIH-sponsored laboratory studies and clinical trials testing the efficacy of stimulation of the immune system after surgical resection for lung cancer, the efficacy of surgery in coronary artery disease, and was a co-principal investigator in the national trials of the Lung Cancer Study Group. He has served on the Commission on Cancer of the American College of Surgeons, the Council of the Society of Thoracic Surgeons, and is presently a Director of the American Board of Thoracic Surgery and Secretary of the American Association for Thoracic Surgery.

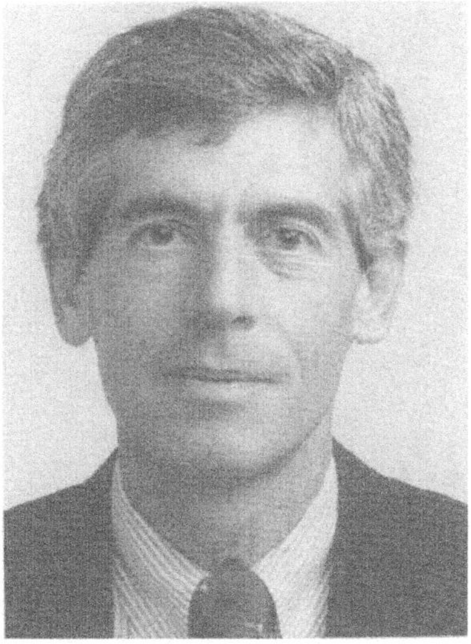

Andrew S. Wechsler, M.D. is the Stuart McGuire Professor of Surgery at the Medical College of Virginia of Virginia Commonwealth University where he serves as Chairman of the Department of Surgery. He is also Professor of Physiology and Head of the Division of Cardiothoracic Surgery. After two years of medical training at the Peter Bent Brigham Hospital in Boston, he spent two years in the laboratory of Dr. Eugene Braunwald, and subsequently, received his surgical training at Duke University Medical Center. He served on the Duke Faculty for fourteen years. He is author or co-author of over two hundred scientific articles and has participated actively in the post-doctoral training of nineteen research fellows who have worked in his laboratory. He is Chairman of the Surgery and Bioengineering Section of the National Institutes of Health, serves on several editorial boards, including those of circulation, the *Journal of Cardiac Surgery*, and the *American Journal of Cardiology*. He has served on the research committee of the American Heart Association and as Vice-Chairman of the Forum Committee of the American College of Surgeons. He serves as a director of the American Board of Thoracic Surgery and is a member of the Research and Education Committee of the American College of Surgeons.

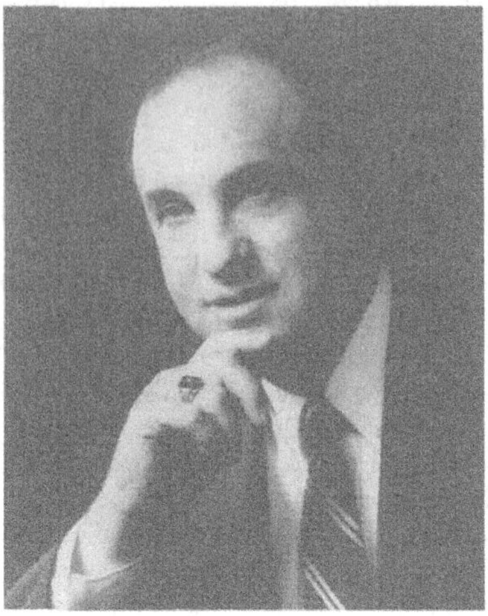

Charles M. Balch, M.D. is Professor and Head, Division of Surgery, at the University of Texas M.D. Anderson Cancer Center. He is also Associate Chairman and Professor of Surgery at the University of Texas at Houston. He received his M.D. degree from Columbia College of Physicians and Surgeons and took his surgical internship at the Duke University Medical Center and his surgical residency at the University of Alabama in Birmingham. He also had a 2-year fellowship in immunology at the Scripps Clinic Research Foundation. Dr. Balch has been the principal investigator of multiple clinical trials involving oncology, including a national surgical trial involving melanoma. He was an Executive Committee member of the Southeast Cancer Study Group for 10 years and is currently chairman of the Intergroup Melanoma Committee. He is also director of both the clinical oncology fellowship training and surgical research fellowship training programs in the Department of General Surgery at the M.D. Anderson Cancer Center. A member of numerous surgical, oncology and research organizations (including the Society for Clinical Investigations), he was President of the Association for Academic Surgery and is President-elect of the Society of Surgical Oncology.

Made in the USA
Monee, IL
18 October 2026

66036441R10328